Neurological Rehabilitation

EDITED BY L. S. ILLIS

MD, BSc, FRCP

Consultant Neurologist, Wessex Neurological Centre,
Southampton University Hospitals (Southampton General Hospital);
Clinical Senior Lecturer in Neurology,
University of Southampton Medical School

FOREWORD BY

LORD WALTON OF DETCHANT

SECOND EDITION

OXFORD

BLACKWELL SCIENTIFIC PUBLICATIONS

LONDON EDINBURGH BOSTON

MELBOURNE PARIS BERLIN VIENNA

© 1982, 1994 by
Blackwell Scientific Publications
Editorial Offices:
Osney Mead, Oxford OX2 0EL
25 John Street, London WC1N 2BL
23 Ainslie Place, Edinburgh EH3 6AJ
238 Main Street, Cambridge
   Massachusetts 02142, USA
54 University Street, Carlton
   Victoria 3053, Australia

Other Editorial Offices:
Librairie Arnette SA
1, rue de Lille
75007 Paris, France

Blackwell Wissenschafts-Verlag GmbH
Düsseldorfer Str. 38
D-10707 Berlin, Germany

Blackwell MZV
Feldgasse 13, A-1238 Wien
Austria

First published 1982
(*Rehabilitation of the Neurological Patient*)
Second edition 1994

Set by Excel Typesetters, Hong Kong
Printed and bound in Great Britain
at the University Press, Cambridge

DISTRIBUTORS

Marston Book Services Ltd
PO Box 87, Oxford OX2 0DT
(*Orders*: Tel: 0865 791155
        Fax: 0865 791927
        Telex: 837515)

USA
Blackwell Scientific Publications, Inc.
238 Main Street
Cambridge, MA 02142
(*Orders*: Tel: 800 759-6102
           617 876-7000)

Canada
Times Mirror Professional Publishing, Ltd
130 Flaska Drive
Markham, Ontario L6G 1B8
(*Orders*: Tel: 800 268-4178
           416 470-6739)

Australia
Blackwell Scientific Publications Pty Ltd
54 University Street
Carlton, Victoria 3053
(*Orders*: Tel: 03 347-5552)

A catalogue record for this title
is available from the British Library

ISBN 0-632-03282-0

Library of Congress
Cataloging-in-Publication Data

Neurological rehabilitation/edited by L.S. Illis;
   foreword by Lord Walton of Detchant. – 2nd ed.
      p.   cm.
      Rev. ed. of: Rehabilitation of
      the neurological patient. 1982.
      Includes bibliographical references and index.
      ISBN 0-632-03282-0
   1. Nervous system – Diseases –
   Patients – Rehabilitation.   I. Illis, L.S. (Leon S.)
   II. Rehabilitation of the neurological patient.
   [DNLM: 1. Nervous System Diseases –
   rehabilitation.   WL 100 N494663   1994]
   RC350.4.N483   1994
   616.8'043 – dc20
   DNLM/DLC
   for Library of Congress

Contents

List of Contributors, v

Foreword, viii
Lord Walton of Detchant

Preface, ix

Acknowledgements, x

1   Introduction, 1
    L.S. Illis

Part 1: The Clinical Background

2   What is Rehabilitation? 7
    H.J. Glanville

3   Communication and Explanation of
    Neurological Disability, 14
    E.M.R. Critchley

4   The Neurological Patient: the Patient's
    View, 25
    Anne and Sean O'Cathasaigh

Part 2: The Scientific Background of Neurological Rehabilitation: Altered Structure and Function

5   Rehabilitation Theory, 33
    L.S. Illis

6   Damage to the Nervous System, 45
    R.O. Weller

7   Plasticity in the Neonatal and Adult Nervous
    System, 59
    M. Devor

8   Clinical Neurophysiology in Rehabilitation, 82
    E.M. Sedgwick

Part 3: Assessment

9   Evaluation and Economics of Treatment in
    Neurological Rehabilitation, 105
    C.N. Martyn and A. Morris

10 Audit in Neurological Rehabilitation, 113
    D.T. Wade

Part 4: The Neurological Patient

11 Rehabilitation: the Role of Remedial
    Therapy, 133
    L.S. Illis

12 Rehabilitation of Traumatic Brain Injury, 141
    C.D. Evans

13 Rehabilitation after Stroke, 157
    R. Langton Hewer

14 Rehabilitation of Parkinson's Disease, 169
    D.E. Bateman

15 Rehabilitation in Epilepsy, 177
    G.A. Baker, D.W. Chadwick and C.A. Young

16 The Rehabilitation of Multiple Sclerosis, 212
    L.C. Scheinberg and C.R. Smith

17 Natural History and Rehabilitation in Spinal
    Cord Damage, 221
    H.L. Frankel

18 Rehabilitation of Progressive Neuromuscular Diseases, 239
M. De Visser

19 Rehabilitation of Peripheral Nerve Disorders, 250
C.B. Wynn-Parry and J. Cowan

20 Management of the AIDS Patient, 269
H. Ochitill and D. McGuire

21 Management of the Chronic Fatigue Syndrome, 282
M. Sharpe and T. Chalder

22 Management of Children with Neuromuscular Disorders, 295
L. Merlini and C. Granata

23 Neurological Rehabilitation in the Elderly, 313
R.C. Tallis

Part 5: Specific Problems

24 Management of Spasticity, 335
L.S. Illis

25 Rehabilitation and Management of the Neuropathic Bladder, 349
K.F. Parsons, R.C.L. Feneley and M.J. Torrens

26 Rehabilitation of Faecal Incontinence, 382
R.I. Hallan, B.D. George and N.S. Williams

27 Rehabilitation of the Patient with Persistent Pain, 394
D.M. Long

28 Management of Communication and Swallowing Disorders, 409
D.P. Fuller, D.B. Pugh and W.M. Landau

29 Management of Sexual Disability, 428
M.A. Jamous

30 Genetic Management in Chronic Neurological Disorders, 438
N.R. Dennis

Part 6: New Concepts in Neurological Rehabilitation

31 Sensory Substitution, Volume Transmission and Rehabilitation: Emerging Concepts, 457
P. Bach-Y-Rita

32 Pharmacological Approaches to Rehabilitation: Noradrenergic Pharmacotherapy and Functional Recovery after Cortical Injury, 469
R.L. Sutton and D.M. Feeney

33 Surgical Rehabilitation in Tetraplegia, 482
A. Ejeskär and A.-G. Dahllöf

34 Engineering Solutions for Patients with Neurological Disability, 504
P.H. Chappell and I.D. Swain

35 Functional Electrical Stimulation (FES) in the Rehabilitation of Patients with Paraplegia and Hemiplegia, 519
A. Krălj, T. Bajd, U. Stanič, R. Ačimović-Janežič and R. Turk

36 Stimulation Procedures, 536
L.S. Illis and E.M. Sedgwick

Appendices, 559

Index, 572

List of Contributors

R. AČIMOVIĆ-JANEŽIČ MD, *University Rehabilitation Institute, Ljubljana, Linhartova 51, 61000 Ljubljana, Slovenia*

P. BACH-Y-RITA MD, *Professor, Department of Rehabilitation Medicine, University of Wisconsin, 1300 University Avenue, Madison, WI 53705, USA*

T. BAJD DSc, *Faculty of Electrical and Computer Engineering, University of Ljubljana, Trzaska, 61000 Ljubljana, Slovenia*

G.A. BAKER BA(Hons), MClinPsychol, CPsychol, AFBPS, *Lecturer in Clinical Neuropsychology, University of Liverpool, Walton Centre for Neurology and Neurosurgery, Liverpool L9 1AE, UK*

D.E. BATEMAN MA, MD, MRCP, *Consultant Neurologist, Royal United Hospital, Combe Park, Bath BA1 3NG, UK*

D.W. CHADWICK DM, FRCP, *Professor of Neurology, University of Liverpool, Walton Centre for Neurology and Neurosurgery, Liverpool L9 1AE, UK*

T. CHALDER SRN, RMN, MSc, *Honorary Lecturer in Health Psychology, Academic Department of Psychological Medicine, Kings College Hospital, London SE5, UK*

P.H. CHAPPELL BSc, PhD, CEng, MIEE, *Department of Electrical Engineering, University of Southampton, Southampton SO9 5NH, UK*

J. COWAN MB, MRCP, *Director of Rehabilitation, Royal National Orthopaedic Hospital, Brockley Hill, Stanmore, Middlesex HA7 4LP, UK*

E.M.R. CRITCHLEY DM, FRCP, *Consultant Neurologist, Royal Preston Hospital, Sharoe Green Lane, Preston, Lancs PR2 4HT, UK*

A.-G. DAHLLÖF MD, PhD, *Associate Professor, Department of Rehabilitation Medicine (Neurological Rehabilitation), Sahlgrenska Sjukhuset, S-41345 Göteborg, Sweden*

N.R. DENNIS MB, FRCP, *Senior Lecturer in Clinical Genetics, University of Southampton; Honorary Consultant in Clinical Genetics, Southampton University Hospitals Trust, Princess Anne Hospital, Southampton SO9 4HA, UK*

M. DE VISSER MD, *Professor, Department of Neurology, Academic Medical Center, University of Amsterdam, The Netherlands*

M. DEVOR PhD, *Professor and Chairman, Life Sciences Institute, Hebrew University of Jerusalem, Jerusalem 91404, Israel*

A. EJESKÄR MD, PhD, *Associate Professor, Division of Hand Surgery, Department of Orthopaedics, Sahlgrenska Sjukhuset, S-41345 Göteborg, Sweden*

C.D. EVANS FRCP, *Consultant in Rehabilitation Medicine, Royal Cornwall Hospital (City), Infirmary Hill, Truro, Cornwall TR1 1LE, UK*

D.M. FEENEY PhD, *Professor of Psychology and Physiology, Department of Psychology, The University of New Mexico, Albuquerque, NM 87131, USA*

R.C.L. FENELEY MA, MChir, FRCS, *Consultant Urologist, Bristol Urological Institute, Southmead Hospital, Bristol BS10 5NB; Senior Clinical Lecturer, University of Bristol, UK*

H.L. FRANKEL OBE, MB, FRCP, *Consultant in Spinal Injuries, National Spinal Injuries Centre, Stoke Mandeville Hospital, Mandeville Road, Aylesbury, Bucks HP21 8AL, UK*

D.P. FULLER PhD, CCC, SPL, *Director, Division of Speech Pathology, Department of Otolaryngology, Washington University Medical School, St Louis, MO 63110, USA*

B.D. GEORGE FRCS, *Senior Registrar in General Surgery, John Radcliffe Hospital, Oxford OX3 9DU, UK*

H.J. GLANVILLE DPhysMed, FRCS, *Emeritus Foundation Europe Professor of Rehabilitation, Medical Faculty, University of Southampton, Southampton SO9 5NH, UK*

C. GRANATA MD, *Professor of Physiotherapy, Physiotherapy Postgraduate Medical School, University of Bologna, Italy; Consultant Physiatrist of the Muscle Clinic, Istituto Ortopedico Rizzoli, Bologna 40136, Italy*

R.I. HALLAN MS, FRCS, *Consultant Surgeon, St Albans City Hospital, St Albans, Herts AL3 5PN, UK*

L.S. ILLIS MD, BSc, FRCP, *Consultant Neurologist, Wessex Neurological Centre, Southampton University Hospitals (Southampton General Hospital): Clinical Senior Lecturer in Neurology, University of Southampton Medical School, Southampton*

M.A. JAMOUS MD, MSc (Oxon), *Associate Specialist in Spinal Injuries, National Spinal Injuries Centre, Stoke Mandeville Hospital, Mandeville Road, Aylesbury, Bucks HP21 8AL, UK*

A. KRĂLJ DSc, *Faculty of Electrical and Computer Engineering, University of Ljubljana, Trzaska 25, 61000 Ljubljana, Slovenia*

W.M. LANDAU MD, *Department of Neurology, Washington University Medical School, St Louis, Missouri, USA*

R. LANGTON HEWER FRCP, *Professor of Neurology, Department of Neurology, University of Bristol, Frenchay Hospital, Bristol BS16 1LE, UK*

D.M. LONG MD, PhD, *Professor and Director, Department of Neurosurgery, Johns Hopkins University School of Medicine, Baltimore, MD 21205, USA*

D. McGUIRE MD, *Director, AIDS Neurology Clinic, San Francisco General Hospital, San Francisco, California 94110, USA; Assistant Professor of Neurology, University of California, San Francisco School of Medicine*

C.N. MARTYN MA, DPhil, FRCP (Ed), *Clinical Scientist, Medical Research Council Environmental Epidemiology Unit, Southampton General Hospital, Southampton SO9 4XY, UK*

L. MERLINI MD, *Professor of Neuropathology, Physiotherapy Postgraduate Medical School, University of Bologna, Italy; Consultant Neurologist, Istituto Ortopedico Rizzoli, Bologna; Muscle Clinic, Istituto Ortopedico Rizzoli, Bologna 40136, Italy*

A. MORRIS MA, *Health Economist, East Anglian Regional Health Authority, Union Lane, Chesterton, Cambridge CB4 1RF, UK*

A. O'CATHASAIGH, *13 Luccombe Road, Upper Shirley, Southampton SO1 2RJ, UK*

S. O'CATHASAIGH, *13 Luccombe Road, Upper Shirley, Southampton SO1 2RJ, UK*

H. OCHITILL MD, *Assistant Medical Chief, Department of Psychiatry, San Francisco General Hospital, San Francisco, California 94110, USA; Associate Clinical Professor of Psychiatry, University of California, San Francisco School of Medicine*

K.F. PARSONS, *Consultant Urological Surgeon, Royal Liverpool University Hospital NHS Trust; Consultant Urological Surgeon, Mersey Regional Spinal Injuries Centre, Southport and Formby District General NHS Trust; Director of Urological Studies, University of Liverpool*

D.B. PUGH MA, CCC, SPL, *Department of Rehabilitation, Barnes Hospital, St Louis, Missouri, USA*

L.C. SCHEINBERG MD, *Professor of Neurology, Mount Sinai Medical School; Attending Neurologist, Mount Sinai Medical Center, New York, NY 10029, USA*

E.M. SEDGWICK BSc, MD, FRCP, *Professor and Consultant in Clinical Neurophysiology, Clinical Neurological Sciences, University of Southampton, General Hospital, Southampton SO9 4XY, UK*

M. SHARPE MA, MRCP, MRCPsych, *Clinical Tutor in Psychiatry, University of Oxford, Warneford Hospital, Oxford OX3 7JX, UK*

C.R. SMITH MD, *Adjunct Associate Professor, Department of Medicine, New York Medical College, Valhalla, New York, USA*

U. STANIČ DSc, *Jozef Stefan Institute, Jamova 39, 61000 Ljubljana, Slovenia*

R.L. SUTTON PhD, *Director of Neurosurgical Research Department of Surgery, Hennepin County Medical Center, 701 Park Avenue South, Minneapolis, MN 55415, USA; and Assistant Professor, Department of Neurosurgery, University of Minnesota, Minneapolis, MN 55415, USA*

I.D. SWAIN BSc, PhD, CEng, MIEE, MBES, *District Physicist, Salisbury District Hospital, Salisbury, Wilts SP2 8BJ, UK*

R.C. TALLIS MA, BM, BCh, FRCP, *Professor of Geriatric Medicine, Department of Geriatric Medicine, University of Manchester, Hope Hospital, Eccles Old Road, Salford M6 8HD, UK*

M.J. TORRENS MPhil, ChM, FRCS, *Holagos 15562, Athens, Greece*

R. TURK, *Faculty of Electrical and Computer Engineering, University of Ljubljana, Trzaska 25, 61000 Ljubljana, Slovenia*

D.T. WADE MD, MRCP, *Consultant in Neurological Disability, Rivermead Rehabilitation Centre, Abingdon Road, Oxford OX1 4XD, UK*

R.O. WELLER BSc, MD, PhD, FRCPath, *Professor of Neuropathology, University of Southampton Medical School; Consultant Neuropathologist to the Wessex Neurological Centre, UK*

N.S. WILLIAMS MS, FRCS, *Professor of Surgery, The Surgical Unit, The Royal London Hospital, Whitechapel, London E1 1BB, UK*

C.B. WYNN-PARRY MBE, MA, DM, FRCP, FRCS, *Director of Rehabilitation, King Edward VII Hospital, West Sussex GU29 0BL, UK*

C.A. YOUNG BSc(Hons), MRCP, *Consultant Neurologist, University of Liverpool, Walton Centre for Neurology and Neurosurgery, Liverpool L9 1AE, UK*

Foreword

Since I began my training in neurology almost 45 years ago, I have witnessed a transformation in my specialty. Developments in neuroimaging, neuropharmacology, neuroimmunology, neurophysiology, neurovirology and molecular genetics, to name but a few fields in which major advances have taken place, have greatly illumined the pathogenesis of many neurological disorders, with consequential advances in treatment and management. Nevertheless, there remain many such conditions in which treatment, whether by pharmacological, physical or psychological means, is only partially successful, and there are still some disorders which remain, in the present state of knowledge, relatively uninfluenced by treatment. Even in those conditions which show a prompt response to treatment, measures which are collectively embraced under the term 'rehabilitation' may be vital in order to enhance the speed of recovery. Equally, in those conditions where treatment is only partially successful or unavailing, rehabilitation in the broadest sense plays a major role in enabling each individual patient to make the best of his or her capabilities and to overcome or adjust to the consequences of on-going disability. As I have regularly taught medical students over the years, there are still many incurable diseases in medicine, not least in neurological medicine, but there are none which are untreatable by pharmacological, physical and psychological means.

Hence, if one accepts the WHO 1969 definition of rehabilitation as extensively modified to meet the needs of the neurological patient, as the editor indicates clearly in his Preface, techniques of rehabilitation are particularly apposite to the management of the neurological patient and have developed by leaps and bounds over the course of the last 30 years. Thus I believe that the publication of the second edition of this book is particularly welcome. As the editor says, it presents a mosaic of basic neuroscience, rehabilitation theory and clinical pragmatism. The individual sections deal with definitions and the importance of communication and of the patient's view, followed by detailed analysis of the scientific background of neurological rehabilitation, a description of methods of assessment, and then issues of particular relevance to the neurological patient. There follow sections on specific problems encountered in neurological medicine and an exciting final section on new concepts, dealing especially with new technology, and developments in pharmacology and in surgery. Hence the book, which I found eminently readable, is a comprehensive compendium written by a series of experts embracing all of the topics which one could think of as being of value in the rehabilitation field. It is relevant not just to the practice of the clinical neurosciences in adults and children, but many doctors working in other branches of medicine, not least rheumatology, as well as those other members of the health care team who play such an important role in rehabilitation, notably physiotherapists, speech therapists and occupational therapists, will, I am sure, find it invaluable not least as a reference source, as will many of those in the population at large who are concerned with the causation and management of disability.

Oxford

John Walton
(Walton of Detchant)

Preface

An improvement in rehabilitation standards could mean more to millions of people than almost any medical advance (Secretary of State for the Social Sciences, UK, 1973). Unfortunately rehabilitation has tended to lack intellectual excitement and fulfilment, and has failed to capture the imagination of medical students.

Rehabilitation means different things to different people. The WHO definition (1969) defines rehabilitation as 'the combined and co-ordinated use of medical, social, educational and vocational measures for training or retraining the individual to the highest possible level of function and ability'. This definition deals only with the final aim of rehabilitation and, for a neurologist, excludes all the important and most interesting areas of neurological rehabilitation.

A wider definition of neurological rehabilitation would include: (i) the application of basic research to the problems of chronic neurological dysfunction; (ii) the determination of the cause and the extent of neurological dysfunction and the way in which *recovery* (as opposed to complications) may be affected by good after care and neuro-modulation techniques; and finally (iii) the WHO interpretation – the way in which the individual can be trained or managed to the highest possible level of functional ability and to cope with residual disability, in the shortest possible time. Rehabilitation in this sense overlaps with diagnosis and treatment, and embraces basic research, and should always be seen in this context.

This book brings together a wide variety of neurological expertise: epidemiologist, pathologist, experimental scientist, clinical physiologist, clinical neurologist, geriatrician, paediatrician, surgeon and engineer are all represented.

The contributors discuss the various ways in which neurological disability may arise, the continuing problems of accurate assessment, treatment, management of specific problems and specific diseases, and look into the future. The underlying concept is that damage to the central nervous system produces a reaction to the lesion or disease, and it is the combination of the damage and the reaction that produces the disability and suggests the means of influencing that reaction, and the management of the patient as a whole person.

The chapters in this book are by authors who bring their own expertise and understanding to the composite whole of neurological rehabilitation. Overlap is intentional and each chapter touches upon the fields of several other chapters and each of these has as many extensions, with the aim that any individual contribution will be given greater interest by the entire work. The book is a mosaic, as is the subject of neurological rehabilitation – a mosaic of basic neuroscience, rehabilitation theory, and clinical pragmatism.

Although overlap and differing emphasis between the disease and the patient is by design, omissions are largely unintentional!

I apologize in advance to international experts who are not represented and offer the consolation that within the next few years many of the contributions will be out of date in this rapidly expanding field of functional neurology and neurophysiology.

L.S. Illis

Acknowledgements

I would like to thank colleagues from various parts of the world who have kindly contributed to this volume and have taken such trouble to prepare up-to-date reviews. They are all experts in their various fields and they have submitted to badgering in a most philosophical way.

It is a pleasure to thank Mrs Sally Allan who has given hours of secretarial work in a most patient and unstinting way.

1: Introduction

L.S. ILLIS

The goal of medicine is the cure of illness but unfortunately the true aim in nearly all branches of medicine is the alleviation of pain and improvement of the quality of life. This is particularly true of neurological rehabilitation. Many of the chapters in this book emphasize the important point that much of rehabilitation is management and not treatment in the sense of cure or complete recovery. But neurological rehabilitation is a many-faceted subject as I hope will be obvious from this book.

As indicated in the preface, rehabilitation means different things to different people. In Part 1 the meaning of rehabilitation and the importance of communicating with the patient are discussed. The whole point of what we are trying to do in this field is brought to the fore with the patient's view of his/her disability and of the treatment he/she receives from the medical profession. These important features form the basis upon which research, treatment and management of neurological disability rests and which dictate whether or not we have achieved any success.

In the individual, diagnosis, treatment of the primary cause where applicable, secondary complications (such as urinary tract infections) and handicap, such as unemployment, lack of mobility and economic problems, are inseparable. These latter features are not strictly the province of the neurologist and need special support services. This admittedly artificial separation is somewhat foisted upon the medical profession by the World Health Organization (WHO) classifications of dysfunction. Teamwork is important but what is equally important is that the neurologist has overall supervision of the facilities to diagnose, treat and manage such a patient.

Neurological rehabilitation should be an equal partner in the context of clinical neurosciences, but sadly it is too often an afterthought or an adjunct to a neurologist's programme, motivated more by what is politically correct than by any true interest. Many neurological rehabilitation meetings resemble a group of society ladies making a token appearance to support a Third World cause. It has even been asserted that existing neuroscience theory may perhaps be abandoned. For example, Shahani & Scheinberg (1987) state: 'the patient and family can only benefit from abandonment of the practice of making a precise anatomic–pathologic diagnosis of impairment' – although to be fair they were highlighting the need for neurological rehabilitation. In a meeting in London in 1990 ('Hither Neurology') the organizer stated: 'to meet the needs of the very large numbers of people affected by neurological disabilities, British neurology would have to undergo a transformation . . . the most important changes would be . . . professional practices (even, perhaps, the nature of the most treasured neurological skill, the clinical examination) would have to change.' The logical outcome of this would be that rehabilitation would be planned *in vacuo*. For example, a patient with gait disability would be treated in a rehabilitation programme, rather than an accurate diagnosis of, say, cord compression or subacute combined degeneration of the cord being made or excluded. Treatment without diagnosis is an almost universal feature of intractable pain, and the result is obvious.

The scope of neurological rehabilitation embraces some of the most interesting and enigmatic problems of neurology, such as the nature of recovery, spasticity and intractable pain. The aim of this book is quite simply to attempt to place neurological rehabilitation in the mainstream of neurosciences: to show that there is a theoretical basis for rehabilitation which is firmly anchored in clinical neurology and the basic neurosciences, and also to demonstrate the exciting intellectual problems posed by chronic neurological deficit. Nobody is attracted to rehabilitation who is not motivated by compassion, but sympathy and caring are not enough, nor is there any reason to assume that high-grade 'academic' research and a sincere desire to help are mutually exclusive, as I hope is apparent in the chapters in this book.

Does neurological rehabilitation have anything to offer the patient? As a neuroscience discipline, does it attract neurologists? Douglas Black, President of the Royal College of Physicians (UK), in *College Commentary*, in January 1980 (p. 7) stated:

> There was much praise for the Alma-Ata resolution of 'Health for all by the year 2000', combined with a tendency to undervalue both biomedical science and high standards of clinical medicine – the two things which give modern medicine its strength. There was much praise for a new type of medical school, which centres the curriculum on public health and discounts such trivia as telling one heart sound from another. My fear is that if these trends prevail, what we will have in the year 2000 will not be health for all, but valetudinarianism for those who don't need medicine, and third-rate medicine for those who do. Unbalanced concentration on what is called 'the delivery of health care' may be a distraction from the real objective, which is to be sure that we have something that is worth delivering. Feeling a little like Daniel, I made some comments at the meeting; the lions turned out to be toothless, or at least dumb, but I don't think I converted them from their addiction to generalising mediocrity.

Are we in danger of promoting third-rate medicine? Unfortunately, some departments of rehabilitation still advocate the abandonment of accurate neurological skills and this would indeed produce a generalized mediocrity. Fortunately, an increasing number of institutes, organizations and individuals are at the forefront of the new approach to neurological rehabilitation. Many of them are represented here.

In all organ systems, damage or disease may result in recovery, which is easily explicable in terms of tissue regeneration and reorganization.

The exception is the central nervous system (CNS). Until the demonstration of sprouting of intact nerve fibres following partial denervation, in the late 1950s and early 1960s, the received wisdom was that a lesion in the CNS produced a fixed neurological deficit. Coming after the discovery of sprouting, there followed theoretical discussions about the nature of recovery, based on simple models of CNS innervation, the demonstration of unmasking, and the pharmacological or neurochemical changes which may occur with partial denervation. Hand in hand with these exciting developments, external stimulation, whether by repetitive electrical stimulation or by pharmacological means, was shown to produce measurable changes in neurological function, possibly by increasing inhibition. The idea of a fixed neurological deficit was no longer tenable and a new concept of neurological dysfunction was born: that the intact CNS reacts to an insult and the clinical syndrome seen in the patient is a combination of the damage caused by the lesion and the often distant effects of the lesion. Recovery of function would then be consequent upon a reorganization of the nervous system directed towards a re-establishment of the function orginally lost, since no regeneration of nerve cells occurs. This would follow Le Chatelier's principle, a principle well known in physical sciences but first applied to biological sciences in an attempt to understand the basis for recovery (Illis, 1967): if a system is in equilibrium and one of the conditions of the system is altered, it will adjust itself in such a way as partially to neutralize the change in condition. Brodal (1973) in his self-observations after his stroke spoke of the far-reaching consequences of a lesion involving a small part of the nervous system. These developments raised neurological rehabilitation out of what, to be honest, is often thought by neurologists to be a sink of despair, to the level of other clinical neurosciences. These concepts, which range across basic neuroscience, neuropathology and neurology, are dealt with in Part 2, which I have, perhaps grandiosely, entitled the scientific background of neurological rehabilitation. In this section are some of the ideas which are altering the view of neurological rehabilitation away from dealing only with complications and towards trying to promote active recovery and to restore function.

There are three main approaches. First, there is

the prevention of secondary pathological events in the hope that not only will this improve the quality of life of the individual but may also influence the chronic state. Second, there is restoration of damaged neuronal connections. Attempts include using some kind of bridge, which may be fetal cells, pieces of peripheral nerve or a collagen matrix. So far, this line has been less than convincing. The repeated failure of regeneration in the adult mammalian CNS produced a disillusionment which has now been replaced by a more optimistic and exciting period. Banyard *et al.* (1991) have discussed some of the discoveries which have led to this change, including Aguayo's demonstration that regeneration was not prevented by factors within the nerve cells themselves, but also depended on the cells they contacted; Schwab's work on inhibitory molecules on the surface of oligodendrocytes, the development of antibodies to the inhibitory molecules, and the genetic engineering of neuroblastoma cells to produce the antibodies; and the search for growth factors which are associated with the ability of fetal nerve cells to grow and find the correct target, but are absent or inhibited in the adult. Third, there is the approach based on how the intact or surviving nervous system reacts to the lesion, and which draws on experimental evidence for plasticity. Here, as stated above, the theoretical premise is that part of the neurological deficit is due to altered function in the intact nervous system, possibly sensory driven, and it is this aspect which is capable of alteration.

Of course, one of the main research drives is to promote successful regrowth of nerve fibres in the CNS. Only fairly recently can such an aim be even mentioned in polite neurological society! For example, in the 1980s a growth-associated protein, GAP-43, was discovered and found to be present only when nerve fibres are growing, such as during embryonic development, but with falling levels in the adult nervous system. After damage to the peripheral nervous system, GAP-43 levels rise not only where peripheral growth occurs, but also in nerve fibre terminals in the spinal cord, and CNS axons grow very short distances in an erratic and perhaps dysfunctional way. In the future, there is a possibility of switching damaged CNS cells to a regenerative mode. Peripheral nervous system Schwann cells promote regeneration, whereas CNS oligodendroglia and astroglia may actively inhibit growth. Implanted peripheral grafts into the injured CNS may stimulate growth into the implant. The hope is that these, and other, experimental studies involving growth-enhancing molecules may lead to true CNS regeneration. When that happy day dawns, we shall be faced with the problems of assessment of neurological deficit, and the long-term effects of deafferentation, which may include cardiovascular alteration, demineralization of bone, wasting and contractures, bladder dysfunction and intractable pain, etc.

In Part 3, assessment – the evaluation of neurological disability – is addressed. All aspects of treatment or management come across the same stumbling-block: assessment of the disability, selection of patients and evaluation of the effects of treatment. Most of the contributors to this book have approached this problem as it relates to their particular field. However, one of the major problems remains that of selection of large enough groups matched for age, sex, type and extent and duration of lesion, etc. and then randomized to control and treatment groups. Furthermore, the assessment should be carried out by workers independent of the therapeutic team. A study which is relatively easy to mount in terms of double-blind drug evaluation is extremely difficult to put into practice in terms of any type of physical therapy. Part 3 overlaps with neurophysiological assessment in Part 2, and leads on to the main sections on the neurological patient, and some of the specific problems of neurological dysfunction. In these sections there is considerable overlap. This is by design, since the aim is to try to avoid a single, dogmatic method, to show how the same problem may be approached in different ways, and to indicate how dysfunction in a specific disease may converge with another disease or with injury.

The final section discusses newer concepts in rehabilitation: newer in terms of a textbook of rehabilitation perhaps, but many of the ideas have been studied for a number of years and are showing promise in selected patients.

The solution to dysfunction caused by damage and disease in the CNS will not be found in the near future. However, the chronic condition is by no means untreatable and in many instances the disturbance sustained can be ameliorated.

References

Banyard P.J., Illis L.S. & Wall P.D. (1991) The amelioration and cure of spinal cord damage: the aim of the International Spinal Research Trust. *Paraplegia* **29**, 143–148.

Brodal A. (1973) Self-observations and neuro-anatomical considerations after a stroke. *Brain* **96**, 675–694.

Illis L.S. (1967) The motorneurone surface and spinal shock. In Williams D. (ed.) *Modern Trends in Neurology*, Chapter 3, pp. 53–68. Butterworths, London.

Shahani B. & Scheinberg L. (1987) Neurological rehabilitation. *Neurological Clinics* **5**, 519–522.

Part 1
The Clinical Background

2: What is Rehabilitation?

H.J. GLANVILLE

Definitions, 8
Potential for improvement, 8
Measurement of function, 10
Communications, 11
Co-ordination, 12

Sommerville (1975) suggested that rehabilitation was first used in common English parlance in the meaning of 'making able' and 'making able again' to denote readoption of denominational dress by transgressors who had been temporarily denied the privilege of wearing it.

Rehabilitation is a word which is used in different contexts; it therefore suggests different things and there is no specific acceptance of its meaning. To some it means reinstatement, or even instatement for the first time in the physical sense; others will interpret it as applying to the reinstatement of offenders, addicts and people suffering from psychiatric disorders. It is within the definition formulated by the Mair Report (1972), *Medical Rehabilitation: the Pattern for the Future*, that the meaning is taken for this book: 'Rehabilitation implies the restoration of patients to their fullest physical, mental and social capability'; and one might add 'in the shortest possible time'.

When we relate this concept to the problem of neurological disability, which is often progressive, which usually affects many rather than single functions and which usually excludes cure as a possible outcome of rehabilitation, the objective will be to help the patient to achieve the best possible quality of life in the circumstances. The patient cannot be considered singly; for example, a wheelchair existence directly affects everyone with whom the sufferer is associated, including family, people at work and many others in society whom he/she regularly meets. In his book, Cooper (1976) intro-duces the concept of the Fourth World of handicapped people who are with us and need the support of family and friends. These people are not two entities, but one organism irretrievably locked together and bound 'by a combination of concern, love, despair, frustration and feelings of guilt'. Parents and loved ones, too, are in a sense citizens of this Fourth World because they are drawn into it. Doctors and others whose role it is to help disabled people must learn to understand these human and social relationships in order to develop the knowledge to counsel and to help them wisely. Cooper rightly points out that the rule for survival has always been 'adapt or perish', and emphasizes that our contribution must be to help victims and their relatives to accept what is inevitable, to correct what is correctable and to build new lives by adapting to new circumstances.

The report on specific technical matters from the 29th World Health Assembly (World Health Organization, 1976a,b) states that rehabilitation is usually defined as the third phase of medicine, prevention being the first and curative care the second. Throughout the report the term is used, as here, to define interactions which in general aim to provide treatment and services for patients who are already disabled or at risk due to an interference with function. In 1969, the WHO expert committee (World Health Organization, 1969a,b) defined rehabilitation as follows: 'the combined and coordinated use of medical, social, educational and vocational measures for training or retraining the individual to the highest possible level of functional ability'. This definition relates mainly to intervention aimed at the individual, with less emphasis upon altering the factors in immediate surroundings or in society, which all bear heavily upon the problem.

An understanding of the word rehabilitation by no means eliminates the confusion surrounding the use of common terms such as impairment, functional limitation, handicap and disability.

Definitions

Impairment, for practical purposes, means 'a missing or defective part, tissue, organ or mechanism of the body' (World Health Organization, 1969a,b).

Functional limitation may or may not result from impairment, as defined above, and such limitations may be regressive or progressive depending upon the cause.

Handicap 'reflects the value attached to an individual's status when it departs from the norm. In the context of health care handicap is the disadvantage that is consequent upon impairment and disability' (Wood, 1975).

Disability 'describes a functional departure from the norm and as such it mediates between impairment and handicap. In the context of health care disability is the loss or reduction of functional ability and activity that is consequent upon impairment' (Wood, 1975).

Obviously impairment, for example the loss of a leg, will be a disadvantage and therefore a handicap to a rock-climber. On the other hand, such loss will little affect a sedentary worker's efficiency at work. Disability consequent upon the same cause will be variously reflected in different individuals consequent upon their attitudes, social status, occupation and so on.

The International Classification of Diseases (ICD) deals with diagnoses but not with their outcome. At the Conference for the Ninth Revision of the ICD, 1975, a resolution recommended a tentative draft classification of impairments and handicaps for trial purposes and the work was undertaken by P.H.N. Wood, ARC Epidemiological Research Unit, Manchester UK. It is an important step because at present there is no standard accepted classification of impairment and handicap, and consequently no common scientific classification of impairment and handicap such as would provide a baseline for research and evaluation by ensuring that like is being compared with like.

Other workers have tackled this problem, for example Agerholm (1975) and Taylor (1977), who draw attention to the interrelationship of physical impairment, functional limitation, disability and social handicap. These attempts at clarification of terms and of coding are particularly important in the field of neurological rehabilitation, which needs a common language as a prerequisite for the measurement of the many factors which, for need of a better word, we describe as function.

WHO has many important functions in relation to rehabilitation. For example, there are probably 380 000 000 disabled people in the world (World Health Organization, 1976a,b), but where do priorities lie for prevention and intervention? With limited resources, where can they be best used? Would it be by providing protein and vitamins for the Third World or are there some areas in which finance should be applied to aid research into neurological disorders, for example, which are responsible for the most severely handicapped people amongst us? For the first time in decades, there is real evidence that such people can begin to hope for a better future through new approaches.

Potential for improvement

The Sherrington concept of neurophysiology no longer explains observed facts. It does not, for example, explain how a man whose sensory apparatus had been destroyed by neurovirus was totally dependent when admitted to our unit and subsequently 'recovered'. The main features were complete absence of proprioception and patchy loss of cutaneous sensation. Eventually, he became totally independent and returned to gainful employment, although at that point routine neurological examination revealed no objective deviation from the pre-recovery state. Similarly, it is usual that, following acute cord or brain damage, stabilization occurs after a period of 2 or more years, but we have no evidence that upper neurons regenerate although they seem to attempt to do so by inexpedient sprouting. What, then, happens? Illis (1973) has postulated how alternative connections would be possible between cell stations. He shows how such interconnections could prevent the total failure of a system if one station were destroyed. On the other hand, failure would follow if alternative pathways did not exist. In this book, Devor states the paradox in recovery of the central nervous system. He puts his finger on the point in the statement that 'among the so called "plastic" changes the physical basis of rehabilitation will be found'.

We do not know enough about the presence of connections of alternative pathways, about how to recruit them or how to influence the 'plastic' changes which undeniably happen. It is interesting to draw an analogy between Victorian engineers (Rolt, 1970), who often found solutions to practical problems before they understood the scientific basis for them, and doctors, who observe the complexity of hand function, for example, and understand the implications of the mechanisms that provide it but not all their details. Control engineers view hand function as a challenge to be reproduced by electronic circuitry and mechanical hardware (Glanville, 1976). Their exciting progress was partly determined by ingenuity in devising sensors and circuitry to perform some of the functions of the interneuron system, so that simple commands would evoke an element of automatic function that is inherent but which is elusive in our comprehension of the human mechanism.

Comparison of the performance of biomechanical and electronic mechanisms leads, not surprisingly, to the observation of differences between them – for example, biological sensors are capable of both coarse and very fine responses according to the requirements of a given movement. Other instances illustrate how normal physiology has been better understood through the need to develop devices to carry out similar functions. For example, computers, calculators and memory banks can carry out, or could be programmed to accomplish, some functions of which the brain is capable. How far the mechanisms are or are not electronically similar is open to conjecture. We do know, however, a good deal about neurophysiological responses in the brain, and computer science now suggests how the brain might handle certain tasks. In another context it was commonly observed that weak muscles from poliomyelitis could be strengthened by exercise. It seemed that perseverance by the rehabilitation team and the patient were of prime importance. If improvement did occur, it tended to continue for about 2 years. When electromyography was used to study action potentials in these patients, recovery seemed to correspond with the appearance of 'giant potentials'. The reason for their appearance and their association with recovery was later explained by the discovery of peripheral sprouting of motor units to innervate adjacent denervated muscle fibres – a hitherto unknown phenomenon. It follows that the organized study of recovery and deterioration of function by qualified personnel at all levels, against the background knowledge of the normal central nervous system, must be rewarding. Imagination as well as the means to develop new diagnostic tools will play an important part.

Our problem is to unravel the complex circuitry of the central nervous system because, until we can do so, a specific approach to its rehabilitation is impossible. The regenerative powers of the peripheral nervous system, improved techniques in nerve and tendon surgery and better orthotic devices have greatly improved the outlook in plexus and peripheral nerve lesions. Wynn Parry (1966) points out here and elsewhere that recovery can be accelerated by good after-care and re-education. He demonstrates through careful serial assessments how motor as well as sensory function can be re-educated in the hand more quickly and completely through training than by a passive approach. He describes, too, how transcutaneous electrical stimulation has proved useful in a number of painful peripheral nerve disorders. His work is supported by carefully compiled evidence which justifies the therapy advised, even if the physiological reasons for the observed effects are not always fully understood. Similarly, Illis and Sedgwick in this book have studied in depth and longitudinally a few patients undergoing spinal cord stimulation, and their work points to the effects that can be expected or at least hoped for. In practice, this means that careful observation makes it possible to advise patients what improvement they can expect and what are the attendant risks. The mechanisms underlying improvement are not known, but Cook's observation that his patients treated for intractable pain by cord stimulation and suffering from concurrent multiple sclerosis showed functional improvement has been confirmed by other workers, and the amount, duration and quality of improvement are being verified, so that cord stimulation in selected cases has passed beyond the stage of 'experimental therapy'.

Unfortunately, in the past, failure to carry out evaluation of outcome to support clinical impression has caused good, or at least useful, forms of intervention to fall into disrepute and useless interventions to be perpetuated. Thus electrical stimulation fell into disrepute and almost rejection in the UK during the three decades after the Second World War on the grounds that it represented a form of passive treatment whilst active treatment, i.e. 'doing exercises', would always achieve a better result. Electrical stimulation, nevertheless, had a few protagonists, some of whom would hold one form of faradic stimulator to be 'better than' another. Certainly, output parameters of faradic stimulators varied wildly, and possibly therefore some did give better results than others, but claims were not supported by real evidence, and it was not until the appearance of square wave stimulators with good output control that serious interest was aroused again. Now electrical stimulation has many uses, including functional electronic stimulation (Dimitrijevic et al., 1968; Glanville, 1972), in which functional motor effects as well as inhibitory effects upon the spastic calf, in hemiplegia, are described.

The ultimate goal will be achieved when control systems and stimulators reach the degree of acceptability and perfection to replace lost function in, for example, paraplegics. It should be possible for them to walk with assist devices, and progress continues. At present, results are encouraging, usually in a limited way, and routine adoption of electronic solutions is probably further off than is generally recognized. In the mean time, unrealistic goals and false hopes have brought disappointment, failure and, indeed, tragedy.

Measurement of function

To measure function accurately, repeatably and objectively is exceedingly difficult because function is compounded by factors which are difficult to identify, isolate and measure. The need to measure in order to compare and to assess the outcome of intervention is not in doubt, and whilst many workers are continually trying to devise and improve methods the clinician will often have to innovate to suit his/her need to test the value and cost-effectiveness of alternative therapies.

The UK armed forces adopted a rough classification for troops in order to measure their suitability for service. During the Second World War a system called PULHEEMS was introduced, which was designed to provide a profile of the individual. Each initial represents a capability which is classified from 1 (perfect) to 8 (nil) for each individual.

P   Physical capacity
U   Upper limbs
L   Lower limbs
H   Hearing
E   Eyesight L
E   Eyesight R
M   Mental capacity
S   Stability (emotional)

It now becomes simple to match the capability of an individual for specific jobs in the services. The score under each heading also gives a rough profile of capability. Obviously a low scorer under H would be a bad choice for a radio operator – motivation, however, does sometimes produce extraordinary exceptions (e.g. a double lower limb amputee who continued a distinguished career as an operational pilot during the Second World War). The system does not give the detail needed for most scientific evaluation, but it probably did influence thinking about scoring systems in common use in daily-living departments of rehabilitation units, where it is necessary to assess the individual as to ability in independence, etc. Most units tend to invent their own systems for this purpose, based upon ability of the individual to carry out essential tasks for independent living without assistance, with aids or with assistance. Some include a time factor because obviously to be able to dress without help is valueless if it takes all day! A seminar at the Northwick Park Hospital dealt with these complex problems (Yates, 1976), including the quality of life (and how to measure it), and amongst other contributions there is a useful description of a move by the British Association of Occupational Therapists to standardize 'activities of daily living' assessment (Jay, 1976). Nichols (1976), however, questioned whether 'activities of daily living' indices were of any value on the grounds that they are subjective and therefore not reliable or repeatable, for a whole variety of reasons. Whiting & Lincoln (1980) discuss an 'activities of daily living' assessment for stroke patients. Evans in this book describes a practical system for the evaluation of progress in brain-damaged patients. The system identifies the point at which improvement stops and therefore when emphasis should change from active to supportive programmes. The decision is always a difficult one for the clinician to make, but clear guidelines are helpful in indicating when to conserve rather than to misapply scarce resources. Lynn and co-workers (1977) describe how a programmed signal can produce a spot tracing or 'target' on a cathode ray screen. The signal can be followed by a patient using a manual device to manipulate in order to maintain a circular marker around the target. Accuracy in following the target can be estimated by scanning and it then becomes possible to show the degree of error, expressed numerically, during the task. Although the actual activity is valueless in terms of usefulness in the life situation, it is nevertheless a valuable measure in assessing accuracy in performing the task, which requires manipulative skill, co-ordination and response in tracking the target. Again, Miller and co-workers (Gandy *et al.*, 1978) demonstrated the electromyogram (EMG) patterns of arm movement and muscle activity in 20 subjects whilst turning a cranked wheel. This activity involves the patterns of muscle activity common to the reaching and retrieving movements of daily living. It was possible to define normals and recognize the effects of learning the task and the abnormalities introduced by spasticity.

There are many complex and sophisticated approaches to the problem of measuring locomotion, for example walkways with multichannel EMG recording, cine-photography in several planes, pressure plate studies and so on, but the case for simple feedback systems is valid both to measure function and as an aid to re-educative procedures. Calibration of such apparatus is a problem, and digital displays are helpful in the clinical use of feedback apparatus. More rational and better therapy will be possible as better techniques for measuring are developed. Sophisticated apparatus in main research centres does not replace the need for the simpler inexpensive tools for making objective measurements in small clinical departments, where much of the remedial work is done.

Communications

Failure to exchange knowledge and experience is an important cause of failure to provide services that could be available for patients. Thus research, teaching and services need to be integrated between main centres and peripheral units for the benefit of both. Special Interest Groups have been set up in the Wessex Region in the UK, largely with the problem of communications in mind. Their functions are:

1 to evaluate, measure and create standards in rehabilitation practice;
2 to improve services through greater efficiency;
3 to promote research where it is seen to be needed;
4 to improve education in rehabilitation; and
5 to share information arising from clinical work.

The model which has been adopted is successful in practice and it lends itself particularly well to neurological disability, which poses severe problems in rehabilitation whose solution does not rest in the hands of any single individual. Such a group must be multidisciplinary, consisting of physicians, surgeons, therapists, ergonomists, psychologists and engineers, to mention only a few. It must be headed by a co-ordinator who is someone with sufficient grasp of the whole field to plan and conduct meetings of good academic and practical standard. The group also requires secretarial support. In practice, the groups in Wessex consist of about 80 regular attenders, who represent district hospitals in the region. Essentially, they are working groups and therefore define needs and allocate tasks, and meetings take place when members of the group have produced something to discuss rather than at regular intervals. In practice, meetings take place two or three times a year. The activities of groups are part research, part teaching and learning and part related to the improvement of practice. The outcome is a general improvement of standards and a means for quick dissemination of new knowledge, for introducing new principles in care and, above all, for evaluating the outcome of rehabilitation activities. There will be other ways of tackling the same problems and the exact organization of any schemes will depend upon local resources, personalities and geography. The objective, however, will remain the same, namely to improve practice based on scientific studies, rather than by reliance on custom or empiricism, and to generate new knowledge. Groups may not carry full competence in all aspects within their membership; therefore access to university departments and faculties is of great value. The support of libraries, teaching media, statistics, ergonomics, mathematics and engineering are needed and are forthcoming from an academic source.

Of great value, too, at an international level are complementary programmes between main centres. Meetings supported by charity have brought workers together from all parts of the world in order to share experience and to effect exchanges of scientific and medical staff.

It is not the purpose of this chapter to describe the organization of rehabilitation units or services. They are described elsewhere (Glanville, 1956, 1976; Cochrane & Glanville, 1975; Nichols, 1980). An important need today is to ensure that new knowledge about neurological disability is communicated to providers of services so that good developments can be incorporated into practice. Unfortunately, much that could be done for patients is not available to them, often through poor communication and lack of awareness.

Co-ordination

Much good would come from a policy to develop research, teaching and services in a few main centres designed to combine both the acute and the rehabilitation phases of care for patients with neurological disorders. Too often, key people in the neurological team are denied the experience of involvement during rehabilitation, which is essential to research and to the growth of knowledge, for the reasons indicated earlier. The study of improvement and the reasons for its taking place have received too little attention but do require increasing study. Academic posts in neurological rehabilitation should be set up to bridge the gap between the acute and restorative phases of care and to ensure that appropriate emphasis is given to the task of harnessing data to increase knowledge and how to use and teach it wisely. The contribution of the paramedical professions to improving the lot of the neurologically disabled is inestimable. These professions require good postgraduate experience and it will be best provided for them in comprehensive centres of the kind envisaged. Centres could not work realistically in isolation for they must stimulate and help to develop community, social and voluntary services as well as public awareness of the

needs of disabled people. So long as professionals consider only their own limited roles in relation to neuropathology and the disability resulting from it, there will be little progress. Unfortunately, neurologists are everywhere in short supply and usually do not find time to lead and co-ordinate services for the rehabilitation of their patients. This is doubly regrettable because their input is essential both to develop the knowledge, skills and attitudes of personnel and to plan and monitor the treatment of their patients. Not the least important is the need to include in neurological medical curricula exposure to the problems of disability and its management. Too often a physically handicapped person seeking advice will be the first exposure of a newly qualified doctor to problems that his training has not prepared him to handle.

Attempting to set standards in the rehabilitation and care of disabled people, the Royal College of Physicians of England published a report: *Physical Disability in 1986 and Beyond* (RCP, 1986). It assessed current practice, discussed the epidemiology of disability and made recommendations to overcome deficiencies. Further, it advised regional disability units on their staffing and emphasized the need for training in disability and rehabilitation in each speciality. Specialists would then be ideally qualified to look after their patients in the rehabilitation phase. This recommendation is particularly apt in the case of neurological disability, but unfortunately neurologists in the UK and other countries are in short supply and do not often enough find time to be leaders in this context. A second report (Edwards & Warren, 1990) followed; this surveys in detail services for adults with physical disabilities at District Health Authority level.

Much effort by voluntary and statutory bodies has been expended and much advice is available (Frank & Maguire, 1988) to help in understanding what physically disabled people, their families and helpers face in order to survive and consequently what measures could be helpful.

Trends should become more favourable as time passes and awareness grows generally. There are factors, however, which make people with neurological disability as a group likely to be disadvantaged in the allocation of resources. Their need should have priority because they are the most severely disabled people in the community. But they are a minority numerically. Unfortunately, their rehabilitation, as evidenced in, for example, brain injury (RCP, 1988), which is only one of many disabling possibilities, is lengthy, labour-intensive in terms of multiprofessional input and disproportionately expensive to managers of health care budgets, whose priorities are to reduce waiting lists, improve bed usage and treat as many patients as possible within financial limits. To them procedures like spare-part surgery, whose costs and outcome are fairly predictable, will look like good use of resources in comparison. In fact, Klein (1991) points out that the amount of money available is not the solution to funding health services. Nevertheless, it is an anomaly that the finance for two totally different kinds of need should come from the same budget at all, for they are incomparable. It is just as impossible to compare outcome and value for money of, for example, a rehabilitation regime given at the right time, which prevented contractures, bed sores and renal failure (although a wheelchair existence was the eventual outcome), with a bypass operation. They should not have to compete in the same market-place and until they do not those entrusted with the treatment of neurological patients must campaign for fair resources. It is arguable that allowances given for spending at the point of need have flexibility and give choice to the sufferer. However, they will never make up for failure of appropriate intervention.

References

Agerholm M. (1975) Handicap and the handicapped. A nomenclature of classification of intrinsic handicaps. *Royal Society of Health Journal* 1, 3–8.

Cantrell E.G., Dawson J. & Glastonbury G. (1983) *Prisoners of Handicap*. Nuffield Provincial Hospitals Trust.

Cochrane G. & Glanville H.J. (1975) Rehabilitation today. *Update* 10, 1357–1372.

Cooper I.S. (1976) *Living with Chronic Neurological Disease*, pp. 11–21. W.W. Norton & Co., New York.

Dimitrijevic M.R., Gracanin F., Prevec T. & Trontelj J. (1968) Electronic control of paralysed extremities. *Biomedical Engineering* 3, 8–14.

Edwards F. & Warren M.D. (1990) *Health Services for Adults with Physical Disabilities: a Survey of District Health Authorities 1988/89*. Royal College of Physicians, London.

Frank A.O. & Maguire G.P. (1988) *Disabling Diseases*, pp. 261–266. Heinemann Medical Books, Oxford.

Gandy M., Lynn P.A., Miller S. & Reed G.A.L. (1978) Quantitative assessment of patterns of muscle activity in the arm. *International Journal of Rehabilitation Research* 1, 356.

Glanville H.J. (1956) A unit for early rehabilitation in a general hospital. *Annals of Physical Medicine* 3, 101–102.

Glanville H.J. (1972) Electronic control of paralysis. *Proceedings of the Royal Society of Medicine* 65, 233–235.

Glanville H.J. (1976) *An Inaugural Lecture. What is Rehabilitation?*, p. 13. University of Southampton, Southampton.

Illis L.S. (1973) Experimental model of regeneration in the central nervous system. *Brain* 96, 47–68.

Jay P. (1976) Association sought a standard way to record assessment. *British Journal of Occupational Therapy* 39, 299–300.

Klein R. (1991) *British Medical Journal* 303, 259–260.

Lynn P., Reed G.A.L., Parker W.R. & Langton Hewer R. (1977) Some applications of human-operator research in the assessment of disability in stroke. *Medical and Biological Engineering and Computing* 15, 184–188.

Mair Report (1972) *Medical Rehabilitation: the Pattern for the Future*. Scottish Home and Health Department, Social Health Services Council, HMSO, London.

Nichols P.J.R. (1976) ADL indices of any value? *Occupational Therapy* 39, 160–163.

Nichols P.J.R. (1980) *Rehabilitation Medicine: the Management of Physical Disabilities*, 2nd edn. Butterworths, London.

Rolt L.J.C. (1970) *Victorian Engineering*. Penguin, Allen Lane.

Royal College of Physicians (RCP) (1988) *The Management of Traumatic Brain Injury*. Medical Disability Society, Royal College of Physicians, London.

Sommerville J.D. (1975) *Workshop on Disablement and Rehabilitation in Developing Countries*, p. 11. Department of Social Studies, Selly Oak College, Birmingham, UK.

Taylor D.G. (1977) Physical impairment social handicap. *Office of Health Care Economics* 60, 6–7.

Whiting S. & Lincoln N. (1980) An ADL assessment for stroke patients. *Occupational Therapy* 43, 44–46.

Wood P.H.N. (1975) *Classification of Impairments and Handicaps*, Doc. No. WHO 1 CD/9 Rev. Conf/7515, p. 2. WHO, Geneva.

World Health Organization (1969a) Technical Report No. 419, p. 7, 1.2 (1).

World Health Organization (1969b) Technical Report No. 419, p. 13, 1.4.1.

World Health Organization (1976a) 29th World Health Assembly. A20 Inf. Doc. 1, p. 13, 1.4.1.

World Health Organization (1976b) A29 Inf. Doc. 1, p. 17, Table 1.

Wynn Parry C.B. (1966) *Rehabilitation of the Hand*, 2nd edn. Butterworths, London.

Yates E. (1976) Measuring the quality of life. *British Journal of Occupational Therapy* 39, 299.

3: Communication and Explanation of Neurological Disability

E.M.R. CRITCHLEY

What a neurological service should offer, 14
Two starting-points, 15
    Communication, 15
    Explanation, 16
Causes of failure, 22
Improvements in management, 23

Communication prompts, promotes and pervades each stage of rehabilitation (Table 3.1). The return of function is impeded unless the patient's understanding can be obtained, his/her will-power reinforced and his/her efforts encouraged. Many negative factors – self-pity, lack of self-esteem, depression, anxiety – have to be overcome. Empathic communication is the key which unlocks the application of medical science to human problems. For rehabilitation to succeed the interchange of information between patient and doctor should be of the highest order. Unfortunately, as stated in the Report of the Royal College of Physicians of London, *Physical Disability in 1986 and Beyond* (RCP, 1986), 'a frequent complaint is the inadequate information given to the disabled person about the nature and the expected course of the underlying condition; about the treatment and the plan of management of the ensuing disabilities; and about the opportunities, services, and help that are available'.

Although individual doctors have a personal responsibility to ensure adequate communication, imperfections within the system also mitigate against the patient receiving, as of right, a full explanation of his/her diagnosis, management and prognosis in a form which he/she can readily understand: thus public attitudes and the organization of services must share much of the blame. Years of neglect, failure to take note of the needs of the disabled and an absence of political will

to implement a succession of reports from 1954 onwards (BMA, 1954, 1968; HMSO, 1967, 1972; RCP, 1986) have left the NHS with the task of implementing an unplanned, underfinanced and unsupported experiment – 'to set up an effective care service for the physically disabled without a substantial speciality of rehabilitation or its equivalent' (RCP, 1986). In practice, since most chronic disability involves either arthritic conditions or a multitude of neurological diseases, neurologists engaged in primary care have a major responsibility to guide the patient through the acute phases of his illness to that of active rehabilitation.

What a neurological service should offer

To achieve the optimum milieu, in which patients with neurological disability are provided with positive activation and encouragement to prepare them to regain their self-esteem and to resume as independent an existence as their disabilities permit, a neurologist must be cognizant of the mix of patients admitted to his/her wards and be prepared to examine his/her own back-up services. Nursing staff and administrators have to be persuaded that neurological patients require more than minimal supportive care and, in fact, require continual motivation as part of a planned programme of recovery. Many patients with multiple neurological disabilities, handicapped by mental and psychological changes – ataxia, hemiparesis or paraparesis, aphasia, dyspraxia and incontinence – require heavy dependency care. Not infrequently, neurological patients have psychiatric reactions to their physical condition. The majority of these reactions take the form of a depressed state, and a cheerful, supportive environment is as essential as

Table 3.1 Stages leading to effective communication

Empathic understanding of the patient's predicament
Explanation and diagnosis
Interchange of information
Explanation of planned action – understanding,
    agreement and co-operation
Continuing support and interchange of information
Encouragement
Practical assessment of progress and prognosis
Discussion and advice on future prospects

any amount of medication. A hospital ward making do with a skeleton staff cannot provide the necessary stimulation. In addition, a small number of neurological patients will need special care and surveillance because they are confused or disruptive and can, at times, become violent. Their needs are often overlooked, early recognition is required, extra staff should always be available, and there should be a clear, predetermined policy to limit the danger of such patients to themselves and to others. Nothing can be more horrifying than to come on to a ward to find frightened, ill patients trying to placate a disturbed, confused patient whilst a junior nurse is trying desperately to summon help from elsewhere.

Such an approach is not one-sided – a blast of indignation against the inadequacies of administration; it is equally essential that the consultant regards as his/her personal responsibility the standard of communication within his/her department and between other staff and the patient. Are the nursing staff confident that the treatment being provided is correct? There may be occasions, when dealing with a violent patient, a new form of therapy or a painful or experimental study, or where life-support measures are being withheld, when he/she should ensure that the nurses – even the most junior – know why a particular approach is being used. The day-to-day responsibility for such explanation falls upon the nursing officer but from time to time the consultant should take it upon him/herself to ensure that the nursing staff are told and are able to question him/her so that their ethical and other doubts are put to rest. The ward officer and nursing staff need to know what has been said to a patient as to his/her diagnosis, prognosis or treatment, and what has been said to

his/her relatives. Indeed, such information should be written clearly in, or at the front of, the patient's file. In a confident situation, the ward officer and senior nursing staff should be enabled to discuss the diagnosis and treatment with the patient, initiate physiotherapy, speech therapy, etc. and liaise as required with the social workers and others. They should be fully aware what they can tell, organize or explain; and their communication skills should be respected and developed. It often happens that a patient may find it easiest to identify and confide in a ward clerk, cleaner or porter. This does not constitute a failure of the system. The ancillary staff should feel that they are part of the team and that, if they are given information that is helpful to the management of the patient, they can talk freely to the ward officer and such information will be passed on, as necessary, to those concerned in the patient's treatment. Lastly, the patients should feel happy that their problems are being dealt with professionally and in confidence, and that there is no idle gossip.

Two starting-points

Communication

Neurological patients may be admitted as an emergency. History-taking and observation may have to be squeezed in between life-saving measures – clearing the airway, putting up a drip, etc. – but should never be squeezed out. However, the patient him/herself may not be able to provide a full history and other means of gaining knowledge of the circumstances – interviewing relatives or eye-witnesses and ringing the family practitioner or chemist – may have to be adopted. Doctors should not regard every friend or bystander who follows a patient into the accident department as just curious. More often than not they are motivated by a desire to impart information that can be crucial. Rather than turn them away, they should be persuaded to wait until they can be interviewed by a doctor or senior nurse. Useful information may include that of previous illnesses, drugs such as insulin, mental or physical handicap, linguistic problems, visual-field defects or speech disorders, or important but mundane information such as broken glasses, lost dentures or a defective hearing-aid.

Patients suffering neurological disability may become aware of their plight as they recover from the initial stage in a hospital bed or intensive care unit (ICU). The majority of these patients will be victims of trauma, strokes, fits or encephalitis. Their first question will be why am I here? Their second, what will become of me? They may not be in a position to ask these questions. They may see themselves as an appendage to a galaxy of monitoring apparatus with unpleasant attachments to their limbs and orifices. Not only may they not be able to speak, they may be unable to move any part of themselves to draw attention to their needs. A strict discipline must be maintained concerning what is said near any patient presumed to be in coma. A placard with the wartime slogan 'Careless Talk Costs Lives' could well be displayed in every ICU. When examining an unconscious patient, removing secretions or changing tubes, it is advisable to keep up a patter of helpful comments: 'This looks fine', 'He's coming lighter', 'There's an improvement'. As soon as a patient is showing ability to listen, a means of communication should be developed even if it is one movement of an eyebrow for 'yes', two for 'no'; and the patient should be told what has happened, what they are doing to him/her and, if possible, what will happen. These statements should be simple but repeated.

An assessment of a patient's ability to communicate is made as part of the routine examination of his/her mental and physical status, recognizing the effects of neurological impairment on the special senses and on higher mental functions and the use of suitable alternative methods of communication. A variety of communication aids are available and should be tried. People may be brought out of coma by tapes of their family, football or other heroes, or olden days in their town. Music can be soothing or invigorating, and radio, television or videos can be helpful in recovery. Explanation is needed with each new stage in their progress, especially when taken off artificial ventilation or with transfer to a general ward from the ICU. Many units report a mortality of around 50% of those transferred from a hard-pressed ICU to general wards at an early stage as a result of budgetary limitations. Among the positive factors enabling a successful outcome is active liaison between the ICU and the wards, gaining the confidence of the patient and relatives before a move is made, and, where communication aids are still needed, encouraging friends and relatives to make full use of these aids.

Explanation

Patients are often told their diagnosis in less than ideal circumstances and fail to comprehend all that is said. Such problems can arise at the initial routine out-patient consultation. Clinicians must be able to sense when the patient's understanding is imperfect even if superficially he or she appears to take in what has been said and its implications. A neurologist is required to adapt his/her professional skills in questioning, examining and explanation to the ability of the patient. However, there are many other factors which impair communication at the initial interview (Table 3.2) and alternative means to ensure that the diagnosis is explained and understood have to be considered.

What the patient is able or is prepared to understand should be a question which the doctor addresses throughout the process of history-taking and examination. Is the patient at ease as he/she gives the necessarily complex history? Are there lessons to be learnt from the patient's behaviour as well as clinical signs to be found during the physical examination? What is his/her emotional state, degree of intelligence, understanding, and insight into his condition? Is the slightly deaf patient lip-reading or merely guessing? Dyspraxia recognized during the examination of the motor system may reflect poor comprehension rather than evidence of motor pathology.

At a consultation the physician's first duty is to obtain as much information as possible, piecing together the patient's story, the GP's letter and further questioning of the relative or friend, acknowledging the patient's fears, and adding to all this his/her own observations throughout the period of history-taking and examination. From this information he/she needs to formulate at least a differential diagnosis and a course of action, be it reassurance to the patient, an immediate explanation, further tests or the need to admit the patient to hospital. The patient will always expect to be given an opinion at this stage, however ill-prepared he/she is to receive it. His/her fears and presumptions about his/her illness rarely lead to a

Table 3.2 Problems that can arise from the initial out-patient appointment

---

Transport to the hospital
By ambulance
    Prolonged wait, several stops made *en route*, ill-fitting times of arrival in relation to clinic times, unable to bring a relative or friend
By public transport
    Expensive and difficult journey, several changes made, long delays, arrival cold and hungry
Own transport
    Difficulty parking, late arrival, fear of a fine for faulty parking

Waiting to be seen
Delays due to inadequate appointment system
Lost notes or letters
Seen by inadequately prepared doctor

Examination
Absence of an interpreter
Absence of friend to add confidence or explanation of the history
Absence of eye-witness, e.g. to a presumed fit
Hearing-aid or glasses left at home by mistake
Exhaustion with the process of history-taking and examination

Explanation
Unable to relate to the doctor
Inadequate explanation
Too nervous to take in what is said
Absence of friend or relative to listen, question and explain later

Follow-up
Not told what will happen next, e.g. follow-up appointment, explanation of tests, letter to GP with full explanation

---

relaxed frame of mind. Despite all vicissitudes, to some extent the patient's uncertainties should have been dispelled by the warmth of the staff and the professional rapport of the doctor. But the inevitable happens. The doctor launches into an explanation and hands the patient an X-ray or laboratory request card with appropriate directions. Before he/she can sit back in self-congratulation, he/she has the humbling experience of observing the patient turn to the clinic nurse asking for the instructions to be repeated.

How can the doctor fully ensure that the patient leaves the clinic satisfied that he/she has understood what has been said? A repeated explanation by another doctor, nurse or social worker before the patient leaves the clinic is more likely to add to the confusion than to clear it. Advice to talk over the diagnosis with his/her GP when the GP has received a letter of full explanation can be helpful; but by far and away the most successful method of ensuring that the patient understands what is said is to ensure that the patient comes to the clinic accompanied by a friend or relative. Economies which prevent a relative or friend accompanying the patient are false ones and mean that more time or even more appointments might be necessary to bring the referral to a successful conclusion.

Even if the 'main helper' suffers from a serious handicap (McAlpine, 1965), his or her presence is stabilizing and reassuring to the patient. The escort may be better prepared than the patient to appreciate and discuss the explanations given and can repeat what has been said later when hopefully the patient will be more relaxed. At least the escort can say that the patient can discuss matters with his/her family doctor when he/she has received a letter from the consultant in a few days.

The outcome of the initial consultation may be a clear diagnosis, reinforced by discussion with a relative. Superficially, this is the most satisfactory outcome, but with neurological disability a programme of further counselling is often required, and needs to be outlined and explained. Alternatively, the diagnosis may be uncertain and is dependent upon further investigation of the patient either as an in-patient or as an out-patient. The purpose of such investigation has to be discussed, albeit briefly. Often, the diagnosis may be abundantly clear to the physician but for one reason or another the time is not opportune for detailed explanations and discussion. A partial, temporizing explanation is still required, but the nature of this is best discussed by examining specific examples.

Motor neuron disease (MND)

Patients with MND retain full mental and intellectual capabilities whilst faced with a progressive motor disability. Most sufferers are all too aware of their bleak prognosis and one of the greatest burdens they and their carers have to bear is the commonly held attitude that nothing can be done. It is vital that they should be helped and advised how to make the fullest use of their abilities to surmount the handicap under which they live.

The physical examination at the initial consultation may leave little doubt as to the diagnosis and the patient may be given some indication that he/she has a potentially progressive wasting disease of muscle resulting from a disorder of the nerve supply. However, the implications of the diagnosis are such that it is always advisable to admit the patient to hospital for a few days:

1 to allow full investigation and the exclusion of any other process, e.g. combined lumbar and cervical stenosis with myelopathy and radiculopathy, which might be potentially treatable;
2 to permit detailed discussion of the diagnosis with the patient and his/her relatives;
3 to advise on physiotherapy and teach postural drainage;
4 to outline and initiate the support services available at home to the patient and carer;
5 to establish a rapport with the patient so that he/she does not feel isolated and knows that the hospital can provide him/her with a back-up service.

Once the diagnosis is established beyond doubt, there must be full discussion with the patient, observing whatever limitations the patient wishes to set to the discussion. That is to say, patients need to know the extent of potential impairment so that they can plan their own arrangements, but all hope need not be closed and it is reasonable to state that some patients do run a longer course and may have to be redesignated as forms of spinal muscular atrophy. However, if the patient asks if the condition is potentially lethal, the answer must be an unequivocal 'yes'. If the reply to this question is ever given in the negative, this is manifestly false information shielding the patient from the grim truth. Few patients really accept this, particularly as they see themselves steadily deteriorating, and they will usually find out the true state of affairs even if this means going or sending someone to the public library. Once this has happened, there is likely to be an instantaneous breakdown of any trust which had previously existed between patient and doctor.

It is essential that the relatives or carers are given a clear indication of the prognosis and eventual outcome. But they should be reassured that with back-up support – essential if the patient has breathing or choking difficulties – most patients can be cared for at home. Despite the enormous physical handicaps endured by sufferers, the actual nursing demands do not, in general terms, present the challenges posed by patients who have lost sphincter control or have established pressure sores. There is no sphincter involvement and the skin does not usually break down over pressure areas. Throughout the illness the patient's intellect, drive and co-operation remain intact. At home the patient has the greatest freedom of activity and is least likely to become bored and introspective. With well-chosen adaptations, the sufferer can lead a fruitful and semi-independent existence manipulating radios, TVs, word-processors, communication aids and POSSUM devices. Few patients become severely depressed, though the possible development of a reactive depression should never be ignored.

Success of home care is dependent upon the active co-operation of support services and training of the carer so that he or she is confident in what they can provide. In the past there have been community therapists who have felt that the provision of aids and appliances for MND patients is an inappropriate use of limited resources because of the progressive course of the disease. To offset any breakdowns in funding or communication, it is essential to seek an early home visit by an occupational therapist or adviser from the MND Association. The patient's mobility can be assisted by the provision of tilt beds, hoists and electric wheelchairs.

Many relatives and friends adapt themselves amazingly well to the task of carer and show greater fortitude than can be expected from even the most dedicated nurses. Such dedication was a central theme of Morris West's novel *Masterclass* (1988). Carers need advice on surmounting communication difficulties, relieving aches and pains by the use of suitable collars, massage and passive movements, help with feeding and the preparation of food to a consistency which the patient manages best, and in the relief of choking or spluttering. Inexpensive foot-powered suckers may be helpful in this respect.

Follow-up consultations are necessary to assess

the need for further appliances, speech therapy, communication aids, or even cricopharyngeal sphincterotomy in selected cases. Patients and carers need continual reassurance and advice especially to overcome psychological pressures (as from other relatives) and fears. Respite care for the patient may be needed. Hospital visits may eventually overtax the patient and consideration should be given to obtaining domiciliary assessments.

Multiple sclerosis

The diagnosis of multiple sclerosis is still made on clinical judgement and there may be delays in obtaining tests such as magnetic resonance imaging (MRI), evoked potentials and oligoclonal bands in the cerebrospinal fluid. Sometimes even the results of these tests may remain equivocal. Thus many years may elapse from the first symptoms before an unequivocal diagnosis of multiple sclerosis can be made. Patients may have been given a series of diagnoses in the past, including hysteria, and when eventually told that they have multiple sclerosis it is not surprising that their first retort is 'why was I not told that earlier?', followed by the comment that they had long suspected the diagnosis. This having been said, it is clear that the doctor must be satisfied in his/her own mind of the diagnosis of multiple sclerosis before discussing its implications with the patient, and it is important that the GP is informed when this has been done. Once a diagnosis can be made, early discussion with the patient is essential, telling the patient that the diagnostic label is helpful in that early treatment can be given in the event of a further exacerbation. Undue delay will only lead to serious difficulties with the longer-term management, and patients will inevitably have assumed the worst possible connotations: that they will become bedridden or wheelchair-bound at an early age.

Thousands of people have multiple sclerosis and continue in gainful employment with reasonable mobility for many years. Others can lead a remarkably full life, despite a degree of handicap, and it must always be remembered that dramatic improvements can sometimes occur. Knowing the diagnosis is an essential first step to the constructive discussion of measures such as special diets, which

are from time to time suggested as being of benefit. An informed patient is better able to adjust to pregnancy, sexual difficulties, incontinence or even depression and feels free to bring up specific problems as they arise.

Epilepsy

An epileptic seizure is a brief and usually unprovoked stereotyped disturbance of behaviour, emotion, motor function or sensation. Other types of stereotyped disturbance include yawns, hiccups, syncopal attacks, migraine, tantrums and panic attacks. To diagnose an epileptic attack there has to be clinical evidence which suggests that the disturbance is a result of cortical neuronal discharge. It is not surprising that four out of every 10 patients referred with a presumed diagnosis of epilepsy after a single episode do not have epilepsy. However, an accurate diagnosis at this stage is essential because:

1 epilepsy is the only disease that causes greater suffering to the patient in terms of social disability than in terms of actual manifestations;

2 the recurrence rate in proven cases after a first seizure is 67–82% and early treatment is nowadays advised (Shovron, 1990);

3 late-onset epilepsy, in particular, may be symptomatic of an underlying neoplasm and investigation is required;

4 pseudoseizures or non-epileptic attack disorders (NEADs) require special and sympathetic investigation (Betts, 1990).

The diagnosis of epilepsy is clinical, based on a detailed description of a series of ephemeral events experienced by the patient and, more importantly, described by an eye-witness. Amplification of the history and investigation does not confirm the diagnosis in every case but from the medicolegal standpoint an unexplained episode of loss of consciousness is regarded as though it were epileptic. It is therefore necessary to stop patients from driving motor vehicles despite uncertainties, until a more authoritative pronouncement can be made. Inevitably, attacks lasting but a few minutes may become of lifelong importance, a fact of which the public is all too aware. Counselling is therefore needed at an early stage to prevent unnecessary stigmatization. The genetic contribution is slight:

apparently absent in 60% of patients, higher in the presence of congenital malformations such as Sturge–Weber disease, with febrile convulsions, generalized *grand mal*, absence seizures or myoclonic attacks, and established as the cause in the 1% of patients with single-gene disorders such as tuberose sclerosis (Shovron, 1990).

Epilepsy is a symptom depending upon a lowering of the threshold of cortical irritation, not a pharmacological exercise in which serum anticonvulsant concentrations are monitored as though they were blood glucose concentrations. The treatment required is that which will both prevent attacks in the short term and reduce the kindling effect which can give rise to refractory epilepsy. The patient expects to know the aetiological diagnosis as far as possible and the forms of treatment available to him/her. Possible trigger factors that may break through medication must be explored and the effect on the patient's lifestyle, occupation, social activities and drinking habits discussed. Continuation of this approach at follow-up may encourage compliance with treatment. The risk of sudden non-compliance can arise from teenage protest and is a potent cause of status epilepticus, which in turn may cause permanent brain damage. If either marriage or pregnancy is contemplated, a discussion with fiancé(e) or partner may help allay fears of possible genetic implications and the risk of drug-induced birth defects minimized.

Genetic disorders

Genetic counselling is usually readily available and neurologists should always be prepared to refer patients with Huntington's chorea, Friedreich's ataxia, muscular dystrophy, etc. to geneticists so that enquiry and counselling can be offered to the whole family. But the neurologist is often called upon to advise upon mental deficiency, neurofibromatosis, brain tumours, muscle disease or a family history of subarachnoid haemorrhage and cannot escape participation.

A cautious approach is often advisable. One cannot always be sure that mental deficiency, for example, is genetically determined and, except with well-recognized syndromes, most cases of genetically determined mental deficiency will arise from autosomal recessive genes. This means that a

child with mental deficiency is not the result of 'bad blood' or 'guilt' of one partner but has developed the condition as a result of a consanguinous marriage or the chance association of two carriers of a recessive gene. If a child is affected by a presumed genetic disorder, it is all the more important to make a diagnosis (including if necessary a brain biopsy) so that the family can be counselled with respect to further pregnancies. A correct diagnosis in an older person is not as essential but increases in importance with the advent of treatments such as elimination diets, if certain drugs have to be avoided or if surgical treatment, e.g. transplantation, can be offered. A neurologist may be able to help patients with muscular dystrophies through respiratory problems or those with Wilson's disease through pregnancies. Patients with presumed dementia should not automatically be diagnosed as having Alzheimer's disease, despite social pressures; isolation or depression can lead to a state of pseudodementia and investigation not uncommonly uncovers a treatable cause, such as a large acoustic neuroma or hypothyroidism.

In some conditions, such as Huntington's chorea, the psychological burden on the whole family is immense and the presence of psychiatric manifestations does not necessarily mean that a particular individual is affected by the disorder. Genetic probes are being developed but as yet diagnostic tests yield too many false positive or false negative results to be ethically justifiable.

Strokes

The stroke victim may regain consciousness and yet remain in a state of confused bewilderment, isolated by the absence of spectacles, hearing-aid or dentures, and exhibiting a mixture of cognitive and physical disarray. The shock of the stroke, especially if accompanied by incontinence, will have shaken his/her self-esteem. Paralysis alone seldom accounts for a patient's incapacity and may contribute little to it. The overriding defect may be a change in intellect or some potentially reversible neurophysiological disturbances. The mental barriers to recovery may include drug effects, mood, perception, memory, attention span and communication disorders. Physical disabilities may include dyspraxia, bulbar problems, visual-field defects and scotomata, and deafness. And speech defects after recovery from bulbar palsy and anarthria can vary from dysarthria to dysphonia, aphasia, including especially comprehension defects, and loss of prosody and gesture. Ability to read may be affected by acquired alexia or paralexic difficulties such as visual-field defects. Loss of sight, as with cortical blindness, may be denied.

This catalogue of disorders is mentioned because there is a danger that comprehension defects, depression and clumsiness may be labelled as dementia, with the false assumption that rehabilitation measures are not indicated. The essential first step is to get through to the patient and to obtain his or her attention. To quote Adams (1971), the treatment of hemiplegia is based on two criteria, one diagnostic, the other an estimate of capacity.

An early diagnosis is helpful. Once a tumour has been excluded, the patient can be reassured that the condition is potentially stable. In the absence of medical expertise, non-vascular disorders such as Parkinsonism and facial palsy can be assumed to be due to strokes. Confusion may result from being in a strange environment and a few objects with which he or she can identify can help to settle the agitated mind. Most hallucinations are probably age-related, e.g. images of a spouse after bereavement or Charles Bonnet's 'philosopher's visions' with failing vision (Berrios & Brook, 1984), some may be due to atropinic drugs and others are a direct result of the cerebrovascular accident. Very rarely do such hallucinations indicate 'madness'.

The estimate of capacity is in part physical and in part cognitive. These factors need to be repeatedly reassessed. Stimulation is important at all stages. The patient needs to be aware of what he/she can and cannot do. Denial of disease (anosognosia) may lead to neglect, lack of recognition and even delusions as to the nature of the affected limb. Patients need to be helped in this respect, as most patients underestimate, deny or are unaware of the extent of their disability and tend to set themselves unrealistic goals, with failure to appreciate their mistakes. An explanation of his or her disability should be accompanied by a simple, personal rehabilitation programme so that a patient knows what is planned for him/her for the coming day and long periods of inactivity are avoided.

Eventually, in-patient care should merge smoothly into home care with the same team advising the patient and his/her relatives. This requires careful discussion with carers, detailed interdisciplinary planning, preliminary home visits with an occupational therapist and/or physiotherapist, and close surveillance by a liaison nurse in the early days of discharge. In the longer term, a regular review of medical problems is essential. Depression can affect 40% or more of those in homes for the elderly. Complications such as pain, fits, constipation and infections need to be recognized and treated, and stimulation and encouragement directed towards realistic goals, which may also require revision from time to time.

Head injury

Although head injury is not the only cause of neurological disability affecting young people, the economic sequelae of head injury are far-reaching. The victim is often the provider for a young wife and family, and the effects of injury often mean that the burden of care falls on those who might have been able to provide an income in default of the injured person. The economic consequences of this are obvious. Much effort has gone into educating the public regarding road safety in recent years. This, coupled with the introduction of seat belts and crash helmet legislation, has led to a reduction in the number of road traffic accident victims with severe head injuries. Despite this, however, accidents still occur, and motor cyclists in particular remain at considerable risk of sustaining head injuries.

Intensive care is required in the acute stage of severe head injury, and head-injured patients are therefore usually managed in either a general or a neurosurgical ward. Local arrangements vary widely and the ideal has been the subject of much discussion. Undoubtedly, many lives are saved in the early stages by the prevention of secondary complications, but a surgical environment rapidly becomes less than ideal as the recovery phase progresses. An acute general surgical ward is not the best place for any head-injured patient requiring active rehabilitation. The physical sequelae may be blatant in cases of major head injury. There may be more subtle changes, particularly when the injury has been less severe. In broad terms, these less obvious changes tend to have psychological implications. Those with frontal damage may show profound behavioural changes; parietal lesions may also impair full rehabilitation. Patients may have problems with learning, language and memory. Emotional difficulties, sometimes with troublesome mood swings, are also often a feature. Active physiotherapy and occupational therapy are crucial in the management of the physical disability. The speech therapist also has an important role in the treatment of those with communication problems. An experienced clinical psychologist is probably the key person in the assessment of cognitive defects, such as those following frontal lobe damage, as scanning techniques are relatively crude measures of brain damage. The psychologist should also initiate the treatment of all those with major behavioural difficulties, which are often the main barrier to successful rehabilitation.

The need will therefore be clear for patients with head injury to be treated in an appropriate environment, i.e. not in a setting where the efforts of the staff are concentrated on saving lives of acutely ill patients. There must be therapists definitely attached to the unit, as well as an active psychological input. Psychiatric help must be readily available. The important contribution of voluntary organizations such as Headway should also be remembered. The availability of separate units for the rehabilitation of head-injured patients attached to all neuroscience units is at present a pipe-dream, but could be forced upon a reluctant society if compensation and legal developments lead to a system of managers for individual head-injury victims ensuring that they obtain the optimum compensation, treatment and rehabilitation.

Causes of failure

Although most clinical colleagues are skilled in the presentation of their initial diagnosis, this is too often inadequately followed up and the patient is left isolated with the comfort or otherwise of a diagnostic label. Unless there is a programme of investigations brought together by a return appointment, the outcome of the first consultation depends heavily on the letter to the GP. Return appointments decrease in value with each different

doctor involved but are reassuring to many with neurological disabilities in so far as they are not forgotten, that they will not miss out on any new treatment and that their particular difficulties will be discussed. The out-patient nursing officer cannot coordinate support in the same way as the ward sister, who is often a key figure in liaison with paramedical services. The ward sister can contact therapists and help to arrange aids and appliances. He or she can also make a link, through the health centre, with district nurses and other community services. Each of these has to be specifically arranged from the out-patient department. The consultant can also arrange hospital services, but the value of physiotherapy and occupational therapy has to be balanced against time spent travelling or waiting for transport. GPs can request the involvement of health visitors, home helps, social services and domiciliary physiotherapy where available. A proper home assessment to adapt the home to the needs of the disabled person requires the co-operation of housing authorities, social services and occupational therapists under the guidance of someone who can organize an overall plan, looking beyond what is available from his/her own department.

Under the Chronically Sick and Disabled Persons Act 1970, local authorities have an obligation to inform themselves of the number of disabled people in their district and to take steps to meet their needs. In pursuit of the requirements of this Act, there should be a system of notification, a dependency register and a monitoring system. There is evidence from the Royal College of Physicians' survey, *Health Services for Adults with Physical Disability* (Edwards & Warren, 1990), that this has not been achieved. Two-thirds of District Health Authorities had made estimates of the number of physically disabled people based on extrapolation from national figures and only 10% kept their own register of such people. There is a partial explanation why this is so. In the present climate notification of disease acquired in adult life is regarded as an invasion of privacy. Attempts to provide a comprehensive handicap and crisis service co-ordinated by a district disability team linked to voluntary services are frustrated due to lack of information. The circumstances of the disabled person can alter rapidly after marital breakdown, progression of the disease and illness or death of the main helper. A formula allowing the notification and regular assessment of the state of all disabled people while respecting their need for privacy is urgently required.

Improvements in management

Over and above the right of each patient to know about his/her condition and to take any vital decisions with respect to his/her state of health, those with disability have a need to understand almost as much about their individual condition as the doctor advising them. A patient with Parkinson's disease who has reached the stage of reduced drug tolerance should be encouraged to experiment in the flexible manipulation of his/her drugs under the guidance of his/her medical advisers to achieve the maximum therapeutic benefit. Too often the provision of a POSSUM apparatus is considered too late in the illness so that the proper advantage cannot be made of it. This also applies to a lesser extent to other aids. There is also often an unsatisfactory delay in the supply of articles after they have been requested by the clinician or therapist. Until such problems can be overcome, an element of anticipation is therefore required. To ensure the provision of such appliances at an optimal stage, one might speak in terms of a 'safety net' in case the 'worst should happen' when first discussing them with the patient in order thereby to avoid undue demoralization.

There are other aspects of management that apply to all disabled people. These include records of drug and other treatments, which provide a rapidly accessible and easily assimilated review of what has been previously done, thus saving unnecessary duplication of effort. It is helpful to record a patient's known drug allergies, sensitivities to drugs taken in normal dosage, abnormal psychological or other reactions to drugs, any genetic disease, and any kidney, heart, chest or liver disease that might affect the distribution and elimination of the drug. The patient could be issued with a card detailing the drugs taken and the dosage regimen, along with precautions to be taken by the patient and an outline of any symptoms which may herald side-effects. This is already done to an abbreviated extent by some pharmacists, but clearly only a limited amount of information can be carried on container labels, and a card could include a space where the patients could list details of possible side-effects that they have noticed themselves.

This approach might be extended to facilitate follow-up consultations. Diary cards and a list of current drugs considerably streamline the review of patients with epilepsy and migraine. Patients should not only be given clear instructions as to what to do if problems develop but, perhaps more importantly, be told what to do if the health centre receptionist suggests an appointment the following week. Drug regimens should be tailored to diurnal fluctuations in disability. This is particularly important in many patients with Parkinson's disease. It is possible that research by non-disabled workers may not suffice and that the desirability of peer-group studies into the needs of other disabled persons should be considered – for example, tetraplegic patients trained in psychology interviewing fellow sufferers (Hohmann, 1966).

Many doctors have been slow to recognize the value and availability of the many excellent guidebooks that have been written for patients and their relatives on living with a wide range of disabilities. Most of these are well written and up to date and provide an honest yet sympathetic account of the disease they describe. They explain the problems that can arise and what can be done to help. The listing of agencies which can help by advising on appliances or supported holidays is particularly useful. Many hospital departments advertise support groups for various disabilities and could help further by retailing books and pamphlets.

One of the most exciting proposals advocated by the Royal College of Physicians (1986) to improve the management of the disabled is the establishment of disabled living centres (DLCs). By 1990 only 23% of District Health Authorities had opened DLCs and several of these were in danger of closure (Edwards & Warren, 1990). DLCs have two principal functions: (i) to provide a permanent standing exhibition of a range of aids and equipment with a supporting information service; and (ii) to act as an education centre for staff, volunteers and patients. Such a centre would occupy rooms 'the size of one or two standard hospital wards' and would bring together voluntary, NHS and social services. Referral would be encouraged from any source, including self-referral by disabled people. With more than 60% of disabled people having a neurological diagnosis, it would be logical for such centres to be developed adjacent to the out-patient clinics of neuroscience units. Neurologists should encourage the therapists in charge of DLCs to exhibit posters, pamphlets and books from the associations concerned with the needs of the physically handicapped and to generate competition in the provision of more efficient and fashionable aids than are currently available.

Acknowledgements

I wish to thank the Editor of the *British Medical Journal* for permission to reproduce excerpts from an article by Dr J.D. Mitchell and myself on 'Explanation and management of neurological disability' (*British Medical Journal*, 1987, **i**, 1203–1205), and Drs J.D. Mitchell and P.H. Merry for further discussion.

References

Adams G.F. (1971) Capacity after strokes. *British Medical Journal* **i**, 91–93.

Berrios G.E. & Brook P. (1984) Visual hallucinations and sensory delusions in the elderly. *British Journal of Psychiatry* **144**, 662–664.

Betts T. (1990) Pseudoseizures: seizures that are not epilepsy. *Lancet* **336**, 163–164.

British Medical Association (BMA) (1954) *The Rehabilitation and Resettlement of Disabled Persons*. BMA, London.

British Medical Association (BMA) (1968) *Aids for the Disabled*. BMA, London.

Edwards F.C. & Warren M.D. (1990) *Health Services for Adults with Physical Disability: a Survey of District Health Authorities 1988/89*. Royal College of Physicians, London.

HMSO (1967) *Report of the Committee of Enquiry on the Rehabilitation, Training and Resettlement of Disabled Persons*. Cmnd 169. HMSO, London.

HMSO (1972) *Rehabilitation (Tonbridge Report)*. DHSS Central Services Council, HMSO, London.

Hohmann G.W. (1966) Some effects of spinal cord lesions on experienced emotional feelings. *Psychophysiology* **3**, 143–156.

McAlpine D. (1965) The problem of diagnosis. In McAlpine D., Lumsden C.E. & Acheson E.D. (eds) *Multiple Sclerosis – a Reappraisal*, pp. 224–257. Churchill-Livingstone, Edinburgh.

Royal College of Physicians (RCP) (1986) Physical disability in 1986 and beyond. *Journal of the Royal College of Physicians* **20**, 160–194.

Shovron S.D. (1990) Epidemiology, classification, natural history and genetics of epilepsy. *Lancet* **336**, 93–96.

4: The Neurological Patient: the Patient's View

ANNE AND SEAN O'CATHASAIGH

Editor's note: Multiple sclerosis (MS) was diagnosed in 1978. Mrs O'Cathasaigh was then aged 25 and had been married 2 years. There has been a gradual and progressive neurological deterioration and Mrs O'Cathasaigh now has severe spasticity, cerebellar and cerebellar pathway signs and bladder problems, and is completely dependent.

Mrs O'Cathasaigh was a successful teacher of English (publication: *Breakthrough in English*, 1985, UTP, Cambridge). Her husband, Sean O'Cathasaigh, is a Lecturer in French and has published works on Pierre Bayle and John Locke. There are no children. Both fathers are dead. Their mothers live in Ireland, but visit regularly.

It is unusual to have a patient's account in a textbook, but it seemed essential to have in the forefront the patient's own experience and the patient's own expectations. For this reason I asked Mrs O'Cathasaigh and her husband to give an account of the effect of severe neurological disability from their point of view.

They have produced a moving and amusing account. Apart from showing the difficulties associated with chronic neurological disturbance, this chapter indicates many neurological aspects which are not only humanitarian and behavioural problems but are also fascinating and difficult research projects, which should provide intellectual stimulation for the most intellectual of doctors and are perhaps the best argument one could put forward to persuade neurologists to undertake neurological rehabilitation: namely, the challenge of such topics as spasticity, intractable pain, fatigue, mechanical and engineering aids, etc.

Anne O'Cathasaigh

I am a Jew. Hath not a Jew eyes? Hath not a Jew hands, organs, dimensions, senses, affections, passions? Fed with the same food, hurt with the same weapons, subject to the same diseases, healed by the same means, warmed and cooled by the same winter and summer, as a Christian is? If you prick us, do we not bleed? If you tickle us, do we not laugh? If you poison us, do we not die? (Shakespeare. *The Merchant of Venice*, III. i. 53)

I was diagnosed in 1978 as having MS. I was then 25, and had been married 2 years. During my Head of Department's absence the previous term I had been working particularly hard. I hadn't managed to shake off a persistent bug. Returning from a long car trip my back seized up. Tests were conclusive: MS.

Since then my illness has developed in ways that I could not have envisaged. It has affected my private and professional relations. On the personal side, there is the burden of care assumed by the family, and the kindness shown to me by many people. On the professional side, I no longer have the social status that having a job confers. But there are positive aspects as well as the negative ones.

Practical help in the form of rehabilitation treatment is essential for someone in my position. A well-founded rehabilitation centre can offer much to alleviate the strains of day-to-day life in the community by offering physiotherapy, counselling and respite care.

Jeffrey Bernard writes the 'Low Life' column for the London *Spectator*. His account of Bohemian activities in Soho includes frequent mention of the progress of his diabetes, a condition which he treats with vodka. It may be the combination of illness and treatment that produced sentiments that will strike a chord in those of us who suffer from neurological disease:

I am so weak now that I could barely get out of the bath this morning. I ended up flapping on

25

the floor like a fish out of water. . . . The bath is no longer a pleasure. Thanks to being so bony it is more than uncomfortable, it is painful. . . . Yes, nearly everything except lying down becomes a mammoth task when you are an invalid. Yesterday I got trapped inside a rollneck jersey when I tried to take it off. It was too small and stuck over my face. It was very claustrophobic and I thought I would suffocate. Even that had me sitting down and panting for ten minutes. And to think that I once had a girlfriend who used to call me 'Tiger'. (*Spectator*, 6 July 1991, p. 42)

Sufferers from neurological disease will empathize. Depending on the illness and how far it has advanced we will understand Jeff Bernard's frustration at not being able to do simple things for himself. We can also understand his nostalgia for the days of physical power, well-being, the capacity to live normally, and the memories of what we used to be able to do. Our lights are no longer 'burning bright'.

Like most people who have neurological illnesses, I used to have a full-time, responsible job. Being unable to continue took a lot of adjustment. My dignity and self-esteem, the feeling of being of value, was taken away, and what fills the void? Being respected and being of value are things that most people take for granted. When one is disabled, these tokens of social value are removed:

> MS meant not just humiliation, stigma, and loss of health, but also loss of income, loss of status, loss of role in the family, loss of work, and loss of the ability to feel part of society.
> (Burnfield A.J. 1989) Multiple sclerosis: an aid to maturity? (*Clinical Rehabilitation* **3**, 75–78)

I was diagnosed as having MS some 13 years ago. At that time I had been teaching English in an upper school (children aged 13–18) for three years. I continued full-time teaching for a further five years while the illness progressed. When full-time employment became impossible, I taught for two years in a special unit for children that schools could not cope with. I loved my job and badly miss being with children.

I have gone through stages in my illness, from walking very badly, to wheelchair use, and, now, to being unable to do anything for myself. I would say

I have learnt quite a lot about myself. I've learnt humility and patience. Humility came quickly when I first got a wheelchair. I felt embarrassed. I also felt humiliated. I didn't want to be seen in it, didn't want people I knew to see me sitting in a chair.

I overcame this unease after a period in a rehabilitation unit, where to my surprise I was one of the most able-bodied people. That was a shock and certainly taught me that there was no point in feeling sorry for myself. Why should I feel embarrassed for something that was not my fault? Having taken that on board, there was no looking back, and thanks to my husband, I think I've been places in a wheelchair that most people would be astonished at.

I have also learnt that people want to help you. I am very independent, but I soon learnt to accept help, graciously I hope. The children I taught were wonderful and would offer assistance. Very often I didn't need their help, but I accepted it knowing that it gave them pleasure. As the MS has progressed I have lost so much but in other ways have gained. I can no longer teach. I can no longer drive. My eyesight is very bad. I cannot move out of the wheelchair.

One thing, however, that is hard to accept is that my speech has deteriorated badly. From being someone who expressed herself articulately, I now speak very slowly, and the speech is laboured and hard to understand. To many people who do not know me, this is taken as mental slowness. Many people are not willing to give me time to say what I want, or they pretend that they have understood; their response shows me immediately that they haven't. It is very difficult to accept being taken for an imbecile.

As well as my speech being very poor I have difficulty in feeding myself, and find this humiliating. I do not like eating with other people who do not know me. I used to really enjoy having people to dinner, meals out in restaurants or in friends' homes, but now feel that my awkwardness is upsetting, not just for me, but an embarrassment for the people I am with.

Tiredness is yet another problem. No longer am I the night person that I was, not for me parties or late evenings, which, I must confess, I do miss.

Tyger! Tyger! burning bright
In the forests of the night . . .
In what distant deeps or skies
Burnt the fire of thine eyes?
(William Blake, *The Tyger*)

But there have been positive elements as well. In adversity, friendship and loyalty show their worth. The old adage that you know who your friends are when something bad happens is true. I owe so much to friends who support me, visit me and ring me up. Because I can no longer drive or get out on my own, their contact keeps me in the world.

So what is a typical day like for me? My husband gets me up and gives me breakfast before he goes to work. Then I am helped by care attendants, from Monday to Friday. They come in, wash me, dress me and get me downstairs. Three afternoons a week home helps come in from one o'clock to three or four, to a total of 8 hours a week. As well as looking after the housework, they give me my lunch and tablets. If I have to go to the toilet they assist me. My husband gets home between four and six. We eat at half past seven, and I try to be in bed by ten.

I have two regular care attendants, three regular home helps, and one husband (who has kept me sane over the years!). The care attendants and the home helps are invaluable. But things can go wrong if there is a mix-up in the programme. I arrange times with both organizations so that I am covered while my husband is at work. It only needs for there to be a small hitch and everything falls apart.

One afternoon, for instance, my regular home help was sick. The office told me they would send a replacement. Five minutes before she was due, I had a phone call to say that no one would be in that afternoon (the replacement had gone sick). My husband came home to give me my tablets and lunch, and helped with toileting. He had a meeting all afternoon, and at tea he came home to check that I was okay. Then back to the meeting, and eventually home. Thankfully this doesn't happen often. My husband is put under pressure and that extends to me, as I worry about his having to cope with his job and having to rush home to make sure that I am all right.

Sean O'Cathasaigh

If it is unusual to have the patient's point of view in a medical textbook, it must be unprecedented to include that of the patient's partner. But common sense tells us that what neurological patients most need is support, and love begins at home. In the 13 years since Anne was diagnosed I have met a wide range of doctors. The ones I found best let me attend consultations, and answered my questions. This meant that I was in a far better position to understand what was happening, to start coping and to help Anne.

The difficulties that partners and carers face are professional, social and personal. They impinge on one another. My good fortune is to have a job that gives me considerable flexibility in setting my working hours. During term, my teaching hours are rigorously fixed. But I can often take time off during the day, as long as I do my research and my admin during the night. We live very close to the university, so if an emergency occurs I can usually rush home for the few minutes it takes to sort it out.

I have never asked for special consideration at work. When my father died three years ago I cancelled a day's teaching in order to go to the funeral, but made up the time later. My colleagues are generally supportive, although I sometimes find their advice unsympathetic – the union representative asked me some time ago if I'd thought of divorce. Luckily I'd heard Lady Runcie's reply to that question: 'Divorce, never! Murder, frequently!'

What *has* suffered in recent years is our social life. The days of preparing six and seven courses for eight are over. We used to share the cooking. Now that I have to do it all, it's much less fun, even if we eat a much more healthy diet. We invite people to dinner much less frequently, and as a result are rarely invited out ourselves by colleagues. That has made us lose touch, and has perhaps made people think we are unsociable. We used to play a lot of bridge, whist and poker, but Anne's difficulty with her fingers has made that impossible with all except the most tolerant of players.

As Anne's condition has developed, I find that I have less time (literally) for others, less time to spend outside the home. I used to write a rock'n'roll column for a local magazine, but it's no longer possible to go out late at night to listen to bands. I was Secretary and then Vice-Chair of the Governing Body of a local school: now I find it difficult to do the work of an ordinary Governor. On the other hand, working at home has allowed me to increase my research output considerably. But somehow Enlightenment philosophical texts don't generate the immediate excitement that the rhythm'n'blues of my local band, Fester and the Vomits, used to produce.

The difficulties that Anne's condition have caused me personally are the most difficult to talk about. In the first place, there is the social pressure on males not to admit to experiencing difficulty in their lives. Dominant images of the 'strong, silent male' encourage society to think of a 'real man' as someone who is self-sufficient and insensitive. And images of the 'new man' insist on his parenting skills: his sensitivity is directed to his children. I'm neither of those: I have cried many times in the past few years, and I don't want to risk having a child that might contract MS – however unlikely the possibility. In the second place, many of these problems are extremely personal. Sexual difficulties are common in neurological patients, and we have had our share. Luckily, we have met some extremely sympathetic counsellors, who advised us with tact and humour. Doctors approaching a neurological patient do well to accentuate the positive. In this as in other matters it is much more important to stress what can be done than to allow the patient to regret what she or he is no longer capable of doing.

What I have found most challenging has been to compartmentalize my life, and to avoid letting worries about Anne affect my work (and vice versa). It seems to me essential to do so, and not only on grounds of productivity. The partner of a neurological patient needs to be able to get out of the house and lead an ordinary life. If she or he doesn't, obsession beckons, to the detriment of both patient and partner. This is why the assistance we get from home helps and care attendants is of such great value and why we appreciate their help so much.

In short, I would recommend that doctors consider the partner as well as the patient. It may take more time in the short term, but over time the extra support the partner can give will make it worth while.

Anne O'Cathasaigh

Another problem is that of getting physiotherapy in the community.

It is unusual for me to see a physiotherapist at home regularly. My physiotherapist has shown my helpers basic passive movements. But I do not have regular professional physiotherapy.

The alternative is to visit the out-patients physiotherapy department in the local hospital. The neurological patient has special difficulties. Typically, the most important is that of transport. How do you get to the hospital?

In some instances it can be done privately. By that I mean you have a car. If not, you depend on taxis or some hospital means of transport. This can be very lengthy. By the time you arrive for the therapy, you are often exhausted.

The dial-a-ride system which operates in several towns will not allow you to book a ride to hospital. So if you haven't private transport you have to pay taxi charges. A friend recently paid £8 for a taxi to the hospital. She lives 2 miles away. A disabled person typically hasn't much money, and this was quite an expense for her.

Getting to the hospital is physically demanding. The problem is carried further when the appointment arrives for you to attend the neurological clinic. For a disabled person, an appointment with a specialist assumes huge importance. It's something that one doesn't want to miss. But the same problems recur – how do you get there? The next problem is, when you do get to your appointment, more often than not you will see a different specialist from the previous one. You will have made all that physical effort, but the person you see will perhaps have had only a few minutes to acquaint himself with your medical history. Why not see the same consultant on each visit? Are these centres undermanned? When members of staff leave, are they replaced?

It is also very off-putting to think that your time is strictly limited. You have to remember any questions or problems that you wanted to discuss. It can be embarrassing to have the room filled with perhaps up to 15 students. This is not particularly conducive to discussing personal problems. The disabled person feels intimidated and quite often will not ask the questions that he or she wanted to.

In short, it may take the whole day to come up to out-patients and return home and all this in order to spend, literally, 2 or 3 minutes talking to a doctor who may not be aware of the medical history.

What can be done, then, to alleviate some of these problems? The establishment throughout the country of well-staffed rehabilitation centres where equipment is first-rate is a priority.

A rehabilitation unit can be beneficial in the early days of a neurological illness. Reassurance is of paramount importance, but this shouldn't end with the early stages. It is on-going; the patient's condition changes, sometimes dramatically, over the years, and help is always needed. Being admitted to such a unit on a regular basis would be of extraordinary value. The carers would have a break and this is important (see below). The doctors would have a chance to see the patient as a whole. The disabled person would feel happy that something concrete was being done.

Who and what would one hope to find in such a unit?

A period of a week or a fortnight in such a centre would allow physiotherapy, counselling and medical treatment. The patient would not be under pressure of time, or be worried about access (either to the building or to toilets). A wide range of services could be provided. Problems for people with neurological diseases cover a huge area.

Being in a rehabilitation unit for a week or a fortnight where your problems are assessed and hopefully dealt with by a trained body of professionals is surely preferable to a once-yearly appointment lasting 5 minutes with an overworked neurologist.

A physiotherapist is crucial. In acute centres, are physiotherapists obliged to treat certain neurological patients as a low priority? Unfortunately, there appears to be a scale indicating which patients would benefit most. I know, however, that for me physiotherapy is helpful and can mean the difference between a day spent getting lots of spasms and a much more comfortable one.

As well as a physiotherapist it is crucial to have a good occupational therapist who can offer advice about practical matters. For instance, advice on choice of wheelchair and the aids that can make you comfortable is vital. Spending your days in a wheelchair is difficult, and can be harmful. An occupational therapist can be a fund of advice on ways to solve problems and where to find the help that you need.

The presence of a speech therapist would also be useful. Many neurological patients have some degree of speech impairment, the social consequences of which can be more disabling than the physical defect. In fact a rehabilitation unit needs the input of so many specialists – people who can give advice on bladder problems, bed sores, how to avoid getting them, and how best to deal with them, diet, sexual counselling, psychological counselling, and the more mundane day-to-day affairs of dealing with laws and regulations, and finding out about available benefits.

But what happens after one's stay in such a unit? We, the disabled, have to come to terms with our diseases before we can go forward:

> What shall I do with this absurdity –
> O heart, O troubled heart – this caricature,
> Decrepit age that has been tied to me
> As to a dog's tail?
>
> (W.B. Yeats, *The Tower*)

Yeats railed against old age, knowing that it could not be averted. For 'decrepit age', substitute any irreversible neurological illness. We cannot shake it off. Are we to ruin our lives and those of the people who love us by being bitter and cantankerous?

> My grandmother, a Victorian, used to say that 'these things are sent to try us'. This sounds rather glib but it is essentially true. Suffering, and MS, can be food for our inner maturity, although most of us no longer seem able to see suffering in this way. (Burnfield, ibid, p. 78)

After the rehabilitation unit do we return home to be confronted with inadequate services? Must we accept the situation where it is difficult to get the kind of help that both we and our carers need? Now that the emphasis is on community care will services – for example, physiotherapy – be expanded so that regular care can be given?

Good respite care centres are desperately needed. Would it be possible for full liaison to happen between the rehabilitation unit and the respite care centre? This would further the work started in the rehabilitation unit, and be much more beneficial than an outpatient appointment which often takes up the whole day for a five minute talk. The

emphasis in the respite care centre must be on
rehabilitation. It is necessary for there to be in-
patient care to a high standard, however far gone
the patient may be: there is always scope for improvement, not only physically but in morale.
Areas to be investigated include speech disturbance,
spasticity, fatigue and pain. Raising public consciousness about disabled people would help too.
Recently I heard of a disabled man who was working
at a supermarket checkout. A woman customer
told him (meaning well) that it was wonderful that
the firm should employ him and wasn't he lucky.
All of us have stories to tell about how we are
perceived in public.

On a holiday in Greece several years ago I was
sitting in my wheelchair while my husband went
off to buy something in a nearby shop. A woman
came past and gave me money. I was really taken
aback but managed to call her and return the
money. It seems to me that even though her action
was done out of kindness it is symbolic of the way
that we are viewed by many people. My husband
thought this was wonderful and that we could pay
for our holiday if he were to take me into town
each day.

Yes, it is amusing, but there is a serious point to
be made. We may look odd and talk funny, but we
do have feelings. Please do not condescend to us. 'If
you prick us, do we not bleed? If you tickle us, do
we not laugh?' The best doctors are those who see
us as neurological patients, not as neurological
diseases. When I was in hospital being diagnosed
the senior registrar brought students around to
examine my legs. He used terms I didn't understand. I asked what they meant. Total shock – the
body had spoken. The registrar told the students to
explain. He ended up having to explain the terms
himself, as none of the students knew. They may
have been furious with me, but they learned about
more than MS that day. A patient is not a dis-
embodied, unfeeling specimen uninterested in what
is happening. On the contrary: she or he is extremely interested in what is happening.

Part 2
The Scientific Background
of Neurological Rehabilitation:
Altered Structure and Function

5: Rehabilitation Theory

L.S. ILLIS

CNS dysfunction, 34
The effect of a lesion in the CNS, 35
Nature of dysfunction and the nature of recovery, 35
    Biological models, 35
    Pharmacological changes, 37
    Sprouting of intact fibres, 39
    Unmasking of existing synapses, 39
    Alteration in synaptic transmission or effectiveness, 39
Spinal shock as an example, 40
Can a general theory of neurological rehabilitation be
    advanced?, 42
Conclusion, 43

Paul Bach-y-Rita has drawn attention to the weak link in neurology, namely neurological rehabilitation (Bach-y-Rita, Chapter 31). Increased survival as a result of medical advances has not been matched by quality of life. Bach-y-Rita rightly points to the absence of a theoretical base. Not only is there no rehabilitation theory but, with few exceptions, questions such as the role of neurotransmitters in recovery and the mechanisms of reorganization and regeneration are not being asked, let alone answers sought. In the neurosciences, diagnosis and treatment are always based on a theoretical concept of neurological function. In rehabilitation, no such theoretical concept exists, even though the problems posed by the patient with neurological disturbance, such as pain or spasticity, not to mention the nature of recovery, are amongst the most difficult and intellectually most challenging which face the neurologist, and these problems have a direct involvement with experimental anatomy and physiology.

The emergence of the concepts of plasticity of the central nervous system (CNS) and its acceptance in the mainstream of neuroscience is described in Chapters 7 and 31 and in other publications. Plasticity and the response of the intact nervous system to damage form the basis of rehabilitation theory.

Abnormal functioning of the nervous system following disease or a lesion cannot be separated from concepts of recovery. There is a continuum of lesion or disease, alteration of the CNS (sometimes discussed under the heading of plasticity or recovery or maladaptation) through to production of the chronic state or so-called fixed neurological deficit. It is only by trying to understand this continuum that logical therapy may be devised.

Where a surgically remediable lesion is found, such as compression of the spinal cord by a meningioma, appropriate therapy usually produces full recovery. Similarly, in medical conditions such as subacute combined degeneration of the cord, early diagnosis and specific treatment should again produce full recovery. However, in many conditions, no specific therapy is as yet available, and the search for treatment, both symptomatic and curative, continues.

The effect of a lesion includes not only a specific neurological deficit, due to loss of the functions subserved by the damaged structures, but, in addition, more widespread and less understood events which may be of great importance. It appears that the CNS responds to a lesion by active reorganization, involving mechanisms which are known to be operative in development and in the maintenance of function in the face of naturally occurring loss of neurons. The lesion triggers a sequence of events which include sprouting of nerve terminals from intact fibres, unmasking of pre-existing but relatively insignificant neural pathways, and changes in neuroactive substances and their receptors. Destruction of a major nerve pathway or major input to a neuron pool will have not only a negative effect, but also the positive effect of making previously minor inputs relatively more important and thus altering the relative density of endings at any particular neuron or neuron pool. This by itself would have a far-reaching effect on neuronal function. There is, therefore, a mechanism by which, even where no structural damage has occurred as a direct result of the lesion, the *intact* CNS has altered and its function has consequently altered.

CNS dysfunction

One of the most extreme examples of breakdown of function is seen in spinal injury in man, where a lesion, often limited in both space and time, produces a disastrous and, at present, incurable effect. In a disease process, such as multiple sclerosis, the disturbed function produced by the lesion is complicated by the ongoing process of the disease. In a static disturbance, such as spinal cord injury, where a single insult is sustained by the spinal cord, the features of spinal cord dysfunction are more easily analysed – though even here a second 'hidden' lesion may have been sustained or there may be a concomitant head injury or there may be late changes. Even in disease processes, each little lesion may produce, in effect, a deafferentation of part of the CNS.

In the chronic state of dysfunction, the management of the patient is conventionally regarded as the management or treatment of complications which arise as a result of dysfunction, and the processes which lead to dysfunction are largely ignored. However, if the clinical picture is seen, not in isolation, but as part of the gradual evolution from the acute phase of the lesion, then the clinical picture becomes less that of the patient who is a burden to the community and more that of the person who is, at least theoretically, amenable to treatment, thus forming a link between academic research based on plasticity of the CNS and clinical neurology. An understanding and investigation of the process leading to dysfunction should lead to attempts to alleviate distress and improve function on a scientific rather than on an *ad hoc* basis.

Formal neurology is concerned largely with integrated function. Here, we are concerned with a nervous system which has become disintegrated and what becomes of importance is not the loss of integrated function but what is preserved, even though it is disintegrated. For example, following a lesion in the spinal cord the clinical picture involves at least three components: volitional mechanisms, postural mechanisms and equilibrium mechanisms. Even if volitional mechanisms are totally absent when the patient is examined lying down, if postural control is present on standing and a withdrawal reflex can be elicited, then this is a different degree of disintegration from that in a patient where postural control is absent.

Before describing the changes which produce dysfunction, the importance of understanding the abnormal processes can best be illustrated by a specific research problem.

Below a spinal lesion, even a complete lesion, there is a relatively normal spinal cord which is potentially capable of central processing of signals, with a normal 'apparatus' of peripheral nerves, muscles, ligaments and limbs simply cut off from higher control. That is, the anatomical and physiological properties which form the circuits contributing to control, say, of walking, exist but the programming remains poorly understood. After spinal transection, lower vertebrates can perform stepping movements, indicating the integrity of neural mechanisms capable of co-ordinating muscle activity over several segments. The groups of nerve cells responsible for this integrated activity are sometimes called neural generators and probably exist for each limb; the overall level of activity in respect of these generators is set by continuous descending stimuli from higher levels of the CNS. The groups of nerve cells are called the central pattern generator (CPG) or spinal pattern generator. In the cat, the CPG can act soon after injury and stepping becomes progressively stronger and may eventually lead to weight-bearing. There appears to be a progressive inhibition of the CPG during ontogeny (the CPG is more readily elicited in a young animal) and phylogeny. The CPG has not been definitely demonstrated in primates and in man. It appears that in higher animals the CPG is more heavily inhibited. Here, then, is a good scientific problem. Why is the CPG not demonstrable in man? Can the CPG be disinhibited and, if so, would this produce stepping and weight-bearing in spinal-injured man? The ability to activate the CPG in man must be basic to any effort to improve spinal cord function and this type of neurological rehabilitation may be essential when spinal cord regeneration becomes a therapeutic possibility. Before such a problem can be approached, the details of dysfunction must be examined.

The effect of a lesion in the CNS

A lesion in the CNS does not consist of a simple matter of destruction of certain pathways which were present in the normal or intact CNS, in that it is not just the removal (by destruction) of various unrelated components but a gradual and dynamic alteration of the CNS as a result of the lesion. To understand this it is necessary to start with the acute phase and follow the changes which occur. For example, trauma disrupts cells with a consequent release of potassium and neurotransmitters into the extracellular environment, which is now hostile. At the same time Ca^{2+} enters the cells, with further deleterious effects. Following acute traumatic damage there is a fall in blood flow in the white matter and the release of potentially toxic agents such as phospholipases, proteinases and lipid peroxides. The study of these changes has led to attempts to improve neurological deficit. For example, Ca^{2+} entry into cells activates phospholipases, interrupts mitochondrial electron transport chains and initiates lipid peroxidation. Lipid peroxidation, in turn, releases free radicals which cause a continuous injury response, resulting in progressive membrane damage, oedema and a further fall in blood flow. Treatment with methylprednisolone may inhibit lipid peroxidation and thus protect against this kind of damage (see Young, 1992).

Cell death leads to axon degeneration but it appears that relatively few axons are needed to support functional activity. Unfortunately, many surviving axons are abnormal and have abnormal conduction properties. If it turns out to be correct that a very small number of surviving axons may be associated with recovery, then this would suggest that sprouting and synaptic replacement may be occurring in order to compensate for the loss.

The fact that the chronic state is different from the acute state must indicate that one of two events has occurred: either the original lesion has progressed or regressed in order to produce the chronic state, or the CNS itself has altered as a result of the lesion. A single insult or lesion is accompanied by changes at the normal–abnormal interface of nervous tissue, producing transient changes in cells, metabolic disturbances and similar changes, and these may be reversible. These changes may be responsible for short-term alterations in the clinical state and they may be of great significance in early management but they are of little importance in the context of a chronic state. Structural changes directly related to the lesions which occur later may be of great clinical importance (e.g. cyst information in spinal cord injury), but these are usually easily recognizable clinically and are complications rather than an alteration in the nervous system.

This means that the evolution of the neurological picture from the acute to the chronic state can only be explained as an evolution of the CNS reaction, and it is this which needs to be analysed in order to put the clinical evaluation of dysfunction into a neurological perspective. The changing picture is, in effect, a reflection of recovery or of maladaptiveness, and can be investigated as a change in anatomy, physiology and neurochemistry. Until recently, nothing could be done about the lesion in terms of recovery, at least in the chronic state, except to teach the patient to live with the disability and to prevent or treat complications. However, more detailed analysis of the altered intact CNS has led to practical methods to improve recovery. In addition, detailed study of the changes throws light on the true nature of the neurological deficit seen after a lesion and will lead to greater understanding of the chronic state of dysfunction. In Chapters 31 and 32, Bach-y-Rita and Sutton and Feeney give greater detail.

Nature of dysfunction and the nature of recovery

Biological models

It is helpful, when considering how the CNS reacts to the lesion and the importance this may have in terms of recovery, to consider biological models of nervous integration. There are two main types of such models – those with a random or diffuse structure and those with a well-localized or specific structure. The rapid association of sensory infor-

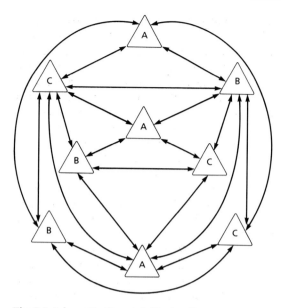

Fig. 5.1 Schematic diagram indicating the connections of nine cells of three types: A, B and C (the lines indicate connectivity and not actual axons). Because of the random connectivity it is possible to have a firing sequence A, B, C, B, A, utilizing any of 99 different pathways. A specific pathway would greatly reduce flexibility.

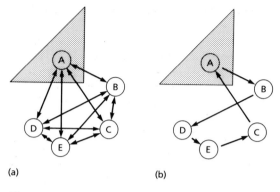

Fig. 5.2 (a) Model of the CNS with random connectivity. A lesion at A does not produce catastrophic effects (unless it is very large) as regards the functioning of the net. For the net to continue functioning, existing pathways are used although some of these may have been little used previously. (The arrows do not represent actual connections but indicate that the chance of any one unit being connected to any other unit is equal.) (b) Model with a specific structure. A lesion at A now produces complete disruption. For the net to continue functioning completely new connections would have to be established. (Reproduced with permission from Illis L.S. (1973) Regeneration in the central nervous system. *Lancet* 1: 1035–1037.)

mation coming from widely different sources and of different modalities obviously requires a richly cross-connected nerve network. The importance of such a cross-connectivity in producing flexibility is indicated in Fig. 5.1. If highly specific inborn circuits were present in the CNS, then this would imply the genetic determination of synaptic connections and would reduce to a minor role the effect of use and disuse on connectivity, and this is contrary to known facts. However, complete randomness of connection is also contrary to known anatomical facts, but genetically rigid connection could not possibly subserve the multitude of genetically unpredictable activities which occur during the lifetime of an organism. In the random type of model, non-specificity of organization produces stability against disturbance but there is a sharp transition from stability to instability as the connectance reaches a critical level (Gardner & Ashby, 1970; May, 1972).

This is probably a general system property since it is so widespread in a variety of systems. It appears

that the larger and more complex a system becomes, the more a change in condition produces either no effect at all, or a sudden and large consequence at one critical level. In the CNS this instability is guarded against, since any specific circuit would reduce the randomness of a structure. If specific circuits only are present, then stability does not exist in the presence of perturbation (see Fig. 5.2).

The simplest form of the diffusely structured nervous system is where the probability of any one unit of the system being connected to any other unit is equal. Assuming the property of synaptic facilitation, such a structure could be altered as a result of the sensory input and made to perform a variety of learned tasks. Some specificity would be established as a result of repetitive stimulation since the effect of such stimulation is to produce a demonstrable structural change in appropriate synapses (Bazanova *et al.*, 1966; Illis, 1969).

The acceptance of this type of random–specific model as a means of studying the functioning of the CNS assumes the relative unimportance of connections, and indeed of the nerve cells themselves, as regards integration at least, and throws into prominence the areas of connectivity or areas of discontinuity of the nervous system. The relative contribution of a pathway to the synaptic zone is not rigid but can be altered by use, by disuse, by degeneration and regeneration and by the effect of toxins (see Illis, 1973a).

In the simplest view, there are three main bodies of opinion regarding the nature of recovery: Von Monakow's (1914) concept of 'diaschisis' (often used as an explanation, although it is purely a description); sprouting and unmasking of nerve terminals, i.e. structural and physiological changes; and alteration of synaptic effectiveness, the area in which investigations of the nature of recovery and possible therapy most overlap. The three groups are not mutually exclusive. Von Monakow's concept of diaschisis was suggested as the explanation for long-delayed spontaneous recovery after a lesion in the CNS. Von Monakow suggested that, if a part of the CNS is destroyed, a distant part with which it was in neuronal contact might stop functioning. After some period of time the 'depressed' area recovers its ability to function. He was unable to explain the mechanism of recovery, but it is clear that recovery of function would be due to removal of 'depression', with no reorganization or regeneration of the CNS taking place. Recent experimental work suggests a possible basis for diaschisis (see Chapters 7 and 32 for a fuller discussion of these aspects).

Pharmacological changes

This important aspect is also dealt with in Chapter 32.

Recent advances in molecular biology have revealed a new insight into the understanding of the functioning of the CNS, but it is essential to remember that the basis of neurological function remains organization, organization at successive levels producing integration and being capable of disintegration. The quintessence of this organization is the synapse — that is, the area of discontinuity of the CNS. This is the unique feature of the CNS and it is because of this discontinuity that integration (and disintegration) can take place. Without this discontinuity the CNS would simply behave as a

kind of complicated telephone switchboard system. The synapse, formed as it is by two cells, is a complex organelle with multiple receptors, the site of release of multiple messengers (primary and secondary) and forming, with other synapses at the cell surface, a synaptic zone. This synaptic zone has multiple sites of origin (the afferent fibres and sources) or multiple sites of control. Functionally there are four main types of communication between nerve cells (see Barker & Smith, 1980).

1 *Point-to-point or fast transmission (conventional neurotransmission)*. This can be split into brief transmission, as at acetylcholine nicotinic synapses, and slow transmission, as at acetylcholine muscarinic synapses. This type of communication is sometimes regarded as cell-to-cell communication.

2 *Neuromodulation*. This involves alteration of postsynaptic membrane conductance. That is, the neuromodulator alters interneuronal communication without itself acting as a neurotransmitter. This modulation of transmission may occur with neuropeptides. This may be regarded as tuning of the transmitter signal.

3 *Neurohormonal communication*. Here there is no anatomical continuity via synaptic contacts, and long-lasting changes of target cells following stimulation of specific peptidergic neurons are involved. This allows activation only of those target cells with appropriate receptors. This can be regarded as a general transmission but with specific reception.

4 *Volume transmission*. The release of 'informational substances', including peptides, which reach target cells by extracellular fluid transmission and thus influence large neuronal arrays, has been implicated in spasticity as well as other pathological states (Bach-y-Rita & Illis, 1993). It may also play a role in functional reorganization after a partial lesion such as damage or elimination of a pathway and its inputs. This could result in hypersensitivity to that volume transmission informational substance by up-regulation of the corresponding receptors. Neurotransmitters and amino acids found in extracellular fluid include dopamine, choline, adenosine, noradrenaline, serotonin and acetylcholine.

The reader is referred to Chapter 31 by Bach-y-Rita, one of the leaders in this field.

However, even this is a simplification since the time course of brief and slow transmission overlaps, as do facilitation and modulation, neurohormonal action and trophic factors. Monoamine release is associated with diffuse neural pathways, with nerve cells localized in the brain stem, and with diffuse ramifications to wide terminal fields, so that very large numbers of target cells may be affected. These anatomical factors suggest that such a system is modulatory and this is a generally accepted view. These transmitter systems include the catecholamines: adrenaline, noradrenaline and dopamine. In the context of possible mechanisms in CNS dysfunction an important system is the noradrenaline system, which ramifies to virtually all areas of the CNS, originating mostly from brain stem nuclei and innervating the cerebral cortex, cerebellum, hippocampus, hypothalamus and spinal cord.

Since 1940 scientists have used drugs to try to influence recovery following experimental lesions in the CNS, but the work is still in its infancy. Endogenous opiates may interact with other physiological systems, particularly in the autonomic nervous system. Opioids are co-stored with catecholamines in sympathetic ganglia and the adrenal medulla, and in some species are released with catecholamines and controlled in the same way as catecholamines. The opioid antagonist, naloxone, has been used as a blocking agent to investigate endogenous opiate function and has been used for a variety of neurological disorders. In experimental spinal injury naloxone has been reported to decrease neurological impairment and to increase spinal cord blood flow (Faden et al., 1981; Young et al., 1981). Improvement has also been reported in the treatment of stroke (Baskin & Hosobuchi, 1981), experimental hemiplegia (Baskin et al., 1982) and subacute necrotizing encephalopathy.

It is possible that opiate receptor blockers may have a beneficial effect in improving neurological deficit following spinal injury. The use of these agents may influence the synthesis and availability of trauma-induced release of substances such as endogenous opioids, catecholamines and serotonin. Spinal cord processes have been pharmacologically manipulated by long-term intrathecal administration of drugs via a catheter connected to a reservoir and pump. Drugs such as morphine, clonidine and baclofen have been used and have been shown to have an effect on pain and spasticity, presumably via an action on specific receptors in the dorsal

horn of the spinal cord, leading to alteration in spinal modulatory systems and central sensory transmission and processing. Intrathecal noradrenaline, morphine and naloxone may alter spinal reflexes (Dhawan & Sharma, 1970) and produce hind-limb extensor posturing and weight support in the cat (see Omeniuk, 1983). Intrathecal morphine in man has been shown to enhance Renshaw inhibition (Roby et al., 1981), reduce polysynaptic flexor reflex activity (Willer & Bussel, 1980) and suppress spasticity (Struppler et al., 1983).

Thyrotropin-releasing hormone (TRH) is present in nerve terminals of motor neurons in the ventral horn of the spinal cord and TRH receptors are present on these neurons. This neuropeptide seems to play an important role in modulating voluntary motor activity. The monoamine, serotonin, and TRH are co-localized in neurons of brain stem origin. Following spinal cord trauma, both substances are depleted and, when administered intrathecally, they have a powerful effect on spinal reflexes. Thus pharmacological reversal or alteration of neurological deficit is a possibility and suggests that some part of the neurological picture is produced by pharmacological methods acting via a neuromodulatory system, indicating perhaps the first correct explanation of the previously purely descriptive concept of diaschisis. That is, the original insult to the CNS produces its effects in two distinct but interrelated ways. On the one hand, there is obvious damage to the CNS, with some recovery at the interface with normal tissue due to reversible damage and circulatory and metabolic effects. This would produce the 'fixed' lesion and fixed deficit of classical and conventional neurology, with a clinical syndrome relating directly to the damaged area of CNS on a simple cause-and-effect basis, narrowing the search for the basis of recovery to the site of the lesion and, not surprisingly, producing decades of somewhat abortive research. On the other hand, there is an as yet unexplained process of recovery which cannot relate to the original insult and must be due to some functional abnormality of areas of the CNS which are necessary for the expression of performance of the behaviour lost as a result of the lesion. The changes must be seen in the context of an abnormal nervous system, i.e. one which has altered structurally and physiologically.

This leads to the second main opinion as to the nature of recovery of function and the nature of dysfunction. This is a corollary of plasticity of the nervous system, so that recovery is consequent upon a reorganization of the nervous system through the sprouting of new synapses or the unmasking of existing synapses.

Sprouting of intact fibres

There are more nerve cells present during embryonic life than in the mature nervous system and it appears that developing neurons must make synaptic contact with appropriate target cells in order to survive. One suggested mechanism for the cessation of nerve growth when appropriate target cells are contacted is contact inhibition, i.e. neurons carry a finite number of terminals and if a proportion of these degenerate due to axonal injury then the uninjured axons sprout to fill the local sites available and consequently expand the synaptic field of the uninjured axons. This has implications in terms of altered physiology since the relative contributions of afferent axons are now altered. Removal or alteration of contact inhibition, possibly by degeneration metabolites, will result in continuous remodelling in the intact nervous system, or regeneration and reorganization of the damaged CNS. Collateral sprouting is recognized as a widespread phenomenon and has been demonstrated in peripheral, central and autonomic systems (Edds, 1953; Murray & Thompson, 1957; Liu & Chambers, 1958; Raisman, 1969; Illis 1973a, b, c; Lynch et al., 1973). However, although the fact of sprouting is largely unquestioned, its significance remains uncertain. Is it regeneration and an attempt to restore normal function, or is it a random response resulting in a haphazard and inappropriate connectivity, or is it a combination of both? Is it initiated by the lesion or is it a natural and continuing process in the normal CNS? The probability is that nerve cells are in a state of continual replacement during development. In adult life this probably does not occur but, when a lesion occurs, there is a response in terms of an increase in the level of amino acids and in protein metabolism, which may be seen within hours. However, sprouting alone cannot explain short-term changes in the nervous system following a lesion and, furthermore, the alteration of the

relative contribution of terminals to the target site will have produced an abnormal connectivity, which, though contributing to the altered clinical state, is not necessarily contributing to recovery. In other words, the sprouting response may of itself produce damaging results. Webb & Hall (1972), writing in another context, produced a memorable sentence: 'When a member of an orchestra gets a few bars out of time, his continued efforts are likely to result in a chaotic disharmony and he would serve the cause of music better if he kept quiet.' The sprouting response may prevent further changes taking place, such as more appropriate reinnervation, and may prevent the appearance of denervation hypersensitivity.

Unmasking of existing synapses

Plasticity does not necessarily mean a change in structure. A new and important field of plasticity in the CNS was opened up by P.D. Wall and colleagues (see Merrill & Wall, 1978) when they described unmasking of synapses. They demonstrated that, when nerve cells lose their normal input, they begin to respond to new inputs which in an intact animal produce no response. This switching from normal to new input may occur immediately and can be switched backward and forward by blocking agents. For the majority of cells the change takes days or weeks to complete. Unmasking may be seen not only after degeneration, but also when there is a change in afferent bombardment without any central degeneration and therefore no sprouting to establish new connections (see Fig. 5.3). The fact that altering peripheral stimulation may alter the receptive fields in the CNS has major implications for the rehabilitation of neurological deficit in humans. For example, in both sprouting and unmasking, previously unused or little used pathways may take on a more significant role. One effect of a lesion, therefore, is to alter the dominance of any particular fibre pathway by sprouting and unmasking of less dominant, but pre-existing, anatomical systems.

Alteration in synaptic transmission or effectiveness

Denervation hypersensitivity or supersensitivity, i.e. the increase in sensitivity of synapses or of

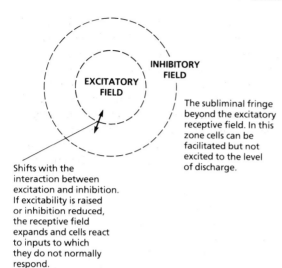

Shifts with the interaction between excitation and inhibition. If excitability is raised or inhibition reduced, the receptive field expands and cells react to inputs to which they do not normally respond.

The subliminal fringe beyond the excitatory receptive field. In this zone cells can be facilitated but not excited to the level of discharge.

Fig. 5.3 Altering afferent stimulation may alter receptive fields. Based on Wall P.D. (1988) Recruitment of ineffective synapses after injury. In Waxman S.G. (ed.) *Functional Recovery in Neurological Disease*, pp. 387–400. Raven Press, New York.

postsynaptic elements following axonal damage, is well documented in muscle and autonomic ganglia. Possibly a similar mechanism exists in the CNS, but the evidence for this is poor.

Alteration of signal traffic may change synaptic transmission and effectiveness. The best-known example of this is post-tetanic potentiation. Repetitive stimulation may alter appropriate synapses anatomically. There is abundant evidence for environmental stimulation and repetitive electrical stimulation producing structural, physiological and behavioural changes in animals and in humans (for review see Illis, 1992). Spinal cord stimulation, a technique which arose directly from the 'gate control' hypothesis of Melzack & Wall (1965), produces clinical and physiological changes and, although the mode of action of repetitive electrical stimulation is unknown, possibly central inhibition is altered and perhaps synapses are unmasked (see Chapter 36). What example is there of investigation of recovery or maladaptiveness in terms of anatomy, physiology and pharmacology? Spinal shock is one such problem.

Spinal shock as an example

Spinal shock is perhaps the best known of all forms of spinal dysfunction and is still very poorly understood. The term 'spinal shock' was first used in 1750 and signifies the effect of sudden injury or transection of the spinal cord. It is characterized by a sensory and motor paralysis and, later, by the gradual recovery of reflexes. Nobody has ever given a convincing explanation of the recovery of reflexes following their complete abolition. Spinal shock occurs at any level of transection below the midpons. Above this level a transection produces decerebrate rigidity. Following transection below the pons, nerve cells in the spinal cord are suddenly cut off from all descending influences and then undergo a dramatic change in their capacity to react. In lower mammals the important descending influences can be identified (reticulospinal and vestibulospinal pathways), whereas in higher animals, including humans, corticospinal connections are probably more important. The intensity and the duration of spinal shock increase as the vertebrate scale is ascended and probably parallel the degree of development of suprasegmental structures. Usually the emphasis is on the destruction of the motor system but it is quite clear that the afferent or sensory system is also important in the production of the clinical picture. This can be compared to the importance of sensory feedback in some of the pharmacological reversals of neurological deficit (see Chapter 32) and the importance of altered signal traffic in altering nervous function.

It is usually assumed that the importance of pathways in producing spinal shock is a reflection of their specificity, but it may equally be argued that the importance lies in their relative contribution to the total spinal cord input: that is, the relative contribution to the descending pathways made by different levels of the neuraxis. This could possibly explain why transection below the pons is more dramatic than transection above the pons. The greater the number of descending pathways interrupted, the more likely that shock will ensue, because the more severely disorganized will be the target area upon which these descending pathways converge. Most theories regarding the first phase of spinal shock (depression of reflexes) include the withdrawal of impulses from descending tracts, but no explanation of spinal shock can be acceptable unless it includes the second phase – that of the return of reflexes in an altered form. There are two further features of spinal shock which are of particular interest. First, it has been commonly assumed that the effects of transection occur in a downward direction only. This is not so, since headward of the transection there is a change in reflex response (Creed *et al.*, 1932). Second, there are experiments which show that, when one limb of a cat is de-afferented by section of posterior roots, electrical stimulation of the brain stem produces no response in the corresponding limb; several days later, however, responses may be evoked more readily in the denervated than in the normal limb (Teasdell & Stavraky, 1953).

This is a similar but reversed state of affairs to that pertaining to spinal shock. Experimental work has led to the suggestion that at the motor neuron surface there is an extremely complex mosaic of nerve terminals from various sources, intermixed with glial cells (Illis, 1963, 1967a, 1973a, b, c). This synaptic zone may be profoundly altered by denervation of a critical number of nerve endings, with the consequences not only of degeneration of those endings which were denervated but also of disorganization of the whole synaptic zone. This would result in the depression of activity of nerve cells. With time, nerve endings with severed afferents would degenerate and those with intact fibres would reorganize. The reorganization would be produced by sprouting and by unmasking and the results of this reorganization would be seen in terms of altered reflexes, such that any reflex-eliciting stimulus would now produce a response which, though more or less specific at any one time, would be changing along with the changes taking place in the reorganization of the network. The abnormal pattern, rather than the abnormal reflex, has been little studied in chronic lesions of the CNS until recently, and more recent work tends to confirm the theoretical concept. Faganel & Dimitrijevic (1982) studied the effect on ankle jerks in patients with clinically complete chronic spinal cord injury after conditioning with noxious electrical stimuli applied to thoracic, lumbar and sacral dermatomes. Painful cutaneous stimulation applied to the skin produces a reflex contraction and withdrawal. The organization includes several segments activated as functional units. In man, in the case of a complete transverse lesion the induced excitation spreads to adjacent and more distal cranial and caudal segments, both ipsilaterally and contralaterally (Sherrington, 1906). This spread of reflexes, not seen in the normal or intact spinal cord, reflects an altered anatomy and physiology. The alteration in anatomy could be explained in terms of sprouting and/or unmasking, since the existence of crossed monosynaptic afferents and the spread over adjacent and distant segments has been demonstrated anatomically (Illis, 1967b). The altered physiology must be on the basis of such altered anatomy. In other words, in the intact animal the anatomical substrate is present but is 'masked' by a dominant system of connections. One effect of the lesion is to alter this dominance by sprouting and by the unmasking of less dominant, but pre-existing, anatomical systems.

Return of reflexes is seen as a progressive change which may begin within 24 hours of injury and varies as one ascends the phylogenetic scale. In the cat, reflexes below the lesion are obtainable after about 1 hour. But not all reflexes are so readily obtainable, and over long periods of time reflexes are still changing in their nature (Sherrington, 1906; Fulton & Sherrington, 1932). Recent techniques in clinical neurophysiology may impose a new interpretation on findings in humans. For example, even in clinically paralysed patients residual and potentially functioning long descending fibres have been demonstrated physiologically (Dimitrijevic *et al.*, 1984) and *post mortem*.

Another important feature of recovery is not only the presence of abnormal reflexes and the time sequence of their return, but also the demonstration of an altered receptive field, so that reflexes may be elicited by minimal stimulation of the skin from a progressively wider area (Wall, 1988). This enlargement of the receptive field is perhaps the most obvious evidence of alteration of the intact nervous system in response to a lesion and is probably due to unmasking of synapses.

As the first stage of spinal shock subsides, afferent impulses from the periphery (skin, tendons, muscles and ligaments, joints, viscera) begin to elicit an excitatory influence. It is as though the process of spinal shock, or, more precisely, the section of sufficient descending pathways, has imposed a resistance on lower spinal cord synapses and in some at present inexplicable way this resistance is now lifted (see Illis, 1963). Reflexes return in a sequential way and not simultaneously. During the early return of reflexes the stimulus must be strong or summated and the response shows easy fatigue. Despite the variability in reflex pattern and the variability in timing of return, there are certain dominant patterns of reflex return. All these abnormal reflex patterns have one thing in common: the stimulus elicits not the usual response, i.e. the response expected in the intact organism, but an abnormal pattern not seen in the undamaged spinal cord. The abnormal pattern of reflexes, therefore, is a reflection of previously existing pathways whose function is normally masked; i.e. these pathways, in the intact nervous system, are structurally intact but play little or no functional part until degeneration of more significant pathways has occurred. Does the unmasking occur simply through the removal of descending control (whatever that precisely means), through chemical hypersensitivity of undamaged endings, or through sprouting of new terminals? This remains a matter of argument and of interpretation. In addition, the abnormal reflex patterns may represent a central alteration of receptive fields secondary to an alteration in afferent input – which itself may be a reflection of partial paralysis. For example, although the neurological syndrome may be primarily motor (e.g. a paralysed limb), the effect on the CNS is a deficit of *sensory* information, not a deficit of motor impulses. The clinical effect is that, when a person with spinal cord damage is examined, one sees a pattern of neurological deficit and abnormal reflex activity which is a reflection not simply of the fact of a lesion being present but also of a CNS adapting to the lesion. Reflex return may fail completely and is then a result of a vertical lesion involving nerve cells in the spinal grey matter.

As mentioned earlier, post-mortem study of patients with spinal cord injury who were thought to have clinically complete lesions during life has shown continuity of nerve fibres and this has been investigated physiologically (Dimitrijevic *et al.*, 1984). The investigations show that residual structures in the injured part of the spinal cord can transmit to segments below the lesion and also that

there is supraspinal activation of motor units during reinforcement manoeuvres. By the use of such techniques it should be possible to categorize patients much more accurately. These residual long descending fibres may have significance in terms of the application of stimulation techniques to relieve spasticity, and in the future through, perhaps, the exploitation of techniques of nerve transplantation.

The pattern of abnormal reflexes reflects anatomical and physiological changes in the spinal cord and pharmacological changes which are a result of the lesion. More detailed study should enable us to influence this process and to influence recovery.

Can a general theory of neurological rehabilitation be advanced?

If neurological rehabilitation can be said to be a scientific discipline in the field of clinical neuroscience, then it should be possible to put forward a series of principles which may influence treatment of a patient, may be tested and may further the development of the subject. Such a system of ideas would include the natural history and evolution of the clinical picture, how natural recovery may take place, how the clinical picture may be theoretically altered and how deterioration may occur:

1 A lesion may have a sudden onset but there is no sudden end, rather a gradual evolution towards a less stable equilibrium.

2 The lesion produces reaction in the intact nervous system, both structurally and functionally.

3 The clinical picture is not a static phenomenon. It is produced partly by the direct destructive effects of the lesion, and partly by the reaction of the intact, undamaged, nervous system.

4 Any natural 'recovery', both beneficial and deleterious, must arise from changes in the undamaged nervous system.

5 The reaction of the intact CNS is theoretically amenable to alteration by external means: by altering afferent stimuli, or by drug therapy producing a similar effect.

6 The corollary is that deterioration may also be produced by external stimuli (e.g. the effect of infection upon neurological signs seen in the

interaction of urinary infection or pressure sores and spasticity).

These ideas are dealt with in more detail and in a different way in Chapter 7 on plasticity, Chapter 31 on emerging concepts and Chapter 32 on pharmacological approaches.

Conclusion

Neurological dysfunction is a complex of several different phenomena. Clinical features are related to the death of nerve cells and the disruption of pathways, reflex arcs and loops. However, the symptomatology and the disturbance of function after a lesion are not simply a matter of disruption of nerve pathways, but are also a reflection of how undamaged parts of the nervous system may react to a lesion. Understanding the symptomatology of dysfunction in terms of disruption of pathways is really only the first step in understanding how the dysfunction actually occurs. Only recently have neurologists begun to investigate the more detailed changes in the intact nervous system. Specific therapy (e.g. removal of compression or treatment of a deficiency disease) may result in complete recovery, but in many patients there is as yet no specific therapy. The increasing understanding of how dysfunction comes about forms the theoretical basis of neurological rehabilitation and should give rise to new ways of management of the patient with neurological deficit.

References

Bach-y-Rita P. & Illis L.S. (1993) Spinal shock: possible role of receptor plasticity and non-synaptic transmission. *Paraplegia* **31**, 82–87.

Barker J.L. & Smith T.G. (1980) Three modes of intercellular neuronal communication. *Progress in Brain Research* **53**, 169–192.

Baskin D.S. & Hosobuchi Y. (1981) Naloxone reversal of ischaemic neurological deficits in man. *Lancet* **ii**, 272–275.

Baskin D.S., Keick C.F. & Hosobuchi Y. (1982) Naloxone reversal of ischaemic deficits in baboons is not mediated by systemic effects. *Life Sciences* **31**, 2201–2204.

Bazanova I.S., Evdokimov S.A., Maiorov V.N., Merkulova O.S. & Chernigovskii V.N. (1966) Morphological and electrical changes in interneuronal synapses during passage of rhythmic impulses. *Federal Proceedings* **25**, T187–T190.

Creed R.S., Denny-Brown D., Eccles J.C., Liddell E.G.T. & Sherrington C.S. (1932) *Reflex Activity of the Spinal Cord.* Oxford University Press, London.

Dhawan B.N. & Sharma J.N. (1970) Facilitation of the flexor reflex in the cat by the intrathecal injection of catecholamines. *British Journal of Pharmacology* **40**, 237–248.

Dimitrijevic M.R., Dimitrijevic M.M., Faganel J. & Sherwood A.M. (1984) Suprasegmentally induced motor unit activity in paralysed muscles of patients with established spinal cord injury. *Annals of Neurology* **16**, 216–221.

Edds M.V. (1953) Collateral nerve regeneration. *Quarterly Review of Biology* **28**, 260–276.

Faden I., Jacobs T.P., Mougey E. & Holaday J.W. (1981) Endorphins in experimental spinal injury: therapeutic effect of naloxone. *Annals of Neurology* **10**, 326–332.

Faganel J. & Dimitrijevic M.R. (1982) Study of propriospinal interneurone system in man: cutaneous exteroceptive conditioning of stretch reflexes. *Journal of Neurological Sciences* **56**, 155–172.

Fulton J.F. & Sherrington C.S. (1932) State of the flexor reflex in paraplegic dog and monkey respectively. *Journal of Physiology (London)* **75**, 17–22.

Gardner M.R. & Ashby W.R. (1970) Connectance of large dynamic (cybernetic) systems: critical values for stability. *Nature* **228**, 784.

Illis L.S. (1963) Changes in spinal cord synapses and a possible explanation for spinal shock. *Experimental Neurology* **8**, 328–335.

Illis L.S. (1967a) The motoneurone surface and spinal shock. In Williams D. (ed.) *Modern Trends in Neurology*, Chapter 3, pp. 53–68. Butterworths, London.

Illis L.S. (1967b) The relative densities of monosynaptic pathways to cells and dendrites in the ventral horn. *Journal of Neurological Sciences* **4**, 259–270.

Illis L.S. (1969) Enlargement of spinal cord synapses after repetitive stimulation. *Nature* **223**, 76–77.

Illis L.S. (1973a) Regeneration in the central nervous system. *Lancet* **i**, 1035–1037.

Illis L.S. (1973b) An experimental model of regeneration in the CNS. I: Synaptic changes. *Brain* **96**, 47–60.

Illis L.S. (1973c) An experimental model of regeneration in the CNS. II: Glial changes. *Brain* **96**, 61–68.

Illis L.S. (1992) Recovery in the central nervous system and the experimental background of central functional stimulation. In Illis L. (ed.) *Spinal Cord Dysfunction III*, pp. 9–37. Oxford University Press, Oxford.

Liu G.N. & Chambers W.W. (1958) Intraspinal sprouting of dorsal root axons. *Archives of Neurology and Psychiatry* **79**, 46–61.

Lynch G., Deadwyler S. & Cotman C. (1973) Postlesion axonal growth produces permanent functional connections. *Science* **180**, 1364–1366.

May R.M. (1972) Will a large complex system be stable? *Nature* **238**, 413–414.

Melzack R. & Wall P.D. (1965) Pain mechanisms: a new theory. *Science* **150**, 971–979.

Merrill E.G. & Wall P.D. (1978) Plasticity of connections in the adult nervous system. In Cotman C.W. (ed.) *Neuronal Plasticity*, pp. 97–111. Raven Press, New York.

Murray J.G. & Thompson J.W. (1957) The occurrence and function of collateral sprouting in the sympathetic nervous system of the cat. *Journal of Physiology* **135**, 133–162.

Omeniuk D.J. (1983) Locomotion induced by intrathecal drug administration in chronic spinal cats. Master's thesis, University of Manitoba.

Raisman G. (1969) Neuronal plasticity in the septal nuclei of the adult rat. *Brain Research* **14**, 25–48.

Roby A., Bussel B. & Willer J.C. (1981) Morphine reinforces post-discharge inhibition of alpha motoneurons in man. *Brain Research* **222**, 209–212.

Sherrington C.S. (1906) *The Integrative Action of the Nervous System*. Charles Scribner's Sons, New York.

Struppler A., Burgmayer G., Ochs G.B. & Pfeiffere H.G. (1983) The effect of epidural application of opioids on spasticity of spinal origin. *Live Sciences* **33**, Suppl. 1, 607–610.

Teasdell R.D. & Stavraky G.W. (1953) Responses of de-afferented spinal neurones to corticospinal impulses. *Journal of Neurophysiology* **16**, 367–375.

Von Monakow C. (1914) *Der Grosshirn und die Abbau-funktion durch Kortikale*. Bergmann, Herde Wiesbaden.

Wall P.D. (1988) Recruitment of ineffective synapses after injury. In Waxman S.G. (ed.) *Functional Recovery in Neurological Disease*. Raven Press, New York.

Webb H.E. & Hall J.G. (1972) An assessment of the role of the allergic response in the pathogenesis of viral diseases. *Symposium of the Society of General Microbiology* **22**, 383.

Willer J.C. & Bussel B. (1980) Evidence for a direct spinal mechanism in a morphine-induced inhibition of nociceptive reflexes in humans. *Brain Research* **187**, 212–215.

Young W. (1992) Therapy of acute spinal injury. In Illis L.S. (ed.) *Spinal Cord Dysfunction II: Intervention and Treatment*, pp. 28–57. Oxford University Press, Oxford.

Young W., Flamm E.S., Demopoulos H.G., Tomasula J.H. & Decrescito V. (1981) Effects of naloxone on post traumatic ischaemia in experimental spinal contusion. *Journal of Neurosurgery* **55**, 209–219.

6: Damage to the Nervous System

R.O. WELLER

Organization of the central nervous system, 45
   Development of the brain and spinal cord, 45
   Cellular organization of the brain, 46
General pathology of the nervous system, 46
   Interference with neuronal function, 46
   Cerebral oedema, space-occupying lesions and raised
      intracranial pressure, 47
The distribution of major neuropathological lesions in the
      brain and spinal cord, 50
Pathology of specific brain diseases, 50
   Head injury, 50
   Stroke, 51
   Parkinson's disease, 51
   Epilepsy, 52
   Multiple sclerosis, 53
   Progressive neuromuscular disease, 54
   Acquired immune deficiency syndrome (AIDS), 57
   Brain damage in the elderly patient, 57
Conclusions, 57

Recovery of function following lesions of the nervous system is still a major problem in neurology. Gradual and progressive recovery of function may occur in some patients but not in others and this has never been adequately explained. The standard procedures used to promote recovery (e.g. rehabilitation techniques and the use of drugs) have little effect on recovery of integrated function, as opposed to preventing development of secondary complications. In other chapters, the physiological, biochemical and pharmacological aspects of rehabilitation are discussed and the problems posed by individual diseases are analysed. The purpose of this chapter is to give a brief account of the structural and cell biological changes that occur following damage to the central and peripheral nervous system, both in general and in relation to specific diseases. Little regeneration, if any, occurs in the central nervous system but, as outlined in Professor Devor's chapter, there is physiological evidence for plasticity and terminal sprouting of axons of preserved neurons. The sequence of pathological changes that occurs in the brain, in particular, has a special relevance to clinicians now that imaging techniques such as computerized tomography (CT) and magnetic resonance imaging (MRI) so clearly reveal the structural changes within the brain. An appreciation of the pathological mechanisms involved in these structural changes is desirable if full use of imaging techniques is to be made in assessing individual patients.

Organization of the central nervous system

Development of the brain and spinal cord

The neural tube develops in the first 5 weeks of gestation and, during the first 20 weeks of gestation, future neurons migrate from the inner lining of the neural tube to their positions in the cerebral cortex, central grey matter of the cerebral hemispheres, brain stem nuclei and grey matter of the spinal cord. Under the influence of growth factors and nerve cell adhesion molecules, axons grow from nerve cell bodies and make connections within the brain, spinal cord and peripheral nervous system. Damage to the nervous system during the first half of gestation often causes severe abnormalities of the brain or spinal cord. Spina bifida, with exposure of the spinal cord on the surface of the fetus, or anencephaly may result from damage in this early period of gestation. Infections, genetic disorders and radiation damage during this period may interfere with the migration of developing neurons and result in severe abnormalities (Weller, 1990).

By 20 weeks of gestation, all the major regions

of the central and peripheral nervous system are
recognizable but the cerebral hemispheres are still
virtually smooth; and gyri and sulci develop in the
second half of gestation. At birth, the brain weighs
approximately 400 g and the gyri and sulci over the
cerebral hemispheres are well developed. Damage
to the central nervous system during the second
half of pregnancy is usually a result of ischaemia, leading to infarction in the cerebral hemispheres. During the perinatal period, ischaemic/
hypoxic damage, intracerebral or intraventricular
haemorrhage may result in permanent neurological damage.

At birth, the cerebral hemispheres contain little
or no myelin and growth in size of the brain during
childhood is accounted for partly by myelination of
the white matter during the first few postnatal
months and partly due to maturation of neurons in
the cerebral and cerebellar hemispheres. Trauma,
meningitis, malnutrition and the effects of genetic
disorders are major factors which damage the nervous system during early childhood.

Cellular organization of the brain

Normal neurological function depends upon a
number of major factors including the biochemical
and pharmacological integrity of neurons, axons
and their synaptic connections. The maintenance
of the internal environment within the brain by
other cell types, such as astrocytes, oligodendrocytes
and capillary endothelial cells, is also essential for
normal brain function.

Figure 6.1 shows the major cell components of
the central nervous system. The axons of neurons
in the cerebral cortex may extend, in the case of
large motor neurons, for 1 m or more from the cell
body. As protein synthesis occurs within the cell
body of the neuron, efficient axoplasmic transport
systems maintain the viability of long large axons.
Oligodendrocytes form and maintain the myelin
sheaths, in both the grey and the white matter;
myelin is a complex, multilamellar lipid-rich sheath
formed by compaction of oligodendrocyte cell
membranes. Rapid conduction of nerve impulses
along the axons depends upon the integrity of the
myelin sheath and the presence of the nodes of
Ranvier regularly spaced along the length of the
axon. Astrocytes are the other major type of glial

cell within the central nervous system; they play a
major role in maintaining the internal environment of the central nervous system, with processes
extending both to the surface of the brain and to
surround blood vessels. Astrocytes also react to
brain damage and are responsible for the scar tissue
(gliosis) formed within the brain. Microglia react
to brain damage by phagocytosing cell debris; in
large lesions the microglia/macrophages are supplemented by monocyte/macrophages from the
blood.

Blood vessels, particularly capillaries, within the
brain have the special function of maintaining the
blood–brain barrier. This is the selective barrier
which allows only certain substances to enter the
brain; it is maintained by the tight adhesion of
neighbouring endothelial cells and the physiological
properties of the cells themselves. It appears that
astrocytes play a role in the blood–brain barrier by
inducing the barrier properties in the endothelium.

Lining the ventricles are the ependymal cells and
within the ventricles is the choroid plexus, which
produces cerebrospinal fluid (CSF) at some 700 ml
per day. The CSF circulates through the ventricular
system and passes into the subarachnoid space
over the surface of the brain and spinal cord. The
majority of the CSF drains back into the blood
through arachnoid granulations, which are particularly prominent in the superior sagittal sinus.
Obstruction to the CSF flow from blockage of either
the ventricular system or the subarachnoid space
results in hydrocephalus, with dilatation of the
cerebral ventricles and, frequently, raised intracranial pressure.

General pathology of the nervous system

Interference with neuronal function

Neuronal function can be disturbed pathologically
by destruction of neurons, damage to the axons or
loss of myelin sheaths – demyelination. A wide
variety of insults to the nervous system may result
in the destruction of neurons or damage to axons.
Such insults include ischaemia, hypoxia, toxins, infective agents, metabolic abnormalities, neoplastic
lesions and trauma. The results of damage to
neurons and axons are expressed diagrammatically

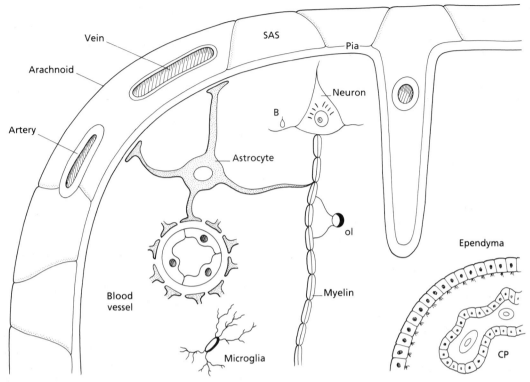

Fig. 6.1 Normal nervous system. The brain and spinal cord are coated by arachnoid and pia mater (leptomeninges). Cerebrospinal fluid occupies the subarachnoid space (SAS) and the arteries and veins supplying the brain lie in the subarachnoid space. Neuron cell bodies lie in the cortex and boutons termineaux (B) from other neurons synapse with their dendrites. Axons ensheathed in myelin, formed by the oligodendrocytes (ol), pass from the cortex into the white matter. Astrocytes extend processes to the surface of the brain, to axons and to blood vessels, in this case a capillary. The capillaries are the site of the blood–brain barrier. Microglia are the resident histiocytes of the brain. Ependyma coats the wall of the ventricles and the choroid plexus (CP) produces cerebrospinal fluid (CSF) in the ventricular system.

in Fig. 6.2. Neither neurons nor axons effectively regenerate in the adult central nervous system, although in the peripheral nervous system axonal regeneration does occur and may lead to the return of some function following axon damage in peripheral nerves.

Demyelination is a process by which the myelin sheaths are destroyed and the axons are preserved. The physiological effect of slowing of conduction and alteration of action potentials along the demyelinated segment of a nerve fibre results in neurological deficit. When compared with the diseases causing neuronal destruction or axonal damage, demyelination is a relatively uncommon event and in man is seen only as a significant pathological feature in multiple sclerosis and in a small number of virus diseases, such as progressive multifocal leucoencephalopathy.

Cerebral oedema, space-occupying lesions and raised intracranial pressure

Cerebral oedema occurs following a wide variety of insults to the brain, including ischaemia, hypoxia, trauma, toxic damage and infections. Furthermore, cerebral oedema may complicate primary and metastatic malignant tumours in the brain.

In the initial stages of cell damage, for example following ischaemia, damaged neurons swell as fluid enters the cells. This initial stage is cytotoxic oedema. Some hours later, vasogenic oedema occurs due to breakdown of the blood–brain barrier

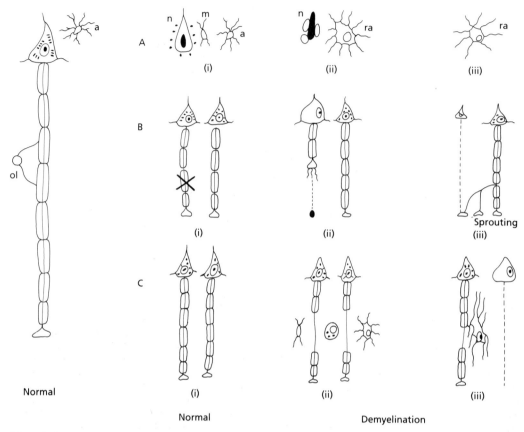

Fig. 6.2 Pathology of neuronal damage. A normal neuron with its axon and myelin sheath formed by oligodendrocytes (ol) is seen on the left-hand side of the illustration; an associated normal astrocyte (a) is depicted top right.

   (A) Neuronal death. (i) Within hours of a neuron being damaged by hypoxia or ischaemia, the cell nucleus shrinks and the neuron loses its Nissl substance (RNA). Boutons termineaux become detached from the neuron (n) and microglia (m) become activated. (ii) After 1–2 days; the neurons (n) are phagocytosed by microglia (neuronophagia) and astrocytes become hypertrophic and reactive (ra). (iii) Once the neurons have been removed, all that remains is the scar tissue formed by astrocyte processes (ra) (gliosis).

   (B) Axonal damage. (i) The neuron on the left has suffered axonal damage (X). (ii) As the distal end of the damaged axon degenerates (Wallerian degeneration), the proximal end of the axon swells to form an axon balloon. Chromatolysis occurs with swelling of the neuron cell body and an increase in protein synthesis. Regenerative axonal sprouting may take place from the distal end of the axon at this time but in the central nervous system such regeneration is ineffective. (iii) If no effective regeneration occurs, the axon and the neuron may degenerate and die. (iv) Sprouting may occur from adjacent axons to take over the field supplied by the degenerated neuron.

   (C) Demyelination in the central nervous system. (i) Two normal neurons have axons ensheathed by myelin. (ii) In demyelinating diseases – especially multiple sclerosis – myelin sheaths are destroyed and the oligodendrocytes often do not survive. Myelin debris is ingested by microglia and macrophages (m) and astrocytes (a) become reactive. (iii) Although some remyelination may occur at the edges of large multiple sclerosis plaques, in many plaques no effective remyelination occurs. The axons remain devoid of myelin with consequent slowing of conduction across the demyelinated gap. Such axons are surrounded by astrocytic scar tissue (a). Axons may degenerate within the multiple sclerosis plaque.

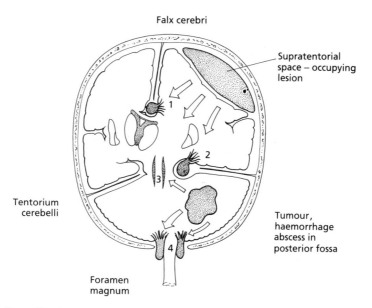

Fig. 6.3 The major effects of focal supra- and infratentorial space-occupying lesions. The intracranial cavity is divided into three compartments by sheets of dura, i.e. the falx cerebri and the tentorium cerebelli. A space-occupying lesion in one of these three compartments may force brain tissue to be displaced into one of the other compartments. A supratentorial space-occupying lesion causes displacement of the midline structures towards the other side and (1) herniation of the cingulate gyrus under the falx cerebri. In addition, such a lesion may result in (2) herniation of the parahippocampal gyrus on the medial aspect of the temporal lobe through the opening in the tentorium cerebelli. Such herniation is particularly common in temporal lobe lesions. Parahippocampal gyral herniation may result in brain stem compression and haemorrhage (3), compression of the third cranial nerve with pupillary dilatation and loss of light reflex in the ipsilateral eye, and compression of branches of the posterior cerebral artery, resulting in temporal and occipital lobe infarction. Space-occupying lesions in the cerebellum may result in (4) herniation of the cerebellar tonsils through the foramen magnum and compression of the medulla. Upward herniation of the cerebellum through the tentorial opening may also occur.

and the passage of oedema fluid into the damaged area of brain. Oedema fluid spreads diffusely through the white matter, greatly expanding the extracellular space; such white matter oedema can be identified as areas of low density on CT scan or can be demonstrated very well by MRI. In the grey matter, oedema fluid resides within astrocytes and the swelling of grey matter areas is not usually as great as the swelling of oedematous white matter. Whether oedema fluid is diffusely spread throughout the brain (as in association with diffuse axonal injury in trauma, or in global hypoxia) or is associated with a focal lesion, displacement of brain tissue may occur, as illustrated in Fig. 6.3, and the intracranial pressure may rise (Miller & Adams, 1992).

Effects of a space-occupying intracranial lesion

The rigidity of the adult skull means that an increase in the volume of the intracranial contents may lead to a fatal rise in intracranial pressure. Furthermore, the division of the intracranial cavity into three major compartments by the falx cerebri and the tentorium cerebelli means that focal space-occupying lesions may cause displacement of the brain from one compartment into another, with consequent further focal brain damage (Fig. 6.3). Apart from the general symptoms of headache, alteration in conscious level and vomiting denoting a rise in the intracranial pressure, focal neurological signs may be present denoting brain shift and herniation. Most notable of these focal signs are those due to damage to structures around the tentorial opening. The third cranial nerve may be compressed and result in pupillary dilatation and loss of its reaction to light on the same side as the space-occupying lesion. Compression of the cerebral peduncle in the brain stem against the tentorium cerebelli may damage the corticospinal tract, producing paresis on the same side of the body as the space-occupying lesion. If the patient survives, the long-term effects may include visual problems due to compression of the arteries supplying the visual cortex on the same side as the space-occupying lesion.

Hydrocephalus

In addition to cerebral oedema and space-occupying lesions, the pressure inside the skull may rise due to an accumulation of CSF within the ventricular system. The circulation of CSF from the lateral ventricles through the third ventricle and aqueduct of Sylvius into the fourth ventricle may be obstructed by tumours within the ventricular system or by scarring following infection. One major cause of hydrocephalus is postmeningitic scarring of the subarachnoid space and interference with the fluid drainage pathways to the arachnoid granulations in the superior sagittal sinus.

The distribution of major neuropathological lesions in the brain and spinal cord

The integrated nature of the central and peripheral nervous system and the length of some of the major tracts, such as the corticospinal tracts and the sensory pathways, mean that certain neurons and axons are liable to be damaged in different parts of their pathways and that the symptomatology of the disease will differ according to the sites of the damage. Figure 6.4 indicates some of the major diseases affecting the central and peripheral nervous system and the areas of the brain, spinal cord and nerves involved. One major difference between the central and peripheral nervous system is that effective regeneration of axons may occur in the peripheral nervous system as long as the site of damage is not too distant from the effector organ and that scarring is minimal, whereas little effective

regeneration occurs in the central nervous system. Similarly, demyelination in the peripheral nerves may be rapidly repaired by remyelination, with consequent return of function, but in the central nervous system remyelination often does not occur or is ineffectual.

Pathology of specific brain diseases

In any treatise on rehabilitation, a large portion of the text is devoted to the practical and often physiological aspects of rehabilitation. The purpose of this part of the chapter on pathology is to outline the basic pathological damage that occurs in the diseases covered in the rest of the book. In the preceding section, the general pathological reactions within the nervous system have been briefly outlined and, in the subsequent pages, the major combinations of damage that occur in specific diseases will be reviewed, thus giving the biological basis from which rehabilitation starts.

Head injury

The majority of head injuries are blunt injuries or injury to the brain due to acceleration without impact (Adams, 1992). Such injuries are mostly the results of falls or road traffic accidents. Figure 6.5 summarizes the types of damage that can occur to the brain from blunt head injuries and the timescale of that damage. Although little can be done to prevent the primary diffuse axonal injury (Adams *et al.*, 1989; Povlishock, 1992) or contusions that occur at the time of the injury, subdural, intracerebral and extradural haemorrhages are potentially treatable; such treatment may prevent death or further brain injury. Cerebral oedema is a result of the traumatic brain damage or a consequence of complications such as hypoxia or hypotension; oedema may result in a rise in intracranial pressure, with death of the patient or further brain damage. If the patient survives the acute stages following the head injury, the brain may be left atrophic and scarred and the patient with neurological deficit.

Injuries to the spinal cord may result from fracture dislocation of the spine or from intraspinal space-occupying lesions such as disc protrusions, extradural haemorrhage, abscess or tumour. Compression of the spinal cord may directly damage

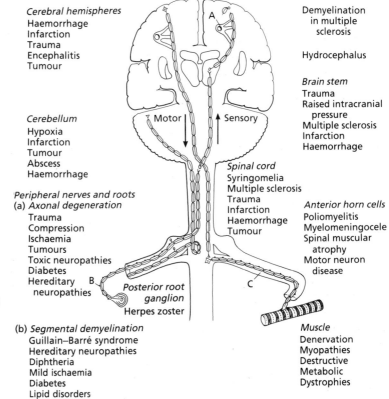

Cerebral hemispheres
Haemorrhage
Infarction
Trauma
Encephalitis
Tumour

Demyelination
in multiple
sclerosis

Hydrocephalus

Brain stem
Trauma
Raised intracranial
pressure
Multiple sclerosis
Infarction
Haemorrhage

Motor | ↑ Sensory

Cerebellum
Hypoxia
Infarction
Tumour
Abscess
Haemorrhage

Spinal cord
Syringomelia
Multiple sclerosis
Trauma
Infarction
Haemorrhage
Tumour

Anterior horn cells
Poliomyelitis
Myelomeningocele
Spinal muscular
atrophy
Motor neuron
disease

Peripheral nerves and roots
(a) *Axonal degeneration*
Trauma
Compression
Ischaemia
Tumours
Toxic neuropathies
Diabetes
Hereditary
neuropathies

*Posterior root
ganglion*
Herpes zoster

(b) *Segmental demyelination*
Guillain–Barré syndrome
Hereditary neuropathies
Diphtheria
Mild ischaemia
Diabetes
Lipid disorders

Muscle
Denervation
Myopathies
Destructive
Metabolic
Dystrophies

Fig. 6.4 The site and nature of major neuropathological lesions. The major diseases affecting the nervous system are placed against the regions of the brain and spinal cord most severely damaged. Within the central nervous system, myelin is formed by oligodendrocytes (A) whereas in the peripheral nervous system axons are myelinated by Schwann cells (B). The blood–brain barrier in the central nervous system has its counterpart in peripheral nerves (the blood–nerve barrier). Capillaries in the nerves are impermeable to many substances and the perineurium (C) surrounding peripheral nerves is also part of the blood–nerve barrier.

axons in the long ascending and descending tracts, or injury may result from ischaemia due to interference with the blood supply of the cord. Trauma and infarction cause axonal degeneration with little ensuing axonal regeneration.

Stroke

Some 85% of strokes are due to cerebral infarction as a result of embolic or thrombotic occlusion of cerebral arteries or their branches (Ramadan *et al.*, 1989). Neurons or their axons are damaged by the infarct and there is little, if any, regeneration. Recovery of function is thought to be largely due to plasticity of the nervous system. Intracerebral haemorrhages cause strokes mainly in patients with hypertension (Weller, 1992); the mortality rate of intracerebral haemorrhage is high, rising to 60% if the haemorrhage extends into the ventricles. The third major type of cerebrovascular disease is subarachnoid haemorrhage, often due to rupture of

a saccular aneurysm on a major cerebral artery or on the circle of Willis. Subarachnoid haemorrhage may also arise from an arteriovenous malformation but, in some cases, the cause of the haemorrhage is not identified. In the acute stages, soon after the haemorrhage, spasm of the arteries bathed in blood in the subarachnoid space may result in cerebral infarction. In the later stages, the haemorrhage becomes organized and fibrosis of the subarachnoid space impedes CSF flow with resultant hydrocephalus.

The major changes within the brain that occur with infarction, intracerebral haemorrhage and subarachnoid haemorrhage are summarized in Fig. 6.6.

Parkinson's disease

The major pathological findings in idiopathic Parkinson's disease are progressive loss of dopamine-producing pigmented neurons from the substantia nigra in the midbrain and the presence of hyaline

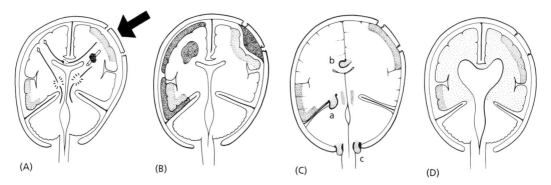

(A)   (B)   (C)   (D)

Fig. 6.5 Head injury. Pathology of a blunt head injury. (a)–(d) can be seen as a progression through time following a blunt head injury.

(A) At the time of the injury, force applied to the head (blunt arrow) may fracture the skull and cause underlying contusion or bruising of the surface of the brain (shaded area) and a contrecoup injury on the opposite side. The brain is suspended in a bath of CSF and swirling of the brain's substance at the time of the injury causes breaks in axons (*diffuse axonal injury*) and may also rupture small blood vessels, causing intracerebral haemorrhage. The *primary brain damage* of diffuse axonal injury and contusions is unrepairable as no significant regeneration of the damaged brain tissue occurs.

(B) Intracranial haemorrhages may be a result of head injury. Such haemorrhages are potentially treatable. *Subdural haemorrhage* (left) may form as a result of bleeding from a contusion or from the tearing of veins on the surface of the brain. The subdural haemorrhage forms a layer of varying thickness over the surface of the brain, causing a rise in intracranial pressure and brain displacement. *Intracerebral haemorrhages* may also enlarge in the hours following the accident. *Extradural haemorrhage* (top right) is usually associated with damage to the middle meningeal artery at the site of the skull fracture. Although the extradural haemorrhage may accumulate very soon after the injury, signs of raised intracranial pressure may only become evident once brain swelling has occurred.

(C) Cerebral oedema occurs in the 12–24 hours following head injury, not only as a result of the primary traumatic damage to the brain but also as a result of any *hypoxic* or *ischaemic damage* that has occurred following the injury. The brain swells particularly in association with contusions but also generally in association with diffuse axonal injury. Herniation of the parahippocampal gyrus (a) may ensue and this may result in fatal midbrain haemorrhage. Displacement across the midline of the cingulate gyrus (b) may ensue and if the cerebellum is damaged, tonsillar herniation (c) may cause fatal medullary compression. The patient may die at this stage from raised intracranial pressure.

(D) The late effects of a head injury are the cumulative results of diffuse axonal injury and contusions at the time of the injury, together with the effects of hypoxia and brain displacement. The overall effect may be loss of neurons and axons with shrinkage and atrophy of the brain leaving shrunken cortical gyri and enlarged ventricles. The patchy scarring or gliosis arising from the diffuse axonal injury is represented by the small dots within the cerebral hemispheres. Reproduced with permission from Fig. 6.1, p. 87, of Weller *et al.* (1983).

Lewy bodies within the cytoplasm of the surviving neurons. Lewy bodies are present in 90% of patients with idiopathic Parkinson's disease and are composed of neurofilaments (Forno *et al.*, 1986) and the heat-stress protein, ubiquitin (Lowe *et al.*, 1988). Little is known about the basic mechanisms of formation of Lewy bodies or their ultimate fate. In addition to the classical Parkinson's disease, parkinsonian signs and symptoms may be due to damage to the caudate nucleus or putamen, frequently following focal infarction.

Epilepsy

The pathology of epilepsy falls into two major categories: the cause of the epilepsy and the brain damage which results from epilepsy. In a large proportion of patients with epilepsy, no pathological cause can be found in the brain. Known causes range from tumours, abscesses and post-traumatic scars to congenital lesions such as tuberous sclerosis and vascular malformations (Lantos, 1990). The regions of the brain that suffer most from the effects of epilepsy are the pyramidal cells in Sommer's sector (CA1) and the CA3 and CA4

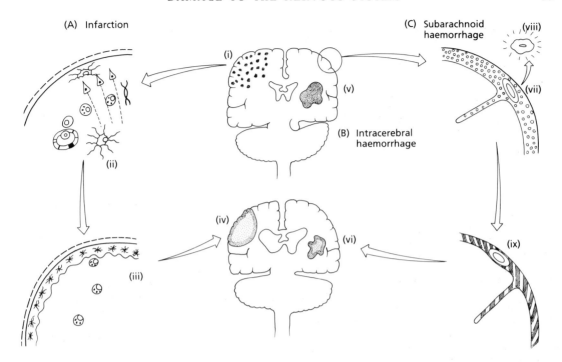

Fig. 6.6 (A) Infarction. Following occlusion of a cerebral vessel, the tissue dies and over the next 12–24 hours the infarcted area swells due to cerebral oedema (i). Histologically (ii) all the cell components, including neurons, astrocytes, oligodendrocytes and blood vessel endothelial cells, die. Within 24–48 hours, microglia in the tissue surrounding the infarct react and, supplemented by monocytes from the blood, phagocytose and remove tissue debris. Astrocytes surrounding the infarct become hypertrophic and form gliotic scar tissue. Once the dead tissue is removed (iii) the area of infarction is left as a cyst surrounded by a layer of gliotic tissue. The removal of debris and the formation of a cyst in an infarct of the size shown in (iv) may take several years. Smaller infarcts become cystic much more quickly.

(B) Intracerebral haemorrhage, associated with hypertension, typically occurs in the region of the basal ganglia and the internal capsule (v) but they can occur in the cerebellum and brain stem, at which sites they are more frequently fatal. If the patient survives, the haemorrhage is resorbed and after many months or years, a blood-stained cystic lesion is all that remains at the site of the haemorrhage (vi).

(C) Subarachnoid haemorrhage is usually concentrated at the base of the brain or surrounds arteries, such as the middle cerebral or anterior communicating artery, bearing the aneurysm that has ruptured. Fresh blood spreads through the subarachnoid space (vii) and surrounds arteries. Spasm of arteries (viii), such as the major middle cerebral or anterior arteries, may result in extensive cerebral infarction. Late complications of subarachnoid haemorrhage include fibrosis and scarring within the subarachnoid space (ix), resulting in obstruction of cerebrospinal fluid flow and consequent hydrocephalus.

regions of the hippocampus, and the Purkinje cells in the cerebellum. Death of these neurons is probably due to the action of excitotoxins (Meldrum & Garthwaite, 1990); astrocytic scarring (gliosis) ensues and, with MRI, the atrophy of the hippocampus may be readily detected. In more severe epilepsy, neuronal loss and scarring may occur in the cerebral cortex, the basal ganglia and the thalamus.

Multiple sclerosis

Multiple sclerosis is the major demyelinating disease in man, in which myelin is destroyed and axons are relatively well preserved. Physiologically, demyelination has the effect of slowing nerve conduction velocities; such slowing can be measured by visual evoked responses (Matthews, 1991). As has been recorded over the last 100 years, the distribution of multiple sclerosis plaques throughout the central nervous system is variable, although there is predilection for certain sites. Most typically, plaques of demyelination are seen in the optic nerves, around the ventricles of the cerebral hemispheres and in the lateral parts of the spinal cord (Weller, 1985). In severe, rapidly progressive multiple sclerosis, large portions of the cerebral white matter may be almost completely demyelinated.

There is a clear progression of the pathology of multiple sclerosis plaques from the *acute stage* of active demyelination, with perivascular and diffuse invasion of the affected white matter by lymphocytes and macrophages and the proliferation of reactive astrocytes to surround the demyelinated axons. As the plaque progresses, its central region becomes devoid of inflammatory cells and lymphocyte and macrophage activity is only seen around the periphery of the plaque (*chronic, active plaques*). Finally, the *sclerotic grey plaques*, which give the disease its name, are left devoid of myelin and inflammatory cells and are composed largely of surviving axons and dense astrocytic scar tissue. The progression of the plaques can be followed by MRI, in which there is gadolinium enhancement corresponding to the acute inflamed demyelinating stage of the plaque and no enhancement of the chronic gliotic plaques. Dynamic MRI studies suggest that episodes of damage may occur more than once in the same plaque site (McDonald *et al.*, 1992). Although some remyelination takes place, particularly at the edges of the multiple sclerosis plaques, the central regions of multiple sclerosis plaques are usually devoid of myelin-forming oligodendrocytes and thus remyelination does not occur. Recovery of function following acute relapses of multiple sclerosis is probably due to physiological adaptation to the slowing of conduction across the plaque rather than to remyelination.

Progressive neuromuscular diseases

There are a large number of diseases that affect peripheral nerves and muscle, many of which cause chronic and progressive neuromuscular disability. It has been emphasized above that little or no regeneration or remyelination occurs in the central nervous system following damage but, in the peripheral nervous system and in muscle, extensive regeneration occurs but may fail due to recurrent damage or due to failure of nerves and muscles to make the appropriate functional connections.

Peripheral nerves exhibit two major pathological reactions (Weller & Cervos-Navarro, 1977; Thomas *et al.*, 1992): axonal (Wallerian) degeneration and regeneration, and segmental demyelination and remyelination. These two pathological reactions are seen to varying degrees in peripheral nerve disorders affecting different parts of the peripheral nervous system (Fig. 6.7).

Axons degenerate if either the neuron cell body is damaged or the axon itself is injured. Anterior horn cells may be killed by virus infections such as poliomyelitis or they may die in motor neuron disease or following infarction or trauma to the spinal cord. Dorsal root ganglion cells, on the other hand, are affected by varicella zoster infections, a variety of toxins and a number of hereditary neuropathies (Fig. 6.7).

Many peripheral nerves run long courses through the subarachnoid space in the spinal column and then along the limbs to the distal parts of the hands and feet. Axons may be damaged by trauma, by ischaemia or by tumours, infections and a variety of metabolic disorders. The longer the course of the nerve, the more likely it is to be damaged. Following injury, the distal part of the axon and its myelin sheath degenerate and the proximal stump of the axon swells; within 2 or 3 days fine *regenerating neurites* sprout from the end of the severed nerve and grow distally at about 1 mm/day. Success of the regenerative process depends upon the distance over which the nerve must regenerate and how intact the pathway is for its regeneration. The longer the distance, the less effective is the regeneration, and the more disrupted the nerve is by, for example, trauma, the less likely is effective regeneration.

Most disease processes affecting peripheral nerves result in axonal degeneration but in a few, especially postinfectious polyradiculoneuropathy (Guillain–Barré syndrome), the major pathological change is *segmental demyelination*. Here, the myelin sheath is destroyed but the axons remain intact. There is slowing of nerve conduction velocity, which accompanies the symptoms and signs of a neuropathy, but *remyelination* and reconstitution of the myelin sheath may begin within a few days and repair of the nerve with return of neurological

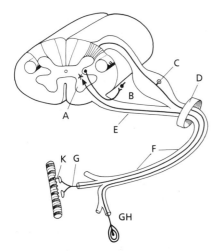

C   *Sensory ganglia*
    Hereditary sensory neuropathies
    Herpes zoster

D   *Spinal canal and intervertebral foramina*
    Trauma
    Nerve or root compression

E   *Nerve roots*
    Post-infectious polyradiculopathy
    (Guillain–Barré syndrome)

F   *Nerve trunks (with or without root involvement)*
    Trauma
    Compression
    Vascular disease
    Demyelination in toxic neuropathies
    Metabolic neuropathies
    Diabetes
    Amyloid
    Guillain–Barré syndrome
    Peroneal muscular atrophy
    Hypertrophic neuropathies
    Disorders of lipid metabolism
    Neuropathies in malignant disease

G   *Distal axonopathies (dying-back neuropathies)*
    Toxic neuropathies
    Porphyria
    Vitamin deficiencies

H   *Leprosy*

KB *Motor end-plate disorders*
    Myasthenia gravis

A   *Anterior horn cells*
    Destructive lesions of the cord
    Motor neuron disease
    Spinal muscular atrophy
    Poliomyelitis

B   *Autonomic neuropathies*
    Diabetes
    Amyloidosis
    Familial dysautonomia
    Fabry's disease

Fig. 6.7 Peripheral nerve diseases. Diagram of the spinal cord, nerve roots, peripheral nerves, muscle and sensory endings to show the anatomical sites of damage in major disorders of peripheral nerves. Reproduced with permission from Fig. 16.12, p. 274, of Weller *et al.* (1983).

function may be complete in 3–6 weeks. Although in severe cases of Guillain–Barré syndrome axons also degenerate, in many cases the intact nature of the axons in demyelinating peripheral neuropathies allows almost complete recovery. Segmental demyelination is also a feature of a number of progressive hereditary neuropathies, for example Charcot–Marie–Tooth disease, in which recurrent demyelination due to a defect in the Schwann cells results in complex onion-bulb whorls around the axons and thickening of the nerves. Such pathology is accompanied by slowing of axonal conduction and sensory and motor deficits.

Normal muscle function depends upon an intact nerve supply, integrity of the neuromuscular junction and anatomical and biochemical integrity of the muscle fibres themselves.

Peripheral neuropathies and motor neuron disease result in atrophy of muscles due to *denervation*, although a variable degree of *reinnervation* may occur. In general, the muscle wasting due to denervation is more marked distally and affects the hands and the feet rather than the more proximal muscles. Interference with the function of muscle motor endplates (neuromuscular junctions) due to antibodies to the acetylcholine receptor proteins is a feature of myasthenia gravis. Sprouting of the distal ends of nerve fibres is seen within the muscle and there may be some muscle fibre atrophy. However, the diagnosis of this disorder is most effectively made by electrophysiology or by pharmacological testing.

There is a wide variety of primary muscle diseases (myopathies) (Dubowitz, 1985; Swash & Schwartz, 1988; Walton, 1988). In some of the more severe myopathies there is destruction of muscle fibres and regeneration (Fig. 6.8). Such features are seen in polymyositis and in dystrophies

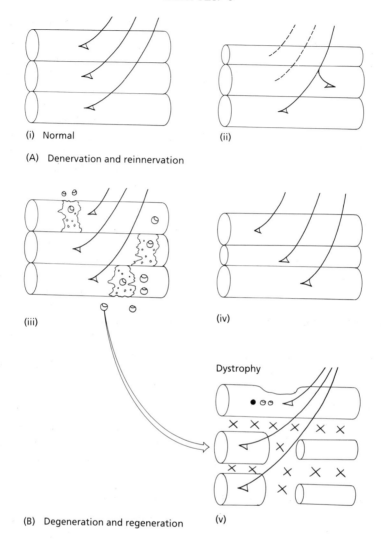

(i) Normal   (ii)

(A) Denervation and reinnervation

(iii)   (iv)

Dystrophy

(B) Degeneration and regeneration   (v)

Fig. 6.8 Muscle disease.

(A) Denervation and reinnervation. When a normal muscle fibre (i) becomes denervated due to damage to the peripheral nerve or death of the motor neuron, the muscle fibre becomes atrophic and the muscle wasted (ii). Reinnervation may occur by sprouting from neighbouring axons (ii), in which case the muscle fibre retains its size and less wasting of the muscle occurs.

(B) Degeneration and regeneration of muscle (e.g. polymyositis and muscular dystrophy). Damage to segments of muscle fibres in diseases such as polymyositis and muscular dystrophy results in death of those segments of fibre and invasion by macrophages, which remove the cell debris (iii). Regeneration of the muscle fibre then occurs and the fibre itself may again become intact. If the myopathy is mild, only a few fibres atrophy (iv). In dystrophies (v) recurrent cycles of muscle fibre degeneration and regeneration are accompanied by fibrous scarring between the muscle fibres (X). There is widespread atrophy of portions of muscle fibres which have become separated from their nerve supply by segments of muscle fibre necrosis. Hypertrophy of muscle fibres is commonly seen in muscular dystrophies and pseudohypertrophy due to the deposition of fibrous tissue and fat is a feature especially of Duchenne muscular dystrophy.

(progressive, hereditary, destructive myopathies). If the disease is mild and regeneration takes place, little muscular atrophy may occur. In severe, progressive dystrophies, such as Duchenne muscular dystrophy, recurrent episodes of muscle cell destruction and regeneration result in fibrous scarring of the muscle and atrophy of those parts of the muscle fibres that have become disconnected from their nerve supply due to segments of muscle cell necrosis (Fig. 6.8).

A variety of congenital myopathies have been described in which there are disorders of mitochondria and their enzymes, or disruption of other intracellular organelles or myofilaments, but without muscle cell necrosis. Such congenital myopathies are distinguished from dystrophies by the lack of muscle cell necrosis and often by the nonprogressive nature of the myopathy.

Acquired immune deficiency syndrome (AIDS)

Most patients with AIDS develop neurological signs and symptoms, particularly in the later stages of the disease. About half the cases develop significant cognitive motor and behavioural problems (AIDS dementia complex) (Navia et al., 1986). Other patients develop neurological signs affecting the spinal cord, muscle or nerves. Damage to the central nervous system arises from several causes. Much of the damage is due to invasion of the brain by opportunistic organisms as a result of immunosuppression; such infections include viruses, bacteria, fungi and protozoa such as Toxoplasma (Esiri & Kennedy, 1992). Lymphomas and vascular disease are also associated with AIDS. Encephalopathies and myelopathy associated with direct invasion of the central nervous system are also relatively common in AIDS patients (Budka, 1991; Budka et al., 1991). Human immunodeficiency virus (HIV) is carried into the nervous system in macrophages and infects microglia and macrophages within the central nervous system (Budka, 1991). Although there is no evidence that the virus infects neurons, it seems probable that substances are released by macrophages or by the virus within the brain that damage neurons and myelin (Lipton, 1991), with the resultant encephalitis and leucoencephalopathy typical of AIDS.

Brain damage in the elderly patient

Although a variety of dementias may occur in the elderly, the two most common causes are Alzheimer's disease and cerebrovascular disease (Tomlinson, 1992).

Alzheimer's disease is characterized by the formation of senile plaques, with a central core of amyloid composed of βA4 protein, and by the development of neurofibrillary tangles within neurons (Probst et al., 1991). The severity of the pathological changes in the brain are broadly proportional to the degree of dementia. As yet, the origins of the abnormal proteins in the brain in Alzheimer's disease have not been fully determined. Cerebrovascular disease may affect the brain in elderly people, either by causing strokes with large infarcts and haemorrhages or by causing dementia due to a large number of small infarcts (multi-infarct dementia) (Tomlinson, 1992). Atherosclerosis of the carotid arteries and myocardial infarction are major sources of emboli for both stroke and multi-infarct dementia. However, hypertensive vascular disease within small arteries in the brain also causes multi-infarct dementia.

A variety of other diseases affect the elderly, such as tumours – particularly metastatic tumours and primary progressive glioblastoma multiforme – hydrocephalus and the rare transmissible dementia, Creutzfeld–Jakob disease.

Conclusions

For almost 150 years, clinicopathological correlation has allowed medicine to advance on a logical basis. With rapid developments in imaging of the nervous system, it is now even more important that the pathological nature of brain lesions is fully investigated so that the images of CT and MRI can be accurately interpreted. Clinicopathological correlation is most satisfactorily carried out if strict audit is instituted through post-mortem examination of the nervous system from patients who have been fully investigated during life.

References

Adams J.H. (1992) Head injury. In Hume Adams J. & Duchen L.W. (eds) Greenfield's Neuropathology, 5th edn, pp. 106–152. Edward Arnold, London.

Adams J.H., Doyle D., Ford I., Graham D.I. & McLellan D. (1989) Diffuse axonal injury in head injury: definition, diagnosis and grading. *Histopathology* **15**, 49–59.

Budka H. (1991) Neuropathology of human immuno-deficiency virus infection. *Brain Pathology* **1**, 163–176.

Budka H., Wiley C.A. & Kleihues P. (consensus report with 23 authors) (1991) HIV-associated disease of the nervous system: review of nomenclature and proposal for neuropathology-based terminology. *Brain Pathology* **1**, 143–152.

Dubowitz V. (1985) *Muscle Biopsy – a Practical Approach*. Baillière Tindall, London.

Esiri M.M. & Kennedy P.G.E. (1992) Virus diseases. In Hume Adams J. & Duchen L.W. (eds) *Greenfield's Neuropathology*, 5th edn, pp. 335–399. Edward Arnold, London.

Forno L.S., Sternberger L.A. & Sternberger N.H. (1986) Reactions of Lewy bodies with antibodies to phosphory-lated and non-phosphorylated neurofilaments. *Neuroscience Letters* **64**, 253–258.

Lantos P.L. (1990) Epilepsy. In Weller R.O. (ed.) *Systemic Pathology: Nervous System, Muscle and Eyes*, 3rd edn, Vol. 4, pp. 360–396. Churchill Livingstone, Edinburgh.

Lipton S.A. (1991) HIV-related neurotoxicity. *Brain Pathology* **1**, 193–200.

Lowe J., Blanchard A., Morrell K. *et al.* (1988) Ubiquitin is a common factor in intermediate filament inclusion bodies of diverse type in man, including those of Parkinson's disease, Pick's disease and Alzheimer's disease, as well as Rosenthal fibres in cerebellar astrocytomas, cytoplasmic bodies in muscle, and Mallory bodies in alcoholic liver disease. *Journal of Pathology* **155**, 9–15.

McDonald W.I., Miller D.H. & Barnes D. (1992) The pathological evolution of multiple sclerosis. *Neuropathology and Applied Neurobiology* **18**, 319–334.

Matthews W.B. (ed.) (1991) *McAlpine's Multiple Sclerosis*, 2nd edn. Churchill Livingstone, Edinburgh.

Meldrum B.S. & Garthwaite J. (1990) Excitatory amino acid neurotoxicity and neurodegenerative disease. *Trends in Pharmacological Sciences* **11**, 379–387.

Miller J.D. & Adams J.H. (1992) The pathophysiology of raised intracranial pressure. In Hume Adams J. & Duchen L.M. (eds) *Greenfield's Neuropathology*, 5th edn,

pp. 69–105. Edward Arnold, London.

Navia B.A., Jordan B.D. & Price R.W. (1986) The AIDS dementia complex: 1. Clinical features. *Annals of Neurology* **19**, 517–524.

Povlishock J.T. (1992) Traumatically induced axonal injury: pathogenesis and pathobiological implications. *Brain Pathology* **2**, 1–12.

Probst A., Langui D. & Ulrich J. (1991) Alzheimer's disease: a description of the structural lesions. *Brain Pathology* **1**, 229–239.

Ramadan N.M., Deveshwar R. & Levine S.R. (1989) Magnetic resonance and clinical cerebrovascular disease. *Stroke* **20**, 1279–1283.

Swash M. & Schwartz M.S. (1988) *Neuromuscular Diseases – a Practical Approach to Diagnosis and Management*, 2nd edn. Springer, London.

Thomas P.K., Landon D.N. & King R.H.M. (1992) Diseases of the peripheral nerves. In Hume Adams J. & Duchen L.W. (eds) *Greenfield's Neuropathology*, 5th edn, pp. 1116–1245. Edward Arnold, London.

Tomlinson B.E. (1992) Ageing and the dementias. In Hume Adams J. & Duchen L.W. (eds) *Greenfield's Neuropathology*, 5th edn, pp. 1284–1410. Edward Arnold, London.

Walton J. (ed.) (1988) *Disorders of Voluntary Muscle*, 5th edn. Churchill Livingstone, Edinburgh.

Weller R.O. (1985) Pathology of multiple sclerosis. In Matthews W.B., Acheson E.D., Batchelor J.R. & Weller R.O. *McAlpine's Multiple Sclerosis*, pp. 301–343. Churchill Livingstone, Edinburgh.

Weller R.O. (1990) Developmental, neonatal and paediatric neuropathology. In Weller R.O. (ed.) *Systemic Pathology. Nervous System, Muscle and Eyes*, 3rd edn, Vol. 4, pp. 309–359. Churchill Livingstone, Edinburgh.

Weller R.O. (1992) Spontaneous intracranial haemorrhage. In Hume Adams J. & Duchen L.W. (eds) *Greenfield's Neuropathology*, 5th edn, pp. 269–301. Edward Arnold, London.

Weller R.O. & Cervos-Navarro J. (1977) *Pathology of Peripheral Nerves*. Butterworths, London.

Weller R.O., Swash M., McLellan D.L. & Scholtz C.L. (1983) *Clinical Neuropathology*. Springer, Berlin.

7: Plasticity in the Neonatal and Adult Nervous System

M. DEVOR

Varieties of neural plasticity, 60
 Diaschisis, 60
 Substitution, 60
 Sprouting, 61
 Synaptic modulation, 61
Plasticity in newborns versus adults, 62
 Critical periods of plasticity, 62
Principles of neural development and plasticity, 65
 Principle 1: Gradients, 65
 Principle 2: Position markers, 65
 Principle 3: Fibre–substrate affinity, 65
 Principle 4: Fibre–fibre interaction, 65
 Principle 5: Timing, 65
 Principle 6: Competition, 65
 Principle 7: Conservation, 66
 Principle 8: Stabilization, 66
 Principle 9: Mutual dependence, 66
 Principle 10: Induction, 66
Plasticity in the adult peripheral nervous system (PNS), 66
 Response to injury, 66
 Regenerative sprout outgrowth, 66
 Target and modality selectivity in regenerating nerve, 68
 Collateral/reactive sprouting, 68
 Arrested regeneration and ectopic neural firing, 69
 Denervation supersensitivity, 69
Plasticity in the adult CNS: sprouting, 70
 Axonal regeneration versus local circuit sprouting, 70
Plasticity in the adult CNS: modulation of synaptic efficacy, 72
 Example 1: Somatotopic remapping in the spinal cord and somatosensory cortex, 72
 Example 2: Spinal shock, cortical blindness and diaschisis, 73
 Example 3: Secondary (neurogenic) hyperalgesia, 74
 Synaptic modulation based on NMDA receptors, 74
 Other mechanisms that modulate synaptic efficacy, 75
Relatively ineffective synapses and their modulation in normal brain function, 75
 Use dependence of synaptic efficacy, 75
 Modulation of synaptic efficacy as a means of adjusting neural representations to the real world, 77
Conclusions, 78

The recovery of functions lost following nervous system injury remains an enigma. On the one hand, the nervous system does not heal itself. With the exception of olfactory receptor cells (Graziadei & Graziadei, 1977), neurons that die are not replaced as are, say, liver cells or cells from abraded skin. On the other hand, as evidenced in many of the chapters in this volume, neural function usually does improve in the weeks and months following injury, sometimes dramatically. The solution, it would seem, is to be found in the accumulating body of data on neuroanatomical and neurophysiological plasticity, i.e. the remodelling that occurs in the nervous system following trauma. The term 'plasticity' deserves some comment. Originally, it was adopted from the field of materials engineering. There, it refers to the middle ground between elasticity and brittleness. Following an impact, an elastic object returns to its original form. A brittle object shatters. A plastic object survives, but it is changed by the experience.

All neural functions – speaking, walking, seeing and the rest – are an expression of neural circuit operation. The functioning of neural circuits, in turn, depends on the intrinsic chemical and electrical properties of the individual neurons, synaptic connections between them, and non-synaptic interactions mediated by non-neural cells, ions and chemicals in the local neuronal environment. None of these is static. Indeed, many are constantly readjusted in the normal course of living. After focal injury, no matter how severe, neural circuits drift into a new functional equilibrium. The new equilibrium, however, is determined by biological rules that operate at the level of the individual cell; there is no guiding hand to nudge it in the direction the patient or his/her physician might have preferred.

This chapter will touch on a broad range of plastic phenomena that may bear on functional restitution following nervous system injury. Particular examples from the experimental literature will be discussed briefly to illustrate the general principles. Early pathophysiological processes such as excitotoxicity, the decline of oedema and recovery from ion imbalances are specifically excluded (see Chapter 6). So also are external interventions such as the use of prostheses or neuroaugmentative devices (see Chapters 34, 35 and 36).

Varieties of neural plasticity

Diaschisis

Neural functions tend to be localized to particular parts of the brain. We can speak, for example, of brain structures that specialize in processing visual information, and others that are particularly important for motivation and emotions. It is a common and fundamental error, however, to stretch the concept of localization of function too far (Teuber, 1974). Brain structures are highly interconnected and interdependent, and the relation of the lesion to the lost function may be non-trivial.

Consider a hypothetical situation in which a particular group of cells is destroyed and as a result a particular behavioural function, say speech, is lost. It cannot be concluded that the speech 'centre' has been destroyed. The functional loss means only that the rest of the brain cannot perform the function (speech) without the contribution normally made by the damaged cells. That contribution might be a minor one, say, setting the level of excitability of a distant group of cells which actually generate speech sequences. Any of a number of the mechanisms to be discussed later in this chapter might be capable of returning the excitability to its prior equilibrium and hence restoring speech. In a sense, speech function was never actually lost; it was only submerged. Early in this century von Monakow (1914) considered this possibility, and gave it the name 'diaschisis'. Diaschisis is a functional loss due to depression of a neural mechanism that was not itself destroyed. As the depression fades, the function gradually re-emerges.

A related recovery mechanism is available for functions dependent on a combination of different sensory (and other) inputs. Each input is normally given a certain weight. A lesion might disrupt the function by removing one of the inputs. In time, the relative weight of the remaining inputs might be readjusted and a functional equilibrium re-established. A specific example of this (see below) is the recovery of control over visual gaze following injury to the vestibular system (Dichgans et al., 1973).

Substitution

On the other hand, somewhere in the central nervous system (CNS) there is a specific circuit that actually generates the impulse sequences of speech. If located in a cluster, the neurons making up this hypothetical cell assembly might properly be called a 'speech centre', and their destruction would surely result in the loss of speech function. In this case, however, recovery will require much more than the fading of a transient inhibition. In the absence of nerve cell replication and replacement, massive and perhaps impossible reorganization of remaining neural aggregates might be required. However, this does not necessarily mean that function will never be restored. It is possible, for example, that another, previously unused neural circuit capable of forming speech sequences could come on line.

Extraordinary as it might seem, there is good reason to believe that such neural substitutions actually occur. It is not that the brain carries a stock of spare parts ready to be installed when needed. Rather, it appears that certain basic kinds of neural circuits are employed widely in the brain, with the same basic circuit module serving a variety of different neural functions. Following injury, these mutually compatible circuit modules may be co-opted from one role to another (Calvin, 1983). For example, in recent work by Metin & Frost (1989), visual information was shunted into the part of the cortex that normally processes somatosensory (touch) information. Their data suggest that, when fed visual information, circuit modules in the somatosensory cortex are able to carry out processing operations similar to those carried out in the visual cortex.

Another type of functional substitution is based on the fact that the brain normally works with several neural processing streams in parallel. If one stream is knocked out by a lesion, remaining ones might readjust and resume the lost function. Parallel processing channels do not necessarily represent redundant capacity. In the intact brain, each channel carries out its own special processing function. However, with one lost, the individual might be able to carry on with remaining ones.

Sprouting

As noted, dead nerve cells are not replaced. But this is not true of axons, dendrites and synaptic connections. As long as the cell soma survives, pathways are capable of regeneration. The renewed growth of neural processes after injury is called 'sprouting', even though it differs markedly from the growth of sprouts in plants. Axonal and dendritic sprouting occurs by protoplasmic extension from the surviving parts of the neuron (Fig. 7.1). When sprouting replaces a lost axon, it is called 'regenerative' sprouting. Sprout outgrowth may also occur from distant, uninjured branches of the injured neuron's axonal tree, in which case it is 'compensatory' sprouting. Finally, axon terminals of completely intact neurons may begin to sprout new connections when nearby neighbours are injured. This is 'collateral' or 'reactive' sprouting. In principle, sprouting is capable of restoring lost functional connections and of creating new ones that never existed before.

Synaptic modulation

The computations carried out by neural circuits depend on the interconnections among individual circuit elements. These interconnections are characterized by a parameter of 'synaptic strength'. A given synaptic contact may yield a large postsynaptic excitation or it may yield a small one. Likewise, the postsynaptic effect may be inhibitory (strong or weak), it may vary in duration (brief or prolonged), it may act alone or be dependent on near-simultaneous activation of neighbouring synapses, and it may vary with the prior history of activation (use dependence). In recent years it has become clear that the effectiveness (efficacy) of synaptic contacts is labile, and that changes in synaptic efficacy are capable of radically changing the functioning of a neural circuit without any change in the 'hardware' of synaptic connectivity. In this way

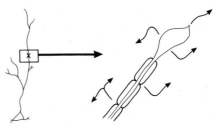

(A)   Regenerative sprouting

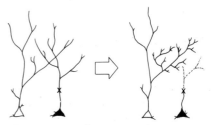

(B)   Reactive (collateral) sprouting

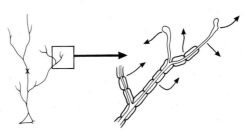

(C)   Compensatory sprouting — the 'pruning effect'

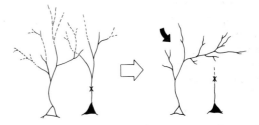

(D)   Compensatory stunting (retraction?)

Fig. 7.1 Various forms of neural sprouting (see text for an explanation of each). The branched figures represent neurons and their axonal arbor. (A)–(C) Sprouting is triggered by transection of axons at the location marked with an (X). (D) Sprouting into a denervated area occasions 'compensatory stunting' of normal growth (arrow).

functional rewiring in the CNS can occur in the absence of sprouting.

Plasticity in newborns versus adults

Critical periods of plasticity

Is age at the time of injury a critical factor in functional recovery? In young animals and children there is often a remarkable degree of functional sparing after CNS injuries that are devastating when they occur in adulthood (Kennard, 1940). On the other hand, recovery after some types of injury is minimal, and in others it may be at a high cost. The sparing of language after early left-hemisphere damage, for example, is accompanied by substantial intellectual and perceptual deficits not seen after equivalent lesions in adults (Woods & Teuber, 1973; Milner, 1974). What are the determining factors?

Experimental studies often find large differences in the physical reaction of the adult and newborn brain to traumatic injury and environmental manipulations. Some point in the direction of greater malleability. For example, Guillery (1972) removed one eye in kittens, thus denying synaptic input to the corresponding layers in the lateral geniculate nucleus. Several months later the connections of the remaining eye were studied. There is normally a sharp border between the geniculate cell layers that receive input from each of the two eyes. However, in kittens enucleated before 9 days of age, the border was breached and sprouts from the intact eye invaded the territory of the enucleated eye. No such cross-layer spread occurs after enucleation at later ages.

In other respects the nervous system of newborns is more vulnerable than that of adults. If a peripheral nerve is crushed in adulthood, for example, injured axons regenerate rapidly and recovery of both sensory and motor function is excellent. However, if the nerve is crushed early in life, most of the parent neurons rapidly die and subsequent regeneration is poor (Devor et al., 1985). In the CNS too, nerve cells in the newborn are extraordinarily sensitive to axotomy (e.g. Allcutt et al., 1984). It turns out that the hour-to-hour survival of neurons in neonates is dependent on a steady flow of 'trophic' molecules that are picked up in the periphery and delivered to the cell soma by retrograde transport in the axoplasm. When nerve injury cuts off this flow, the parent neuron cannot survive long. Neurons in older animals are less acutely dependent on trophic support from the periphery (Yip et al., 1984).

Even given such qualifications, the relative lability of the newborn brain is impressive. What are the reasons? In the following three experimental preparations, the effect of age at the time of injury was studied specifically.

Example 1: The superior colliculus (SC)

Our first case study is axonal reorganization in the superior colliculus (SC) of the golden hamster. Most fibres of the left optic nerve cross at the optic chiasma and make synaptic terminals in the right forebrain (diencephalon). Of these, many continue on into the midbrain (mesencephalon), where they terminate in a map-like fashion in the superficial cell layers of the SC. Schneider (1973) found that, if the superficial SC on the right is destroyed at birth, recently arrived and/or newly ingrowing fibres from the left eye change their normal connections in three ways: (i) The density of termination in the right diencephalon increases; (ii) anomalous synaptic connections are formed in the deep layers of the right SC; and (iii) most surprisingly, optic fibres (re)cross the midline and terminate on the medial edge of the left SC. The left SC, of course, is normally fully occupied by axon endings from the right eye. Thus, normal input from the right eye is forced to yield part of its territory to the invader. If, in addition to the right SC, the right eye is also removed, anomalous fibres of the left eye spread out and occupy the entire left SC. This indicates that adjacent axon populations compete for the exclusive occupation of terminal space.

The various anomalous neural connections resulting from neonatal SC damage have favourable or unfavourable functional consequences depending on the nature of the new connections formed. For example, anomalous visual input directly to the deep layers of the damaged SC provide a substrate for the sparing of visual target acquisition. In the same animals, however, fibres that cross to the contralateral colliculus cause wrong-direction turning to targets presented in the part of the visual field corresponding to the abnormal (re)crossing fibres. Presentation of a food target on the right triggers obviously maladaptive orientation to the left! This wrong-direction turning can be eliminated by 'corrective surgery', cutting the anomalous re-crossing fibres (Schneider & Jhaveri, 1974).

The ability of optic fibres to make abnormal connections is limited in time. Extensive left-eye connections in the 'wrong' SC occurred if competition from the right eye was removed on or before the 10th day after birth, but they no longer formed after the 14th day (So & Schneider, 1978). Such 'critical periods' for synaptic remodelling occur in most neural systems, although their exact timing varies from system to system.

Several aspects of neural reorganization after SC lesions are noteworthy. First, optic sprouts invade not only areas that lose their normal input as a result of the lesion, but also areas not denervated. Second, they can make anomalous connections in regions they do not normally enter. Finally, the amount of anomalous growth in one part of the optic projection depends on the amount of anomalous growth in other parts. For example, the more invasion of the left SC, the less sprouting occurs in the right diencephalon. Thus, developing neurons appear to conserve their total axonal arborization. When distal branches are 'pruned' off, remaining axonal branches grow in excess ('compensatory sprouting', Fig. 7.1).

Example 2: The lateral olfactory tract (LOT)

The lateral olfactory tract (LOT) originates in the olfactory bulb as a tight caudally running bundle, but its axons soon fan out to terminate in a thin superficial sheet throughout most of the pyriform (olfactory) cortex. In contrast to the map-like distribution of the optic tract, LOT fibres form a widely branched and essentially non-topographic projection (Devor, 1976a).

Consider first experiments in which the whole LOT was cut across leaving the (target) cortex distal to the cut intact (Devor, 1976b). When this was done shortly after birth, many fibres simply grew over the cut and continued on their way (Fig. 7.2, upper right). These successful fibres were probably newly outgrowing ones that had not actually been severed, since fibres no longer crossed the cut when the experiment was repeated 3 days after birth, the age at which the last outgrowing fibres normally arrive at the level of the cut (also see Kalil & Reh, 1982).

LOT injury on day 3 caused a tremendous build-up of axonal arbor proximal to the cut. This involved both (i) sprouting of synaptic terminals deeper into the cortex at the expense of intracortical association fibres, and (ii) lateral and medial spread beyond the normal borders of olfactory cortex (Fig. 7.2, upper). In addition, some LOT fibres grew around the medial edge of the cut to partially

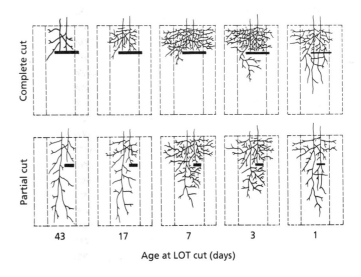

Fig. 7.2 Schematic representation of rearrangements in lateral olfactory tract (LOT) axon branches following complete (upper) or partial (lower) transection in hamsters 1–43 days of age. (From Devor, 1976b, reprinted with permission, *Journal of Comparative Neurology*.)

Age at LOT cut (days)

reinnervate olfactory cortex behind the cut (Fig. 7.2).

When the LOT lesion was made in ever older animals, one by one these anomalous connections failed to appear. By the 7th day reinnervation of the distal cortex ceased, although there was still sprouting proximal to the cut and spread into non-olfactory cortex. By the 17th day spread ceased, though excess proximal growth remained. LOT section on or after the 43rd day did not induce anomalous axon growth (Fig. 7.2, upper). Reinnervation of cortex distal to the cut in the two youngest surgical groups supported partial sparing of olfactory function. Similar lesions at later ages resulted in more severe olfactory loss (Devor, 1975).

Partial LOT section yielded different results (Fig. 7.2, lower; Devor, 1976b). The fibres that were cut responded with proximal sprouting, just as after complete LOT section. However, the fibres left untouched did not simply continue to make their normal diffuse connections in the distal olfactory cortex. Rather, they formed relatively dense connections in the zone just behind the cut, and failed altogether to reach the most distal cortical fields ('compensatory stunting', Fig. 7.1). The result was foreshortening of the LOT projection zone, i.e. failure of fibres that had not themselves been injured to form normal connections in the distal olfactory cortex.

Compensatory stunting, and consequent foreshortening of the cortical olfactory distribution, occurred only when the partial cut was made in hamsters less than 17 days of age. In older animals the severed LOT fibres were affected, but the surviving ones were not rearranged. That is, they continued to form their normal connections all the way to the caudal edge of the olfactory cortex. As a consequence of foreshortening, early partial LOT section proved to be more disruptive of olfactory functioning than partial LOT section performed in adulthood (Devor, 1975). Thus, in this system, an answer to the question of whether neonatal brain injury carries a more favourable prognosis than the same injury in adulthood depends on the nature of the lesion.

Both the proximal sprouting and distal foreshortening of LOT fibres are explained by the 'principle of conservation of axon arbor' (Devor & Schneider,

1975). As in the SC, the 'pruning' of distal branches of cut LOT fibres triggers excess proximal growth. The spared fibres find reduced competition for terminal space just behind the cut and therefore make more than their normal number of synaptic terminals there. However, since the total amount of arbor they can make is limited, growth into the most distal part of the cortex is sacrificed (Fig. 7.2, lower).

Growth rules such as competition and conservation of arbor predict axonal rearrangements in areas completely unrelated to sight and smell. The foreshortening of the olfactory projections into the distal olfactory cortex after partial LOT cut, for example, triggers expansion of neighbouring intracortical association fibres into this vacated zone (Price et al., 1976). This, in turn, probably causes compensatory stunting of other, distant parts of the association system. There, too, neighbouring systems must find a new equilibrium. Thus, a focal lesion in the neonate can have a cascade of otherwise unexpected effects across many synapses. Might this be the reason why functional sparing in the neonate tends to exact a cost of otherwise unrelated deficits (Woods & Teuber, 1973; Milner, 1974)?

Example 3: The visual cortex

The perturbation that brings about a reordering of axonal and synaptic arrangement need not be a physical lesion. Altered neural activity, as expressed in sensory experience, may be sufficient. Studies in monkeys (Hubel et al., 1977; Rakic, 1977) have shown that, in the normal course of development, geniculocortical fibres representing the two eyes terminate in the primary visual cortex in alternating stripes. Early in development adjacent stripes overlap broadly. Beginning in the late prenatal period, the afferent axons move away from one another until the stripes of alternating input are segregated — right eye, left eye, right eye. None the less, because of dendritic spread and intracortical connections, most cells receive input equally, or nearly equally, from the two eyes.

Segregation of inputs proceeds with or without visual stimulation. However, abnormal visual input such as results from blocking one eye (monocular occlusion) severely disrupts connectivity. Thus, in animals reared with a patch over one eye, cortical afferents driven by the open eye come to dominate the cortex at the expense of the interdigitated stripe from the closed eye. Most cortical cells then respond to visual stimuli delivered through the opened eye, but sluggishly or not at all to stimuli delivered through the eye that had been occluded. Functionally, the deprived eye is all but blind.

Suppression of the covered eye ('occlusion amblyopia') occurs only if the eye is occluded during an early 'critical period'. If the occluded eye is given visual experience before the end of the critical period, these effects can be partly or fully reversed. However, even extended monocular occlusion in adulthood does not cause amblyopia, nor does visual experience correct an existing amblyopia (Blakemore *et al.*, 1978). The adult cortex has lost its lability.

Principles of neural development and plasticity

The genome does not determine the fate of each of the roughly 10^{11} CNS neurons individually. Rather, it defines a relatively small number of fundamental rules of cell–cell interaction. Diversity results from the genetic programme of individual cells being played out in a complex and continuously varying milieu. Analysis of orderly changes in neural connectivity following discrete insults, such as those discussed above, has provided clues as to the general properties of these rules. Some have even begun to be understood at the molecular level.

It is important to stress that structural reorganization after injury is regulated at the level of the single cell. If an axon sprouts new processes and forms new synapses, it is because of intrinsic changes and/or local influences from neighbouring neurons, not because of a centrally orchestrated rehabilitation schema. Indeed, as noted, new connections formed may well be abnormal and detrimental. What follows is a brief inventory of some of the principles that shape both normal organization and plastic reorganization in the developing nervous system. Interestingly, with appropriate modifications, most also apply to the adult nervous system (see below).

Principle 1: Gradients

Outgrowing axons are partially directed by pre-existing chemical 'fields' or gradients. These almost certainly involve differential affinities between cell and substrate elements, but it is also likely that there are important diffusible substances in the intercellular spaces to which growing axonal tips are sensitive.

Principle 2: Position markers

Axons and cells may recognize their proper target by means of specific cytochemical position markers made up of specific tissue-target recognition molecules.

Principle 3: Fibre–substrate affinity

Neurons and their processes tend to move in 'mechanical' adherence to pre-existing axonal or glial processes, presumably determined by cell-surface recognition molecules such as NCAM (nerve cell adhesion molecule). However, they can be deflected from their normal trajectory by abnormal tissue configurations. Deflected axons can sometimes form synaptic connections at anomalous locations.

Principle 4: Fibre–fibre interaction

Individual axons in an outgrowing population may interact with one another, each constraining the growth of its neighbour, by mutually attractive and/or repulsive influences. This may result in the axons distributing in a fixed relation to one another within their terminal area.

Principle 5: Timing

The establishment of axonal terminations may be subject to temporal factors. For example, the earliest arriving axons may form connections to the exclusion of later arriving ones.

Principle 6: Competition

Axonal systems compete for the exclusive occupation of available terminal space, that left vacant by the degeneration of neighbouring axons and that arising naturally from the expansion of the neuropil during growth.

Principle 7: Conservation

Members of at least certain axonal populations tend to conserve the total amount of their axonal arborization (or synaptic complement). If growth in one part of the tree is limited or stopped, branches in another part tend to sprout extra collaterals. If exaggerated growth occurs in one part of the axonal tree, growth in another part may be stunted in compensation.

Principle 8: Stabilization

In many systems neurons, neuronal processes and/ or synaptic connections are produced in excess. Those that form 'functional' connections are stabilized, while those that fail to do so are eliminated. Functionality, in this context, is probably determined by impulse activity and/or the uptake of trophic factors which sustain the successful connections.

Principle 9: Mutual dependence

Neural elements may be mutually dependent. Thus, in the absence of one element, a second may fail to differentiate or may change or atrophy. The dependence may involve physical contact, chemical signals, impulse activity, etc.

Principle 10: Induction

The differentiation of neurons and their processes may be altered by the milieu through which they pass on their way to their final target.

Plasticity in the adult peripheral nervous system (PNS)

With maturity the CNS loses a good deal of its early lability, but not so the PNS. Indeed, because neurons in adults better tolerate injury to their axon (see above), recovery of function may be superior in the adult.

Response to injury

In all but the most minimal forms of nerve injury, there is disruption of nutritive contact between the nerve cell body and the axon distal to the injury site. This triggers macrophage-mediated degeneration of the distal part of the axon, along with its myelin sheath ('anterograde' or 'Wallerian' degeneration; Beuche & Friede, 1984). In contrast, in many invertebrates glial cells can maintain the severed axon for months (Bittner & Johnson, 1974). In the distal nerve segment, Schwann cells survive, proliferate within the basal lamina tubes that surrounded the intact axons before injury and become aligned in strands (bands of Bungner). These Schwann cell strands will serve as guides along which regenerating sprouts later grow (Cajal, 1928).

Looking centrally from the point of injury, the axon dies back a short distance, but the rest remains functional. The survival, in adults, of the cell soma and proximal axonal branches sets the stage for regenerative growth if circumstances are favourable, and for ectopic neural firing if they are less so (see below).

The cell body undergoes retrograde 'chromatolysis', changes in central synaptic endings (especially in sensory neurons) and the stripping of some afferent synapses off dendrites of axotomized motor neurons. Once considered degenerative, these retrograde reactions are now thought to reflect metabolic mobilization in preparation for axon repair (Lieberman, 1971; Fawcett & Keynes, 1990). Retrograde neural changes are largely reversed upon successful regeneration, but tend to be progressive in its absence. If regeneration is delayed or prevented, some cells eventually die.

Regenerative sprout outgrowth

As with initial axon outgrowth in the developing brain, the severed axon stump emits sprouts, anywhere from one to as many as 20 of them, each led by a growth cone (Cajal & Ramon, 1928; Shawe, 1955). The growth cones advance by addition of structural and membrane molecules delivered by axoplasmic transport from the cell soma. Elongation begins after a latent period of 1–2 days, the time required for modification of biosynthetic activity in the cell body. If a second more proximal axotomy is made at the end of the latent time, the delay before sprout outgrowth from the new cut is reduced (Gutmann, 1942; McQuarrie et al., 1977).

The fate of outgrowing sprouts depends upon their success at entering the distal nerve stump and reaching the peripheral target. Regeneration is most satisfactory after crush injury where the nerve sheaths remain intact and axons have easy access to the distal stump. It is least satisfactory when proximal and distal stumps are separated by a large gap. Attempts at surgical repair of severed nerves concentrate on closing or bridging the gap while minimizing tissue obstructions and maintaining as good a fascicular alignment as possible (Sunderland, 1978).

In the process of crossing the zone of injury, fibres are strongly influenced by local mechanical and chemical factors. Errant axons may grow in a retrograde direction back into the proximal nerve stump, often forming spirals around parent axons or blood vessels. Others are arrested or escape from the nerve bundle (Cajal & Ramon, 1928; Fried et al., 1991). Sprouts that do reach the distal nerve stump enter the basal lamina tubes that housed mature axons before the injury. They then track down the strands of Schwann cells that fill the tubes. Once constrained within a basal lamina tube, each elongating axon is guided inevitably toward that tube's peripheral ending. Growth proceeds at a rate of up to about 4 mm/day for sprouts of large-diameter parent fibres, somewhat less (about 1 mm/day) for sprouts of fine-diameter parent axons (Sunderland, 1978).

It is not easy to know what proportion of parent fibres successfully send a sprout across the defect to elongate distally. Anatomically, it is impractical to trace single axons and their sprouts for substantial distances. The usual approach, comparison of the number of axon profiles proximal and distal to the lesion, is grossly misleading as individual parent fibres often cross many sprouts. Routine electrophysiological measures are also uncertain. Because of retrograde changes in axon calibre, etc., measurement of the size of the electrical nerve response (compound action potential) elicited by stimulation distal to the injury gives only a crude indication of the number of crossing fibres.

The best method available, applicable only in experimental preparations, involves recording from large numbers of single axons in appropriate spinal roots and asking what percentage of axons that respond to electrical stimulation just proximal to the point of injury also respond to stimulation distally. For crush injury in rat sciatic nerve, this method indicates that 100% of myelinated fibres eventually regenerate (Devor & Govrin-Lippmann, 1979). For rat sciatic nerve section with ideal and immediate end-to-end resuture, the value ranges from 40% to 70%. Under clinical conditions lower percentages of regeneration are expected (Ashur et al., 1987).

Although there is massive overproduction of sprouts at first, most fibres are thought to maintain to maturity only one regenerated branch. The mechanism for culling the 'unsuccessful' sprouts may be like that involved in the culling of excess neurons and synaptic endings in developing organisms (Oppenheim, 1991). In both cases, the first outgrowing sprout to become stably connected signals this fact by means of trophic molecules picked up in the periphery and transported back to the cell body by retrograde axoplasmic flow. The cell soma responds by shunting structural metabolites towards the connected sprout, speeding its maturation and eliminating its sisters.

In addition to gross structural changes, growth and maturation entail a complex symphony of cytoplasmic and membrane changes in the neuron and its accompanying glia. For example, as in developing nerves, regenerating sprouts conduct impulses in the continuous (non-saltatory) mode of normal unmyelinated axons. In neurons with large-diameter parent fibres, even before the regenerating sprouts reach the periphery, a wave of diameter increase and myelinization sweeps over the outgrowing axon from the point of injury distalward. As this occurs, conduction changes from continuous to saltatory and conduction velocity accelerates. These changes involve radical revision of the electrical properties of the axon membrane (Waxman & Ritchie, 1985). In particular, the molecules responsible for saltatory conduction, especially voltage-dependent Na^+ channel proteins, become concentrated at nodes of Ranvier. Likewise, the growth cone must be replaced with a sensory receptor apparatus in afferents and an apparatus for neurotransmitter release in efferents.

Target and modality selectivity
in regenerating nerve

Do regenerating sensory and motor axons in the PNS return to their original target, and, if so, how do they find it? The most clear-cut data on target selectivity are from invertebrates, where individual neurons can be identified from preparation to preparation. Following nerve crush in the leech, for example, almost all regenerating cutaneous fibres were found to return precisely to their original location (van Essen & Jansen, 1977). Following nerve section, on the other hand, there were about 50% location errors, and, after section with avulsion of the distal stump, the errors rose to 70%. In contrast, the stimulus selectivity of regenerated fibres, i.e. whether they responded to touch, pressure, noxious force, etc., was always appropriate to the cell type, even if the fibre ended far from its original target.

In mammals, although the data are less unequivocal, the basic result is the same. Nerve crush is followed by highly accurate regeneration, presumably because sprouts formed by each parent fibre are constrained within the same basal lamina tube used by the parent fibre before injury. Like a train on a single-line track, the sprouts simply grow forward within the tube with little chance of error.

When the continuity of the basal lamina tubes is disrupted, the picture is very different. Sprouts do show an affinity for the distal nerve stump (Kuffler, 1989). Not only are Schwann cells permissive of sprout growth, but they release trophic molecules which apparently attract and promote growth cones. Among these are nerve growth factor (NGF) and platelet-derived growth factor (PDGF), and perhaps also ciliary neurotrophic factor (CNTF) and fibroblast growth factor (FGF; Fawcett & Keynes, 1990). However, beyond a preference for growing into them, axons appear to show little selectivity for particular basal lamina tubes. Errors are numerous, and topographic maps are not re-established. For example, when muscle nerve fibres are given a choice in Y-tube regeneration experiments, they exercise little preference for the distal stump of a muscle versus a sensory nerve (Brushart & Seiler, 1987). Likewise, afferent axons do not divert toward their original skin if a patch of it has been transplanted elsewhere, and they successfully rein-

nervate foreign skin when directed into it (Jacobson, 1991).

Indeed, the capacity for heterotypic reinnervation is impressive. Schiff & Loewenstein (1972), for example, found that cat hypogastric nerve can reinnervate mesenteric Pacinian corpuscles even though its normal target, the bladder, does not contain any Pacinian corpuscles. Similarly, hair follicles are reinnervated when transplanted to hairless skin on the soles of feet of mice and guinea-pigs (Kadanoff, 1925), and taste-buds from the tongue can be reinnervated by lumbar dorsal root ganglion cells (Zalewski, 1973). One of the most remarkable examples is the reinnervation of slow-muscle blocks by nerves that previously served fast muscle. Following this anomalous reinnervation, the slow muscle actually changes its properties and takes on the biochemical and functional characteristics of fast muscle (Hnik *et al.*, 1967). Of course, there are limits to heterotypic cross-reinnervation. Motor fibres will not form sensory endings; sensory fibres will not form motor endplates (Zalewski, 1970; Jacobson, 1991).

Some selectivity is shown in the short-range (micrometres) choice of terminal site. In motor nerves, regenerating sprouts recognize and favour sites where junctions originally occurred. Their cue is molecular markers left on the basal lamina tube by the axon that originally occupied it (Letinsky *et al.*, 1976). Sensory fibres of a particular class tend to return to the correct cutaneous cell layer (e.g. dermis versus epidermis), and seek out appropriate local non-neural cell aggregates (e.g. Merkel domes, Pacinian onion-bulb cells, etc.; Burgess & Horch, 1973). Indeed, in some systems, reinnervation induces the redifferentiation of non-neural receptor structures that have atrophied following denervation (Burgess *et al.*, 1974).

Regenerated sensory fibres in mammals, as in invertebrates, usually 'reacquire' their original sensory modality even if they end up in abnormal locations (e.g. Burgess & Horch, 1973). In both cases the reason is that sensory modality is largely determined by the sensory neuron itself, rather than the non-neural sensory apparatus. In most cases the role of the non-neural receptor structure is to fine-tune the afferent terminal's intrinsic responsiveness.

Finally, as in the developing CNS, the functional

outcome of nerve regeneration depends on the number of fibres that regenerated and on their target accuracy. Regeneration after nerve crush typically restores completely normal sensation and motor control. On the other hand, the frequent location errors made by sensory and motor fibres regenerating after nerve cut can cause disturbing and anomalous function, such as sensory mislocalization and poor motor control (Sunderland, 1978). An extreme example is the reconnection of salivatory parasympathetic fibres to lacrimal glands in Bell's palsy. This may cause 'crocodile tears' on viewing appetizing food.

Collateral/reactive sprouting

Even when regenerating sprouts are free to advance without obstruction and at maximal speed, it usually takes weeks or months before they arrive back in the target tissue. During this time, intact fibres spared by the lesion and fibres in neighbouring nerves tend to sprout into the denervated area (Fig. 7.2). This process, known as 'collateral' (or, by some, 'reactive') sprouting, has been well documented in skin, muscle and autonomic ganglia. Diamond et al. (1976), for example, found that, after cutting the middle of three cutaneous nerves in salamanders, the remaining two sprouted into the denervated skin. Interestingly, sprouts advanced only until they reached a new common boundary. This suggests a competitive interaction between the invading sprouts. Within the reinnervated zone, the normal complement of receptor 'spots' was reformed, but no more. Sprouting also occurred after blocking axoplasmic flow in the middle nerve. However, since this does not destroy the nerve's own terminals, the result was hyperinnervation. Typically, when regenerating sprouts finally arrive back in their original territory, the collateral invaders withdraw (Weddell & Zander, 1951; Devor et al., 1979).

Not all fibre types react with collateral sprouting. For example, in the rat, transection of the sciatic nerve denervates the foot except for a narrow dorsomedial strip of skin served by the saphenous nerve. Over the next few weeks, the saphenous nerve distribution expands and sensation returns to much of the denervated foot. However, only high-threshold mechanoreceptive fibres grow, not fibres

responsive to light touch (Devor et al., 1979; Horch, 1981). This could partly explain the dysaesthesias and pain seen at the borders of skin denervation (Sunderland, 1978; Inbal et al., 1987).

Arrested regeneration and ectopic neural firing

As noted, regeneration is never complete if the nerve sheath is breached. Some fibres, often most, become trapped in a tangled mass in the region of the injury and their continued growth is arrested. It might reasonably be presumed that these axons cease to play a role in functional recovery. This, however, is probably not the case. Rather, arrested sprouts often actively disrupt function by introducing spurious impulses into the CNS (Devor, 1994). Immediately upon transection, axons produce an intense 'injury discharge' lasting seconds to minutes and then they fall silent. Over the next few days, a storm of abnormal neural impulses begins to appear in the nerve. This spontaneous ectopic firing originates alternatively in the region of the nerve injury and in axotomized sensory neurons in dorsal root ganglia. Ectopic impulse generation is also known to occur in patches of demyelination in nerves, sensory roots and spinal tracts (reviewed in Devor, 1994).

In addition to firing spontaneously, ectopic neural discharge sites are sensitive to a range of mechanical, chemical and metabolic stimuli. Thus, for example, forces applied during movement or neurotransmitters released during sympathetic nervous system activity may exacerbate the abnormal discharge. Ectopic neural discharge is known to contribute to the abnormal paraesthesias and dysaesthesias often associated with neural injury (Nordin et al., 1984; Devor, 1994).

Denervation supersensitivity

A final important category of plastic change secondary to axonal damage is the increase in chemo-sensitivity of denervated postsynaptic elements. The best studied example of this 'denervation supersensitivity' is in striated-muscle fibres, but it clearly occurs also in autonomic ganglia, viscera, blood vessels, etc. (Sharpless, 1964; Purves, 1976). It is less well established to what extent it occurs in the CNS (Sharpless, 1975; Macon, 1978). Denervation supersensitivity can alter the responsiveness of muscles, blood vessels, glands and neurons to residual synaptic inputs, and introduce abnormal responses to substances in the systemic circulation.

Plasticity in the adult CNS: sprouting

Axonal regeneration versus local circuit sprouting

In lower vertebrates, including some fish and amphibians, CNS fibre trunks such as the optic nerve and spinal tracts are capable of regeneration much as in the mammalian PNS (Jacobson, 1991). The mammalian CNS has essentially lost this ability. A great deal of anatomical evidence from the last century, culminating in Cajal's (1928) monumental work, showed that central fibres usually begin to sprout, but that growth is soon arrested and damaged tracts are not replaced. The only well-established examples of residual axonal regeneration in the mammalian brain are the hypothalamohypophyseal tract (Adams *et al.*, 1969) and, in a limited sense, several fine-fibre systems (see below).

The evolutionary reasons for this lost lability are unclear, but the fact itself suggests that regeneration is the more primitive state, and that some active suppressive process has been superimposed in more advanced species. This, in turn, suggests that suppression of regenerative ability in the mammalian CNS provides some hidden performance benefit. That is, we may be better off without it.

Recent studies have substantiated this hint of a growth-suppressive overlay in mammals. Specifically, it has been found that glial cells in the CNS, particularly oligodendrocytes, produce molecules which cause the collapse of growth cones and prevent the elongation of outgrowing sprouts (Schwab, 1990). These studies raise hopes that in the future one might be able to promote CNS regeneration by blocking growth suppression. The complementary approach, supplementing growth-promoting molecules, is also being investigated intensively, as is the idea of replacing lost CNS

tissue by neuronal grafts. It is possible that in the future these lines of research will change the face of rehabilitation medicine.

In the mean while, we may be consoled by the knowledge that, despite the lack of long tract regeneration in the unaided CNS, the status of neural connectivity after injury is not static. On the contrary, there is substantial structural re-organization of residual circuits. These changes, which mostly occur at short range within the neuropil, very probably contribute importantly to functional recovery following CNS injury and disease in adults. CNS sprouting will be illustrated in three experimental examples.

Example 1: Local circuit sprouting in the spinal cord

One of the earliest studies of synaptic rearrangement in the adult mammalian CNS was based on the 'spared-root preparation' in cat spinal cord (Liu & Chambers, 1958). In their study, Liu & Chambers cut all dorsal roots caudal to T_9 except for the L_7 root, which was left intact. When traced about 9 months later, synaptic terminals of the residual L_7 afferents were reported to have increased in density within their normal territory, and also to have extended for up to five spinal segments (about 5 cm) beyond the normal limits. Correspondingly dramatic indications of short- and long-distance collateral sprouting were also reported following spinal cord hemisection. Unfortunately, Liu & Chambers's (1958) claim of long-distance inter-segmental sprouting has not held up well in replications using modern axon tracing methods. However, the local increase in terminal density has been confirmed and extended to a number of other neural systems (Bernstein & Goodman, 1973; Illis, 1973; Raisman, 1977; Goldberger *et al.*, 1986).

As in the neonatal CNS and the adult PNS, sprouting in the adult CNS can have favourable or disruptive functional consequences depending on what connections are formed. For example, Goldberger & Murray (1974) found that, after hindlimb deafferentation in cats, locomotor and postural use of the limbs was lost and, along with it, reflexes dependent upon descending pathways such as the vestibular reflex and the (ear) scratch reflex. Each of these reflexes returned over the first postoperative month, with the degree and rate of return proportional to synaptic proliferation observed in local and descending pathways. Likewise, in experiments involving spinal cord hemisection, there was a correlation between the return of suppressed reflexes mediated by peripheral input and the sprouting of ipsilateral dorsal root fibres (Murray & Goldberger, 1974). On the other hand, McCouch and co-workers (1958), also basing themselves on correlated anatomical, electrophysiological and functional changes, concluded that abnormal sprouting and synapse formation in injured spinal cord can result in spasticity.

Example 2: Sprouting in cortex and cortical projections

Rose and his co-workers (1960) used a focused nuclear particle beam to make lesions restricted to discrete layers of (rabbit) neocortex. Silver-stained sections taken at intervals after the irradiation revealed axonal invasion of the damaged layer and, perhaps more surprisingly, the extension of dendritic processes from neighbouring intact cell layers. Dendritic sprouting has been seen in other systems as well, but it has received little attention compared with axonal sprouting.

Where it occurs, axonal and dendritic rearrangement on the borders of cortical defects may be related to functional restitution after focal injury. Glees & Cole (1950) reported rapid recovery of limb movements after localized damage in the sensorimotor cortex in monkeys. Excision of cortex immediately surrounding the original lesion recalled the deficit, suggesting a role for this tissue in the initial recovery. More recently, electrophysiological studies have documented remodelling of synaptic connectivity in regions adjacent to cortical lesions (Jenkins & Merzenich, 1987; Doetsch et al., 1990).

The most labile cortical system described to date is the hippocampus (Cotman & Lynch, 1976). The dentate gyrus of the hippocampal formation receives a number of different classes of afferent input, each arranged along the length of the pyramidal cell dendrite in a largely non-overlapping layered arrangement. This stratification permits investigation of changes in the various inputs when

any particular one is eliminated. One closely studied example is elimination of input from the ipsilateral entorhinal cortex (perforant pathway). When this is done, terminals of most of the remaining afferent systems sprout and replace up to 80% of the synapses lost as a result of the lesion.

Here, too, synaptic reorganization supports functional restoration. In rats, unilateral entorhinal cortex injury disrupts spontaneous alternation behaviour. This recovers in parallel with the sprouting of surviving (contralateral) entorhinal fibres in the dentate gyrus. Secondary destruction of the contralateral entorhinal cortex and elimination of its now expanded input into the dentate gyrus reinstate the deficit, this time permanently (Loesche & Steward, 1977).

Example 3: Sprouting in the fine-fibre pathways

Because of the small diameter of their axons, near the resolution limit of optical microscopes, the classical anatomists knew relatively little about unmyelinated fibre pathways in the brain. Some of these have since become accessible with the development of histo- and immunocytochemical procedures capable of labelling them on the basis of their individual neurochemical signature. Examples include the cholinergic fibre system on the banks of the third ventricle, noradrenaline-containing fibres originating in the locus ceruleus, serotonin-containing fibres of the brainstem raphe, and dopamine-containing fibres of the substantia nigra and scattered brain sites (see Nieuwenhuys, 1985).

The fine-fibre pathways have proved remarkably labile in response to injury. The widely branched adrenergic system is a prime example. When central adrenergic fibres are severed in the hypothalamus, spinal cord and elsewhere, the axon stump rapidly swells. Over the next week or two this swelling fades and large numbers of fine, intensely fluorescent varicose processes, outgrowing sprouts, begin to appear proximal to the lesion. Many of these skirt the edges of the scar and some have been followed for substantial distances along local blood vessels and myelinated fibre tracts. Because the sprouts appear to emerge from near the severed axon stump they are usually called regenerative sprouts (Fig. 7.1). Under favourable circumstances they return to their original sites of termination, and presumably participate in functional recovery (e.g. Stenevi *et al.*, 1973). On the other hand, it has been argued that catecholamine fibre sprouting at cortical insults can induce foci of epileptic activity (Bowen *et al.*, 1975).

Dramatic examples of fine-fibre sprouting come from experiments in which bits of peripheral tissues are implanted alongside central aminergic and/or cholinergic pathways. An elegant example is an experiment by Svendgaard *et al.* (1976), who implanted fragments of dissected iris into the caudal diencephalon in adult rats. The iris normally receives peripheral adrenergic and cholinergic innervation. Within 2–4 weeks of implantation, central fibres of both types invaded the implant. In many cases these tracked along pre-existing neural sheaths, and made terminal plexes characteristic of the normal sympathetic and parasympathetic iris innervation respectively. Destruction of the locus ceruleus on the side of the implant eliminated the anomalous adrenergic input, but did not affect the cholinergic fibres. Stimulation of the regenerated fibres was able to cause contractions in iris smooth muscle.

Finally, as in the developing CNS, damage to one part of a cell's axonal arbor may evoke sprouting in distant intact parts, even if no nearby terminal space has been freed. An example of such 'compensatory sprouting' (Fig. 7.1) was reported by Pickel *et al.* (1974). They partially severed the superior cerebellar peduncle in adult rats, thus cutting ('pruning') the cerebellar branch of locus ceruleus neurons. This resulted in an increase in the density of locus ceruleus projections to the cerebrum (hippocampal formation). The phenomenon of compensatory sprouting in the fine-fibre systems may be particularly important for adult CNS plasticity because of the wide-ranging branch pattern characteristic of these systems. Through the 'pruning effect', a lesion in one part of the brain can trigger sprouting and functional readjustment in distant parts of the brain.

Plasticity in the adult CNS: modulation of synaptic efficacy

In the previous sections, sprouting and the formation of new synaptic contacts were discussed as a mechanism for remodelling damaged neural circuits. These are 'rewiring' or 'hardware' changes. Functional remodelling also occurs through changes in 'software programming', i.e. through modulation of the strength of synaptic contacts within the circuit. In the following section, several examples will be presented in which functional remodelling is thought to depend on this process. Specific neural mechanisms of synaptic modulation will be discussed subsequently.

Example 1: Somatotopic remapping in the spinal cord and somatosensory cortex

Many somatosensory neurons in the CNS respond to electrical stimulation of dorsal roots and skin far outside the cells' cutaneous receptive field. This indicates that, in addition to the complement of afferent synaptic contacts that define the receptive field, there are a large number of contacts from far afield that are relatively ineffective (Wall, 1977). The strengthening or uncovering of these latent contacts, through one or another of the modulatory mechanisms noted below, is thought to account for the changes in receptive fields and the remodelling of somatotopic maps that occur after peripheral nerve injuries (Fig. 7.3).

Briefly, the skin surface is represented centrally in a series of topographic (somatotopic) maps. Each neuron in a map responds to stimulation within a restricted receptive field, with the map forming in the manner of a mosaic. In experiments carried out on cats and rats, severing nerves to the toes and foot rendered cells in the toe–foot part of the dorsal horn map unresponsive to any skin stimuli. However, after only a few weeks in cats (Devor & Wall, 1981a) or a few days in rats (Devor & Wall, 1981b), these same cells once again responded, but now to stimulation of the thigh, perineum and lower back (Fig. 7.3). This functional reconnection resulted from a change in the CNS, not abnormal peripheral regeneration. And it occurred in fully mature animals. The failure to observe sprouting, the existence of positive evidence of subliminal unexpressed input from proximal skin in normal animals and the rapidity of remodelling in some maps combine to suggest that the underlying mechanism is synaptic modulation (Wall, 1977; Devor & Wall, 1981a, b).

Somatotopic remapping analogous to that seen

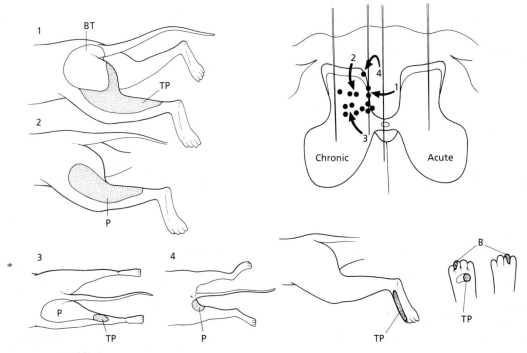

Fig. 7.3 Results of a typical experiment illustrating functional remodelling in the adult spinal cord. Neurons in the medial dorsal horn normally respond to touch and pressure on the toes and foot (lower right). After acute transection of the hindlimb nerves, all response is lost. Later, however, the cells acquire novel responses on the thigh, lower back and perineum. The location and receptive field of four such rewired cells is shown on the left. These four responded to pinch (P), touch and pressure (TP) and light brushing or touching (BT) in different parts of their receptive field. (Modified from Devor & Wall, 1981a, with permission, *Journal of Comparative Neurology.*)

in the dorsal horn also occurs in the trigeminal complex, the dorsal column nuclei, the ventrobasal thalamus and the somatosensory cortex in many mammalian species, including primates (Kaas *et al.*, 1983). Moreover, the sorts of sensory anomalies expected on the basis of the animal remapping experiments are seen in humans who have suffered denervation of extremities (especially amputees). Touching the skin of the proximal stump, for example, evokes sensation locally and also in the phantom (Cronholm, 1951).

There is some uncertainty as to whether remapping in the cortex simply reflects changes that occurred in lower somatosensory relays, or whether there is an additional, intracortical effect. One of the strongest arguments used by advocates of intracortical remodelling is that map shifts in monkeys

never went beyond the distance that corresponds to the length of cortical dendrites (e.g. Jenkins *et al.*, 1990). However, in a recent study of monkeys that had been deafferented for several years, map shifts were observed to have gone far beyond this limit (Pons *et al.*, 1991). It is unlikely that remodelling of this extent could have occurred solely within the cortex.

Example 2: Spinal shock, cortical blindness and diaschisis

Nervous system lesions sometimes dramatically reduce excitability in related surviving structures. A well-known example is 'spinal shock'. Sudden transection of the spinal cord in humans results in immediate areflexia below the level of the lesion, which passes off over several weeks or months. In monkeys, spinal shock lifts in days or weeks, in cats, hours or days, and in rodents it is barely manifest at all (Fulton, 1949). Shock probably results from the removal of tonic descending excitation. The mechanism of its passing has not been determined.

A related phenomenon was described by Sprague (1966) in cats with unilateral visual cortex injury. These animals showed a permanent failure to attend to stimuli presented in the contralateral visual field ('cortical blindness'). However, when the superior colliculus (SC) on the side opposite the cortical lesion was subsequently destroyed or if the intercollicular commissure was split, visual attention instantly returned! Clearly this is not a case of sprouting. Existing evidence suggests that the 'Sprague effect' results from an imbalance of SC excitation. Specifically, the SC ipsilateral to the lesion is normally excited by the ipsilateral cortex and inhibited by the contralateral SC. Removal of the ipsilateral cortex results in unbalanced inhibition and hence visual neglect. Reduction of crossed inhibition by removal of the opposite SC or transection of the commissure restores the equilibrium of excitation and, with it, collicular function (Berman & Sterling, 1976).

The 'extinction' phenomenon in cortically injured humans (Denny-Brown et al., 1953) may have a similar basis. These patients fail to 'see' one of two objects presented simultaneously in the two visual fields, even though when presented separately the objects are equally visible.

A final example was reported in nerve-injured rats (Devor et al., 1979). Some rats have a completely anaesthetic foot 24 h after sciatic nerve transection even though the saphenous nerve innervating the medial edge of the foot is intact. By 48 h sensitivity returns to the medial foot. Once again, it would appear that functional recovery is based on the fading of a lesion-evoked inhibition (diaschisis, von Monakow, 1914).

Example 3: Secondary (neurogenic) hyperalgesia

Prolonged ache and tenderness often develop after an injury to skin or deep tissue. Part of this is due to sensitization of fine-diameter nociceptive afferents in the area of the injury (primary hyperalgesia).

Surrounding this, however, is an area of 'secondary hyperalgesia', in which pain is thought to be evoked by impulse activity in fast-conducting, large-diameter Aβ fibres, the kind that normally produce light-touch sensation (Campbell et al., 1988). The synaptic change that renders CNS pain-signalling neurons abnormally sensitive to input from Aβ touch fibres apparently occurs in the dorsal horn. A specific modulatory mechanism has been proposed that is based on the remarkable properties of N-methyl-D-aspartate (NMDA) receptors (Woolf & Thompson, 1991).

Synaptic modulation based on NMDA receptors

A large proportion of the synapses in the brain are thought to employ the excitatory amino acid glutamate as neurotransmitter, with the post-synaptic membrane employing one of several different kinds of glutamate receptors. One of these, the NMDA receptor, appears to play a special role in mediating long-term plastic phenomena (Brown et al., 1988).

Under normal circumstances NMDA receptors are insensitive to glutamate released from the presynaptic terminal because of an Mg^{++} plug blocking their ion-conducting central pore. However, if the postsynaptic cell is somewhat depolarized, the Mg^{++} plug comes off and the receptor is enabled. When glutamate binds to an enabled NMDA receptor, Ca^{++} ions flow into the cell and once inside they are capable of producing a broad range of long-term changes in the activity and responsiveness of the cell. The beauty of this system is that the Ca^{++}-evoked long-term changes can only occur if two things happen in the correct sequence: a small, enabling depolarization and release of glutamate from presynaptic terminals. This type of contingency requirement recalls classical (Pavlovian) conditioning where the sound of a bell comes to evoke salivation, but only if it was previously paired with the presentation of food. Indeed, many investigators believe that NMDA receptor activation may be the biological substrate of this and other forms of simple learning (Brown et al., 1988).

Woolf & Thompson's (1991) model of injury-induced secondary hyperalgesia takes advantage of these special properties of NMDA receptors as follows. According to Woolf & Thompson, the initial tissue injury excites nociceptive afferents, which release the neurotransmitter substance P (SP) from their synaptic terminals. The SP produces a small, but prolonged depolarization of pain-signalling dorsal horn neurons. This depolarization is sufficient to displace the Mg^{++} plug from NMDA receptors on these neurons. Thus enabled, the neurons are subject to excitation by glutamate released from previously ineffective synaptic endings of Aβ touch fibres. In addition, the Ca^{++} that enters the cells through the NMDA receptor channels may render them sensitive to Aβ input for a prolonged period of time. If the original injury caused nerve damage and triggered ectopic ongoing discharge (see above), the process could be self-sustaining. In this way, pain and hyperalgesia provoked in a single event of trauma could persist indefinitely (Devor et al., 1991).

Other mechanisms that modulate synaptic efficacy

NMDA receptor activation is only one of many different processes capable of altering the efficacy of synapses for extended periods of time. To illustrate, 12 additional modulatory mechanisms are shown in Fig. 7.4. These are divided into two categories: those involving changes in the presynaptic neuron (sketches 2–7) and those involving changes in the postsynaptic neuron (sketches 8–13). The 12 mechanisms are not mutually exclusive. Moreover, they are only a sample out of a potentially much longer list.

Sketch 1. The basic sketch (Fig. 7.4, panel 1) shows a round nerve cell with a tapering dendrite and a presynaptic terminal. Neurotransmitter molecules released from the terminal act on the postsynaptic membrane, causing a change in ion permeability. This generates a de- or hyperpolarizatory signal, which spreads down the dendrite toward the cell body, attenuating as it goes. If the signal is large enough when it reaches the impulse-initiation zone (double line near the junction of cell soma and axon), one or more impulses form and propagate down the axon. If not, it decays and vanishes. 'Synaptic efficacy' is a measure of the downstream influence of the synaptic signal.

Sketch 2. Enlargement of the presynaptic terminal may increase the strength of the signal it generates.

Sketch 3. Single synaptic terminals may sprout twins (Raisman, 1977).

Sketch 4. The synaptic terminal may shift position along the dendritic shaft. When a synapse is closer to the impulse-initiation zone, its signal attenuates less, retaining more of its initial strength.

Sketch 5. The width of the synaptic gap, or the concentration of transmitter-degrading enzymes within it, may change. Likewise, if the synaptic ending is on a dendritic spine, this could swell or contract.

Sketch 6. The presynaptic terminal may be under the control of interneurons (e.g. presynaptic inhibition).

Sketch 7. The amount of neurotransmitter released is intrinsically variable. Likewise, there may be co-release of two synergistic transmitters.

Sketch 8. The sensitivity of the postsynaptic site may increase, e.g. by the addition of neurotransmitter receptor molecules. This could result, for example, from a change in receptor gene expression in the postsynaptic neuron.

Sketch 9. The 'leakiness' (permeability) of the dendritic membrane may change, resulting in greater or lesser attenuation of the synaptic signal as it travels down the dendrite.

Sketch 10. There may be simultaneous activation of other synapses on the dendrite. Even if such a synapse caused depolarization, its net effect could be inhibitory because of current shunting.

Sketch 11. Injury to the axon can cause dendrites to become excitable (e.g. by the addition of voltage-sensitive ion channels). Some dendrites produce partial or full action potentials.

Sketch 12. Likewise, the impulse-initiation zone may become more excitable. A smaller synaptic signal would then suffice to evoke propagating impulses in the axon.

Sketch 13. The dendrite may shrink, bringing the synapse closer to the impulse-initiation zone (see sketch 4).

Relatively ineffective synapses and their modulation in normal brain function

Use dependence of synaptic efficacy

Why is the brain constructed with masses of relatively ineffective synapses? Perhaps, as Wall (1977)

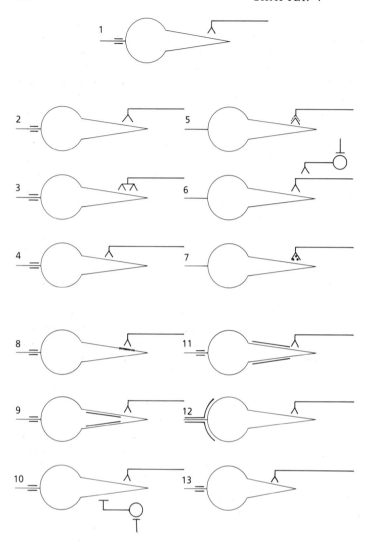

Fig. 7.4 A variety of mechanisms capable of modulating synaptic efficacy. See text for an explanation. (Reprinted from Devor, 1987, with permission, Alan R. Liss, Inc.)

suggested, they are 'ghosts' left over from an early stage of development. It was noted above that the overproduction and subsequent culling of excess neurons and neuronal connections are one of the fundamental strategies of neural development. Might excess connections sometimes be suppressed rather than being eliminated?

A quite different possibility is that modulation of the strength of relatively ineffective synapses plays a previously unappreciated role in the normal physiology of nervous systems. A hint of such a role is provided by the evidence noted above that blocking afferent input into the CNS by nerve section triggers

central synaptic reorganization (Fig. 7.3). Might afferent activity shape CNS connectivity in an ongoing way in the adult, much as it does in the developing brain (Edelman & Finkel, 1984)?

There is substantial evidence in the literature that synaptic efficacy may be dependent upon use, integrated over long periods of time (Wolpaw et al., 1991). For example, in experiments in which impulse traffic from muscle spindle afferents was chronically reduced by transection of muscle nerves, the monosynaptic reflex evoked in corresponding motoneurons declined (Eccles et al., 1959). This decline was not simply a result of cutting the motor axon as it also occurred in agonist motoneurons that were not axotomized. Unfortunately, in these experiments axons of the muscle spindle afferents were also cut, with potential effects beyond simply reducing impulse traffic. This problem was avoided in subsequent series of experiments in which proprioceptive inputs were silenced by severing tendons (tenotomy), fracturing bones or blocking nerve conduction with tetrodotoxin (Spencer & April, 1970; Gallego et al., 1979). These procedures yielded an increase in the efficacy of chronically underused synapses.

Returning to sensory neurons in the spinal dorsal horn (Fig. 7.3), long-term alterations in afferent input might change the relative strength of synapses, and hence the shape and characteristics of receptive fields of postsynaptic neurons. This would ultimately affect sensation. However, it is still uncertain whether remodelling of spinal maps can be ascribed to changes in impulse traffic alone. Some of the many structural and neurochemical changes that occur in the spinal cord following nerve injury probably result from disruption of trophic (chemical), rather than impulse, interactions between centre and periphery (Devor et al., 1991). In cortical maps, on the other hand, there is good evidence in favour of the impulse traffic interpretation. For example, Jenkins et al. (1990) recently showed that repetitively brushing the skin of the fingertip for several months caused the size of the cortical map devoted to the exercised finger to increase. Perhaps the reason why CNS maps reflect the relative use of different parts of the body (e.g. the finger–hand part of the sensory 'homunculus' is particularly large) is that they are constantly being updated by actual sensory use.

Modulation of synaptic efficacy as a means of adjusting neural representations to the real world

A similar principle may operate in the establishment of functional balance in systems that operate with two complementary sensory input channels. An interesting example comes from experiments on the control of head–eye co-ordination during visual target acquisition in primates (Dichgans et al., 1973). When a visual target appears, the eyes rapidly move toward it. Then, as the head begins to turn toward the target, the eyes counter-rotate in the head so that the gaze remains fixed on the target. In normal animals, counter-rotation of the eyes is accomplished mostly by vestibular input, with only a small contribution from neck muscle proprioceptive afferents. If the vestibular feedback is destroyed by labyrinthectomy, compensatory head–eye co-ordination is lost and visual gaze cannot be kept on target. However, within a few weeks, co-ordination is restored. The basis for the restoration proved to be an increase in the efficacy (gain) of the previously ineffective proprioceptive feedback channel.

Gain adjustment in this example followed a lesion. The adjustment mechanism, however, appears to have evolved as part of a normal physiological calibration process. This is illustrated in an example from normal eye–hand co-ordination. Say a visual target is presented +20° to the left. Normal subjects are able to extend the arm at this same angle and point accurately at the target. If the subject is now fitted with prism goggles that displace the visual field by +10°, the object will now be seen at +30° and the corresponding arm extension will be to +30°. This, of course, is +10° off the real target. Remarkably, it takes only a brief period of experience wearing such goggles for the gain of the hand–eye co-ordination system to compensate for this error and for on-target pointing to return. Moreover, prism adaptation does not require an intellectual effort ('I see the target at +30°, therefore I must point at +20°'). After adaptation, the 'feel' of the arm's position (i.e. the interpretation of proprioceptive feedback from the arm) is recalibrated. On the other hand, for prism adaptation to occur the subject must actively move about his/her environment; passive experience wearing the goggles does not work (Held, 1965).

Whenever there is an interaction between an organism and the real world, grasping a seen object or pointing at a sound source, for example, there must be some process to adjust the internal representation of the world to the co-ordinate system and scale of the real world. Otherwise the grasping and pointing would be inaccurate, and ultimately the organism would not survive. Such calibration occurs at at least three distinct levels. At the most primitive level, co-ordination is set by intrinsic brain connectivity, determined by genetic instructions shaped in the process of evolution and natural selection. A finer degree of co-ordination is achieved during early postnatal development, when neural populations are culled and synaptic connections stabilized on the basis of their functional suitability. Finally, in some systems at least, this calibration process appears to be ultimately fine-tuned on an ongoing basis by the modulation of synaptic efficacy in adulthood. The importance of these three levels is different in different systems, but each, including the third, can be powerful indeed. A dramatic example is adaptation to prism goggles that invert the visual world, making up down and down up. Humans readily adjust their sensory-motor co-ordination to this inversion, and indeed their very perception, within a few days. Again, no conscious calculation is involved (Melvill-Jones, 1977).

Conclusions

Could the evolutionary process have produced a nervous system with better capacity for functional recovery? The answer is undoubtedly yes, but that it never 'tried'. Evolution proceeds by the differential propagation of individuals with favourable traits. Faster, stronger or smarter individuals have an advantage over their competitors. However, this is not necessarily so for individuals with better chances of recovery after CNS injury. The reason is that in natural animal populations, it is unlikely that an individual that had suffered a crippling nervous system injury would ever be able to compete successfully for mates etc. against healthy individuals. Thus, a tendency for better regeneration would not have had the opportunity to become translated into more offspring with this improved trait. Only if crippling injuries were very common, and injured individuals competed against one another, would functional recovery be strongly selected for. This and related considerations argue against recovery of function being a capability that has evolved and improved over time. The brain evolved to avoid injury, not to recover from it.

What capacity we do have for functional recovery after CNS injury appears to be an unintended side-effect of plastic mechanisms designed to serve other ends, the most prominent being: (i) neural development; (ii) the ongoing calibration of internal representations; and (iii) the learning of new skills. These are the pillars upon which efforts at rehabilitation need to be built, and in these spheres the brain is intrinsically and exquisitely labile.

References

Adams J.H., Daniel P.M. & Pritchard M.M.L. (1969) Degeneration and regeneration in the neurohypophysis after pituitary stalk section in ferret. *Journal of Comparative Neurology* **135**, 121–144.

Allcutt D., Berry M. & Sievers J. (1984) A quantitative comparison of the reactions of retinal ganglion cells to optic nerve crush in neonatal and adult mice. *Developmental Brain Research* **16**, 219–230.

Ashur H., Vilner Y., Finsterbush A., Rousso M., Weinberg H. & Devor M. (1987) Extent of fiber regeneration after peripheral nerve repair: silicone splint vs. suture, gap repair vs. graft. *Experimental Neurology* **97**, 365–374.

Berman N. & Sterling P. (1976) Cortical suppression of the retino-collicular pathway in the monocularly deprived cat. *Journal of Physiology (London)* **255**, 263–273.

Bernstein J.J. & Goodman D.C. (eds) (1973) *Neuromorphological Plasticity. Brain, Behaviour and Evolution.* Karger, Basel, **8**.

Beuche W. & Friede R.L. (1984) The role of non-resident cells in Wallerian degeneration. *Journal of Neurocytology* **13**, 767–796.

Bittner G.D. & Johnson A.L. (1974) Degeneration and regeneration in crustacean peripheral nerves. *Journal of Comparative Neurology* **89**, 1–21.

Blakemore C., Farey L.J. & Vital-Durand F. (1978) The physiological effects of monocular deprivation and their reversal in the monkey's visual cortex. *Journal of Physiology, London* **238**, 223–262.

Bowen F.P., Karpiak S.E., Demirjian C. & Katzman R. (1975) Sprouting of noradrenergic nerve terminals subsequent to freeze lesions of rabbit cerebral cortex. *Brain Research* **83**, 1–14.

Brown T.H., Chapman P.F., Kairiss E.W. & Keenan C.L. (1988) Long-term synaptic potentiation. *Science* **242**, 724–728.

Brushart T.M.E. & Seiler W.A. IV (1987) Selective reinnervation of distal motor stumps by peripheral motor axons. *Experimental Neurology* **97**, 289–300.

Burgess P.R. & Horch K.W. (1973) Specific regeneration of cutaneous fibres in the cat. *Journal of Neurophysiology* **36**, 101–114.

Burgess P.R., English K.B. & Horch K.W. (1974) Patterning in the regeneration of type 1 cutaneous receptors. *Journal of Physiology, London* **236**, 57–82.

Cajal S. & Ramon Y. (1928) *Degeneration and Regeneration of the Nervous System* (trans. May, R.M. 1968). Hafner, New York, 1968 reprint of 1928 edition.

Calvin W.H. (1983) A stone's throw and its launch window: timing precision and its implications for language and hominid brains. *Journal of Theoretical Biology* **104**, 121–135.

Campbell J.N., Raja S.N., Meyer R.A. & MacKinnon, S.E. (1988) Myelinated afferents signal the hyperalgesia associated with nerve injury. *Pain* **32**, 89–94.

Cotman C.W. & Lynch G.S. (1976) Reactive synaptogenesis in the adult nervous system: the effects of partial deafferentation on new synapse formation. In Barondes S. (ed.) *Neuronal Recognition*, pp. 69–108. Plenum Press, New York.

Cronholm B. (1951) Phantom limb in amputees: study of changes in integration of centripetal impulses with special reference to referred sensations. *Acta Psychiatria et Neurologica* **Suppl. 72**, 1–85.

Denny-Brown D., Meyer J.S. & Horenstein S. (1953) The significance of perceptual rivalry resulting from parietal lesion. *Brain* **75**, 433–471.

Devor M. (1975) Neuroplasticity in the sparing or deterioration of function after early olfactory tract lesions. *Science* **190**, 998–1000.

Devor M. (1976a) Fiber trajectories of olfactory bulb efferents in the hamster. *Journal of Comparative Neurology* **166**, 31–48.

Devor M. (1976b) Neuroplasticity in the rearrangement of olfactory tract fibres after neonatal transection in hamsters. *Journal of Comparative Neurology* **166**, 49–72.

Devor M. (1987) On mechanisms of somatotopic plasticity. In Pubols L.M. & Sessle B.J. (eds) *Effects of Injury on Trigeminal and Spinal Somatosensory Systems*, pp. 215–225. Liss, New York.

Devor M. (1994) The pathophysiology of damaged peripheral nerves. In Wall P.D. & Melzack R. (eds) *Textbook of Pain*, 3rd edn, pp. 79–100. Churchill-Livingstone, London.

Devor M. & Govrin-Lippmann R. (1979) Selective regeneration of sensory fibres following nerve crush injury. *Experimental Neurology* **65**, 243–254.

Devor M. & Schneider G.E. (1975) Neuroanatomical plasticity: the principle of conservation of total axonal arborization. In Vital-Durand F. & Jeannerod M. (eds) *Aspects of Neural Plasticity*. Les Colloques de L'Institut National de la Santé et de la Recherche Médicale (INSERM) **43**, 191–200.

Devor M. & Wall P.D. (1981a) The effect of peripheral nerve injury on receptive fields of cells in the cat spinal cord. *Journal of Comparative Neurology* **199**, 277–291.

Devor M. & Wall P.D. (1981b) Plasticity in the spinal cord sensory map following peripheral nerve injury in rats. *Journal of Neuroscience* **1**, 679–684.

Devor M., Schonfeld D., Seltzer Z. & Wall P.D. (1979) Two modes of cutaneous reinnervation following peripheral nerve injury. *Journal of Comparative Neurology* **185**, 211–220.

Devor M., Govrin-Lippmann R., Frank I. & Raber P.

(1985) Proliferation of primary sensory neurons in adult rat DRG and the kinetics of retrograde cell loss after sciatic nerve section. *Somatosensory Research* **3**, 139–167.

Devor M., Basbaum A.I., Bennett G.J. *et al.* (1991) Mechanisms of neuropathic pain following peripheral injury. In Basbaum A.I. & Besson J.-M. (eds) *Towards a New Pharmacology of Pain*, pp. 417–440. Dahlem Konferenzen, Wiley, Chichester.

Diamond J., Cooper E., Turner C. & MacIntyre L. (1976) Trophic regulation of nerve sprouting. *Science* **193**, 371–377.

Dichgans J., Bizzi E., Morasco P. & Tagliasco V. (1973) Mechanisms underlying recovery of eye–head coordination following bilateral labyrinthectomy in monkeys. *Experimental Brain Research* **18**, 548–562.

Doetsch G.S., Johnston K.W. & Hannan C.J. Jr (1990) Physiological changes in the somatosensory forepaw cerebral cortex of adult raccoons following lesions of a single cortical digit representation. *Experimental Neurology* **108**, 162–175.

Eccles J.C., Krenjevic K. & Miledi R. (1959) Delayed effects of peripheral severance of afferent nerve fibres on the efficacy of their central synapses. *Journal of Physiology, London* **145**, 204–220.

Edelman G.M. & Finkel L.H. (1984) Neuronal group selection in the cerebral cortex. In Edelman G.M., Gall W.E. & Cowan W.M. (eds) *Dynamic Aspects of Neocortical Function*, pp. 653–695. Wiley, New York.

Fawcett J.W. & Keynes R.J. (1990) Peripheral nerve regeneration, *Annual Review of Neuroscience* **13**, 43–60.

Fried K., Govrin-Lippmann R., Rosenthal F., Ellisman M.H. & Devor M. (1991) Ultrastructure of afferent endings in a neuroma. *Journal of Neurocytology* **20**, 682–701.

Fulton J.F. (1949) *Physiology of the Nervous System*, 3rd edn. Oxford University Press, London.

Gallego R., Kuno M., Nunes R. & Snier W.D. (1979) Disuse enhances synaptic efficacy in spinal motoneurons. *Journal of Physiology, London* **291**, 191–205.

Glees P. & Cole J. (1950) Recovery of skilled motor functions after small repeated lesions of motor cortex in macaque. *Journal of Neurophysiology* **13**, 137–148.

Goldberger M.E. & Murray M. (1974) Restitution of function and collateral sprouting in cat spinal cord: the deafferented animal. *Journal of Comparative Neurology* **158**, 37–54.

Goldberger M.E., Gorio A. & Murray M. (eds) (1986) *Development and Plasticity of the Spinal Cord*, Fidia Research Series Vol. 3. Livinia, Padua.

Graziadei P.P.C. & Graziadei G.A.M. (1977) Continuous nerve cell renewal in the olfactory system. In Jacobson M. (ed.) *Handbook of Sensory Physiology*, Vol. 9, pp. 55–78. Springer-Verlag, Berlin.

Guillery R.W. (1972) Experiments to determine whether retinogeniculate axons can form translaminar collateral sprouts in the dorsal lateral geniculate nucleus of the cat. *Journal of Comparative Neurology* **146**, 407–420.

Gutmann E. (1942) Factors affecting recovery of motor function after nerve lesions. *Journal of Neurology, Neurosurgery and Psychiatry* **5**, 81–95.

Held R. (1965) Plasticity in sensory-motor systems. *Scientific American* **213**, 84–94.

Hnik P., Jirmanova I., Vyklicky L. & Zelena J. (1967) Fast and slow muscles of the chick after nerve cross-union. *Journal of Physiology, London* **193**, 309–325.

Horch K. (1981) Absence of functional collateral sprouting of mechanoreceptor axons into denervated areas of mammalian skin. *Experimental Neurology* **74**, 313–317.

Hubel D.H., Wiesel T.N. & Levay S. (1977) Plasticity of ocular dominance columns in monkey striate cortex. *Philosophical Transactions of the Royal Society of London, Series B* **278**, 377–410.

Illis L.S. (1973) Experimental model of regeneration in the central nervous system. *Brain* **96**, 47–60.

Inbal R., Rousso M., Ashur H., Wall P.D. & Devor M. (1987) Collateral sprouting in skin and sensory recovery after nerve injury in man. *Pain* **28**, 141–154.

Jacobson M. (1991) *Developmental Neurobiology*, 3rd edn. Plenum, New York.

Jenkins W.M. & Merzenich M.M. (1987) Reorganization of neocortical representations after brain injury: a neurophysiological model of the bases of recovery from stroke. In Seil F.J., Herbert E. & Carlson B.M. (eds) *Progress in Brain Research*, Vol. 71, pp. 249–266. Elsevier, Amsterdam.

Jenkins W.M., Merzenich M.M., Ochs M.T., Allard, T. & Guic-Robles E. (1990) Functional reorganization of primary somatosensory cortex in adult owl monkeys after behaviorally controlled tactile stimulation. *Journal of Neurophysiology* **63**, 82–104.

Kaas J.H., Merzenich M.M. & Killackey H.P. (1983) The reorganization of somatosensory cortex following peripheral nerve damage in adult and developing mammals. *Annual Review of Neuroscience* **6**, 325–356.

Kadanoff D. (1925) Untersuchungen über die Regeneration des sensibelen Nervenendigungen nach Vertauschung verschieden innervierten Haustucke. *Archiv für Entwicklungsmechanik der Organismen* **106**, 249–278.

Kalil K. & Reh T. (1982) A light and electron microscopic study of regrowing pyramidal tract fibers. *Journal of Comparative Neurology* **211**, 265–275.

Kennard M.A. (1940) Relation of age to motor impairment in man and in subhuman primates. *Archives of Neurology and Psychiatry* **44**, 377–397.

Kuffler D. (1989) Regeneration of muscle axons in the frog is directed by diffusible factors from denervated muscle and nerve tubes. *Journal of Comparative Neurology* **281**, 416–425.

Letinsky M.S., Fishbeck K.H. & McMahan U.J. (1976) Precision of reinnervation of original postsynaptic sites in frog muscle after a nerve crush. *Journal of Neurocytology* **5**, 691–718.

Lieberman A.R. (1971) The axon reaction: a review of the principle features of perikaryal responses to axon injury. *International Review of Neurobiology* **14**, 49–124.

Liu C.-N. & Chambers W.W. (1958) Intraspinal sprouting of dorsal root axons. *Archives of Neurology and Psychiatry* **79**, 46–61.

Loesche J. & Steward O. (1977) Behavioural correlates of denervation and reinnervation of the hippocampal formation of the rat: recovery of alternation performance following unilateral entorhinal cortex lesions. *Brain Research Bulletin* **2**, 31–39.

McCouch, G.P., Austin, G.M., Liu, C.N. & Liu C.Y. (1958) Sprouting as a cause of spasticity. *Journal of Neurophysiology* **21**, 205–216.

Macon J.B. (1978) Neuronal responses to amino acid iontophoresis in the deafferented spinal trigeminal nucleus. *Experimental Neurology* **60**, 522–540.

McQuarrie I.G., Grafstein B. & Gershon M.D. (1977) Axonal regeneration in the rat sciatic nerve: effect of a conditioning lesion and of dbcAMP. *Brain Research* **132**, 443–453.

Melvill-Jones G. (1977) Plasticity in the adult vestibulo-ocular reflex arc. *Philosophical Transactions of the Royal Society of London, Series B* **278**, 241–436.

Metin C. & Frost D.O. (1989) Visual responses of neurons in somatosensory cortex of hamsters with experimentally induced retinal projections to somatosensory thalamus. *Proceedings of the National Academy of Science (USA)* **86**, 357–361.

Milner B. (1974) Hemispheric specialisation: scope and limits. In Schmitt F.O. & Worden F.G. (eds) *The Neurosciences: Third Study Program*, pp. 75–89. MIT Press, Cambridge, Mass.

Murray M. & Goldberger M. (1974) Restitution of function and collateral sprouting in cat spinal cord: the partial hemisected animal. *Journal of Comparative Neurology* **158**, 19–36.

Nieuwenhuys R. (1985) *Chemoarchitecture of the Brain*, Springer, Berlin.

Nordin M., Nystrom B., Wallin U. & Hagbarth K. (1984) Ectopic sensory discharge and parasthesiae in patients with disorders of peripheral nerves, dorsal roots and dorsal columns. *Pain* **20**, 231–245.

Oppenheim R.W. (1991) Cell death during development of the nervous system. *Annual Review of Neuroscience* **14**, 453–501.

Pickel V.M., Segal N. & Bloom F.E. (1974) Axonal proliferation following lesions of cerebellar peduncles: a combined fluorescence microscopic and autoradiographic study. *Journal of Comparative Neurology* **155**, 43–60.

Pons T.P., Garraghty P.E., Ommaya A.K., Kaas J.H., Taub E. & Mishkin M. (1991) Massive cortical reorganization after sensory deafferentation in adult macaques. *Science* **252**, 1857–1860.

Price J.L., Moxley G.F. & Schwob J.E. (1976) Development and plasticity of complementary afferent systems to the olfactory cortex. *Experimental Brain Research* **Suppl. 1**, 148–154.

Purves D. (1976) Long-term regulation in the vertebrate peripheral nervous system. In Porter R. (ed.) *Neurophysiology II*, Vol. 10. University Park Press, Baltimore.

Raisman G. (1977) Formation of synapses in the adult rat after injury: similarities and differences between a peripheral and a central nervous site. *Philosophical Transactions of the Royal Society of London, Series B* **278**, 349–359.

Rakic P. (1977) Prenatal development of the visual system in rhesus monkey. *Philosophical Transactions of the Royal Society of London, Series B* **278**, 245–260.

Rose J.E., Malis L., Kruger I. & Baker C.P. (1960) Effects of heavy ionizing monoenergetic particles on the cerebral cortex. II. Histological appearance of laminar lesions and growth of nerve fibres after laminar destruction. *Journal of Comparative Neurology* **115**, 243–295.

Schiff J. & Loewenstein W.R. (1972) Development of a receptor on a foreign nerve fibre in a Pacinian corpuscle. *Science* **177**, 712–715.

Schneider G.E. (1973) Early lesions of superior colliculus: factors affecting the formation of abnormal retinal projections. *Brain, Behaviour and Evolution* **8**, 73–109.

Schneider G.E. & Jhaveri S.R. (1974) Neuroanatomical correlates of spared or altered function after brain lesions in the newborn hamster. In Stein D.G., Rosen J.J. & Butters N. (eds) *Plasticity and Recovery of Function in the Central Nervous System*, pp. 65–109. Academic Press, New York.

Schwab M.E. (1990) Myelin-associated inhibitors of neurite growth and regeneration in the CNS. *Trends in Neuroscience* **13**, 452–456.

Sharpless S.K. (1964) Reorganisation of function in the nervous system: use and disuse. *Annual Review of Physiology* **26**, 357–388.

Sharpless S.K. (1975) Supersensitivity-like phenomena in the central nervous system. *Federation Proceedings* **34**, 1990–1997.

Shawe G.D.H. (1955) On the number of branches formed by regenerating nerve fibres. *British Journal of Surgery* **42**, 474–488.

So K.F. & Schneider G.E. (1978) Abnormal recrossing retinotectal projections after early lesions in Syrian hamsters: age related effects. *Brain Research* **147**, 277–295.

Spencer W.A. & April R.S. (1970) Plastic properties of monosynaptic pathways in mammals. In Horn G. & Hinde R.A. (eds) *Short-term Changes in Neural Activity and Behaviour*. Cambridge University Press, Cambridge.

Sprague J.M. (1966) Interaction of cortex and superior colliculus in mediation of visually guided behaviour in the cat. *Science* **153**, 1544–1547.

Stenevi U., Bjorklund A. & Moore R.Y. (1973) Morphological plasticity of central adrenergic neurons. *Brain, Behaviour and Evolution* **8**, 110–134.

Sunderland S. (1978) *Nerves and Nerve Injuries*, 2nd edn. Churchill Livingstone, London.

Svendgaard N.-A., Bjorklund A. & Stenevi U. (1976) Regeneration of central cholinergic neurons in the adult brain. *Brain Research* **102**, 1–22.

Teuber H.-C. (1974) Recovery of lesions of the central nervous system: history and prospects. *Neurosciences Research Program Bulletin* **12**, 197–211.

van Essen D.C. & Jansen G.K.S. (1977) The specificity of reinnervation by identified sensory and motor neurons in the leech. *Journal of Comparative Neurology* **171**, 433–454.

von Monakow C. (1914) *Das Grosshirn und die Abbaufunktion durch Kortikale*. Bergmann, Herde, Wiesbaden.

Wall P.D. (1977) The presence of ineffective synapses and the circumstances which unmask them. *Philosophical Transactions of the Royal Society of London, Series B* **278**, 361–372.

Waxman S.G. & Ritchie J.M. (1985) Organization of ion channels in the myelinated nerve fiber. *Science* **228**, 1502–1507.

Weddell G. & Zander E. (1951) The fragility of non-myelinated nerve terminals. *Journal of Anatomy* **85**, 242–250.

Wolpaw J.R., Schmidt, J.T. & Vaughan T.M. (eds) (1991) Activity-driven CNS changes in learning and development. *Annals of the New York Academy of Sciences* **625**, 1–400.

Woods B.T. & Teuber H.-L. (1973) Early onset of complementary specialization of cerebral hemispheres in man. *Transactions of the American Neurological Association* **98**, 113–117.

Woolf C.J. & Thompson S.W.N. (1991) The induction and maintenance of central sensitization is dependent on N-methyl D-aspartic acid receptor activation: implications for the treatment of post-injury hypersensitivity states. *Pain* **44**, 293–299.

Yip H.K., Rich, K.M., Lampe, P.A. & Johnson E.M. (1984) The effects of nerve growth factor and its antiserum on the postnatal development and survival after injury of sensory neurons in rat dorsal root ganglia. *Journal of Neuroscience* **4**, 2986–2992.

Zalewski A.A. (1970) Reinnervation of denervated skeletal muscle by axons of motor, sensory and sympathetic neurons. *Physiologist* **13**, 354–360.

Zalewski A.A. (1973) Regeneration of taste buds in tongue grafts after reinnervation by neurons in transplanted lumbar sensory ganglia. *Experimental Neurology* **40**, 161–169.

8: Clinical Neurophysiology in Rehabilitation

E.M. SEDGWICK

Why neurophysiology?, 82
  Assessment, 83
  Progress, 84
  Research, 84
What neurophysiology?, 84
  Polyelectromyography (pEMG), 84
  Inhibition in the spinal cord, 86
Which neurophysiology?, 89
  Plasticity of somatotopic maps, 89
  Trophic factors, 90
  The motor unit, 91
  Axons, 91
  Muscle spindles, 92
  Walking, 93
Movement, 95
  Corticospinal tract, 95
  Magnetic stimulation, 95
  Anatomy of movement, 96
Higher nervous function, 99
Whither neurophysiology?, 100

There are those who see no need for neurophysiology in rehabilitation and no need for research, or at least for technical methods of research. By implication these people must either be satisfied with the existing state of neurological rehabilitation or regard the situation as hopeless. The aim of this chapter is to disenchant the former and encourage the latter.

It is difficult to begin without admitting that clinical neurophysiology has contributed rather little to the rehabilitation of the central nervous system (CNS)-damaged patient in the past. Perhaps this has been because the only widely applied technique has been electroencephalography (EEG), which relates only distantly to the rehabilitation process. Electromyography (EMG), on the other hand, and nerve conduction studies have been successfully used by rehabilitation specialists themselves to observe denervation, reinnervation and other changes. There are many excellent texts available which the interested reader may consult.

In this chapter some ideas and lines of research which are being pursued in clinical departments or in laboratories devoted to animal work and which seem pertinent to rehabilitation are summarized and discussed. In many cases, direct application of the ideas or techniques into rehabilitation practice may seem remote, but remote ideas have been developed into important practices by gifted persons, often in a rather short space of time. Should none of this happen, neurophysiology still offers objective methods for studying the function of a damaged nervous system and how it changes as the CNS adapts to damage. Just as the function of the heart is to pump blood, so the function of the nervous system is to adapt to changing circumstances. Even though the dead nerve cells are not replaced, the CNS still adapts to injury – imperfectly to be sure, but it changes none the less, and one role of the neurophysiologist is to observe and understand these changes. Another role is to measure carefully any beneficial or harmful change which might have been wrought by treatment and to suggest possible procedures which may alleviate particular problems.

Why neurophysiology?

It might be asked why neurophysiology should be thought at all relevant to rehabilitation, as it is a study of events within the nervous system, whereas rehabilitation is concerned with the restoration of capabilities which lie outside the nervous system. We all possess a nervous system which is more or less the same as that of our fellows in terms of anatomy and physiology. This applies whether our lives have developed the skills of force (labouring, physical sports), the skills of dexterity and aestheticism (artist, musician) or merely the skills of daily living. Whatever the skills, the same neurophysiological processes are common to all. Impairment can therefore be expressed in physiological terms, while functional limitation, handicap and disability are all compounded concepts developed from the interaction between impairment and lifestyle, social status, ideas of normality and premorbid skills.

Assessment

The first meeting point of neurophysiology and rehabilitation could be in the neurological assessment of a patient entering a course of rehabilitation. The diagnosis has been firmly established, all appropriate acute treatments have been applied and the prognosis is known to an acceptable level of probability. One begins with an evaluation and assesses degrees of paralysis, spasticity, lack of co-ordination, etc. It is here that neurophysiological techniques allow a more detailed evaluation than clinical methods. Readers of this book are no doubt aware of the need for better, more thorough and more relevant methods of assessment. It must be appreciated that the clinical neurological signs probably will not change, but the immutability of signs such as extensor plantar responses and brisk tendon reflexes does not preclude significant functional changes which can favourably alter lifestyle.

Assessment of patients at the beginning of a programme of rehabilitation is a fundamental activity of the rehabilitation team and must extend across all aspects of human function and behaviour, from an assessment of a person's financial status, his/her family and home circumstances through to personal activities such as sexual, physical and vegetative functions, sometimes going into extreme details such as whether a particular muscle can produce any tension and how much. The team frequently have to take decisions which have moral implications that often colour one's approach to a particular patient. There is a need to assess an apparent lack of function as due to fear of pain, to hysterical overlay, to malingering or to over-emphasis on matters of legal compensation, and to separate such factors from more organic problems.

Table 8.1 The place of neurophysiology in the rehabilitation process

	Disease	Neurophysiology
Rehabilitation	Damaged nervous system	Neurophysiology
Rehabilitation	Pathophysiology	Neurophysiology
Rehabilitation	Impairment	Neurophysiology
Rehabilitation	Disability	
Rehabilitation	Handicap	

In this area objective tests of function can be very valuable in helping to restore confidence.

Table 8.1 helps to clarify where neurophysiology fits into the rehabilitation process. Neurophysiological tests come early in the scheme, assisting the understanding of the pathophysiology of the neurological impairment and perhaps the resulting disability. Neurophysiological tests are measurements; they allow some degree of quantification of physiological processes and the resulting deficits. They are therefore a basic measurement technique for assessing pathophysiology and any natural or therapeutically induced changes (Tallis, 1991).

Phrenic nerve

One example of a simple assessment which would profoundly affect rehabilitation management is the function of the phrenic nerve in apnoeic quadriplegia. Movement of the diaphragm may be tested by measuring vital capacity or by radiological screening but, if there is no diaphragmatic activity, it is important to know whether the phrenic motor neurons and axons have survived the injury or have degenerated. Experience shows that in apnoeic tetraplegia functional activity in the diaphragm may begin to return up to 4 months after injury. In the absence of functional recovery the use of electrical stimulation of the phrenic nerve to provide respiratory excursions may be considered but the integrity of the phrenic nerves must be established first.

The phrenic nerve can be stimulated by surface electrodes at the posterior border of the midpoint of sternomastoid. The M response of the diaphragm can be recorded by electrodes placed in the 7th–9th intercostal spaces in the anterior axillary line.

Normally a response amplitude of up to 1 mV can be expected, but the diaphragm undergoes disuse atrophy like other muscles, so a very low-amplitude response may be expected (Newsom Davis, 1967). Higher-amplitude responses may be obtained from oesophageal electrodes placed near the cardiac sphincter, where they lie between the crura of the diaphragm. Needle EMG of the diaphragm is not attempted. It may easily lead to pneumothorax.

Implantation of phrenic nerve electrodes can be a useful aid to respiration (see Chapter 36). Once correctly placed around the phrenic nerve, the stimulating electrodes function for many years and fears that fibrosis may eventually impede the stimulating current are unfounded. After implantation, a careful programme of stimulation needs to be implemented in order to reverse the disuse atrophy of the diaphragm before it becomes fully functional as a respiratory muscle.

Progress

Having made a thorough assessment of a patient, one must selectively reassess certain functions from time to time to measure progress and the effects of treatment. One of the major problems in rehabilitation is to know just what effect, if any, treatment has and what changes are due to the natural history of the repairing progress. To an outsider the unquestioned acceptance of very expensive and prolonged treatment regimes administered by physiotherapists is a continuing surprise. If the techniques of physiotherapy were subjected to rigorous assessment, like new drugs, then the services of well-trained physiotherapists could be used to greater effect and with more confidence. Neurophysiological techniques should be able to aid in showing the effectiveness, or otherwise, of different physical, pharmacological and surgical treatments.

Research

There has been so little use of neurophysiological techniques in rehabilitation that almost any series of investigations has a research element to it in the sense that similar work will not have been reported previously. That a project 'has not been done before' is not, however, sufficient reason for doing

it. One has to construct a hypothesis which is testable by applying the techniques available in such a way that the results will unequivocally support or refute the starting hypothesis. All of this must be accomplished within the framework of ethical considerations for the patients. The role of neurophysiological techniques in research into the rehabilitation of the neurological patient is self-evident, especially as nearly all the techniques are non-invasive and risk-free.

What neurophysiology?

Table 8.2 lists neurophysiological techniques all of which involve the measurement of factors which are relevant to neurological rehabilitation. A lesion of the nervous system can alter the parameters of one or several of the functions listed. In this section a few of the more generally applicable techniques are described. The techniques are mostly non-invasive and risk-free and the majority require little co-operation by the patient.

The list gives a good indication of the range of neurophysiological techniques and measurements at present available. It is beyond the scope of this chapter to explain how each is performed or in which cases they should be used. Rather, one would wish to encourage those proposing a course of treatment, whether physical or pharmacological, to identify and describe patients' problems in physiological terms as well as in medical and social terms. Then some objective test of the physiological process to be influenced is applied before, during and after treatment. An analogy might be the treatment of anaemia, which one would not begin without a haemoglobin measurement; in rehabilitation, however, extensive treatments are given for spasticity without any objective measure of spasticity and without any objective measure of the outcome. Only by detailed studies will rehabilitation be able to establish rational bases for treatment and show that they work.

Polyelectromyography (pEMG)

Polyelectromyography (pEMG) consists of recording many channels of EMG through surface electrodes on the arms or legs of a subject. An ink-jet EEG recording machine is almost ideal for the

Table 8.2 List of neurophysiological investigations available

Test	CNS level
Conduction velocity of muscle fibre	Muscle
Neuromuscular transmission	Motor endplate
Motor unit:	Motor unit
Firing pattern	
Force generation	
Territory	
Recruitment number	
Nerve conduction velocity	Nerve
Single-fibre conduction velocity	
Sensory nerve function	
Automatic fibre activity	
Muscle spindle activity	Motoneuron
F response	Motoneuron and ventral root
Monosynaptic reflex excitability	Spinal
Flexor reflex	Spinal
Cutaneous and other reflexes	Spinal
Autonomic bladder reflexes	Spinal
Presynaptic inhibition	Spinal
1a interneuron inhibition	Spinal
1b interneuron inhibition	Spinal
Renshaw cell inhibition	Spinal
Conduction times in central tracts	Long tracts
Brain stem − auditory pathway	Brain stem
Brain stem reflexes:	
Blink	
Pinna	
Stapedius	
Respiratory centre − CO_2 response	Brain stem
Long-loop reflexes	Rostrocaudal tracts
Sensory evoked responses	Sensory pathways
EEG	Cortex
Motor potentials	Cortex
Magnetic stimulation	Corticospinal tract

purpose, but pen recorders can also be used. The EMG is a high-frequency signal and much of the artefact produced by movement is of low frequency and can be reduced by adjustment of the amplifier bandwidth characteristics. Bipolar recordings from disc electrodes stuck 20−40 mm apart over the muscles are used, and low-noise cable, together with arrangements to prevent lead sway and friction, help to cut down movement artefact. We follow a similar convention to that used in EEG; the first channels at the top of the paper record from the most proximal muscles on the right side and the last channels will therefore record the most distal muscles on the left.

A standard recording protocol is used, but the physician and an experienced technician will add to it according to their findings and the idiosyncrasies of the subject. It is essential to record from normal subjects in order to learn the normal responses and to recognize artefacts and 'crosstalk' from muscles deep to the one immediately beneath the electrodes. An outline of a protocol is given in Fig. 8.1. Each procedure is repeated three times to get an estimate of habituation. In the course of 1 hour a very detailed and semiquantitative estimate of spasticity and the response of motoneuron pools to various centripetal and centrifugal influences can be determined and recorded for comparison with later pEMGs. The initial recording can assist in planning therapy and subsequent ones help to determine if treatment has been effective. Of course, techniques can be refined with quantitative forms of stimulation, i.e. constant-force tendon hammers, goniometers and devices for moving joints at constant rates, and the resultant EMG can be quantified by signal analysis, such as integration. pEMG can be used as an adjunct to drug trials in spasticity and in trials of physiotherapeutic regimes, but, more fundamentally, it can be used just to observe the natural history of conditions, as Twitchell (1951) did for hemiplegia.

It has been mainly the use of pEMG in patients with spinal cord trauma that has led to the demonstration by Dimitrijevic *et al.* (1977) that many patients with clinically complete spinal cord lesions do, in fact, have some preserved descending pathways which can influence motor unit and reflex activity caudal to the lesion. It is rare for a spinal cord to be severed completely; there is usually some tissue bridge across the region and this may contain surviving nerve tracts, possibly propriospinal or small reticulospinal fibres. The demonstration of surviving pathways is of extreme theoretical importance as it maintains the possibility of using impulses in these pathways to trigger some of the automatic functions in the distal cord. The concept of dyscomplete spinal cord lesions has now become accepted.

We have used pEMG to assess changes in motor

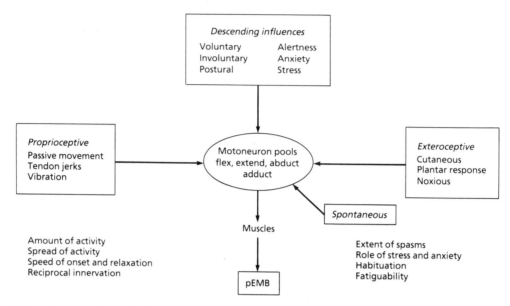

Fig. 8.1 The diagram indicates the different central and peripheral influences on the motoneuron pools of flexor, extensors etc. which can be tested during a pEMG examination for their part in the production of spasticity. The record is examined also for the features noted in smaller type.

function of patients with multiple sclerosis who were undergoing a trial of spinal cord stimulation. The technique is extremely valuable for assessing fatiguability of repetitive movements and the speed and regularity with which they can be carried out. Figure 8.2 is an example of a portion of the pEMG record of the muscles of one leg of a patient with an apparently clinically complete traumatic spinal cord lesion. All the muscles become active during a short period of breath-holding and continue active after exhalation. The second trial gives a small response, indicating some degree of habituation.

pEMG is only semiquantitative and it only re-cords 45–60 minutes of a patient's day. Other techniques are necessary to follow fluctuations in spasticity throughout the day and according to medication. Small tape recorders are available which will monitor 24 hours of electrocardiography (ECG) or EEG over one to eight channels, and these could, with minimal modification, be used to record EMG. One principle for artefact-free recording is to have the amplifier as close to the pickup electrode as possible, and pickup electrodes which are an integral part of a small first-stage amplifier are now

commercially available (Oxford Medical Systems Ltd, Oxford, England).

Interpretation is facilitated by considering a pEMG as measuring the responsiveness of moto-neuron pools to different inputs and Fig. 8.1 gives an outline of how to organize a pEMG recording and how to interpret the findings. A series of pEMG observations very pertinent to spasticity have been made by Dimitrijevic & Nathan (1967a, b, 1968, 1970, 1971). Modern computer-based signal-processing techniques now make display and quantification of recordings easier.

Inhibition in the spinal cord

Workers in animal physiology have shown very clearly the existence of three important groups of inhibitory interneurons in the spinal cord. They are: the Renshaw cell, which is excited by collaterals from motoneurons and which inhibits motoneurons of the same pool; the 1a inhibitory neuron (1aIN), which is excited by incoming volleys from muscle spindles and inhibits motoneurons of the antagonist muscle; the Golgi inhibitory neuron,

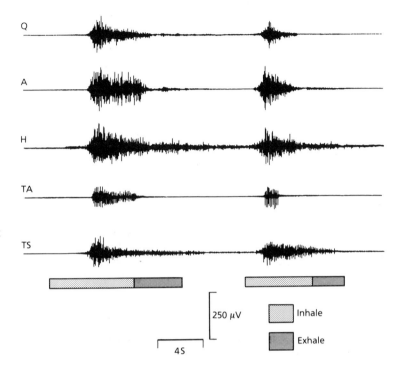

Q

A

H

TA

TS

250 μV

⬜ Inhale

⬛ Exhale

4 S

Fig. 8.2 Part of a pEMG recording of the activity in muscles of one leg of a patient with traumatic paraplegia: Q, quadriceps; A, adductors; H, hamstrings; TA, tibialis anterior; TS, triceps surae. Muscle spasm was triggered by a deep inhalation after a 3 second delay and continues after exhalation. (Kindly supplied by Professor M.R. Dimitrijevic.)

which is excited by impulses from Golgi tendon organs (tension receptors) and inhibits moto-neurons of the same muscle. These neurons are shown diagrammatically in Fig. 8.3. Their existence in a similar form in human spinal cord is assumed, and recently indirect methods of studying their functions have been devised.

Use of the size of the H reflex as a test of monosynaptic reflex excitability has permitted a study of no less than four different spinal segmental inhibitory mechanisms. The H reflex, so called after Hoffmann (1918), who first described it, is a reflex muscle twitch of soleus produced by electrical stimulation of the low-threshold muscle afferent fibres of the tibial nerve; these are large-diameter, fast-conducting class 1a fibres from muscle spindles. Electrical stimulation of the muscle nerve therefore gives a precisely controlled afferent volley which monosynaptically excites the motoneurons in the same way as a tap on the Achilles tendon. At rest, the H reflex occurs only in soleus, but it can also be obtained in arm and hand and other muscles which are actively contracting.

Under favourable conditions a single volley in the tibial nerve will excite 30–80% of the soleus motoneurons activated. Two closely spaced volleys, say up to 10 ms apart, will temporally summate to produce a larger response. With more widely spaced volleys the second shock fails to elicit a response until the shocks are 50 ms or so apart, when a complex 'recovery' cycle begins and goes on for up to 3–5 s. This recovery cycle has been extensively studied and is of different forms in hemiplegic spasticity, extrapyramidal disorders and cerebellar disease (Matthews, 1970). Interesting though these findings are, they have led to no significant insight into the pathophysiology of these neurological syndromes. The real interest in the H reflex now lies in its use in studying spinal segmental mechanisms. The segmental mechanisms to be mentioned here are shown diagrammatically in Fig. 8.3.

An interesting series of experiments by Tanaka and colleagues (Mizuno et al., 1971; Tanaka, 1972, 1974; Simoyama & Tanaka, 1974; Yanagisawa et al., 1976) used the size of the H reflex of soleus after stimulation of the tibial nerve as an indication of monosynaptic excitability of soleus moto-

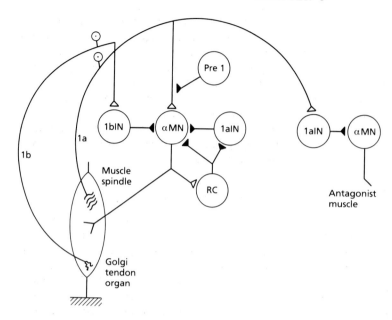

Fig. 8.3 Spinal segmental inhibitory mechanisms. The alpha motoneuron (α MN) is excited by 1a afferent fibres from muscle spindles of its own muscle which also inhibit the α MN of the antagonist muscle by activating the 1a inhibitory interneuron (1a IN). The Golgi tendon organs inhibit their own MN by way of the 1b interneuron (1b IN) and there is recurrent inhibition by the Renshaw cell (RC). The presynaptic inhibitory interneurons (Pre I) have not been anatomically or physiologically identified.

neurons. A preceding stimulus to the peroneal nerve, which supplies tibialis anterior, an antagonist of soleus, should, they argue, excite the 1aIN, which projects on to soleus motoneurons and the soleus H reflex should therefore be reduced in size. By careful timing of the conditioning stimulus to the peroneal nerve and by adjustment of the stimulus strength so that it gave a maximal 1a volley and minimally excited other fibres, they were able to explore the nature of inhibition mediated by the 1aIN. It is thought that the process of reciprocal innervation (relaxation of the antagonist muscle while the agonist contracts) is mediated by the 1aIN and, as reciprocal innervation fails in spasticity, study of its mechanism is of great interest in clinical neurophysiology.

The studies show that, at rest, a single peroneal nerve volley fails to activate the 1aIN as the soleus H reflex remains unchanged. If, however, a small voluntary contraction of tibialis anterior is made, the 1aIN receives excitatory synaptic bombardment from two sources. First, there is an excitatory input from the corticospinal tract and possibly from other descending motor pathways (Janowska & Tanaka, 1974); the second excitatory input is from the muscle spindle afferents which are excited by contraction of the muscle (tibialis anterior in this case). Under these conditions an additional electrically

induced volley in the peroneal nerve produces an inhibition of the soleus H reflex of about 30%.

Studies on neurological patients are incomplete and await confirmation, but the following pattern of 1aIN activity has emerged. In athetosis the 1aIN is active even at rest, while in spastic hemiplegia there is some evidence that the activity of the 1aIN is unbalanced. It seems that the 1aIN can be activated by the extensor muscle to inhibit the dorsiflexor but not by the flexor to inhibit the extensor; the normal reciprocal innervation is therefore disrupted. This could be one factor underlying the weakness of ankle dorsiflexors seen in hemiplegia.

Further alteration of the timing and strength of the conditioning stimulus to the peroneal nerve reveals another period of inhibition of the H reflex, lasting from 7 to 30 ms after arrival of the peroneal nerve volley. Tanaka (1972, 1974) suggests that this is presynaptic inhibition because it has characteristics similar to presynaptic inhibition seen in animals. He and El-Tohamy & Sedgwick, (1983) have demonstrated motoneuron inhibition in man similar in time course to presynaptic inhibition by using an experimental protocol equivalent to that used in animals. There is evidence that this inhibition is still present in spinal shock and spasticity due to spinal cord injury but is altered in hemiplegic spasticity (El-Tohamy & Sedgwick, 1983; Benfield *et al.*, 1988; Sedgwick *et al.*, 1992).

A third inhibitory system, that from the Golgi tendon organs on the homologous and synergist muscles, has been studied in normal subjects by Pierrot-Deseilligny *et al.* (1979), again using the H reflex as a test of motoneuron excitability. It is not yet known whether this type of inhibition is altered by upper motoneuron lesions.

Finally there is the recurrent inhibition provided by the Renshaw neurons – so called after the man who, on the basis of physiological experiment, postulated their existence. These neurons are excited by discharges of motoneurons and feedback inhibition into the homologous motoneuron pool. Their precise role and even the extent of distribution of their axons are unknown. Control engineers have been quick to point out, however, that they appear to form part of a negative feedback loop which would regulate and stabilize the firing of the motoneurons, perhaps matching the rate of firing to the physical properties of the muscle and smoothing recruitment of motoneurons to make for evenly regulated muscle tension. Bussel & Pierrot-Deseilligny (1977) and Hultborn & Pierrot-Deseilligny (1979) have demonstrated presumed Renshaw neuron inhibition in normal man, but no studies of disease states are yet available.

There are, then, four spinal segmental inhibitory mechanisms which can be studied non-invasively in man: the IaIN, presynaptic inhibition, Golgi tendon organ inhibition and Renshaw inhibition. We teach students that spasticity is caused by a release of motoneurons from inhibitions; now there is an opportunity to demonstrate whether these four types of inhibition are the ones from which the motoneuron is released. If they are involved, as seems likely, in movement disorders and if their neurotransmitter mechanisms can be elucidated by animal experiments, then a sensible pharmacological strategy for the treatment of spasticity could be evolved, tried and monitored objectively.

Which neurophysiology?

Scientific neurophysiology is a notoriously difficult field for the non-specialist. The literature is a bewildering collection of technical terms borrowed from control engineering, chemistry and physics, with added abbreviations conspiring to make papers read like a foreign language. In this section some of the recent advances in neurophysiology are briefly reviewed. These topics have been selected for their potential importance to rehabilitation of the neurological patient. Nearly all the experimental work was done on animals, so that interspecies assumptions have to be made; nevertheless, a small but highly significant proportion of the work derives from human studies.

Plasticity of somatotopic maps

Neuroanatomical teaching implies that the somatotopic representation in the sensory cortex is 'hardwired', that is, one skin area projects to one cortical area. Indeed, the somatotopic organization has been explored in detail in primates and other animals. Mapping experiments performed after deafferentation have shown that new functional connections are formed (Wall & Egger, 1971). The extent of the plasticity of the sensory and motor maps has been reviewed by Kaas (1991). Most work has been done after peripheral nerve injury so that complications due to lesions within the CNS are avoided.

After a nerve lesion on digit amputation, the cortical area normally responding to that area very quickly – within the space of a few hours – begins to respond to stimulation of neighbouring areas. In the case of nerve crush, the area re-establishes its normal responsiveness once the peripheral axons have reinnervated the skin. The initial changes are so rapid that the change is thought to be due to unmasking of already present but non-functional synapses: an unmasking of pre-existing connections. Subsequent changes in the nature of responsiveness of the 'denervated' cortex may be due to axonal sprouting but evidence is so far lacking.

To date, no precise behavioural or perceptual changes can be attributed to this plasticity. An interesting experiment in man was to employ microstimulation of a nerve fascicle from a previously amputated finger. The subjects perceived sensations in their phantom fingers of the same quality and intensity as those perceived from 'real' fingers (Schady & Braune, 1993). Again, no convincing evidence has shown increased sensitivity in the areas near to amputations.

The importance of these experiments has been to

demonstrate a degree of plasticity in adult animals in a projection system whose gross anatomy is genetically programmed. If we can begin to understand the process of plastic change we may be able to influence it for the benefit of patients. The process can be studied in humans by evoked-potential methodology. Similarly, motor maps may be studied by magnetic stimulation.

Trophic factors

The close relationship between nerve and muscle is dramatically illustrated by the effects of denervation. The immediate result is paralysis as impulses no longer reach the muscle. The sarcolemma of muscle fibres begins to change immediately after denervation, and alteration in ionic permeability and sodium pump activity soon result in a lowered resting membrane potential. From the region of the endplate, acetylcholine (ACh) receptors spread along the fibre. The endplate itself becomes unstable and spontaneously generated action potentials – fibrillation potentials – appear. The fibres lose contractile protein and a large number of histological atrophic changes begin, culminating in replacement of muscle bulk by fibrous tissue, but small atrophic muscle fibres survive for many years. Subsequent contraction of the fibrous tissue results in contractures. If the denervation is partial, the remaining nerves will sprout collaterals, which will innervate neighbouring denervated fibres.

To what extent are the atrophic changes attributable to disuse of the muscle and which, if any, can be attributed to the absence of a trophic substance? If there is a trophic substance, is it ACh or some other chemical? Disuse of a muscle results in wasting, which is mainly loss of contractile protein, and this well-known clinical phenomenon is reversible. Other changes, such as fibrillation potentials and sprouting of innervating nerves, do not occur in disuse atrophy, but these changes are not prevented by direct electrical stimulation of denervated muscle. These long-established facts lead to the idea that nerve has a trophic or sustaining effect on muscle. Could this effect be simply the liberation of ACh at the endplate? Liberation continues even during disuse as there is always some leakage of ACh from the endplate even in the absence of impulses which evoke miniature endplate poten-

tials. If not ACh, could there be a specific trophic substance, or group of substances, liberated at the same time as ACh or perhaps leaking out continually? It is well established that axonal transport carries a considerable quantity of material down the axon. Much of this is protein and enzymes as these can only be manufactured in the perikaryon. Amino acids, prostaglandins and protein are known to leak out of the nerve at the motor endplate.

The cross-reinnervation experiments beginning with those of Buller et al. (1960) boosted interest in trophic substances. They showed that a nerve taken from a fast-twitch muscle (e.g. flexor digitorum longus of the cat) would innervate a previously denervated slow-twitch muscle (soleus) and convert it into a fast-twitch muscle. The speed of muscle contraction depends on two factors, the speed of liberation and uptake of Ca^{2+} by sarcoplasmic reticulum and the rate of a reaction controlled by a calcium-dependent enzyme, myosin adenosine triphosphatase, which is involved in the formation of cross-bridges between actin and myosin. The cross-reinnervated muscles showed appropriate biochemical changes in their myosin adenosine triphosphatase and in the speed of movement of Ca^{2+} as well as other changes.

Slow muscles serve postural functions and tend to be excited by long steady trains of impulses at 10 Hz or so, while fast muscles are only activated occasionally by fast short bursts of impulses (20–60 Hz). It has been shown that the speed of twitch of muscle can be altered by imposing upon it a particular firing pattern; this can be done experimentally by implanted stimulators. The trophic influence in this case seems to be a pattern of excitation and not a trophic substance (Buller & Pope, 1977).

Another aspect of trophic function which has come under close scrutiny in recent years is the production and distribution of ACh receptors on muscle fibres. Normally these are present in a high concentration only at the motor endplate. Shortly after denervation, an increase in synthesis of these protein receptors has been observed in the muscle fibre. The receptors are transported to, and incorporated in, clusters or hot spots along the whole of the length of the muscle fibre membrane. Here they survive for 6–36 hours before being destroyed by the usual lysosomal mechanisms but they are replaced by continuing synthesis. Denervation therefore stimulates genetically controlled protein synthesis.

Direct electrical excitation of muscle early after denervation will prevent the increase in ACh receptors. The complete blocking of action potentials in the nerve by local anaesthetics or by botulinum toxin, which prevents most ACh release, results in some increase in Ach receptors. Muscle activity therefore seems to be the major regulator for production of ACh receptors and this is possibly mediated by the adenylcyclase system or by the concentration of intracellular Ca^{2+}. Changeux (1991) has argued that the liberation of ACh at the endplate results in gene activation of those genes in nearby nuclei which are responsible for synthesis of ACh receptors.

Acetylcholinesterase (AChE), normally associated with ACh receptors at the motor endplate, does not appear at the newly formed ACh receptor hot spots unless the hot spot becomes innervated by a regenerating nerve. Reinnervation is independent of nerve or muscle activity but cannot occur in the absence of ACh receptor hot spots. When the muscle fibre is reactivated, ACh receptor synthesis is turned off and receptors concentrate and stabilize at the new endplate. The fibre begins synthesis of AChE, which also concentrates at the endplate.

Despite 30 years of vigorous investigation, no trophic substance has been discovered, but the importance of muscle activity has been emphasized and Drachman (1974) points out that, in the absence of ACh, any other trophic substance that may be released from a nerve is incapable of preventing degenerative change. Detailed molecular mechanisms such as these may seem remote from rehabilitation, but an understanding of the processes of disuse and denervation degeneration are fundamental to rehabilitation.

The motor unit

The concept of the motor unit as a functional and anatomical entity has been established for many years. The recruitment of more and more motor units into activity to give greater muscle tension is well known and the size principle of Henneman is now widely accepted. This principle, arising first from animal experiments (Henneman *et al.*, 1965), is that, during graded muscular activity, units producing small tensions are recruited first and those producing large tensions are recruited later. The organization within the CNS to produce such an orderly pattern seems quite simple. The small motor unit consists of anatomically few muscle fibres, which are innervated by a relatively small-diameter axon, which in turn arises from a small motoneuron. The membrane of motoneurons behaves electrically as a resistor and capacitor in parallel and therefore the larger the area of membrane the lower is its electrical resistance. A standard excitation will therefore produce a higher-voltage excitatory postsynaptic potential in small motoneurons than in large ones. In the large ones the excitation current flows through the low-resistance membrane and a high voltage cannot build up. The small neurons, therefore, will be the first to be depolarized to their excitation threshold. It has also been established that all the muscle fibres innervated by one motoneuron are of the same biochemical type and therefore have common mechanical properties, such as twitch speed and fatigue resistance. With such a wealth of detailed physiological and biochemical knowledge about motor units, the time is ripe to study them in man in health and disease. Fortunately, recent technical developments enable exploration of new areas in man with usually no more inconvenience than the insertion of a needle.

Axons

Axons in the CNS have been regarded by neurologists as passive transmission lines, which work normally unless physically disrupted or demyelinated. The importance of the myelin sheath for rapid transmission of impulses has long been appreciated and the way impulses jump from node to node has been well established. Recent work, however, on experimentally demyelinated fibres in animals has revealed details of the relationship of axons and their myelin which allow explanations of certain clinical phenomena seen in demyelinating disease and indicate possible avenues for the search for therapeutic strategies.

Conduction of the action potential is a sequence of depolarization and repolarization of the axon membrane. Depolarization occurs when sodium channels in the axonal membrane open and permit sodium ions to flow into the fibre. The sodium channels are lipoprotein structures, which, it is believed, can be visualized by the electron microscope after preparation of the specimen by a freeze–fracture technique. Their numbers can be estimated because they bind securely with certain toxins which can be isotope-labelled. Using these methods, it can be shown that there are about 500 times more sodium channels at nodes of Ranvier than on the internodal axon (Meiri *et al.*, 1989; Black *et al.*, 1990). It is thought that the paucity of sodium channels in a demyelinated segment would produce a small depolarization insufficient to trigger an action potential in the next part of the fibre. If demyelination is partial or the demyelinated segment very short, the action potential may be conducted across the lesion at a slowed rate. The computer models show that such fibres exist on a knife-edge between conduction and block. Conduction can be blocked by a slight rise in temperature, and it is thought that this is the basis of Uhthoff's phenomenon, seen in MS, where a patient's functional abilities decrease markedly if body temperature is raised by exercise, fever or climatic change. Reduction in Ca^{2+} can improve conduction and the clinical state of patients with MS.

It has been suggested (Schauf & Davis, 1974) that drugs which increase the time for which a sodium channel remains open, or decrease or delay the time of opening of potassium channels, would facilitate conduction of action potentials through areas of demyelination. So, too, would an increase in the number of sodium channels, and we are beginning to acquire knowledge of how these are produced, although it is very probable that the oligodendrocytes which produce CNS myelin play a role in arranging the distribution of the sodium channels to concentrate at the nodes. Attempts to manipulate ion channels in multiple sclerosis have shown changes in patients' functional states but they have not proved beneficial (Stefaski *et al.*, 1987; Kaji *et al.*, 1990).

The altered function of demyelinated fibres underlies the use of evoked potentials in clinical diagnosis of multiple sclerosis. The visual evoked potential can be delayed in this condition, thereby revealing a previously unsuspected lesion of the optic nerve; the demonstration of multiple lesions is fundamental to the diagnosis of multiple sclerosis. Few workers have yet studied the evolution of evoked potentials during the course of multiple sclerosis (Robinson & Rudge, 1978; Matthews & Small, 1979; Sedgwick *et al.*, 1980), but this is a simple procedure which could give valuable information about the state of the axons operating on a knife-edge. Such studies would be mandatory if an attempt were made to rehabilitate patients by modifying the sodium channels in their axons.

Muscle spindles

Since the discovery of the role of these end organs in the stretch reflex, they have been central to any consideration of spasticity, movement disorder or tremor. It is here that human studies have added so much to our understanding of muscle tone.

At rest the muscle spindle is not stretched and sends no impulses to the spinal cord. During contraction, however, the spindle shortens at the same rate as the muscle, due to discharges in its own motor fibres (γ fibres), and sends a moderate barrage of impulses into the spinal cord, where they contribute to the excitation of the motoneuron (α motoneuron). At the beginning of contraction both the α and γ motoneurons are excited simultaneously, called αγ co-activation.

In any arresting disturbance of a planned movement, the muscle spindle continues to attempt to shorten by stretching its elastic central region, where the afferent fibre terminates; an increased barrage of afferent impulses is therefore induced and, on reaching the cord, will increase the activity of the α motoneurons, thereby increasing the force of contraction and tending to overcome the arresting force. This mode of action is called the load compensation reflex, because it provides the first immediate (30 ms or less) response to a disturbance (Phillips & Porter, 1977).

Because, in spasticity, the muscles are so sensitive to slight manipulation, it has been proposed that the γ motoneurons are overactive, thereby enhancing the afferent discharge of the muscle spindles. The limited experimental data so far available show that the γ motor system of spastic subjects at rest is not overactive (Vallbo *et al.*, 1979).

Muscle spindle function has been so central to physiological thought that it has come as a surprise to learn of a man who has lost all proprioception and yet can function well. J.D. Cole (1991) describes vividly the trials and triumphs of a man who lost all touch and proprioception, but not other modalities, up to the neck as a result of a postinfective neuropathy. This book illustrates very well how neurophysiology and rehabilitation can interact.

Walking

Recent neurophysiological work on the coordinated act of walking or stepping has induced a move away from the old idea of successive reflexes coming into action, the 'chain reflex' hypothesis, and forced a re-examination of a much older idea called the 'reciprocal half-centre hypothesis', which was first proposed in 1914. This latter hypothesis has been refined and modelled by Miller & Scott (1977) and their half-centre or stepping generator is a simpler and more testable proposal than the 'ring' hypothesis set forth by Shik & Orlovsky (1976). The importance of recent work on stepping lies in the clear demonstration that the neurons of the spinal cord can act as generators of stepping movements within a limb and also, by propriospinal pathways, stepping generators of each limb can be co-ordinated to produce gait. Even spinal animals can produce co-ordinated stepping activity in certain circumstances (Shik & Orlovsky, 1976). All the experimental work has been on cats and it remains to be shown that a similar organization is present in primates and, indeed, in man.

The simplest effective model of a stepping generator is that proposed by Miller & Scott (1977), which involves just three types of neuron for each muscle group. The α motoneuron, the 1aIN and the Renshaw cell make up a 'half-centre' and are known to be anatomically connected in the manner shown in Fig. 8.4. The 1aIN and Renshaw cell both send projections to the antagonist half-centre and both half-centres receive simultaneous tonic excitation, which raises the extensor 1aIN to firing point. This will inhibit the flexor α motoneuron and the flexor 1aIN, which results in disinhibition

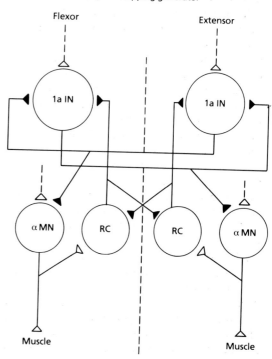

Fig. 8.4 The smallest assembly of neurons necessary to generate stepping movements according to Miller & Scott. For a functional description see text.

of the extensor motoneuron. The extensor motoneuron fires, producing limb extension, and the impulses are fed back on to the Renshaw cell, which is excited. The connections of the Renshaw cell, which are inhibitory, are to the 1aIN of the extensor centre and to the Renshaw cell of the flexor group. The Renshaw cell activity reduces or turns off the extensor 1aIN and thereby disinhibits the flexor 1aIN, which is now able to become active and permit the flexor half of the cycle to begin. This very simple model can explain alternating flexion and extension of a limb. The necessary anatomical connections are known to exist and the neurons involved are known to be inhibitory, except for the α motoneuron. Two, four or more generators can be modelled by computer and coupled together, when they show co-ordinated activity between the generators within a limb or between limbs.

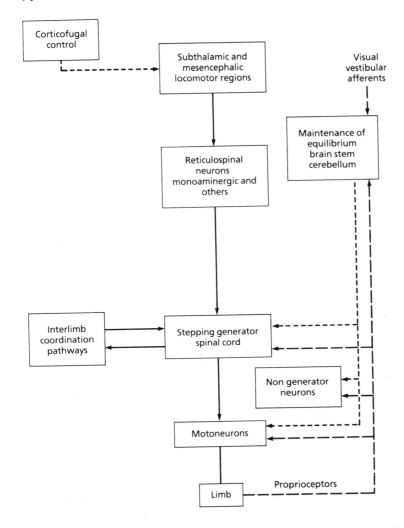

Fig. 8.5 Diagram of the organization of the locomotor system as revealed by experiments on stepping in cats.

Previously afferent input was regarded as essential for stepping, but this is not so; hence there was no need to include the gamma system or skin and joint sensors in the model. This must not be taken to imply that afferents play no part; rather, they provide for maintenance of posture by modulating muscle force so that the body is carried smoothly even over rough ground.

Supraspinal control of the stepping generators appears to involve fine reticulospinal fibres, some of which release noradrenaline, some 5-hydroxytryptamine and some other unspecified transmitters. The reticulospinal neurons are activated by a midbrain locomotor area, which seems co-terminous with the nucleus cuneiformis in the cat. Electrical stimulation of this region of a cat after removal of its forebrain (a mesencephalic animal) will produce co-ordinated stepping activity. A subthalamic locomotor region has also been described (Fig. 8.5).

This work on mesencephalic cats has emphasized the importance of the spinal stepping generator and the slow-conducting reticulospinal systems. The role of the traditional motor pathways, corticospinal, vestibulospinal, cerebellum, etc., has been relegated to subsidiary modulation. These fast-conducting pathways are active during walking, but the effect of their impulses is dependent on the state or setting of the spinal locomotor generator. The afferent pathways have also been relegated, as has the gamma motor system. Future work will examine the relationships between the different systems during walking and no doubt will investigate to what extent the walking mechanisms of primates, including man, are similar to those of quadrupeds and also to what extent to organization of a stepping centre can survive upper motoneuron lesions.

There have been many studies of gait in man; forces, speeds, accelerations and numerous other mechanical parameters have been measured accurately by sophisticated computerized systems and this is of great value in orthopaedic specialities. Observation of the step-by-step data shows that no two steps are exactly alike. Each step depends to some extent upon the previous one, two or more steps. This is an example of how self-correcting mechanisms allow balance to be maintained on uneven ground. An attempt by Knutsson & Richards (1979) to classify gait disorders in hemiplegia deserves mention. They found three types of abnormality:

1 premature activation of calf muscles in the stance phase;

2 cases where two or more muscles were relatively more paralysed than others;

3 those in which inappropriate co-contraction of several or all muscle groups in the leg occurred.

It was necessary to have a fourth group to accommodate unclassifiable varieties of gait disorder.

Group 1 is interesting; it includes the common problem of foot drop due to upper motoneuron lesions. These patients could be fruitfully studied in the light of the work of Yanagisawa et al. (1976), who indicated that the 1aIN from the flexor (tibialis anterior) to the extensor (gastrocnemius−soleus) is inactive in hemiplegia. If one set of neurons can be identified as responsible for a particular type of deficit, then the challenge to rehabilitation is to find a means of facilitating the action of those neurons by drugs, by training, by electrical stimulation or by any other means.

Movement

In recent years it has been possible to study movement with more accuracy than previously and the findings have been interpreted using ideas and concepts borrowed from control engineering. Germinal to most modern work were the papers by Hammond et al. (1956), who proposed that muscle spindles operated as a feedback device for a follow-up length servo system. Earlier pioneers analysed movement in some detail and photographed and described locomotion accurately; Holmes (1922) carefully analysed the defects of movement following cerebellar lesions; the work of Bernstein (1966) deserves to be better known in the West.

Corticospinal tract

Generations of students have been confused by the use of the word 'pyramidal' as an adjective for a type of neuron, a tract and a set of clinical manifestations of a cerebral lesion. The clinical terms pyramidal lesion, pyramidal hemiplegia, pyramidal syndrome, upper motoneuron lesion of pyramidal type and pyramidal pattern of weakness are so well entrenched that it will be years before alternative terms are introduced. There seems to be no reason to continue to refer to the corticospinal tract as pyramidal as it leads to the assumption that a lesion of it will produce a pyramidal syndrome.

Magnetic stimulation

One of the exciting recent advances in neurophysiology has been the development of magnetic stimulation of the brain, the corticospinal tract in particular, and deep peripheral nerves and spinal roots (Barker et al., 1985, 1987). The principle is simple; a large capacitor is made to discharge a brief very high current (1000 amp) through a low-impedance insulated coil held over the head. The sudden change in magnetic flux induces a current in the secondary conductor, in this case the brain, which is sufficient to stimulate the corticospinal tract axons. A muscle twitch in the hand or leg follows.

Magnetic stimulation is proving safe. It does not trigger fits in non-epileptics and no important untoward effects have been reported. Muscle, as well as nerve, beneath the coil is stimulated so one would need to be circumspect about using it in the vicinity of unstable spinal vertebrae. The force generated by a single twitch of the paraspinal muscles is mainly dissipated in the viscous and elastic components of the muscle. Crush fractures are not thought likely and none have been reported.

Delays in conduction have been shown in myelopathies of numerous aetiologies (Sedgwick, 1988). Development of a delay appears to follow closely the development of the clinical upper motor neuron syndrome and the extensor plantar response in particular. There have been instances where a delay has given evidence for a clinically unsuspected lesion in multiple sclerosis and it is common to find a delay to a muscle which is clinically strong. With increasing delay and severity of lesion, the amplitude of the response decreases and is eventually lost. In most spinal injury patients, the response is absent below the lesion.

Interest has focused on apparent reorganization of the corticospinal pathway after cord injury (Levy *et al.*, 1990; Topka *et al.*, 1991). Careful placement of and searching by the stimulating coil over the scalp enable definition of an excitability map showing areas from which a set of muscles can be excited by stimuli of different strengths. A comparison of the excitability maps for muscles just proximal to a cord lesion appears to show enhanced excitability compared with normal. Just how to interpret these findings is not at all clear, and the time over which they develop is not known. Whether it is some change in the motor cortex or an expression of the Schiff–Sherrington phenomenon, operating at the spinal cord level, has yet to be determined. Any explanation would need to take into account the now extensive knowledge of the corticomotoneuronal projections, recently reviewed by Lemon (1990).

In order to estimate the corticomotoneuronal conduction time, it is necessary to measure the latency from cortex to muscle and subtract from it the latency from motoneuron to muscle. The latter measure may be made by placing the coil over the spinal column, where the stimulus excites the motor fibres in the region of the intervertebral foramen (Conway *et al.*, 1988; Ungawa *et al.*, 1989; Cross *et al.*, 1990; Evans *et al.*, 1990; Schmid *et al.*, 1990). Subtraction of the latencies from one another gives the 'central' conduction time for the impulses to travel from the brain to motor neuron to motor root.

Fries *et al.* (1991) recorded muscle twitches in patients following stroke where pyramidal tracts (in the internal capsule) had undergone Wallerian degeneration. The implication was that corticoreticulospinal pathways carried the volley. As the patients all made good functional recoveries, it is possible that the Wallerian degeneration inferred from magnetic resonance imaging (MRI) scans was not the true pathology. Experience with stroke patients shows that a muscle twitch may still be obtainable even during the acute phase of paralysis. If a muscle twitch is present during the first 72 hours, one can expect a reasonable degree of recovery. Patients with no motor twitch recover poorly. After the initial 3 days, the twitch response declines and may become absent for the next 14 days or so.

It will be of considerable interest to determine the conduction across spinal injuries, by whatever tracts. Unfortunately, the poor conductivity of bone means that the spinal cord cannot be stimulated directly, but it may be possible to do so in patients who have had a laminectomy.

If stimulation of the spinal cord directly is critical for testing a hypothesis, one could use cutaneous electrical stimulation or percutaneous electrical stimulation through an electrode placed in the epidural space. These techniques are uncomfortable and the second is invasive.

Anatomy of movement

Voluntary movements can be divided into two main types, which are quite different in their organization. These are the ramp movement and the ballistic movement. Ramp movements are slow and sustained and are under visual and proprioceptive feedback control, which regulates the force developed to minimize external disturbances and to maximize accuracy. Ballistic movements are rapidly executed and there is no time for feedback control; the movement is planned as a whole in the CNS, where local conditions, e.g. posture and ongoing movement, are taken into account with experience and the whole motor command is given with precise timing. If the outcome is inappropriate, nothing can be done to correct it. An incorrect ballistic movement is experienced when one quickly picks up a suitcase which was thought to be heavy and is not.

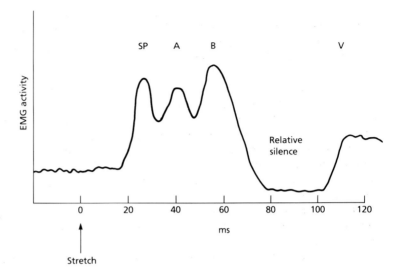

Fig. 8.6 Diagram compiled from the work of Marsden showing increased EMG activity after sudden unexpected muscle stretch during a tracking task. SP, spinal stretch reflex; A, probable transcortical reflex; B, a 'long-loop' reflex of uncertain origin; V, a voluntary contraction to overcome the stretch.

Ramp movements

Ramp movements have been profitably studied by a very ingenious method by Marsden *et al.* (1972, 1973). The subject's thumb was attached to a frame which allowed measurement of angle of the interphalangeal joint and force of flexion. A motor, attached to the frame, provided a resistance to movement and could produce a sudden increase or release of resistance. The subject was required to track a target on an oscilloscope by flexing his thumb slowly while the EMG activity of flexor pollicis longus was recorded.

The findings of this type of experiment are summarized in Fig. 8.6. When the ramp movement is disturbed by a sudden stretch, four phases of muscle response can be identified. The first, labelled SP, has a short latency of 23 ms and is the spinal segmental stretch reflex equivalent to a tendon jerk. Next are two peaks of EMG activity at 40 and 55 ms, labelled A and B respectively. These are reflex events because they cannot be voluntarily suppressed and their size depends upon the magnitude and velocity of the displacement. There is then a short period of relative silence of EMG followed by a final EMG burst, labelled V. This burst is under voluntary control and its size depends upon prior instruction to the subject, i.e. the 'set of the motor system'. When told to resist stretch as vigorously as possible, V was large; when told to let

go as soon as stretch occurred, V was absent. At its earliest, the latency of V was about 80 ms. The second response to stretch at 40 ms, A, could be a transcortical stretch reflex. This hypothesis was proposed by Marsden *et al.* (1973) and is supported by a large body of circumstantial evidence. The latency time is appropriate; it is known that muscle spindles project to the cortex and can almost certainly excite pyramidal tract neurons in primates; lesions in the dorsal columns, sensory or motor cortex or internal capsule all abolish this response.

These precisely measured responses to muscle stretch are beginning to be made in patients with CNS disease. As mentioned above, the 'A' response is abolished by lesions of the dorsal column, cortex and cerebrospinal tract, but Lee & Tatton (1978) describe a case where the response recovered after a surgical lesion of cortex. In extrapyramidal disease the findings are equivocal and publication of further work is awaited. In cerebellar disorders, where there is no pyramidal disturbance, the 'A' response occurs, but its latency is prolonged, whereas the initial 'SP' response is normal. These interesting experimental findings are still at an early stage, but it is clear that such precise measurements of the behaviour of the motor system will be relevant to rehabilitation, where an accurate assessment of a disability is required and an equally accurate assessment of whether time and therapy can restore normal responses.

Ballistic movements

When a ballistic movement is executed, the first event is a relaxation of the antagonist muscle if that is active. The agonist muscle gives a short burst of activity, followed by a silent period and then a second burst. During the silent interval of the agonist, there is a short burst of activity in the antagonist (Fig. 8.7). The initial agonist burst of activity is of short and invariable duration; accuracy of movement is provided by variation in the amplitude rather than duration of muscle activity. The antagonist burst is important for arresting the movement but is not of variable amplitude. The final part of the movement is a second burst of activity in the agonist of variable size; this burst is probably feedback-controlled and corrects any misalignment remaining after the initial burst. The timing of the bursts seems to be preprogrammed,

and their amplitude depends on experience and the expected force required.

Peripheral conditions must be taken into account in programming a ballistic burst, but some experiments suggest that the transcortical stretch response does not operate for a time after the initial burst of activity in the agonist muscle, but a stretch occurring just before the movement results in a higher-amplitude initial EMG burst. The brain updates the ballistic movement programme with respect to peripheral conditions, but just before movement the updating ceases and the programme is put into effect. The onset and timing of the bursts of activity during ballistic movement are severely disturbed by cerebellar disease. The initial contraction of the agonist is delayed and sometimes occurs before appropriate inhibition of the antagonist. The durations of the agonist and antagonist bursts are prolonged. With these disturbances one can see how many of the clinical manifestations of abnormal movement of cerebellar disease can be explained.

These novel ways of examining willed movement have supported a model of motor control first proposed by Kornhuber (1971, 1974). The model proposes that there are generators in the brain for ramp and ballistic movements. The motor area simply executes the movement planned by the generators. Kornhuber identifies the posterior association cortex of the parietal lobe as the assessor of the movement required, e.g. 'the hand should not be too close to the table top or it will knock over the glass'. Lesions here produce loss of skill or apraxias. Ramp generation is thought to be a role of the basal ganglia and this is supported by the clinical picture of parkinsonism; akinesia is the absence of ramps and athetosis is continuous uncontrolled ramps. Ballistic movements are organized by the cerebellum, and cerebellar failure results in dysmetria, which can be interpreted as a disturbance of ballistic movement.

The novel feature of this model is that the basal ganglia and cerebellum are involved in the planning of a movement and are 'upstream' of the motor cortex. This role does not obviate their traditional role in responding to changing circumstances during a movement. These structures therefore become the repository of learned and skilled movement. The model may seem to be a remote con-

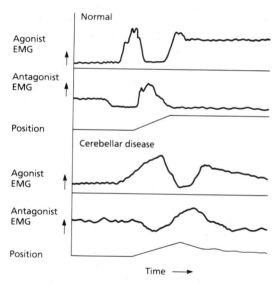

Fig. 8.7 The diagram shows the main features of an EMG recorded during a ballistic movement. In normal subjects, the antagonist muscle relaxes prior to agonist contraction. Movement follows a short burst of agonist activity and is arrested by a burst of the antagonist. Both muscles then become active to hold the new position. In cerebellar disease the events are much slower and the antagonist relaxation may not occur until the agonist is contracting. The level of contraction is not always appropriate for the task and the final position is not held.

ceptual affair of little relevance to the rehabilitation clinic. It is too recent a development to have had any impact on physical therapy techniques, but it is an important model for anyone intending to study the control of movement, whether in the disabled or in the dancer or sportsman who wishes to achieve ultimate perfection in muscle control.

An ingenious method for studying the electrical events in the brain preceding a motor act has revealed a set of potentials which are generated by the motor system. The technique is similar to averaging evoked potentials, but the trigger for averaging is the onset of a prescribed movement and the electrical events preceding the movement are averaged – a process called opisthochronic averaging.

The potentials associated with movement have been identified as: the bereitschaftspotential (BP) or readiness potential, the pre-motion potential (PMP) and the motor potential (MP). The first, BP, is a slowly developing surface negativity beginning 800 ms before a rapid finger movement or as long as 1300 ms before a ramp movement. It reaches 7 µV in amplitude over the anterior parietal area and is bilateral even when only one finger is to be moved, but it eventually becomes higher in amplitude over the hemisphere contralateral to the moving side. The BP also precedes saccadic eye movements and speech as well as brisk finger movement. The PMP is not easily detected as it is less than 2 µV in amplitude and cannot be seen in all subjects. It appears bilaterally, is spread widely over the scalp and begins 90 ms before the movement. The MP is also a small potential of less than 2 µV, beginning 60 ms before movement and located rather precisely over the contralateral motor cortex. It is believed to correspond to discharges of neurons in the motor cortex.

It is of some interest that BP and MP occur over those areas of cortex and in the order predicted by the Kornhuber model. It has also been reported that the BP is reduced over the affected hemisphere in unilateral parkinsonism with a lesser reduction over the unaffected hemisphere when the normal hand is moved. Both the MP and PMP were reduced when moving the affected side.

Higher nervous function

It is in the area of higher mental function that advances in rehabilitation are most hoped for and yet least likely to be achieved. Experimental physiologists have elaborated an operational policy or belief which may appear sterile and unduly mechanistic to many rehabilitationists. It is based on the idea of psychoneuronal identity, which is that the total neural events within the brain are, of themselves, the items we call sensation, perception, consciousness and behaviour. Mind, consciousness and their contents are physicochemical neural events occurring in reactive structures (brain) and cannot be separated from the material of the nervous system. The neural events obey physical laws and are not subject to interference from gods, ghosts or free will.

Behaviour is based on the perceived environment and not on the real environment. Mountcastle (1975, 1978) forcibly explains how our image of the world depends upon a set of imperfect sensory maps drawn with the ink of action potentials on the sensory cortices. Abstractions and interferences from these maps give a perception of the environment on which behaviour is based. Work on the visual cortex has shown how groups of neurons respond to particular abstractions of a stimulus: edge, orientation, corner, direction of movement, colour, etc. Mountcastle has begun to identify the abstractions represented by activity in neurons of the parietal cortex and has been able to indicate the positive features of neural activity which correspond reasonably well with the negative symptoms of the parietal lobe syndrome of spatial inattention, seen not uncommonly after strokes.

If a behaviour pattern is identified as depending upon certain features in the environment and if the neurons which normally abstract that feature of the environment from the sensory map are damaged, then that particular behaviour pattern will never follow, regardless of the state of drive or need of the individual. The organism may develop alternative strategies and thereby achieve the same ends on some occasions, but the total behaviour pattern will be degraded to a greater or lesser extent.

One of the first questions to which a rehabilitation neurologist requires an answer is whether, given destruction of one group of abstracting neurons, another group of neurons may take on that function as a result of learning, training, drugs, insight into the problem or any other means. If, then, a group of neurons can take on a new function, what happens to their previous function? Neurophysiologists are beginning to provide some insight into these problems; it seems that the CNS is more plastic than once thought.

There are large areas of neurological rehabilitation where necessity demands attention but where the neurophysiologist can offer little or no help. Perhaps the most pressing area is that of aphasia, where the only advance since Broca and Wernicke has been the demonstration of an anatomical asymmetry of the hemispheres. Psychological and linguistic studies have proceeded apace, but perhaps it has been the lack of an animal model which has retarded the study of the brain in relation to speech. Evoked-potential and EEG techniques are being applied to the subject, but there are serious methodological problems to be overcome (Wanner *et al.*, 1977).

Whither neurophysiology?

The answer to the question of whether to involve neurophysiologists in neurological rehabilitation is a self-evident affirmative. The prospect of attempting to advance rehabilitation without neurophysiology is gloomy indeed. There are certain areas in which rehabilitationists could actively involve neurophysiologists and vice versa. First there is the problem of monitoring long-term changes to establish in greater detail the natural history of diseases and the effects of treatment. Neurophysiological parameters are largely objective and many can be made numerical, while some assess very specific changes relating to only one cell group. Many techniques already devised are relatively simple to apply from the point of view of the patient and the doctor.

Very practical assistance can be rendered to those using forms of electrical stimulation for treatment. Biocalibration of stimulators and the assessment and diagnosis of malfunction are essential for an electrical stimulation programme, and a neurophysiologist's familiarity with electrical matters enables him to play a useful part in such activities.

The course neurophysiology should take in the field of rehabilitation is not self-evident, but the directing force must be a spirit of enquiry into the detailed mechanisms underlying neurological deficit. There is a strong argument for directing one's efforts entirely towards studying animal models, which, compared with human neurological disease, are compellingly simple and offer many advantages. The needs of society and individuals and humanitarian instincts, however, give human work a necessary attraction but can also detract from the basic scientific requirements of neurophysiology. The great intellectual challenge to neurophysiology in rehabilitation is to explain the clinical phenomena of neurological deficit within the framework provided by basic preclinical science. Such an exercise is destined to undergo an unexpected convolution whenever it is found that accepted animal models or frameworks are not entirely adequate and the rehabilitation neurophysiologist has to ask his/her colleagues in animal laboratories to re-examine their concepts. When a lively intellectual intercourse develops along these lines, understanding of the problems moves ahead apace with the inevitable revelation of useful strategies for treatment.

References

Barker A.T., Jalinous R. & Freeston I.L. (1985) Non-invasive magnetic stimulation of the human motor cortex. *Lancet* i, 1106–1107.

Barker A.T., Freeston I.L., Jalinous R. & Jarratt J.A. (1988) Magnetic and electrical stimulation of the brain: safety aspects. In Bossini P.N. & Marsden C.D. (eds) *Non-invasive Stimulation of Brain and Spinal Cord: Fundamentals and Clinical Applications*, pp. 131–144. Alan R. Liss, New York.

Benfield J., Russell J. & Sedgwick E.M. (1988) The H reflex and D1 inhibition during spinal shock in man. *Journal of Physiology* **406**, 155P.

Bernstein N. (1966) *The Co-ordination and Regulation of Movements*. Pergamon Press, Oxford.

Black J.A., Kasis J.D. & Waxman S.G. (1990) Ion channel organisation of the myelinated fibre. *Trends in Neuroscience* **13**, 48–54.

Buller A.J. & Pope R. (1977) Plasticity in mammalian skeletal muscle. *Philosophical Transactions of the Royal Society, London, Series B* **278**, 295–305.

Buller A.J., Eccles J.C. & Eccles R.M. (1960) Interactions between motoneurones and muscles in respect of their characteristic speeds of their responses. *Journal of Physiology, London* **150**, 417–439.

Bussel, B. & Pierrot-Deseilligny E. (1977) Inhibition of human motoneurons, probably of Renshaw origin, elicited by an orthodromic motor discharge. *Journal of Physiology* **269**, 319–339.

Changeux J.-P. (1991) Compartmentalized transcription of acetylcholine receptor genes during motor end plate epigenesis. *New Biology* **3**, 423–429.

Chokroverty S. (1989) *Magnetic Stimulation in Clinical Neurophysiology*. Butterworths, London.

Cole J.D. (1991) *Pride and a Daily Marathon*. Duckworth, London.

Conway R.R., Hof J. & Backlow S. (1988) Lower cervical magnetic stimulation: comparison with C8 needle root stimulation and supraclavicular stimulation. *Muscle and Nerve* **11**, 977–984.

Cross D., Chiappa K.H., Gominak S., Fang J., Santamaria J., King P.J. & Shahani B.T. (1990) Cervical magnetic stimulation. *Neurology* **40**, 1751–1756.

Dimitrijevic M.R. & Nathan P.W. (1967a) Studies of spasticity in man. 1. Some features of spasticity. *Brain* **90**, 1–30.

Dimitrijevic M.R. & Nathan P.W. (1967b) Studies of spasticity in man. 2. Analysis of stretch reflexes in spasticity. *Brain* **90**, 333–357.

Dimitrijevic M.R. & Nathan P.W. (1968) Studies of spasticity in man. 3. Analysis of reflex activity evoked by noxious cutaneous stimulation. *Brain* **91**, 349–368.

Dimitrijevic M.R. & Nathan P.W. (1970) Studies of spasticity in man. 4. Changes in the flexion reflex with repetitive cutaneous stimulation in spinal man. *Brain* **93**, 743–768.

Dimitrijevic M.R. & Nathan P.W. (1971) Studies of spasticity in man. 5. Dishabituation of the flexion reflex in spinal man. *Brain* **94**, 77–90.

Dimitrijevic M.R., Spencer W.A., Trontelj J.V. & Dimitrijevic M. (1977) Reflex effects of vibration in patients with spinal cord lesions. *Neurology* **27**, 1078–1086.

Drachman D.B. (1974) The role of acetylcholine as a neurotropic transmitter. *Annals of the New York Academy of Sciences* **288**, 161–176.

El-Tohamy A. & Sedgwick E.M. (1983) Spinal inhibition in man – depression of the soleus H reflex by stimulation of the nerve to the antagonist muscle. *Journal of Physiology* **337**, 497–508.

Evans B.A., Daube J.R. & Lilcky W.J. (1990) A comparison of magnetic and electrical stimulation of spinal nerves. *Muscle and Nerve* **13**, 414–420.

Fries W., Danek A. & Witt T.N. (1991) Motor responses after transcranial electrical stimulation of cerebral hemispheres with a degenerated pyramidal tract. *Annals of Neurology* **29**, 646–650.

Hammond P.H., Merton P.A. & Sutton G.G. (1956) Nervous gradation of muscular contraction. *British Medical Bulletin* **12**, 214–218.

Henneman E., Somjen G. & Carpenter D.O. (1965) Functional significance of cell size in spinal motoneurones. *Journal of Neurophysiology* **28**, 560–580.

Hoffmann P. (1918) Über die Beziehungen der Schnenreflexe zur willkurlichen Bewegung und zum Tonus. *Zeitschrift Biologie* **68**, 351–570.

Holmes G. (1922) The Croonian Lectures on the clinical symptoms of cerebellar diseases and their interpretation. *Lancet* **100** (1), 1177–1182, 1231–1237; (2) 59–65; 111–115.

Hultborn H. & Pierrot-Deseilligny E. (1979) Changes in recurrent inhibition during voluntary soleus contractions in man studied by an H reflex technique. *Journal of Physiology* **297**, 229–251.

Janowska E. & Tanaka R. (1974) Neuronal mechanism of the disynaptic inhibition evoked in primate spinal motoneurones from the corticospinal tract. *Brain Research* **75**, 163–166.

Kaas J.H. (1991) Plasticity of sensory and motor maps in adult animals. *Annual Review of Neuroscience* **14**, 137–167.

Kaji R., Heppel L. & Sumner A.J. (1990) Effect of digitalis on clinical symptoms and conduction variables in patients with multiple sclerosis. *Annals of Neurology* **28**, 582–584.

Knutsson E. & Richards C. (1979) Different types of disturbed motor control in gait of hemiplegia patients. *Brain* **102**, 405–430.

Kornhuber H.H. (1971) Motor functions of cerebellum and basal ganglia. *Kybernetik* **8**, 157–162.

Kornhuber H.H. (1974) Cerebral cortex, cerebellum and basal ganglia: an introduction to their motor functions. In Schmitt, F.O. & Worden F.G. (eds) *The Neurosciences, Third Study Program*, pp. 267–280. MIT Press, Cambridge, Mass.

Lee R.G. & Tatton W.G. (1978) Long loop reflexes in man: clinical applications. In Desmedt J.E. (ed.) *Cerebral Motor Control in Man: Long Loop Mechanisms*, Vol. 4, pp. 320–333. Karger, Basle.

Lemon R.N. (1990) Mapping the output functions of the motor cortex. In Edelman G.M., Gall W.E. & Cowam W.M. (eds) *Signal and Sense, Local and Global Order in Perceptual Maps*, pp. 315–356. Wiley-Liss, New York.

Levy W.J., Amassian V.E., Traad M. & Cadwell J. (1990) Focal magnetic coil stimulation reveals motor cortical system re-organised in humans after traumatic quadriplegia. *Brain Research* **510**, 130–134.

Marsden C.D., Merton P.A. & Morton H.B. (1972) Servo action in human voluntary movement. *Nature, London* **238**, 140–143.

Marsden C.D., Merton P.A. & Morton H.B. (1973) Is the human stretch reflex cortical rather than spinal? *Lancet* **i**, 759–761.

Matthews W.B. (1970) The clinical implications of the H reflex and other electrically induced reflexes. In

Williams D. (ed.) *Modern Trends in Neurology*, Vol. 5, pp. 241–253. Butterworths, London.

Matthews W.B. & Small D.G. (1979) Serial recording of visual and somatosensory evoked potentials in MS patients. *Journal of the Neurological Sciences* **40**, 11–21.

Meiri H., Baum Z. & Rosenthal Y. (1989) Dynamic changes in sodium channels at demyelinated axons. *Progress in Neurobiology* **32**, 159–179.

Miller S. & Scott P.D. (1977) The spinal locomotor generator. *Experimental Brain Research* **30**, 387–403.

Mizuno Y., Tanaka R. & Yanagisawa N. (1971) Reciprocal group I inhibition on triceps surae motoneurones in man. *Journal of Neurophysiology* **34**, 1010–1017.

Mountcastle V.B. (1975) The view from within: pathways to the study of perception. *Johns Hopkins Medical Journal* **136**, 109–131.

Mountcastle V.B. (1978) Brain mechanisms for directed attention. *Journal of the Royal Society of Medicine* **71**, 14–28.

Newsom Davis J. (1967) Phrenic nerve conduction in man. *Journal of Neurology, Neurosurgery and Psychiatry* **30**, 420–426.

Phillips C.G. & Porter R. (1977) *Corticospinal Neurones: Their Role in Movement*. Academic Press, London.

Pierrot-Deseilligny E., Katz R. & Morin C. (1979) Evidence for 1b inhibition in human subjects. *Brain Research* **166**, 176–179.

Robinson K. & Rudge P. (1978) The stability of the auditory evoked potentials in normal man and patients with multiple sclerosis. *Journal of the Neurological Sciences* **36**, 147–156.

Schady W. & Braune S. (1993) Changes in somatosensory function after nerve injury. *Electroencephalography and Clinical Neurophysiology* **86**, 17p.

Schauf C.L. & Davis F.A. (1974) Impulse conduction in multiple sclerosis: a theoretical basis for modification by temperature and pharmacological agents. *Journal of Neurology, Neurosurgery and Psychiatry* **12**, 152–161.

Schmid U.D., Walker G., Hess C.W. & Schmid J. (1990) Magnetic and electrical stimulation of cervical motor roots: technique, site and mechanisms of excitation. *Journal of Neurology, Neurosurgery and Psychiatry* **43**, 770–777.

Sedgwick E.M. (1988) Neurophysiology of the spinal cord. *Current Opinion in Neurology* **1**, 585–591.

Sedgwick E.M., Illis L.S. & Bentfield J. (1992) Spasticity. In Illis L.S. (ed.) *Spinal Cord Dysfunction II: Intervention and Treatment*, pp. 94–100. Oxford University Press, Oxford.

Sedgwick E.M., Illis L.S., Tallis R.C., Thornton A.R.D., Abraham P., El-Negamy E., Docherty T.B., Soar J.S., Spencer S.C. & Taylor F.M. (1980) Evoked potentials and contingent negative variation during treatment of

multiple sclerosis with spinal cord stimulation. *Journal of Neurology, Neurosurgery and Psychiatry* **43**, 15–24.

Sedgwick E.M., El-Tohamy A. & Frankel H. (1983) Spinal D1 inhibition in paraplegia and hemiplegia. *Electroencephalography and Clinical Neurophysiology* **56**, 70P–71P.

Sedgwick E.M., Illis L.S. & Benfield J. (1992) Spasticity II. In Illis L.S. (ed.) *Spinal Cord Dysfunction: Intervention and Treatment*, pp. 94–100. Oxford University Press, Oxford.

Shik M.L. & Orlovsky G.N. (1976) Neurophysiology of locomotor automation. *Physiological Reviews* **56**, 465–501.

Simoyama M. & Tanaka R. (1974) Reciprocal Ia inhibition at the onset of voluntary movements in man. *Brain Research* **82**, 334–337.

Stefaski D., Davis F.A., Faut M. & Schauf C.L. (1987) 4-Aminopyridine improves clinical signs in multiple sclerosis. *Annals of Neurology* **21**, 71–77.

Tallis R.C. (1991) Assessing outcome in rehabilitation. In Seymour C.A. & Summerfield J.A. (eds) *Horizons in Medicine*, No. 3, pp. 128–138. Transmedia Europe Ltd, Eastbourne, UK.

Tanaka R. (1972) Activation of reciprocal Ia inhibitory pathway during voluntary motor performance in man. *Brain Research* **43**, 649–652.

Tanaka R. (1974) Reciprocal Ia inhibition during voluntary movements in man. *Experimental Brain Research* **21**, 529–540.

Topka H., Cohen L.G., Cole R.A. & Hallett M. (1991) Reorganisation of corticospinal pathways following spinal cord injury. *Neurology* **41**, 1276–1283.

Twitchell T.E. (1951) Restoration of motor function following hemiplegia in man. *Brain* **74**, 443–480.

Ungawa Y., Rothwell J.C., Day B.L., Thompson P.D. & Marsden C.D. (1989) Magnetic stimulation over the spinal enlargements. *Journal of Neurology, Neurosurgery and Psychiatry* **52**, 1025–1032.

Vallbo A.B., Hagbarth K.E., Torebjörk H.E. & Wallin B.G. (1979) Somatosensory, proprioceptive and sympathetic activity in human peripheral nerves. *Physiological Reviews* **39**, 919–957.

Wall P.D. & Egger M.D. (1971) Formation of new connections in adult rat brains after partial denervation. *Nature* **232**, 542–545.

Wanner E., Teyler T.J. & Thompson R.F. (1977) The psychobiology of speech and language – an overview. In Desmedt J.E. (ed.) *Language and Hemispheric Specialization in Man: Cerebral ERPS*, Progress in Clinical Neurophysiology, Vol. 3, pp. 1–27. Karger, Basle.

Yanagisawa N., Tanaka R. & Ito Z. (1976) Reciprocal Ia inhibition in spastic hemiplegia of man. *Brain* **99**, 555–574.

Part 3
Assessment

9: Evaluation and Economics of Treatment in Neurological Rehabilitation

C.N. MARTYN AND A. MORRIS

Efficacy, effectiveness and efficiency, 106
Clinical trials in rehabilitation, 106
Generalizing from the results of clinical trials, 107
Implementing effective treatments, 108
Economic evaluation, 108
　The range of costs and benefits, 109
　Cost−benefit and cost-effectiveness analysis, 110
　Cost−utility analysis, 110
Conclusions, 111

Over the last few decades there has been a striking change in the sort of evidence that we require before we are prepared to introduce a new drug into clinical practice. We tend to be dissatisfied with anything less than unequivocal results from a large, prospective, randomized clinical trial; and we feel happier if these results have been replicated on several occasions. While a few have railed about the intellectual tyranny that such a viewpoint imposes (Dudley, 1983), there is a general belief that only this methodology is rigorous enough to provide a reliable and objective assessment of a drug's efficacy. Those who lament any loss of clinical freedom need to be reminded that the history of therapeutics is crammed with examples of treatments that we now know to be useless, if not actually inimical. Our laughter when we hear of fever being treated by venesection or peptic ulcer by milky diets should be tempered by the realization that only the randomized controlled trial stands between us and similar acts of credulity.

More recently, we have also become aware that establishing the efficacy and safety of a particular form of treatment is no more than a first step along the route to delivery of that treatment to the people who might benefit from it. If an example is needed, think how long it took to institute any half-way systematic strategy to identify and treat asymp-tomatic hypertensive people in the community, following the clear demonstration that drug treatment of mild to moderate hypertension significantly reduced the risk of stroke. We are being forced to realize, too, that health care resources have always been, in one way or another, rationed. There is a sharper perception that the basis for rationing must become more explicit and more widely discussed. This has inevitably focused attention on the costs of medical intervention and the need to add economic considerations to any evaluation of treatment.

The main theme of this chapter is that there is an urgent requirement to operate these standards in the appraisal of treatments used in rehabilitation. They must be applied not just to the evaluation of new treatments; we also need to examine the efficacy of many current practices and investigate how effectively they are made available to those who might benefit. To avoid any confusion about our aims, it may be as well to point out that this chapter is not primarily about audit – the process of setting targets for quality of medical care and assessing performance in terms of meeting these targets – but about the way in which the effectiveness of treatments and interventions must be evaluated to enable targets to be set in the first place.

As a subtext, the chapter also carries a message about the need for a rational foundation for rehabilitation. Many regimens of rehabilitation exist because of tradition or because of the enthusiasm of their proponents, rather than as a result of any objective assessment of their worth. In the course of a polemic about whether rehabilitation should be a key area in the UK government's strategy for health, McLellan (1991) drew attention to the profound ignorance of most medical graduates of rehabilitation and the low level of funding for research in the subject. We agree that a positive response is required and have tried to sketch out how a more critical evaluation of treatments used in rehabilitation might be part of this response. An implicit part of our argument is that there is an ethical obligation to measure the effectiveness of the health care that we offer. We also suggest that, to an increasing extent, the future of rehabilitation will depend on the use and development of economic techniques to assess efficiency.

Efficacy, effectiveness and efficiency

In everyday use, the meanings of the three words efficacy, effectiveness and efficiency are so close that they are almost interchangeable. But these terms have been hijacked by those concerned with the evaluation of health care (Cochrane, 1971) and, in this specialized context, each has come to mean something quite different. Efficacy is used to indicate whether, and by how much, medical or surgical intervention alters (for the better) the outcome of a particular disease in a set of defined circumstances, usually a clinical trial, where compliance with the treatment can be assumed to be complete or very nearly so. Effectiveness refers to how completely that outcome can be achieved when the treatment or intervention is translated into the usual conditions of clinical practice; that is, the extent to which the treatment can be expected to benefit those to whom it is offered. Efficiency is a measure that relates effectiveness to the amount of resources used up in implementing the treatment. An example may help to make these distinctions plainer. Numerous experiments in metabolic balance have shown that individuals whose calorie intake is less than their energy expenditure lose weight. We can agree therefore, that dietary restriction is an efficacious treatment for obesity. On the other hand, most physicians will know from personal experience that advising overweight people to eat less is not generally an effective treatment for their condition. It inevitably follows that giving such advice cannot be an efficient use of medical resources. None of this, of course, implies that obesity is a trivial problem or that efforts to find useful treatments or to understand how they work are not worth while. We are simply trying to make the point that, no matter how sound their

physiological basis, we should desist from offering treatments that are found to be ineffective and inefficient in clinical practice. Rehabilitation, like the rest of clinical medicine, should be an intensely practical business. As Asher wrote: 'One of the most important things about treatment is that it should *be* effective – not merely that it *ought* to be effective. A remedy that is known to work, though nobody knows why, is preferable to a remedy which has the support of theory without the confirmation of practice' (Asher, 1961).

Clinical trials in rehabilitation

McPherson (1984), in a short and clearly argued piece about the design and interpretation of clinical trials, categorized the reasons why, in a clinical trial, one group of patients might fare better than another, independently of any intrinsic merits of the treatment they received, under three headings: chance, patient selection and ancillary factors associated with a particular treatment. The first of these – chance – requires little discussion. The main purpose of statistical analysis is to estimate the likelihood that an observed effect associated with a particular treatment was a chance result and to argue for the application of statistical methods to clinical trials would be to refight a battle that has already been won.

The effects of patient selection and the value of random allocation of treatment in eliminating them are less well appreciated. Until quite recently, few randomized controlled trials of treatments used in rehabilitation were carried out. Some of the reasons for this are obvious; the difficulty of organizing randomized trials and the expense of performing them, especially when any benefits are likely to be apparent only in the long term, mean that many aspects of health care, including rehabilitation, are hard to evaluate in this way. In the absence of evidence from randomized trials, evaluations of rehabilitation treatments have often depended on making formal or informal comparisons with historical controls. A new treatment is assessed by comparing the outcomes of a group of patients so treated with the outcomes of a group of apparently similar patients who had been cared for before the new treatment became available. The central logical weakness of this design is that changes other than the institution of treatment may have occurred between the two times. There are good examples of circumstances in which reliance on comparisons with historical controls has been misleading (Christie, 1979). A series of patients admitted to the Royal Melbourne Hospital with stroke during 1978 and who had been computerized tomography (CT)-scanned were matched for age, diagnosis and level of consciousness at admission to a series of similar patients who had been admitted to the same hospital in 1974 before a CT scanner had been installed. Survival amongst patients in the later series, who had had the benefit of a CT scan, was better by an amount that was statistically significant and it appeared that the introduction of CT scanning had much improved the chances of survival in patients admitted with stroke. The investigator was unsatisfied with this remarkable result; using the same matching technique, he carried out a similar study on patients admitted with stroke in 1978 who, despite the availability of the technique, had not had a CT scan. The improvement in survival in the later series of unscanned patients was even greater than in the patients who had been scanned. The explanation is that the change in survival was independent of the introduction of the CT scanner and reflected time trends in the case fatality of stroke. The experience of this investigator shows the dangers of historical comparisons even when the time period over which the comparison is made is short. When eagerly seeking therapeutic advances, it is only too easy to persuade oneself that an improvement in outcome is due to the introduction of a new treatment.

The reason why it is essential for patients to be allocated at random to different treatments in clinical trials is not always fully appreciated, even by some of the investigators who carry out these trials. It is not that randomization ensures that the groups being compared will be identical. Indeed, the fact that treatments are allocated at random makes chance differences between groups likely and modifications of the randomization procedure, such as stratification and minimization, may be necessary to ensure that such differences are small. The overwhelming advantage of randomization is that the allocation of patients to the treatments being compared is unbiased, not only with respect to features that can be identified or measured,

such as age or degree of disability, but, equally important, with respect to features that cannot be so readily identified but that may none the less have an effect on outcome. Randomization eliminates the possibility that the whims, prejudices and unconscious biases of the investigators or the subjects recruited into the trial have affected who gets which treatment.

The last of McPherson's three reasons why one group of patients may enjoy a better outcome than another in a clinical trial is that it was a result of some ancillary factor associated with treatment. One way in which this can happen, even in randomized controlled trials, is if the person assessing outcome is aware of which treatment the patient received. Expectations of a treatment effect may then bias the way in which the assessment is carried out. While more difficult to arrange than in drug trials, it is important to minimize this potential difficulty in trials of treatments in rehabilitation. This can often be achieved by having the assessment of outcome carried out by someone not involved in the day-to-day care of the patient or the running of the trial and who can therefore remain blind to which treatment the patient is receiving.

Generalizing from the results of clinical trials

Inclusion and exclusion criteria for clinical trials, particularly when innovative treatments are being evaluated, tend to select patients who have the highest risk of suffering the most severe consequences of their disorders and who are most likely to respond to the intervention being tested. This may cause difficulty when trying to extrapolate from the results of a clinical trial. Sometimes the limited applicability of the results of a trial is fairly clear; more often, the answer to the question of whether other, more mildly affected patients would also benefit is a matter of judgement.

There may also be problems in gaining acceptance of the results of a trial if the findings challenge long-held beliefs about the efficacy of a treatment. It is part of human nature that we demand higher standards of evidence against a cherished hypothesis than we would readily accept in support of it. Investigators who publish results that show the failure of a treatment that everyone knows ought to work are invariably criticized. Any readers who think themselves free of such prejudice might find it interesting to consider why speech therapy continues to be so widely used in the treatment of dysphasic stroke patients in spite of the paucity of evidence that it is effective. They should contrast this state of affairs with the general attitude of physicians, neurologists and specialists in rehabilitation towards chiropractic treatment of chronic low back pain in spite of evidence from a well-designed randomized controlled trial that it is of benefit.

A fall-back position frequently adopted by those confronted with results from a clinical trial that they are unwilling to accept but whose correctness is hard to challenge is that the results of the trial as a whole might fail to identify a subgroup of patients who derive particular benefit. Unfortunately, such a suggestion is unlikely to prove helpful. Experience indicates that, even in very large clinical trials, analysis of subgroups is not worth while. The authors of the report of the ISIS-2 trial of intravenous streptokinase and oral aspirin in the treatment of acute myocardial infarction, into which 17 187 patients were recruited, demonstrated the unreliability of trying to identify subgroups in which treatment was especially advantageous or in which it was ineffective (ISIS-2, 1988). They found that, when patients were subdivided by their astrological birth signs, there was a slightly adverse effect of aspirin on mortality for those born under Gemini or Libra, while for those born under all other astrological signs there was a strikingly beneficial effect. They pointed out that, in a trial with a clearly positive overall result, when many subgroup analyses are considered, false negative results in some subgroups must be expected. The converse is also true for trials that fail to show an overall positive result. The best estimate of the real size of the treatment effect in each subgroup is given not by the results in that subgroup alone but by the overall results in all subgroups combined.

Implementing effective treatments

There is increasing concern over the haphazard geographical variations that exist in the way in which patients with similar diseases and disabilities are treated (Warlow, 1992). Part of this variation can be attributed to lack of firm evidence about which treatments are most effective. If the relative merits of different treatments have not been established, patients become vulnerable to the individual preferences of their physicians. But part of the variation also derives from the fact that clinicians do not have the time, and may not possess the skills or inclination, to search the literature for trials of many different treatments and evaluate them critically. In any case, it would be an absurd reduplication of effort for all clinicians to do this for themselves. There is a desperate, though largely unperceived need for some systematic way of making available information about which treatments are most effective to those who most require it—the clinicians who spend their working hours looking after patients.

The model for comprehensive reviews of therapeutics in a clinical discipline is the *Oxford Database of Perinatal Trials*, edited by Iain Chalmers (1992). As a recent editorial in the *British Medical Journal* stated uncompromisingly, 'perinatologists now have no need or excuse for being out of date' (Haynes, 1992). But Chalmers's systematic and exhaustive critical review achieves more than the highlighting of effective treatments. Therapeutic interventions are divided into four categories:

1 Forms of care of proven benefit.
2 Forms of care that appear promising, but require further evaluation.
3 Forms of care with unknown effects, which require further evaluation.
4 Forms of care that should be abandoned in the light of the available evidence.

This provides a framework not only for rational modification of current strategies of treatment but for establishing priorities for further research. Can someone be persuaded to take on the task of coordinating a similar endeavour for the treatments used in neurological rehabilitation?

Economic evaluation

Economic analysis is sometimes misconceived as being concerned with the costs rather than the value of services. In fact, the process has much more to offer to those who have to make decisions about resource allocation than simply estimating the cost of a treatment. By the identification of measures of benefit or outcome that incorporate quality as well as quantity of life, economic analyses highlight the importance of taking a long-term view and so can contribute to protecting the investment in resources needed in rehabilitation.

We have already alluded to the increasing demand for decisions about allocation of health care resources to become more widely discussed. It is inevitable that choices must be made in the way the resources available for health care – which include time, skills, people, buildings and equipment as well as money – are deployed. Only some organized consideration of the different factors involved in which all assumptions are made explicit can lead to effective decisions being made. The central questions are whether a particular treatment is worth while when judged by a yardstick of what else could be done with the same resources and whether the resources which are required to make the treatment available to those who stand to benefit are best spent in this rather than some other way.

The range of costs and benefits

In attempting to answer such questions, the first task of any economic evaluation is to identify the costs and benefits of the treatment under scrutiny and the second to compare their relative magnitudes.

1 What are the costs of rehabilitation?

2 On whom do they fall?

3 When do they fall?

4 What is the range of costs that must be included in the evaluation?

5 How are these costs to be measured?

6 What are the benefits to be gained from rehabilitation?

7 Who will benefit: patients, their families or society?

8 How are these benefits to be measured?

9 Are these benefits to be evaluated only in clinical terms?

10 Can these benefits be expressed in terms commensurate with costs?

Consideration of the costs and benefits associated with rehabilitation requires a wider-angle view than that often applied to the treatment of acute

illness. Within cost–benefit analysis of acute treatments, the main, if not the only, focus is on the direct cost to the unit that provides the treatment. This approach is usually justified as these direct costs represent the largest change in resource use associated with treatment. Within rehabilitation, the network of relevant costs is larger, and care should be taken in deciding the limits of the range of costs to be taken into account. The costs that the patient and society must bear in rehabilitation are very significant and they should not be allowed to disappear from view.

The costs of rehabilitation treatment to the patient and their family include the time involved in travel to and from treatment, time spent in nursing and caring for the patient at home and the contingent loss of income, adaptations to the patient's home, special diets, heating and laundry. Most of these are borne by the patient's family. Even when a person is not in paid employment or the treatment is carried out during time that would not be spent at work, time is not costless. Leisure time has alternative uses and something must be forgone or sacrificed when a consultation with the patient's general practitioner or a hospital outpatient appointment is kept. Even if the sacrifice is not evaluated in terms of money or no payment has to be made for the use of the time, it is likely to be an important factor in decision-making by the patient and the patient's family. Other costs falling on the patient and family are the psychic costs of worry, pain and stress.

Costs associated with health care programmes also fall on areas of society outside the health service and the patient. These costs, although hidden, may be substantial. A study that analysed the costs of a national outbreak of salmonellosis found that the non-direct notional health service costs – i.e. those to families and society – constituted 80% of the total costs of the outbreak and its control (Roberts et al., 1989).

Benefits from health care can also be specified in different ways. Only one of these is the gain in health to the individual patient – increased mobility, greater ability in the activities of daily living, greater independence and choice. The wider benefits that may accrue to patients and their relatives include keeping their jobs, maintaining ability to work at a higher level, improved quality of life and lower levels of stress. Wider still are effects on friends, the local community and society generally. Direct benefits may include cost savings within health services. One study which examined the impact of early input of therapy, information and counselling to neurological patients found that the investment paid off both in terms of improved benefits to patients and their families and in terms of reduced need for acute intervention later (Oxtoby et al., 1988).

A study is continuing in which the effects of early and later support for neurological patients and their families are being compared (Morris, unpublished). Costs and benefits are being examined in several ways. The costs of early intervention include the salaries of the individual workers, their travel and necessary administration. These are being balanced against benefits, which include savings in acute medical interventions and fewer or more appropriate calls on support agencies.

The fragmentation that exists between providers of health and social care has done little to assist availability of treatment. There have been few incentives for any provider agency to change its method of working to increase the overall availability of care to patients unless it was able to reap direct cost savings even if an overall gain in health would have resulted. Perhaps the recent requirement for joint working between health and social services specified in the NHS and Community Care Act will allow the organization of a more unified strategy of care in England and Wales.

Cost−benefit and cost-effectiveness analysis

Once the problems of deciding the range of costs and benefits that are to be considered have been resolved, the second part of any economic evaluation is deciding the most appropriate technique with which to compare them. Cost-effectiveness analysis is most useful when comparing different ways of achieving a single result. Where alternative methods are directed towards one main objective, their relative success is measured in terms of the cost of achieving that end, given that the different methods achieve the outcome equally well. No value is assigned to the benefit or outcome to be achieved; cost-effectiveness analysis simply

examines the costs associated with the different ways of achieving it. The technique has the merit of simplicity but its application is limited to circumstances in which there is no doubt that the outcome is both worth while and measurable.

Cost−benefit analysis attempts to express all costs and all benefits explicitly in the same units of account − usually money − to enable direct comparison. Unlike cost-effectiveness analysis, this approach contains an evaluation of the value of achieving the objective in that the benefits of the treatment are measured. Here, the decision rule is expressed either as a cost/benefit ratio or in terms of net benefits (that is, benefits − costs) over the life of the project. But neither cost-effectiveness nor cost−benefit analysis sheds any light on the question of the extent to which the objective under consideration should be met as compared with any others.

A particular drawback of cost−benefit analysis is the difficulty of expressing all the benefits in monetary terms. This may lead to benefits being undervalued. In such cases, those involved in making decisions about allocation of resources must weigh up the extent of the undervalued benefits. Economic appraisals should be seen as an aid to decision-making; they do not constitute the whole of it.

Cost−utility analysis

It is in cases where benefits are measured in health terms and then valued in monetary terms that most opprobrium has been heaped on economic evaluations. Many have expressed repugnance at attempts to quantify the value of human life and health in terms of money. Although at least part of such criticism may represent unease about making explicit what was previously implicit, rather than any fundamental objection to thinking about such matters in terms of money, cost−utility analysis provides a way of circumventing such difficulties. Cost−utility analysis focuses on the quality of the health outcome associated with treatment. The incremental cost of treatment is compared with the additional improvement in health as measured in quality-adjusted life-years (QALYs) gained. Results are usually expressed in terms of the costs of achieving a QALY. The quality adjustment is made by applying a set of weights to particular health states (utilities) in a way that reflects their relative desirability. The weighting is derived from a variety of sources: from measurements taken directly from a sample of subjects, from published sources and from judgements made by the analyst.

Whilst QALYs allow a measure of outcome that takes into account both quality and quantity of life, they are not without disadvantages. In the early work using QALYs, the weightings applied to the various states of disability were derived from very small samples (Rosser & Watts, 1978). Further, the measures of morbidity most frequently used to adjust life-years for quality are pain and immobility. Not all patients and families would agree that these are the only, or even the most important, factors that determine quality of life. The advantages of cost–utility analysis emerge in three sets of circumstances: where quality of life is the sole or the dominant outcome of treatment; where the treatment affects both mortality and morbidity and a common unit of account that combines both outcomes is required; and where the treatments being compared have disparate outcomes and some common currency is needed on which to base the comparison.

Whatever method of economic analysis is used, consideration must be given to the time at which costs are incurred and at which benefits are likely to accrue. Generally, costs of treatment must be borne early while benefits may continue in the long term. Some treatments, including many used in rehabilitation, require resources to be committed over the life of the patient. Account must be taken of the differential timing of costs and benefits; a given sum spent or received now is not the equivalent of the same sum spent or received 5 years hence. As a general rule, when we lend money we expect a premium even when we perceive no risk because, by lending the money, we have to postpone our own spending until it is returned. In economists' jargon this is known as a positive rate of time preference. The difficulty is to incorporate this concept into evaluations of health services in a sensible way. One way to do this is by discounting – a process that is essentially the reverse calculation of compound interest. Discounting can make a large difference to the result of the cost–benefit comparison, especially in circumstances where the timing of the costs and benefits of different treatments vary greatly. High discount rates will favour projects whose benefits occur early.

Conclusions

We argued earlier that the future of rehabilitation will depend upon our willingness to measure the effectiveness of the treatments that we offer and our ability to demonstrate their efficiency. All would surely agree with the principle that rehabilitation should be effective. Disagreement arises over which treatments are effective and the best way of implementing them. In this chapter we have tried to show how this disagreement can be used as a stimulus to improving the quality of rehabilitation and to point out some of the economic considerations that have to be taken into account. Many of the potential benefits of rehabilitation ripple out into the community and become lost from view. There is a danger that the difficulty of estimating these benefits will lead to an undervaluation of rehabilitation.

References

Asher R. (1961) Apriority. Thoughts on treatment. *Lancet* **ii**, 1403–1404.

Chalmers I. (ed.) (1992) *Oxford Database of Perinatal Trials*. Oxford Electronic Publishing, Oxford University Press, Oxford.

Christie D. (1979) Before-and-after comparisons: a cautionary tale. *British Medical Journal* **2**, 1629–1630.

Cochrane A.L. (1971) *Effectiveness and Efficiency: Random Reflections on Health Services*. Nuffield Provincial Hospitals Trust.

Dudley H.A.F. (1983) The controlled clinical trial and the advance of reliable knowledge: an outsider looks in. *British Medical Journal* **287**, 957–960.

Haynes R.B. (1992) Clinical review articles. *British Medical Journal* **304**, 330–331.

ISIS-2: Second International Study of Infarct Survival Collaborative Group (1988) Randomised trial of intravenous streptokinase, oral aspirin, both or neither among 17 187 cases of suspected acute myocardial infarction: ISIS-2. *Lancet* **ii**, 349–360.

McLellan D.L. (1991) Rehabilitation. *British Medical Journal* **303**, 355–357.

McPherson K. (1984) The evaluation of treatment. In Warlow C. & Garfield J. (eds) *Dilemmas in the Management of the Neurological Patient*, pp. 277–285. Churchill Livingstone, Edinburgh.

Morris A. (unpublished) Work on the evaluation of two models of support for people with neurological conditions and their families in Suffolk.

Oxtoby M., Findley L., Porteous A., Kelson N., Thurgood S., Pearce P. & Wood A. (1988) *A Strategy for the Management of Parkinson's Disease and for the Long-term Support of Patients and Carers.* Parkinson's Disease Society, London.

Roberts J.A., Sockett P.N. & Gill O.N. (1989) Economic impact of a nationwide outbreak of salmonellosis: cost—benefit of early intervention. *British Medical Journal* **298**, 1227–1230.

Rosser R.M. & Watts V.C. (1978) A scale of valuations of states of illness. *International Journal of Epidemiology* **7**, 347–358.

Warlow C.P. (1992) Hither neurology: research. *Journal of Neurology, Neurosurgery and Psychiatry*, **55** (suppl.), 26–31.

10: Audit in Neurological Rehabilitation

D.T. WADE

The aims of rehabilitation, 113
Audit, 115
   Structure, 115
   Process, 116
   Outcome, 117
Case-mix measures, 118
Audit in practice, 119
   Clinical audit (case-note review), 119
   Service audit, 119
Measures, 120
   Pathology (diagnosis), 120
   Impairment, 120
   Disability, 122
   Handicap, 122
Conclusion, 122
Appendix 1: Sources of measures mentioned in text, 122
Appendix 2: Tests, 123

Audit is (or should be) an integral part of rehabilitation. Rehabilitation is a reiterative process starting with assessment and ending with evaluation (i.e. reassessment), which should then lead to further or different action adjusted to take account of the reassessment. This feedback loop should apply not only to the management of individual patients but also, in an adapted way, to the service(s) offered; audit is then the term applied. This chapter focuses on the process of evaluation and in doing so it necessarily discusses both assessment of individual patients and the assessment of case mix. The chapter does not prescribe what corrective actions should be undertaken as a result of audit, or how such actions are themselves checked, but it is important that audit itself is checked and that actions initiated after audit are themselves evaluated.

The chapter starts by discussing the aims of rehabilitation. The aims will determine the outcomes to be audited. Without agreement on the aims of the process being subjected to audit, it is impossible to carry out audit. Next the nature of audit is discussed, emphasizing that three aspects of a service can be subjected to audit: structure (what is there available?); process (what happens?); and outcome (so what?). Each aspect will be discussed with respect to rehabilitation. Interpretation of any data collected is difficult because, in rehabilitation especially, so much depends upon the case mix of patients seen. Therefore the measurement of case mix is discussed next.

Little has been written about audit of neurological rehabilitation in practice. This chapter itself is written largely from a theoretical basis but throughout there is an emphasis on practical ways of undertaking audit, and the next section discusses this in more detail. This includes a discussion on the context of audit, emphasizing that rehabilitation relates to communities, and that audit must consider all potential patients, not simply those seen in a particular service.

Finally, there is a section on measurement. Audit depends upon measurement (quantification) and so the various measures available which should be of clinical use are discussed. More detailed information is available elsewhere (Wade, 1992).

The aims of rehabilitation

Rehabilitation is a team activity and all clinicians involved in the team must agree on the aims of rehabilitation (Davis *et al.*, 1992; McGrath & Davis, 1992). This is the vital first step in any clinical audit. Agreement is often difficult and clinicians may have widely differing views. For example, a recent informal survey in one centre found one nurse believing the aim was 'to provide terminal care' whereas another person felt the aim was 'to assess the patient for a wheelchair'. Moreover, clinicians often confuse the process of rehabilitation with its aims; for example, a therapist might consider that rehabilitation ended when his/her own specific therapeutic input was complete, while the social worker might expect finding suitable housing and helping adaptation to be valid components of rehabilitation.

The usual (and common) conflict is between those who see rehabilitation as primarily concerned with achieving independence (usually in activities of daily living), and those who consider that the wider issues of housing, daytime occupation and life satisfaction are a legitimate concern of rehabilitation services. A second common conflict is between people who believe that only patients suitable for the service in question should receive rehabilitation and those who believe that the service should respond to the needs of the patients and the community.

Although discussing aims can be a touchy topic, it is vital to consider it because ultimately having different aims will lead to conflict within the team. This conflict can often be stark: one or more professions can consider that a patient should leave 'as they are no longer benefiting from rehabilitation', but others may be trying to improve social support, etc. It is especially important to consider the aims in relation to the needs of the community. For example, some spinal injury centres (or other specialist centres) may refuse to accept patients who do not have any home or hospital to return to, or may refuse to accept patients with non-traumatic spinal cord disease. Being homeless after spinal cord injury might be considered by purchasers a legitimate problem to be resolved by the service, and the patient aged 70 years with a spinal artery thrombosis may not appreciate the reason for being denied specialist care.

Conflicts can arise not only within a service, but also between different services and between purchasers and providers. For example, a service might see itself as offering only 'specialist assessment and advice' but the users might expect more, such as arranging the interventions advised and reassessing. The conflict may arise in future between purchasers and providers.

These conflicts arise primarily because the services have not considered and discussed the aims of their service in any detail, perhaps because they consider them self-evident. Aims are never self-evident. Audit can only be carried out in relation to the stated aims of the service. Therefore it is necessary for all team members of a service to discuss and contribute towards the overall aims.

The following definitions of the general aims of rehabilitation are offered, and form the basis for the rest of this chapter.

1 The *aims* of rehabilitation are to minimize the handicap, dissatisfaction and emotional distress arising from disease or as part of illness behaviour, within any limitations imposed by availability of resources and by underlying pathology.

2 *Handicap* refers to limitations in an individual's freedom to:

    (a) live in any surroundings;

    (b) live independently of personal support;

    (c) achieve and maintain wished positions within his/her own social networks;

    (d) partake in social relationships to the extent he or she wishes;

    (e) occupy time in a personally meaningful way;

    (f) adapt to changes.

3 Consequently the *objectives* of rehabilitation are to:

    (a) maximize the patient's independence within any environment;

    (b) optimize the patient's physical environment;

    (c) provide the level of personal support needed;

    (d) achieve the widest range of role behaviours possible;

    (e) optimize the level of social interaction;

    (f) provide the patient with opportunities to occupy him/herself;

    (g) maximize the patient's ability to adapt to change;

    (h) modify the patient's expectations in terms of future positions;

    (i) modify behaviour and expectations of family and significant others.

4 The *methods* (or *processes*) involved in rehabilitation are:

    (a) assessment (diagnosis, measurement, interpretation);

    (b) planning (discussion and the setting of goals);

    (c) intervention (none, care, treatment);

    (d) evaluation (reassessment).

Audit

Anyone involved in the rehabilitation of brain-damaged patients will appreciate the important contribution self-monitoring and self-awareness make to a patient's successful behaviour. Therefore it should be no surprise that the same applies to rehabilitation, only the word used is audit. Unfortunately, the word audit (like rehabilitation) carries many meanings and implications. Here it is used to refer to any process which monitors other processes or services in order to improve their quality and/or cost-effectiveness. Much has been written about audit (Hopkins, 1990) and most readers will already be involved in audit, and so only an outline will be given, stressing some important points.

Most texts on audit refer to structure, process and outcome as being the three most important aspects of a service amenable to audit. However, in rehabilitation the importance of the case mix ('patient characteristics') cannot be overstated. The use of resources and a patient's long-term morbidity will often depend upon a host of factors, many outside the control of the rehabilitation service. For example, the length of stay in hospital after stroke is determined both by the extent of disability and by social factors (Wade & Langton Hewer, 1985; Epstein et al., 1988). The diagnosis itself is of relatively little importance (Rondinelli et al., 1991).

Therefore, any process auditing rehabilitation must have accurate information about all relevant prognostic factors relating to resource use and outcome if any rational interpretation and subsequent actions are to occur. Unfortunately, at present we are unable to predict either resource use during or outcome after rehabilitation with any accuracy whatsoever (Rondinelli et al., 1991).

Lastly, it is vital to remember that audit is intended to improve clinical practice. Therefore some mechanism is needed to agree as to what action is needed, to check that it is carried out and to monitor its effect. Further discussion of this vital area is outside the scope of this chapter, but it is none the less pointless to start audit without an agreed mechanism to act on the findings.

Next the areas of the rehabilitation service which could be subject to audit will be discussed, using the three headings of structure, process and outcome. Much of this is shown in Tables 10.1 to 10.4.

Structure

The aspects of structure worthy of audit are given in Table 10.1. Of course the precise questions asked will depend upon the nature of the service being audited.

The relevant physical structures in rehabilitation are the buildings and other facilities such as hydrotherapy pools or computers. The most important attributes are not related to the presence of high technology or capital-intense equipment but to the environment patients live in. All in-patient rehabilitation settings should be as home-like as possible, given the nature and severity of the disabilities being managed. A further important aspect of structure is transport, either to bring the patient to the centre or to take the team to the patient's home.

The most important 'structure' in rehabilitation is the team providing the service. The nature and composition of the team will obviously depend upon the service being offered, but in neurological rehabilitation it is vital to always have easy access to almost all professions, even if they are not a regular part of the team. For example, from time to time one may need an orthopaedic surgeon,

Table 10.1 Audit of rehabilitation: structure

Buildings (in-patient services)
As home-like as possible?
Easy access to shops and community facilities?
Easy access for relatives and others?

Matériel (in- or out-patient services)
Adequate range of equipment for assessment and
　treatment?
Budget for unusual or specialist aids/equipment?

Personnel
Easy access to all specialists needed?
Sufficient staff to care for levels of disability seen?
Sufficient and appropriately experienced staff to assess
　and treat?
Adequate support staff?

Miscellaneous
Availability of transport, e.g. for home visits?

an orthoptist, an orthodontist or an authority on gastrostomy management. Of equal importance, staff must have sufficient experience for the job.

Lastly, the importance of excellent secretarial support cannot be overstated. The most vital component of good rehabilitation is communication. Although this is especially so in complex cases, it applies even in relatively simple cases. Indeed, audit itself can only occur if secretarial help is good.

Table 10.2 Audit of rehabilitation: processes

Assessment
Is there a structured approach ensuring cover of all areas?
Are standard, reliable measures used?
Are measures used and interpreted appropriately?
Are unnecessary assessments avoided?
Are the results recorded, readily available and
   understandable?

Goal-planning
Has this occurred and been documented?
Was its timing appropriate?
Did it involve (or take into account) all relevant parties?
Are there both long-term aims and medium-term
   objectives?
Are the short-term targets measurable?
(Is it distorted because goal achievement determines
   payment for the service?)

Care
Are avoidable complications occurring?
Are relatives and/or other carers being involved and
   taught?
Is the patient being made overdependent?
Is there sufficient care available?

Treatments
Are acceptable treatments being used?
Are expected treatments absent?
Are relatives and other carers involved?
Is the duration and frequency appropriate?
Has the environment been adapted?

Evaluation
Is there evidence of reassessment?
Are changes in goals documented?
Are reasons for changes in goals given?

Miscellaneous
Length of stay (or length of involvement)
Patient activity during the day

Process

Rehabilitation is a problem-solving educational process focused on disability (Wade, 1990). The steps involved are: assessment – the identification and analysis of all significant problems; goal-planning; intervention, which may be care or treatment; and evaluation (reassessment). The questions one might ask are given in Table 10.2.

Sometimes assessment is seen as an end in itself, but this trap should be avoided. The purposes of initial assessment are: (i) to identify all major problem areas; and (ii) to acquire the relevant additional information needed to determine prognosis and action. As far as possible, assessments should use valid, reliable measures or tools. Further, assessment should always be limited to those necessary at the time.

Goal-planning in rehabilitation is difficult (Davis *et al.*, 1992; McGrath & Davis, 1992), and it is particularly difficult when managers or purchasers use the achievement of goals as an outcome measure for payment. Goal-planning should only be part of the rehabilitation effort and process, and good goal-planning will often involve setting high targets, in part as a motivation to the patient. Once payment (or provision of resources) becomes dependent upon actually achieving the goals, then the whole process of rehabilitation is distorted, to the detriment both of the patient and ultimately of society. Goals are then set at a much lower level and are often not particularly related to the patient's real needs or interests.

Interventions can conceptually be subdivided into *care*, actions needed to preserve the status quo, and *treatments*, which influence change. Many interventions in practice achieve both aims; for example, passive stretching of joints may both prevent contractures and increase range of movement. Furthermore, therapists giving treatment often give care and nurses giving care may well also give treatment. The two types of intervention are closely intertwined. Many of the audit measures relating to intervention properly refer to observed outcome, but a few intervention process measures will be given.

Care at some level is necessary and must be available and sufficient for the patient's level of disability. However, a rehabilitation service should aim to teach the patient and the likely long-term carers to undertake care themselves. Secondly, it is as important to avoid too much care as it is too little care.

An audit of the process of treatment itself is difficult. Audit which monitors process is common in many medical specialities, and is based on the (often untested) assumption that certain processes inevitably improve outcome. In rehabilitation (as in most medicine) there is rarely any evidence that specific treatments definitely and uniquely achieve a better outcome than other treatments (including no treatment), and so one cannot equate failure to deliver a specific treatment with a poor service (or vice versa). Consequently it is necessary to rely on professional consensus, never a happy option. However, one can monitor what patients are doing during the day within a centre (Tinson, 1989).

The last stage of the rehabilitation process is to reassess, evaluating change against expectations. As stated earlier, it is expected that some goals will not be achieved, but one part of reassessment is to determine the reason for failure, which might be, for example: an unidentified impairment (e.g. depression); goal conflicts between team members or others; poor knowledge about natural history and prognosis; or overambitious goals being set.

It is important to stress that in fact all five processes will be occurring simultaneously rather than in sequence. Certainly this applies when there are several different problems, and also to an extent within a problem. For example, when teaching someone to walk after a stroke, the therapist is likely to assess, intervene and reassess within a single 30-minute session. The therapist might also deliver care (e.g. changing soiled clothes or taking to the toilet); give counselling and information; educate carers; and contact other agencies involved.

Outcome

Measurement of outcome after rehabilitation should relate to the expressed aim of the service, and the broad areas are given in Table 10.3. If the aim given earlier is accepted, then it should ideally concentrate upon a patient's handicap, a patient's satisfaction with his/her new lifestyle (in contrast to satisfaction with the service) and a patient's emotional state. Although not explicitly stated

Table 10.3 Audit of rehabilitation: outcome – handicap, satisfaction, emotion, carer

Handicap (all measured in relation to patient's viewpoint)
Accommodation achieved
Support required and provided
Satisfying occupation of time
Level of social integration and interaction
Roles within society

Satisfaction with new lifestyle

Level of emotional distress

Stress on carer
Physical
Emotional
Social/financial

among the aims of the service given earlier, in reality one must also be concerned about the carers and almost certainly there should also be some measure of stress on unpaid carers.

In practice, measurement of handicap is difficult and it is reasonable to concentrate upon disability, which is more easily measured. Again, the measures chosen will depend upon the expressed aim of the service. Some of the many available measures are given later (Appendix 1), and Table 10.4 outlines some broad areas of concern.

Table 10.4 Audit of rehabilitation: outcome – disability measures

Social independence
Personal ADL independence
　Mobility
　Dexterity
Domestic ADL independence
Community ADL independence

Occupation of time
Work, ability and achievement
Leisure, ability and achievement

Social interaction
Communication (speech, etc.)
Interpersonal interaction

Cognitive independence
Bureaucratic independence
Memory, planning, initiative

Interpretation of outcome measures requires two cautions. Firstly, there needs to be a clear distinction between the measurement of outcome after rehabilitation (or any other medical process) as part of audit on the one hand and, on the other hand, planned scientific research into whether the process is effective. In other words, audit should record what the outcome was and neither the clinicians nor the purchasers should consider that the results prove any cause and effect between process and outcome. Sometimes there will be external proof of a relationship, but this is rare. Audit is not a substitute for research.

The second caution is that outcome measures can only be interpreted in relation to many variables. The diagnosis is one, and its importance is that it usually determines which 'field' of natural history applies. However, there is no other connection between pathological diagnosis and either the use of resources or the eventual outcome. The second major determinant is the severity of the presenting illness in the individual patient. This is usually best measured using impairments. For example, after stroke prognosis relates to the extent of motor loss, the presence of hemianopia and the extent of cognitive impairment (neglect or aphasia).

While both the above determinants of outcome and resource use are sometimes recognized (though not often by purchasers) and both can be measured, the third and probably major determinant is outside the influence of the health service. It is the patient's social setting: the family, finances, housing, employment, etc. Much research shows that variations in length of stay are strongly influenced by factors beyond the immediate diagnosis and disability (Wade & Langton Hewer, 1985; Rondinelli et al., 1991).

Therefore, in order to interpret outcome measures in audit, it is vital to have accurate information on case mix, including diagnosis, severity of initial impairment or disability (and severity on admission to service, if later) and as many social items as possible, especially whether or not the patient lives alone.

Case-mix measures

In any audit on rehabilitation information about case mix is of vital importance for several reasons.

Economically, the resources used by a rehabilitation service depend vitally upon the case mix, and the diagnosis itself is of minor importance. This is especially the case for in-patient rehabilitation. The major resource implications of disabled patients are the use of personnel, especially for providing care. This is a fixed cost. In practice, there are few identifiable variable costs (specific consumables or pieces of equipment or procedures). Simply counting numbers of patients and/or lengths of stay is of no value because patients vary so greatly.

Of equal importance is the use of information on case mix to interpret outcome data. For example, if a service specializes in treating patients with multiple, complex problems, its outcomes will appear much worse than a second centre which only accepts 'easy, straightforward' cases.

Lastly, and of concern to purchasers responsible for ensuring equity in the distribution of resources, information about case mix allows the specific service to be set in the context of the total needs of its community. Rehabilitation is or should be equally appropriate and available to all those in need in the community, but this can only be checked using epidemiological information coupled with information on the patients seen in each component service within the community.

This aspect of audit, referred to by Hopkins (1990) as 'system characteristics', covers such areas as relevance to the community, equity in delivery of service and the accessibility the acceptability of

Table 10.5 Audit of rehabilitation: case-mix information

Diagnosis
To determine expected natural history, prognosis, etc.

Severity of initial/admission impairments
Especially prognostic items

Severity of initial/admission disability
Same measures as outcome
Pre-existing disability

Social background
Living alone or with carers
Type of house and housing
Financial resources
Employment status
Family status

the service provided. Some possible questions of interest are shown in Table 10.5.

Audit in practice

Undertaking audit is still a new activity, and most experience relates to acute medical conditions, often with well-defined outcomes such as death. Relatively little has been published on audit in rehabilitation. Therefore this section will largely outline personal ideas, which themselves need testing.

Clinical audit (case-note review)

As usually discussed, clinical audit consists of review of one or more sets of case notes by professional colleagues, usually concentrating upon some specific aspect of management. Much of this type of audit consists of checking that the process undertaken in the individual cases complies with generally accepted standards for the process of rehabilitation.

Traditional clinical audit is difficult for several reasons. There is little agreement even on what constitutes rehabilitation, let alone what constitutes a reasonable standard. There is little evidence to guide clinicians in their management, and many decisions are based purely upon opinion (otherwise known as prejudice). Rehabilitation is a team effort, and it is not sensible to restrict audit to intra-professional audit; an excellent physiotherapy department scoring highly on national criteria might still be part of a very poor service not helping patients. Also, there is one major practical problem in medical circles: the rarity of people who are sufficiently specialized, experienced and well recognized to undertake review of case notes. Lastly, clinical audit is extremely time-consuming.

None the less, clinical audit is perhaps the easiest place to start, and is probably especially useful when the service is relatively small and isolated, because there is less informal peer review in that setting.

As an extension of this approach, one can select some special aspect of the service for audit. This might be a group of patients (e.g. stroke patients, patients with amnesia) or a specific procedure (e.g. use of ankle–foot orthoses) or a component of the process (e.g. documentation of goal-planning).

A random or complete sample of patients' notes would then be surveyed.

Service audit

On a larger scale, one could audit the whole service, documenting the case mix and the outcome. We have done this at Rivermead Rehabilitation Centre. Diagnosis is recorded using International Classification of Diseases (ICD) codes, which have been tested for reliability (Wood et al., 1989). Other demographic information is recorded, especially whether or not they have a carer – 15% do not. The major impairments recorded are motor loss, using the motricity index; trunk control, using the trunk control test; memory and orientation, using the short orientation memory concentration test; neglect, using the star cancellation test; and post-traumatic amnesia (PTA), assessed clinically. The major disabilities measured are independence in activities of daily living (ADL), using the Barthel index; mobility, using gait speed and the Rivermead mobility index; communication, using the Frenchay aphasia screening test (FAST); and dexterity, using the nine-hole peg test (NHPT). The information is collected routinely on admission and discharge by the doctor.

The main lessons learned so far are as follows. It is quite possible and easy to collect the information, but good guidelines are needed because the junior doctor changes every 3 months, and most have no experience of neurological disability or measurement. The audit system needs close monitoring. Secondly, although many patients did show improvement, particularly in mobility, we did not show improvement in many patients because we did not use measures able to detect the improvement. Consequently, we are now using a measure of extended ADL, and we may in future use a measure of life satisfaction in a postal follow-up questionnaire.

So far we have discussed audit of rehabilitation in relation to individual patients, but in practice most good services do more than simply treat the patients referred. For example, most services will be involved in education and training, and a (disappointingly) small number will be involved in research. Other legitimate activities include supporting voluntary services and support groups (such

Table 10.6 Audit of the rehabilitation service

Is there evidence of:
Continuing education of staff within service?
Involvement in research?
Providing education to other staff?
Responding to new information/research?
Change in response to previous audit?
Clinical audit?
Explicit aims for the service?

In relation to community served, is there evidence of:
Efficiency?
   Appropriate length of involvement?
   Non-excessive use of resources?
Effectiveness?
   Involvement with all appropriate patients?
Equity?
   Equally easy access to service?
   No bias in acceptance/refusal?
Relevance?
   Are there more important problems to address?
Acceptability?

In its running, does the service have:
Easy referral to the service?
Monitoring of patients not seen?
Explicit, reasonable prioritization?

as Headway), hosting specialist meetings and being involved in service planning. Therefore any audit of a service should consider the questions shown in Table 10.6.

Next, as stressed earlier, the service must not only consider the patients referred and accepted but also patients never referred but who might benefit, and patients referred but rejected for some reason. This must be considered in any audit.

Measures

An audit involves giving an (oral) account of resources used, which requires quantification. Measures are vital at all stages of audit, and should be used throughout clinical rehabilitation. This last section discusses measures, giving examples of measures found useful in normal clinical practice. It can only outline possible measures, and more details about measurement are available elsewhere (Wade, 1992). The measures fall into the four areas of pathology, impairment, disability and handicap.

Table 10.7 shows the measures recommended (with references), and most are shown in the Appendix at the end of this chapter. There are many measures available and readers are strongly advised to review existing measures before developing new ones.

Pathology (diagnosis)

Although the medical diagnosis is not the major determinant of resources needed, it is none the less of vital importance both in planning rehabilitation and in evaluating outcome, because the natural history and prognosis are determined by pathology. The traditional method of recording the diagnosis is the ICD, but this is probably inaccurate and unreliable (Wood *et al.*, 1989). Moreover, it is often inappropriate in rehabilitation.

Personal experience shows that the rehabilitation diagnosis of 'head injury' is rarely recorded as such. The systems used try to be far too specific (e.g. giving subdural haematoma or skull fracture as the primary diagnosis). Stroke, as a second example, is subdivided into several categories, whereas the rehabilitation requirement is simply to identify a vascular disease, giving focal damage which is likely to improve over the first 6 months. Spinal cord injuries can also have several possible ICD codes. Rehabilitation services should develop and use their own diagnoses, reflecting the level of precision relevant to their needs. Of course, the system should relate to the ICD to allow comparisons to be made.

Impairment

Measures of impairment usually relate well to the severity of the initial pathology. For example the extent of motor loss is a good prognostic measure for stroke (Wade & Langton Hewer, 1987), and the duration of PTA is the best prognostic measure for head injury (but not very good).

In clinical practice, the most important measures of impairment are likely to be motor loss (including trunk control); neglect; aphasia; memory loss; and (in head injury) PTA. There are, of course, many other impairments seen. Some, such as abnormal control of eye movement or abnormal sensation, are common and important but difficult to measure; others, such as apraxia or dystonia, are less common

Table 10.7 Measures for use in service audit

Audit item	Measure	Reference
Demography		
Gender		
Age		
Living arrangements		
Alone/carers?		
Ownership of accommodation		
Structure of accommodation		
History and process		
Delay: onset → admission		
Length of stay/involvement		
Complications		
Pathology		
Diagnosis	ICD, limited detail	
Impairments		
Motor loss	Motricity index	Collin & Wade, 1990
Trunk control	Trunk control test	Collin & Wade, 1990
Orientation and memory	Short orientation−memory−concentration test	Katzman *et al.*, 1983
	Rivermead behavioural memory test (RBMT), if detail needed	Wilson *et al.*, 1989
Neglect	Star cancellation test	Halligan *et al.*, 1989
Aphasia	Frenchay aphasia screening test	Enderby *et al.*, 1986
Hemianopia, other sensory loss	Clinical	
Disability		
Personal ADL	Barthel ADL index	Collin *et al.*, 1988
Domestic and community ADL	Nottingham EADL index	Nouri & Lincoln, 1987
	Frenchay activities index	Wade *et al.*, 1985
Memory	RBMT	
Mobility	Gait speed	Wade *et al.*, 1987; Collen *et al.*, 1990
	Rivermead mobility index	Collen *et al.*, 1991
Dexterity	Nine-hole peg test (NHPT)	Heller *et al.*, 1987
Handicap		
Possible measures	WHO ICIDH	WHO, 1980
	Glasgow outcome scale	Jennet *et al.*, 1981
Miscellaneous		
Satisfaction	Life satisfaction index	Viitanen *et al.*, 1988; Fugl-Meyer *et al.*, 1991
Emotional distress	General health questionnaire	Goldberg & Hillier, 1979
	Hospital anxiety and depression scale (HADs)	Zigmond & Snaith, 1983
Carer stress	General health questionnaire	

although they may be vital when present. In the routine collection of data, one has to concentrate upon the common, measurable and relevant impairments; in individual patients one must concentrate upon the relevant impairments for that person with his/her disease. The two will not always coincide but should usually overlap.

Disability

There are very many measures of disability, but most are poorly developed. In practice, fortunately, one can choose relatively few for routine use, and one rarely needs disease-specific measures. Most measures used will concentrate upon independence in the activity (i.e. they are qualitative) but some measure speed or some other aspect of performance.

The measures need to cover the broad areas of personal ADL, mobility, dexterity, domestic and community ADL, communication and social interaction (i.e. the 'behaviour' problems seen sometimes). There are reasonable measures for some of these areas, but not all.

Handicap

Measurement of handicap is at present very difficult, not least because there is no real agreement on the definition of handicap. The WHO (1980) *International Classification of Impairments, Disabilities and Handicaps* (ICIDH) does offer six areas, each with a scale, and these can be used relatively easily. However, there have been no studies on validity and reliability of the whole group; the physical independence scale has been used and developed.

Conclusion

Audit in neurological rehabilitation has scarcely started in a formal way, and may be difficult. However, the principles of audit should be second nature to anyone involved in rehabilitation, as the processes involved are identical. The most important steps to take include defining the aims of the service, so that appropriate outcome measures can be chosen, and collecting information relevant to case mix. There are now acceptable measures for most outcomes of interest, although better ones can always be developed.

Appendix 1: Sources of measures mentioned in text

Frenchay aphasia screening test (FAST)
General health questionnaire (GHQ)
From: NFER-Nelson, Darville House, 2 Oxford Road East, Berks SL4 1DF.

Rivermead behavioural memory test (RBMT)
Behavioural inattention test (BIT)
From: Thames Valley Test Company, 7–9 The Green, Flempton, Bury St Edmunds, Suffolk IP28 6EL.

Copies of test sheets shown in Appendix 2 (and others) can be obtained from: Test Department, Rivermead Rehabilitation Centre, Abingdon Road, Oxford OX1 4XD.

Appendix 2: Tests

Barthel ADL index

Bowels   ....
0 = Incontinent
1 = Occasional accident
2 = Continent

Bladder   ....
0 = Incontinent or catheterized and unable to manage
1 = Occasional accident (max 1 per 24 hours)
2 = Continent (for over 7 days)

Grooming   ....
0 = Needs help
1 = Independent, face / hair / teeth / shaving

Toilet use   ....
0 = Dependent
1 = Needs some help but can do something
2 = Independent (on and off, dressing, wiping)

Feeding   ....
0 = Unable
1 = Needs help cutting, spreading butter, etc.
2 = Independent

Transfer   ....
0 = Unable
1 = Major help (1–2 people, physical)
2 = Minor help (verbal or physical)
3 = Independent

Mobility   ....
0 = Immobile
1 = Wheelchair independent including corners, etc.
2 = Walks with help of 1 person (verbal or physical)
3 = Independent (but may use any aid, e.g. stick)

Dressing   ....
0 = Dependent
1 = Needs help, but can do half unaided
2 = Independent

Stairs   ....
0 = Unable
1 = Needs help (verbal, physical, carrying aid)
2 = Independent up and down

Bathing   ....
0 = Dependent
1 = Independent

Total   _____

Life satisfaction questionnaire

How satisfactory are these different aspects of your life?

Circle the number which best suits your situation.

1: Very dissatisfying
2: Dissatisfying
3: Rather dissatisfying
4: Rather satisfying
5: Satisfying
6: Very satisfying

Life as a whole is	1	2	3	4	5	6
My ability to manage my self-care (dressing, hygiene, transfers, etc.) is	1	2	3	4	5	6
My leisure situation is	1	2	3	4	5	6
My vocational situation is	1	2	3	4	5	6
My financial situation is	1	2	3	4	5	6
My sexual life is	1	2	3	4	5	6
My partnership relation is	1	2	3	4	5	6
My family life is	1	2	3	4	5	6
My contacts with friends and acquaintances are	1	2	3	4	5	6

Rivermead mobility index

Name: ....

Score: **No = 0**   **Yes = 1**

Date:

1   Do you turn over from your back to your side
    without help?

2   From lying in bed, do you get up to sit on the edge
    of the bed on your own?

3   Do you sit on the edge of the bed without holding on
    for 10 seconds?

4   Do you stand up (from any chair) in less than 15 seconds,
    and stand there for 15 seconds (using hands,
    and with an aid if necessary)?

5   Observe standing for 10 seconds without any aid

6   Do you manage to move from bed to chair and back
    without any help?

7   Do you walk 10m, with an aid if necessary,
    but with no standby help?

8   Do you manage a flight of stairs alone, without help?

9   Do you walk around outside alone, on pavements?

10 Do you walk 10m inside with no caliper, splint or
    aid and no standby help?

11 If you drop something on the floor, do you manage
    to walk 5m, pick it up and then walk back?

12 Do you walk over uneven ground (grass, gravel,
    dirt, snow, ice, etc.) without help?

13 Do you get in/out of bath or shower unsupervised
    and wash yourself?

14 Do you manage to go up and down four steps with no rail,
    but using an aid if necessary?

15 Do you run 10m without limping in 4 seconds
    (fast walk is acceptable)?

Total

Short orientation, memory and concentration test

Name: ....

		Date:				

Instruction   Possible scores

1 What year is it now?   0,4

                                       Answer ___ ___ ___ ___

2 What month is it now?   0,3

                                       Answer ___ ___ ___ ___

3 Repeat this address:

   (a) Arthur / Jones   (b) Joe / Smith   (c) Tom / White   (d) Philip / Winter
        42 / West Street   34 / Church Road   26 / Station Road   18 / North Way
        Witney   Banbury   Aylesbury   Oxford

   Try and remember this, I'll ask you at the end of the test to recall it.

4 About what time is it?   0,3
   (within one hour)

                                       Answer ___ ___ ___ ___

5 Count backwards 20 to 1   0,2,4

   20 19 18 17 16 15 14 13 12 11 10 9 8 7 6 5 4 3 2 1

6 Say months in reverse order   0,2,4
   Dec Nov Oct Sept Aug July June May April Mar Feb Jan

7 Repeat the address given   0,2,4,6,8,10

                                   Address given ___ ___ ___ ___
                                   (a,b,c,d)

   Total score (/28)

Motricity index and trunk control test

Name: ....   **Date:**

Side (L or R)

Arm (to be conducted in sitting position)

1 Pinch grip
   2.5cm cube between thumb and forefinger

2 Elbow flexion
   from 90, voluntary contraction/movement

3 Shoulder abduction
   from against chest

Leg (to be conducted in sitting position)

4 Ankle dorsiflexion
   from plantar flexed position

5 Knee extension
   from 90, voluntary contraction/movement

6 Hip flexion
   Usually from 90

Arm score $(1 + 2 + 3) + 1$

Leg score $(4 + 5 + 6) + 1$

Side score $(Arm + Leg) / 2$

Trunk control test (to be conducted on the bed)

1 Rolling to weak side

2 Rolling to strong side

3 Sitting up from lying down

4 Balance in sitting position (on side of bed)

Trunk score $(1 + 2 + 3 + 4)$

Scoring
   Test 1   (Pinch grip)
      0   No movement
     11   Beginnings of prehension (any movement of finger or thumb)
     19   Grips cube, but unable to hold against gravity
     22   Grips cube, held against gravity, but not against weak pull
     26   Grips cube against pull, but weaker than on other side
     33   Normal pinch grip

   Tests 2–6
      0   No movement
      9   Palpable contraction in muscle, but no movement
     14   Movement seen, but no full range / not against gravity
     19   Movement; full range against gravity, not against resistance
     25   Movement against resistance, but weaker than other side
     33   Normal power

   Trunk control test
      0   Unable to do on own
     12   Able to do, but only with non-muscular help — pulling on bedclothes, using arms to steady self
          when sitting, pulling up on monkey pole, etc.
     25   Able to complete normally

Nottingham extended ADL assessment

Answers:
0 = Not at all
1 = With help
2 = *Alone* with difficulty
3 = *Alone* easily

Questions

Mobility
Do you:

walk around outside? _____

climb stairs? _____

get in and out of the car? _____

walk over uneven ground? _____

cross roads? _____

travel on public transport? _____

Total _____

In the kitchen
Do you:

manage to feed yourself? _____

manage to make yourself a hot drink? _____

take hot drinks from one room to another? _____

do the washing up? _____

make yourself a hot snack? _____

Total _____

Domestic tasks
Do you:

manage your own money when you are out? _____

wash small items of clothing? _____

do your own shopping? _____

do a full clothes wash? _____

Total _____

Leisure activities
Do you:

read newspapers or books? _____

use the telephone? _____

write letters? _____

go out socially? _____

manage your own garden? _____

drive a car? _____

Total _____

Frenchay activities index

Score	Activity	Code (score)

In the last three months

———————	Preparing main meals	0 = Not at all
———————	Washing up	1 = Under once weekly
		2 = 1–2 times/week
		3 = Most days
———————	Washing clothes	0 = Never
———————	Light housework	1 = 1–2 times in three months
———————	Heavy housework	2 = 3–12 times in three months
———————	Local shopping	3 = At least weekly
———————	Social occasions	
———————	Walking outside > 15 mins	
———————	Actively pursuing hobby	
———————	Driving car/going on bus	

In the last six months

———————	Travel outings / car rides	0 = Never
		1 = 1–2 times in 6 months
———————		3 = 3–12 times in 6 months
		4 = At least twice weekly
———————	Gardening	0 = Never
———————	Household/car maintenance	1 = Light
		2 = Moderate
		3 = All necessary
———————	Reading books	0 = None
		1 = One in 6 months
		2 = Less than one in fortnight
		3 = Over one each fortnight
———————	Gainful work	0 = None
		1 = Up to 10 hours/week
		2 = 10–30 hours/week
		3 = Over 30 hours/week
———————/45	Total	

References

Collen F.M., Wade D.T. & Bradshaw C.M. (1990) Mobility after stroke: reliability of measures of impairment and disability. *International Disability Studies* **12**, 6−9.

Collen F.M., Wade D.T., Robb G.F. & Bradshaw C.M. (1991) The Rivermead mobility index, a further development of the Rivermead motor assessment. *International Disability Studies* **13**, 50−54.

Collin C. & Wade D.T. (1990) Assessing motor impairment after stroke: a pilot reliability study. *Journal of Neurology, Neurosurgery and Psychiatry* **53**, 567−569.

Collin C., Wade D.T., Davis S. & Horne V. (1988) The Barthel ADL index: a reliability study. *International Disability Studies* **10**, 61−63.

Davis A.M., Davis S., Moss N., Marks J., McGrath J., Hovard L., Axon J. & Wade D.T. (1992) First steps towards an interdisciplinary approach to rehabilitation. *Clinical Rehabilitation* **6**, 237−244.

Enderby P.M., Wood V.A., Wade D.T. & Langton Hewer R. (1986) The Frenchay aphasia screening test: a short, simple test for aphasia appropriate for non-specialists. *International Rehabilitation Medicine* **8**, 166−170.

Epstein A.M., Stern R.S., Tognetti J. *et al.* (1988) The association of patient's socioeconomic characteristics with the length of hospital stay and hospital charges within diagnosis-related groups. *New England Journal of Medicine* **318**, 1579−1585.

Fugl-Meyer A.R., Branholm I. & Fugl-Meyer K.S. (1991) Happiness and domain-specific life satisfaction in adult northern Swedes. *Clinical Rehabilitation* **5**, 25−33.

Goldberg D.P. & Hillier V.F. (1979) A scaled version of the general health questionnaire. *Psychological Medicine* **9**, 139−145.

Halligan P.W., Marshall J.C. & Wade D.T. (1989) Visuo-spatial neglect: underlying factors and test sensitivity. *Lancet* **ii**, 908−910.

Heller A., Wade D.T., Wood V.A., Sunderland A., Langton Hewer R. & Ward E. (1987) Arm function after stroke: measurement and recovery over the first three months. *Journal of Neurology, Neurosurgery and Psychiatry* **50**, 714−719.

Hopkins A. (1990) *Measuring the Quality of Medical Care*. Royal College of Physicians, London.

Jennett B., Snoek J., Bond M.R. *et al.* (1981) Disability after severe head injury: observations on the use of the Glasgow outcome scale. *Journal of Neurology, Neurosurgery and Psychiatry* **44**, 285−293.

Katzman R., Brown T., Fuld P., Peck A., Schechter R. & Schimmel H. (1983) Validation of a short orientation−memory−concentration test of cognitive impairment. *American Journal of Psychiatry* **140**, 734−739.

McGrath J.R. & Davis A.M. (1992) Rehabilitation: where are we going and how do we get there? *Clinical Rehabilitation* **6**, 225−235.

Nouri F.M. & Lincoln N.B. (1987) An extended activities of daily living scale for stroke patients. *Clinical Rehabilitation* **1**, 301−305.

Rondinelli R.D., Murphy J.R., Wilson D.H. & Miller C.C. (1991) Predictors of functional outcome and resource utilisation in inpatient rehabilitation. *Archive of Physical Medicine and Rehabilitation* **72**, 447−453.

Tinson D.J. (1989) How stroke patients spend their days. *International Disability Studies* **11**, 45−49.

Viitanen M., Fugl-Meyer K.S., Bernspang B. & Fugl-Meyer A.R. (1988) Life satisfaction in long-term survivors after stroke. *Scandinavian Journal of Rehabilitation Medicine* **20**, 17−24.

Wade D.T. (1990) Neurological rehabilitation. In Kennard C. (ed.) *Recent Advances in Clinical Neurology*, Vol. 6, Ch. 5, pp. 133−156. Churchill Livingstone, London.

Wade D.T. (1992) *Measurement in Neurological Rehabilitation*. Oxford University Press, Oxford.

Wade D.T. & Langton Hewer R. (1985) Hospital admission for acute stroke: who, for how long, and to what effect? *Journal of Epidemiology and Community Health* **39**, 347−352.

Wade D.T. & Langton Hewer R. (1987) Motor loss and swallowing difficulty after stroke: frequency, recovery and prognosis. *Acta Neurologica Scandinavica* **76**, 50−54.

Wade D.T., Legh-Smith J. & Langton-Hewer R. (1985) Social activities after stroke: measurement and natural history using the Frenchay activities index. *International Rehabilitation Medicine* **7**, 176−181.

Wade D., Wood V., Heller A., Maggs J. & Langton Hewer R. (1987) Walking after stroke: measurement and recovery over the first three months. *Scandinavian Journal of Rehabilitation Medicine* **9**, 25−30.

Wilson B.A., Cockburn J., Baddeley A.D. & Hiorns R.W. (1989) The development and validation of a test battery for detecting and monitoring everyday memory problems. *Journal of Clinical Experimental Neuropsychology* **11**, 855−870.

Wood V.A., Wade D.T., Langton-Hewer R. & Campbell M.J. (1989) The development of a disease classification system based on the International Classification of Disease, for use by neurologists. *Journal of Neurology, Neurosurgery and Psychiatry* **52**, 449−458.

World Health Organization (WHO) (1980) *The International Classification of Impairments, Disabilities, and Handicaps*. World Health Organization, Geneva.

Zigmond A.S. & Snaith R.P. (1983) The hospital anxiety and depression scale. *Acta Psychiatrica Scandinavica* **67**, 361−370.

Part 4
The Neurological Patient

11: Rehabilitation: the Role of Remedial Therapy

L.S. ILLIS

The untreated patient, 133
Does rehabilitation improve functional ability?, 134
Physiotherapy, 134
    Early intervention, 134
    Types of physiotherapy, 135
    Specific physiotherapy procedures, 136
Family and social care, 138
Counselling, 138
Occupational therapy, 139
Stimulation techniques, 139
Conclusion, 139

Rehabilitation, as is often stated, implies the use of medical, social, educational and vocational measures for restoring the individual to the highest level of physical, mental and social ability in the shortest possible time. In most instances, rehabilitation must involve a continuing programme, although the degree of involvement may vary from time to time.

Physiotherapy is the core of rehabilitation, but family and social care and occupational therapy are essential parts of the rehabilitation process. In the best departments, occupational therapists and social workers work in close liaison with physiotherapists and, indeed, in many hospitals the physiotherapists themselves instigate family care and occupational therapy.

The fact that physiotherapy lies at the centre of most rehabilitation programmes, and that physical disability is not only the most obvious problem but the easiest in which to observe improvement, has meant that this has become the focus of attention of patient, family and staff. Physical progress usually dictates the timing of discharge and this has tended to produce neglect of the psychological consequences of neurological disability. Clearly early improvement in physical disability will itself be part of psychological care, but the long-term emotional and social as well as physical care should be planned at the onset.

Although the future must lie in the fields of regrowth and connection of nerve fibres, in the development of genetic engineering techniques to encourage growth connection and in the use of pharmacological techniques, any improvement produced will give only limited benefit if physical therapy measures are not utilized as well. It is essential that the highest level of functional ability is maintained: for example, regrowth of nerve fibres will not suffice to restore function if the patient cannot sustain weight-bearing or joint movement or if contractures have occurred. Even where specific medical treatment is available, e.g. in Parkinson's disease or subacute combined degeneration of the cord, physiotherapy has a definite and considerable role.

All rehabilitation measures must rely upon accurate assessment. This is essential in order to plan rehabilitation programmes and to delineate goals, and also as a means of monitoring progress and validating therapy. Clinical and physiological assessment are dealt with in other chapters in this volume.

The untreated patient

Completely untreated patients are rare. However, it is worth bearing in mind that untreated patients with neurological involvement affecting respiratory muscles and who are unable to cough effectively will drown in their own secretions. Patients may develop ileus or dilatation of the stomach, and may die of inhalation of vomit. Patients who are untreated will almost certainly develop severe pressure sores with secondary infection and urinary tract infections. Osteomyelitis and septicaemia will ensue, and patients who survive this will die of urinary tract complications on a background of increasing contractures and spasticity.

Does rehabilitation improve functional ability?

Many of the earlier reports of functional improvement with rehabilitation programmes were uncontrolled. However, the development of specific stroke units allowed better trials which showed more definite benefit, although most of these trials still remain poorly controlled. These trials indicate that in specialized stroke units, compared with treatment on general medical wards, the benefits include:

1 Improved outcome for patients with moderate disability (McCann & Culbertson, 1976).

2 Better hospital discharge rate and better functional result (Dow *et al.*, 1974; Feigenson *et al.*, 1979).

3 Faster improvement in early stages (not sustained) (Garraway *et al.*, 1980a, b; Hamrin, 1982a, b; Smith *et al.*, 1982).

These good results must be set against reports that it is natural recovery and not intensive physical therapy which is most important (Lind, 1982), and negative or inconclusive reports (Feldman *et al.*, 1962; Gordon & Kohn, 1966; Brockelhurst *et al.*, 1978).

There are many patients who are considered unsuitable for rehabilitation because of poor facilities or restricted access to facilities, or the patient is thought to be too old, etc. O'Neill and colleagues (1987) reported an interesting study of 'slow-stream' rehabilitation and showed that, of 52 patients admitted to the unit, 45 were eventually discharged home or to nursing homes. Before slow-stream rehabilitation was introduced, only three patients would have been discharged. Unfortunately, this potentially important study, like so many in this field, was not randomized or controlled and the actual therapy used is not described.

The fact remains, unfortunately, that, although most clinicians and perhaps all physiotherapists think that physiotherapy definitely aids functional recovery, the statistical evidence is lacking. This is of particular interest in the case of specific physiotherapy procedures (see below). However, the lack of statistical significance should not detract from

some very obvious advantages of physiotherapy treatment, such as prevention of complications, improvement in posture and retraining of muscles, as well as an often overlooked benefit: the marked improvement in patient and family morale.

Physiotherapy

The modern physiotherapist is concerned with the whole patient and the maintenance of total body function and not just joint range and muscle power. Most clinicians and therapists believe the patient with a neurological problem needs physiotherapy early and needs it frequently. The choice of the type of therapy is usually left to the physiotherapist but, if the clinician is to keep some kind of control over treatment (and a glance at specific therapeutic procedures later in this chapter should alert the clinician to this need), then it is essential to have a working knowledge of the types of therapy available. The quality of physiotherapy will determine the outcome and the quality of therapy depends on the quality of the physiotherapist. A good physiotherapy department can transform a neurological unit.

Early intervention

The precise stage of mobilization depends on the presence or otherwise of specific limitations, such as fracture. Where there is no such disturbance, the aim is nearly always to mobilize the patient as early as possible. In those cases where bedrest is essential, nursing on a special turning bed should avoid the occurrence of pressure areas. Improvement is most likely to occur during the first 3 months, but therapy should continue to prevent the occurrence of complications and deterioration.

Posturing and positioning are carried out in such a way as to keep muscles, joints and limbs in a neutral position in order to avoid contractures, with frequent corrections of the patient's position. It is a truism that rehabilitation starts as soon as the injury or lesion occurs, and the importance of this is best seen in the care of joints and muscles, since contractures are likely to become pronounced within the first few weeks if treatment is delayed. This is particularly important in patients with spinal problems. But passive movements also have a major role, not only in the early stages, but in the late stages of many conditions, such as when spasticity is marked in patients with multiple sclerosis.

Passive and active movement is not only necessary from the point of view of preventing pressure areas and improving cardiovascular function, but also in the prevention of para-articular ossification. Such therapy early on in the condition also has a marked effect on the patient's morale.

Eventually, paralysed limbs will begin to demineralize, and as a result paralysed patients are more prone to fracture, sometimes from relatively minor trauma. The progress of demineralization can be prevented to some extent by regular weight-bearing. In specific cases, such as a high spinal cord lesion, blood-pressure control may be impaired or abolished, and it is then necessary to mobilize the patient very slowly into the sitting position, with careful monitoring of blood pressure. Sometimes it may be necessary to use limb cuffs.

More specific aspects of rehabilitation should be a joint effort by the therapist and the patient. Important aspects, such as spasticity, the management of cardiovascular abnormalities, bladder management, the treatment of pain, etc., are dealt with in detail in specific chapters, and these accounts will not be reiterated here.

The treatment of skin care is a good example of the importance of the involvement of both patient and therapist. The patient must be fully aware of the fact that lack of sensation is likely to produce pressure sores. The patient must be taught to alter posture and to lift the body for short periods and at regular intervals. Daily inspection of skin over pressure areas is an important part of prophylaxis, and this must be explained to the patient and to relatives or carers.

Early introduction of rehabilitation, particularly by skilled therapists, may be more beneficial than the actual duration of treatment. This was well demonstrated by Smith et al.'s (1982) controlled trial of rehabilitation. In this study a total of 307 stroke patients were randomly assigned to treatment in a designated rehabilitation unit or to an ordinary medical unit. The cut-off point was 16 weeks after admission. Patients in the rehabilitation unit received less therapy over a shorter period of time but achieved independence much earlier than those in the non-specialized medical units.

Types of physiotherapy

Physiotherapy procedures are conventionally described as active and passive. The following account is a summary and the reader is referred to physiotherapy manuals for further details.

Passive

Heat

For many painful conditions, heat, using any source of heat, including hot-water bottles, wax baths and electromagnetic radiation, has a palliative effect.

Short-wave diathermy

This is said to produce deep heat, but there is little objective evidence for this.

Ultrasound

High-frequency ultrasound is said to produce mechanical heating and possibly chemical effects, and there is some experimental evidence for accelerated healing.

Ice

Ice therapy is used in the treatment of spasticity (see Chapter 24) and also in the alleviation of acute pain.

Electrotherapy

Electrical stimulation of muscles may be helpful in retraining of muscles after surgical transplantation or in maintaining poorly used muscles.

Massage

This is soothing and palliative. Combined with aromatic oils, it is a form of therapy which has entered the realms of fantasy.

Active

Exercise therapy

This is the major part of a physiotherapist's work. The types of exercise and the number of their proponents are legion. They include exercises for muscle strength, speed of contraction and co-ordination, isometric and isotonic exercises, exercises with apparatus, free exercises, etc. They all have some benefit, not only physically. Even apparently minor benefit in posture and gait may have a profound effect on the patient's confidence and thus on function.

Traction

Continuous or intermittent traction may be applied to limbs, neck or back in the treatment of painful conditions. Therapeutic trials are nearly always uncontrolled and claims for treatment often unsubstantiated.

Specific physiotherapy procedures

Physicians are often baffled by the wide range of physiotherapy techniques, mostly named after the original describer and sometimes with a rather questionable scientific basis. The role of these techniques is sometimes questioned. Trials of physiotherapy and rehabilitation programmes are frequently uncontrolled and the results have ranged from improvement which could not be attributed to spontaneous recovery, to no benefit for mild or severely affected patients but significant benefit for those with moderate disabilities, to definite improvement in those patients who had rigorous physiotherapy and rehabilitation programmes carried out by specially trained staff. One of the problems in this field is that the selection criteria are not uniform. The type of rehabilitation or physiotherapy procedure tends to differ and is also applied by personnel with different training, sometimes in specialized units, sometimes in normal medical wards and sometimes as a cottage industry. Most trials seem to agree that rehabilitation produces recovery which is greater than that which can be expected from spontaneous return of function. Most trials also agree that rehabilitation should begin as soon as possible after the acute event and that the most marked improvement is achieved during the first few months but that rehabilitation should be continued for a much longer period in order to prevent any further deterioration.

Ernst (1990) has compared various types of physiotherapy procedure and he comes to the conclusion that 'all trials seem to convey the same message: the type of treatment does not matter as long as the stroke patient gets some sort of physiotherapy'. He adds the sobering thought that, if an optimal physical therapy exists, it has not yet been identified.

Modern physiotherapy not only includes the prevention of complications in limbs which are not functioning or are poorly functioning, and training normal muscles to compensate for loss of function, but also involves attempts to overcome the neurological disability in paralysed limbs. These newer techniques are often called 'facilitation therapy' or 'inhibition therapy', and are as much a part of modern physiotherapy as passive movements, massage and active exercises. Many of the facilitation and inhibition techniques were based, or were intended to be based, upon neurophysiological studies, and they were all developed as treatments for patients with cerebral problems, although the techniques can be used for patients with other types of neurological dysfunction (although not all proponents would agree with that last statement). Many of the techniques suppress spasticity, alter abnormal reflex activity and relieve spasm and pain, and are clearly applicable to patients with those particular symptoms even if the origin of the symptoms does not lie in a stroke illness.

Although the followers of particular schools emphasize the differences between them, the general principles are actually much the same.

The major facilitation techniques were described by Fay (1948), Kabat (1952), Rood (1954), Knott (1967), Brunnstrom (1970) and Bobath (1978) (Table 11.1).

The *Bobath* method and variations of it are based on the premise that movement is continuously modulated by afferent information. Neurological lesions alter the control exerted by afferent systems and unmask abnormal reflex activity. Stimulation of afferent systems, by adjustment of posture, by skin stimulation and by joint movement, are thought to suppress spasticity and pathological reflexes. The patient is then taught simple repetitive exercises which gradually build up to a return to controlled movement. Wagenaar *et al.* (1990) describes the *neurodevelopmental treatment* as a modernized version of the Bobath method. The description

Table 11.1 Specific physiotherapy procedures

Facilitation and inhibition techniques
Bobath
Fay
(Kabat)
Rood
(Knott)
Brunnstrom
Neurodevelopmental

Proprioceptive neuromuscular facilitation
Kabat
Knott

Electromyography (EMG) biofeedback

Conductive education (Peto)

includes the emergence of basic synergies as pathological manifestations of spasticity. The patient is taught to overcome these by using reflex inhibitory patterns or positions and thus to exert conscious control of muscle tone.

In the *Brunnstrom* approach, abnormal reflex patterns are broken down using facilitation techniques or sensory stimulation, such as the stretching and tapping of muscles. Proponents of this method describe the emergence of successive stages or patterns during the natural evolution of hemiplegia, from paralysis to 'flexion and extension synergies' and then to 'basic synergy patterns' plus 'associated movements'. Adherents deny any similarity to the Bobath method although both schools claim their techniques are based on the same neurophysiological principles. The similarities become closer, as each school, other than purists, appears to use similar aids.

Since the Bobath and neurodevelopmental approach, on the one hand, and the Brunnstrom method, on the other, apparently have such a different physiological rationale, one would expect to find a significant difference in outcome in patients treated with these techniques. Wagenaar *et al.* (1990) compared the effect of these methods in a small group of stroke patients and found no clear difference.

The *proprioceptive neuromuscular facilitation* school of Kabat and Knott is again based on the precept that motor behaviour is continuously modulated by sensory information, and not many people would

argue with that (see earlier chapters). Kabat designed patterns of movements which were intended to re-establish normal agonist–antagonist muscle action. Knott went a little further: the physiotherapist assists the patient's initial attempts at movement, so theoretically this would produce an afferent barrage from muscle spindles and Golgi tendon organs, i.e. 'proprioceptive neuromuscular facilitation'. As power and control improve, further training includes the application of resistance.

EMG *biofeedback* methods, sometimes called integrated behavioural physical therapy, consists of persuading the patient to be an active participant in treatment rather than a passive recipient. The biofeedback seems to consist of cutaneous electrodes, which are used to either recruit or inhibit specific muscles. The patient is taught EMG feedback goals and how to direct skills.

Basmajian *et al.* (1987) compared EMG biofeedback techniques with the neurofacilitatory technique of Bobath and could demonstrate no statistically significant difference between any of the variables measured. It should be noted here that not only is there no clear evidence of benefit of one technique versus another, the actual differences in techniques are far from clear. Wagenaar *et al.* (1990), for example, describe the neurodevelopmental treatment as a modernized version of the Bobath method: 'neurodevelopmental treatment being a modernized version of Bobath', while Basmajian *et al.* (1987) equate neurofacilitatory techniques with Bobath: 'strictly adhered to the principles described in Bobath's text'. Wagenaar *et al.* (1990) seem to list proprioceptive neuromuscular facilitation as a separate technique.

Is proprioceptive neuromuscular facilitation the same as the neurofacilitatory techniques? Is it the technique of Kabat or Knott or Bobath? If proprioceptive neuromuscular facilitation is the same as neurofacilitatory techniques, and neurofacilitation is the same as Bobath, and Bobath is the same as neurodevelopmental techniques and in any case there is no difference in outcome, it suggests that physical therapists need to get their house in order.

The Peto Institute in Budapest has developed a further approach to neurological disability which is called *conductive education*. This was developed about 40 years ago by a Hungarian physician,

Andras Peto. The thesis is the development or establishment of what is termed 'orthofunction'. This term is meant to signify a dynamic development and progression of adaptation which considers the changing biological and social requirements of the individual – or what the rest of the world presumably means by the restoration of patients to their fullest physical, mental and social capability (in the WHO definition).

In conductive education the individual is guided ('conducted') to 'realize his own will' (see Cottam & Sutton, 1986), and educated in terms of the education philosophy upon which the whole framework rests. Not surprisingly, this method has met with a degree of scepticism. However, it is claimed that the primary aims of stimulating development is based on neural plasticity and on learning theory, that is, on the re-establishing of new patterns of connection or the opening up of paths which are not normally used. The neuroanatomy and the neurophysiology is well established in experimental work (see earlier chapters). There are many anecdotal accounts of the effectiveness of this kind of treatment, but there are no properly structured trials at the time of writing.

Shields (1989) carried out a clinical evaluation of conductive education and concluded that there was improvement in the initiation of movement and independence as tested in a variety of tasks, and 'immeasurable yet important changes' were reported 'in the form of improved communication, a positive environment, positive expectations' – a conclusion which produces a wave of despair in a neurologist's environment, a failure of communication and a foundering of expectations.

All the above techniques, and variations of them, are widely used both by idealist adherents of a particular technique and, more commonly, by therapists using a combination of various facilitation techniques adapted to the individual patient and the specific neurological disability. Controlled trials which evaluate these different techniques or compare the facilitation techniques with a more traditional approach have not shown any definite benefit. This, however, should not detract from the fact that the techniques may actually produce a certain degree of restoration of function, but much more needs to be done in the form of rigorous assessment and controlled trials.

Family and social care

As indicated earlier, family and social care should not be separated from physiotherapy. Both the clinician in charge of the patient and all therapists should be aware of potential as well as actual problems. The degree of family and social care which can be provided and which is necessary depends partly on the type of disability, but also on factors which include financial status of the patient, the presence or absence of family members, and the presence of available social security. The failure of family support and the failure of social security are perhaps the greatest reason for institutional care and this should be borne in mind early on in the illness. Domiciliary services are available in most countries and should be instigated as early as possible, since structural adaptation in terms of handrails, alteration of bath and lavatory accommodation, etc., may be necessary.

Counselling

Counselling should include practical information both for the patient and for the family or carers. Counselling involves continuous advice and guidance and, where necessary, support. Obviously time must be set aside for communication between the doctor in charge of the case, the patient and the family. However, the need for continual counselling must be recognized by all members of the therapeutic team. Counselling is at various levels and includes, for example, the need for skin care, the management of bladder disability, advice about social security, and sexual counselling.

Group discussions between disabled patients are often useful, and in some instances groups of relatives or families may give active support to each other as well as to patients. Most disability groups have support associations and addresses of these associations are readily available in hospital outpatients and in social services departments. Holebrook (1982) has put forward a model for the adjustment to disability which is similar to models which have been put forward for bereavement. He identifies four stages which describe the reaction of families to patients with stroke illness, but the stages really apply to any kind of severe neurological disability. In the first stage, which is called *crisis*, the reactions of shock, confusion and anxiety are seen. In the second stage or the *treatment stage*, the patient and family often have a very high expectation of recovery, they tend to deny the possibility of permanent disability, fears for the future begin to surface and this includes the future as regards mobility, lifestyle, the ability to cope and employment. In the third stage, that of *realization of disability*, the reactions turn to anger, rejection, despair, frustration and depression. The final stage in this model is that of *adjustment*. It is important that the doctor in charge of the patient and the whole therapeutic team recognize these stages and the reactions that occur from the patient and from the family. With this recognition, counselling of the patient and the family is likely to be more logical and more successful.

Occupational therapy

There is usually some degree of ignorance as to the true role of occupational therapists in the management and treatment of patients with neurological disability. This is not entirely the fault of the clinician since many units have no access to occupational therapists. Perhaps the best way of summarizing the occupational therapist's role is to say that the therapist is involved in assessing not so much the functional disability as the patient's capability after a lesion or neurological insult has occurred. This assessment includes that of disability and handicap, together with the training of the patient in various techniques. It also involves collaboration with physiotherapists and with clinicians. The occupational therapist is involved in the application of aids and various tools for living and the training of patients to use them, together with education of the patient's family and carers in the use of such techniques.

At the Wessex Neurological Centre the occupational therapy service aims are:
1 To develop and maintain functional independence.
2 To help patients and carers to adjust to their change in circumstances.
3 To assess for specialist equipment and services in preparation for discharge.
4 To assist with discharge planning and carry out home assessments.

5 To link with the patient's local occupational therapist and other appropriate services outside the district.

As with physiotherapy, the aim of occupational therapy is to enable the patient to return home and to live as independently as possible.

Stimulation techniques

This is a large and gradually increasing field which started with the use of functional electrical stimulation some 30 years ago. This complex and wide field of therapy is dealt with in separate chapters and the reader is also referred to Illis (1992).

Conclusion

This short résumé of physiotherapy and remedial therapy should be seen in conjuction with the other specific chapters outlining treatment and interventional techniques. Rehabilitation cannot be separated from treatment as though it were an isolated speciality, but should be planned from the onset of the neurological insult and continued for as long as the neurological disability continues.

The fact that there is so much uncertainty about the types of physical therapy and the benefit which can be obtained is no fault of the therapists themselves. It is only recently that clinicians have become seriously interested in neurological rehabilitation. Good rehabilitation requires time and careful organizing. Ideally, neurological rehabilitation should be an integral part of every neurological/neurosurgical unit and all clinical neuroscience specialists should play some part in the rehabilitation of their patients. The overall organization and running of the department of neurological rehabilitation should be under a designated consultant in that speciality with an interest in and an obligation to both clinical and basic research.

For further details the reader is referred to the excellent book *Rehabilitation Medicine* by Dr P.J.R. Nichols (Butterworths).

References

Basmajian J.V., Gowland C.A., Finlayson A.J., Hall A.L., Swanson LR., Stratford P.W., Trotter J.E. & Brandstater M.E. (1987) Stroke treatment: comparison of integrated behavioural–physical therapy vs traditional physical therapy programs. *Archives of Physical and Medical Rehabilitation* **68**, 267–272.

Bobath B. (1978) *Adult Hemiplegia: Evaluation and Treatment.* Heinemann, London.

Brockelhurst J.C., Andrews K., Richards B. & Laycock P.J. (1978) How much physical therapy for patients with stroke? *British Medical Journal* **1**, 1307–1311.

Brunnstrom S. (1970) *Movement Therapy in Hemiplegia.* Harper & Row, New York.

Cottam P.J. & Sutton A. (1986) *Conductive Education: a System for Overcoming Motor Disorders.* Croom Helm, London.

Dow R.S., Dick H.L. & Crowell F.A. (1974) Failures and successes in a stroke program. *Stroke* **5**, 40–47.

Ernst E. (1990) A review of stroke rehabilitation and physiotherapy. *Stroke* **21**, 1081–1085.

Fay T. (1948) The neurological aspects of therapy in cerebral palsy. *Archives of Physical Medicine* **29**, 327–331.

Feigenson J.S., Gitlow H.S. & Greenberg S.D. (1979) The disability orientated rehabilitation unit: a major factor influencing stroke outcome. *Stroke* **10**, 5–8.

Feldman D.J., Lee P.R., Unterecker J., Lloyd K., Rusk H.A. & Toole A. (1962) A comparison of functionally orientated medical care and formal rehabilitation in the management of patients with hemiplegia due to cerebrovascular disease. *Journal of Chronic Diseases* **15**, 197–310.

Garraway W.M., Akktar A.J., Prescott R.J. & Hockey L. (1980a) Management of acute stroke in the elderly: preliminary results of a controlled trial. *British Medical Journal* **1**, 1040–1043.

Garraway W.M., Akktar A.J., Hockey L. & Prescott R.J. (1980b) Management of acute stroke in the elderly: follow-up of a controlled trial. *British Medical Journal* **2**, 827–829.

Gordon E.E. & Kohn K.H. (1966) Evaluation of rehabilitation methods in the hemiplegic patient. *Journal of Chronic Diseases* **19**, 3–16.

Hamrin E. (1982a) Early activation in stroke: does it make a difference? *Scandinavian Journal of Rehabilitation Medicine* **14**, 101–109.

Hamrin E. (1982b) One year after stroke: a follow-up of an experimental study. *Scandinavian Journal of Rehabilitation Medicine* **14**, 111–116.

Holebrook M. (1982) Stroke: social and emotional outcome. *Journal of the Royal College of Physicians of London* **16**, 100–104.

Illis L.S. (1992) *Spinal Cord Dysfunction II: Intervention and Treatment.* Oxford University Press, Oxford.

Kabat H. (1952) Studies on neuromuscular dysfunction: the role of central facilitation in restoration of motor function in paralysis. *Archives of Physical Medicine* **33**, 521–523.

Knott M. (1967) Introduction to and philosophy of neuromuscular facilitation. *Physiotherapy* **53**, 2–5.

Lind K. (1982) A synthesis of studies on stroke rehabilitation. *Journal of Chronic Diseases* **35**, 133–149.

McCann C.T. & Culbertson R.A. (1976) Comparison of two systems of stroke rehabilitation in a general hospital. *Journal of the American Geriatrics Society* **24**, 211–216.

Nichols P.J.R. (1980) *Rehabilitation Medicine.* Butterworths, London.

O'Neill T.J., McCarthy K. & Newton B.M. (1987) Slow-stream rehabilitation: is it effective? *Medical Journal of Australia* **147**, 172–175.

Rood M.S. (1954) Neurophysiological reactions as a basis for physical therapy. *Physical Therapy Review* **34**, 444–449.

Shields R. (1989) A practical application of aspects of conductive education. *Australian Journal of Physiotherapy* **35**, 159–165.

Smith M.E., Garraway W.M., Smith D.L. & Akktar A.J. (1982) Therapy impact on functional outcome in a controlled trial of stroke rehabilitation. *Archives of Physical and Medical Rehabilitation* **63**, 21–24.

Wagenaar R.C., Meijer O.G., Van Wieringen P.C.W., Kuik D.J., Hazenberg G.J., Lindeboom J., Wichers F. & Rijswijk H. (1990) The functional recovery of stroke: a comparison between neuro-developmental treatment and the Brunnstrom method. *Scandinavian Journal of Rehabilitation Medicine* **22**, 1–8.

12: Rehabilitation of Traumatic Brain Injury

C.D. EVANS

Definitions, 141
  Classification of severity of traumatic brain injury, 142
  Other definitions, 142
Who gets traumatic brain injuries?, 142
Causation, 143
The acute phase, 144
The post-acute phase, 144
Processes of rehabilitation, 145
Relevant disciplines, 145
  Doctors, 145
  Occupational therapists, 145
  Physiotherapists, 145
  Clinical psychologists, 146
  Speech therapists, 146
  Social workers, 146
  Nursing staff, 146
  Case managers, 147
  Carers and relatives, 147
  Disablement resettlement officers (DROs), 147
  Technical instructors, 148
  Voluntary organizations, 148
Discharge home, 148
Community rehabilitation teams, 148
Long-stay care, 148
Assessments, 149
  Relevance, 149
  Repeatable, 150
  Recordable, 150
  Retrievable, 150
Outcomes, 150
  Employability, 150
  Financial status, 151
  Accommodation, 151
  Aids and adaptations, 152
  Dependency, 152
Specific problems, 152
  Epilepsy, 152
  Behavioural problems, 152
  Memory and concentration, 153
  Post-traumatic syndrome, 154
  Pre-injury personality, 154
Prognosis, 154
The need for research, 155

Management and rehabilitation after traumatic brain injury (TBI) has taken place over at least the last century. Unfortunately, very little change has happened until recently. Even now, most management of TBI is done indifferently and there are few places where there are clear policies, adequate space and staffing in hospital and competent community follow-up.

Definitions have become clearer over the last 10 years and there is a better understanding of the acute management of TBI and an increased awareness of problems that brain damage causes for the victim and their families. There has been an increasing realization that the long-term problems are rarely confined to physical handicap. The problems of impaired memory, concentration and cognition and altered behaviour are the biggest causes of distress to both patients and carers.

In 1988 in Great Britain the Medical Disability Society (MDS) (now renamed the British Society for Rehabilitation Medicine) commissioned a working party to produce a report on the management of TBI. This report was published in the same year. Many of the definitions in this chapter are from that monograph (McLellan *et al.*, 1988). Most of the others are from World Health Organization (1989).

Definitions

The definitions of impairment, disability and handicap are all to be made within the 'context of health experience'.

Impairment is any loss or abnormality of psychological, physiological or anatomical structure or function. (Note: 'Impairment' is more inclusive than 'disorder', in that it covers losses – e.g. the loss of a leg is an impairment, but not a disorder.)

Disability is any restriction or lack (resulting from an impairment) of ability to perform an activity in the manner or within the range considered normal for a human being.

Handicap is the social consequences of the disability, i.e. it will limit or prevent fulfilment of the role that is normal for the individual. For example, a torn cartilage is an impairment, a stiff, painful knee is the disability and the handicap may vary according to the victim. It may be an inconvenience to a sedentary worker but loss of career for a footballer.

Classification of severity of traumatic brain injury

Minor. An injury causing unconsciousness for 15 minutes or less.

Moderate. An injury causing unconsciousness for more than 15 minutes, but less than 6 hours, or a post-traumatic amnesia (PTA) of less than 24 hours.

Severe. An injury causing unconsciousness for 6 hours or more, or a PTA of 24 hours or more.

Very severe. An injury causing unconsciousness for 48 hours or more, or a PTA of 7 days or more.

Disaster. An injury causing unconsciousness for 14 days or more. This is a personal interpolation in the classification which is relevant for prognosis.

Other definitions

Unconsciousness. A condition which lasts until meaningful responses can be made which are better than 'Yes' or 'No' but which allow for diffi-culties caused by tracheotomies, wired jaws, etc. The use of the duration of unconsciousness as a predictor is made more difficult where other factors have contributed to its duration, such as alcohol or operation for causes unrelated to the head injury. In recent years the intubation and ventilation of

most severely brain-damaged patients confuses the issue, and reduces the predictive value of the measure.

Unconsciousness is now defined by the Glasgow coma score (GCS) (Teasdale & Jennett, 1974). This is a summation of the scores of best motor response, best verbal response and eye opening. Patients are said to be unconscious when they score 9 points or less out of a total of 15. This can occasionally mislead, since it is a summation of the scores of three assessments. If there is a distorted response (e.g. instead of being 3, 3, 3, it is 1, 3, 5), then prognosis is difficult.

Post-traumatic amnesia (PTA). The loss of memory from the time of the original injury to the time when continual day-to-day memory has been re-established. This has been the standard measure of severity of the injury. It was in the forefront after the paper by Russell & Smith (1961). Information from Glasgow and Chessington suggest that the duration of unconsciousness is roughly a quarter of that of PTA, though by the time unconsciousness has been present for 2–3 months the establishment of normal memory may never appear.

Who gets traumatic brain injuries?

Field's report (1975) identified twin peaks of in-cidence of head injury: those between the ages of 15 and 19 years of age and those over 75. He also showed that young men are more at risk than young women, though by the time the second peak is reached the difference has all but disappeared. Kraus *et al.* (1984) also demonstrates this. Evans (1989) reported on the cohort of patients examined from Chessington. In this highly selected group there was a bias towards the younger age range. Wade & Langton Hewer (1987) and the MDS report (McLellan *et al.*, 1988) drew similar conclusions. (See Fig. 12.1.)

Cornwall (UK) has a managed population of 400 000. In 1990 there were about 900 patients discharged from Cornish hospitals with the diag-nosis of head injury. Only 15 were admitted to the Cornwall Stroke and Rehabilitation Unit (CSRU); all had severe or very severe TBI. The outcomes of mild and moderate injuries do not appear in these

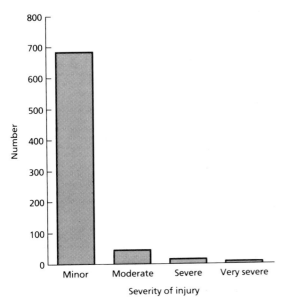

Fig. 12.1 Incidence of traumatic brain injury per 250 000 population.

figures, as there is no system yet for identifying or assessing them.

A record has been kept since October 1983 of all patients seen by the rehabilitation service in Corn-wall. This has just been analysed. Figure 12.2 shows the number and ages of survivors of severe and very severe TBI in the county. Despite the expected higher incidence in youth, the prevalence evens out as the population ages.

The expectation of life after surviving TBI has been recorded, in US veterans, by Corkin *et al.* (1984) and they confirm a relatively normal life expectancy, unless epilepsy has supervened. There-fore facilities to help people recover from, or cope with, brain damage must cover all age-groups.

If the MDS estimates are extrapolated for the managed population for Cornwall of 400 000 this would predict a total of 480 disabled survivors in the county. Only 145 have been seen in the rehabilitation service. This is because only severe and very severe patients are seen. Mild and mode-rate injuries are rarely presented to the rehabili-tation service.

Causation

Road accidents cause the majority of head injuries (Fig. 12.3). This has been observed ever since there has been traffic. The cause of the injury is of greatest importance in planning rescue services. The improvement in the skills of paramedical

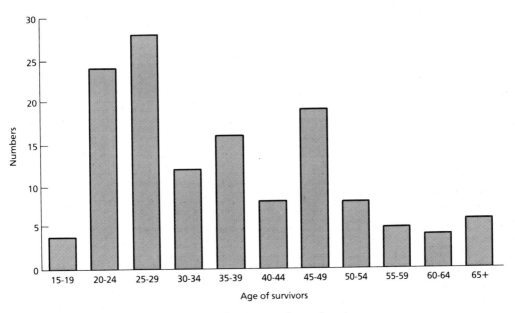

Fig. 12.2 Traumatic brain injury patients in Cornwall: point prevalence of survivors.

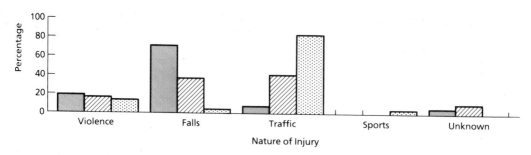

Fig. 12.3 Causes of traumatic brain injury over a century. Traffic injuries rose from 7% in 1886 to 82% in 1988.

crews of rescue vehicles, the use of rapid-response vehicles and the use of helicopters have led to better management during the first hours after the injury. A better understanding of the need to prevent 'secondary injury' has helped to minimize long-term damage.

The cause of the injury only affects rehabilitation if a claim for compensation can provide extra services. Only a small percentage of victims have a prima facie case as the law stands, and this will not change until 'no-fault compensation' becomes law. In any event, settlements are often delayed for years and this may make it impossible to look to the courts for funds for anything other than long-term care.

The acute phase

This lasts from admission to medical stability. In Cornwall, as in most other places, there is an element of chance about which route is taken through the acute service. Clinical management may be from general surgeons, orthopaedic surgeons, anaesthetists or neurosurgeons. It is not usually a matter of conscious choice but more a matter of local expediency and practice. The wise patient will take care both where and when to have the head injury. (The wiser still would avoid it!)

The post-acute phase

This follows the acute stage. Probably the least satisfactory situation for the patient with a TBI is to be the unwanted guest in a surgical or neuro-surgical ward. It is a costly option and, as even

minimally disruptive behaviour may be intolerable, it sometimes leads to inappropriate sedation.

In Cornwall patients with severe or very severe TBI are usually sent from resuscitation unit, intensive treatment unit or the neurosurgical unit to the CSRU at City Hospital in Truro, so bypassing the acute surgical or medical ward. The CSRU takes patients who are still unconscious, but are detached from all monitors and intra-arterial lines. Tracheotomies, nasogastric tubes or urinary catheters are not a bar to admission.

It is difficult to justify a unit for just 15–20 patients a year, which is the number expected in a district of average size. It might be possible to expand this by screening for the moderately and mildly injured. It is more realistic to link the management of TBI with cerebrovascular accident (CVA) and the after-effects of subarachnoid haemorrhage or other form of intracranial insult. The disciplines required will be common to all.

The value of a unit geographically remote from the patients' homes is debatable (Evans & Skidmore, 1989). If the patient is ultimately to be managed in the community, the closer that contact is kept with family and friends, the easier it will be to get home. In practice, only two patients could not be managed on the CSRU in the last 8 years.

In more populated areas, then, a specialized unit drawing from a population of over one or two million could be viable and specialize in TBI only, especially those who have behaviour problems.

Processes of rehabilitation

These can be broadly divided into three. The first is the efforts made to alter and improve a patient's ability, whether physical, psychological or behavioural. This is perhaps the most conspicuous aspect of rehabilitation, as it usually involves therapists and others while the patient is in hospital and diminishes when he/she returns to the community.

The second is to do with altering the environment if the problems the patients are left with cannot be improved. This stage will include modifying housing, transport and clothing. It is often the lot of occupational therapists to plan this form of environmental manipulation.

Finally, the third process is to make a concerted attempt to alter and improve 'behaviour'. Memory, concentration and socializing are embraced by this rather diffuse term. Part of the process is to help patients, their families and carers to come to terms with residual problems, be they physical or psychological, and part is a wider role to educate the general public in tolerating this group of handicapped citizens better.

Relevant disciplines

Doctors

There seems no alternative but that a doctor should be, and in most centres is, legally responsible for the general care and direction of the rehabilitation while the patient is in hospital. It is not always clear which doctor has this task. For example, during the acute stage, the overall management might be the responsibility of the neurosurgeon, general surgeon or any consultant in whose department the patient has been admitted.

When the patient has left the acute phase, he/she may go to another ward or hospital, attend a rehabilitation centre or go back into the community. Whatever stage the patient is in, there should be a consultant or specialist with clear responsibility, and easy access to other opinions.

Often the nature of the original doctor's work will involve much routine but pressing work, and because of this there is too little time to take a direct interest in rehabilitation after the acute stage. The

responsibility is often delegated, formally or informally, to junior medical staff, who will have little experience in the field, or to therapists. If this is to be done, it needs to be formal so that, in the event of medical advice being required, the channel to get it is clear.

Occupational therapists

Occupational therapists have traditionally had a working knowledge of anatomy, physiology and relevant medical conditions. They were originally employed to provide what their name suggests, i.e. therapeutic occupation. They have now specialized in assessment of activities of daily living (ADL), provision of aids, appliances and wheelchairs and alteration of environment both at home and at work. They often work in the community with social service departments.

The Association of Occupational Therapists runs courses to train occupational therapists to administer basic psychological tests. This is a most constructive development since only a few hospitals have clinical psychologists as part of the rehabilitation team, nor will they have for the foreseeable future. Most hospitals have occupational therapy departments. Some departments not only assess perceptual problems, but try to retrain patients with such deficits as early as possible.

Physiotherapists

This profession also has a working knowledge of general anatomy, physiology and relevant medical conditions, and a specialist cover of the musculoskeletal and nervous systems. Over the last few years this profession has spent a great deal of time trying to develop reliable assessments of physical ability. Both in the UK and overseas, physiotherapy departments have been responsible for developing many different systems of physical rehabilitation. In some of the systems, the neurophysiological basis now seems somewhat sketchy.

As to which system is best, the conviction of the therapist that what he or she is doing is correct is probably of more significance than the actual technique. This is another subject on which research is urgently needed. However, when a specific technique is agreed by a unit, all the other disciplines should be aware of this decision and respect it. The introduction of such a system necessitates close collaboration between all staff, and this in itself helps a team approach.

Clinical psychologists

They have expertise in assessing and managing the after-effects of TBI. The clinical psychologist is expected to be able to make formal assessments of such qualities as memory, mood, intellect, comprehension and expression. All are of great moment to both the attendants and the relatives of those who have suffered brain damage. Clinical psychologists can help patients, staff and carers to identify important issues and either manage them or come to terms with them. If, as may often be the case, there is no realistic therapy to put damage right, then coping strategies can be used.

Unfortunately, there are too few clinical psychologists, so that frequently they can assess but are not able to give any therapy the assessments might suggest. They can advise on setting realistic goals, behaviour modification and introducing suitable incentives for patients (and sometimes for their relatives and the staff). It has been interesting to note the transfer from the management of physical aspects of TBI by physiotherapists to the management of behavioural problems by the psychology services over the last few years. For most patients, a genuine multidisciplinary team is needed.

Speech therapists

Like other therapies, for wide areas of the UK, the number of staff available is very small. When this is the case, the most useful role for the therapist may be to assess at what level communication with the patient exists and how the relatives and nursing staff may use it. If there is neither a speech therapist nor a clinical psychologist, the responsibility for this particular function may devolve upon the occupational therapist, but rest somewhere it must, for establishment of any method of communication as early as possible with the brain-damaged survivor seems to be of crucial importance. Speech therapists are developing a special expertise in assessing the problems of swallowing, often in conjunction with ear, nose and throat (ENT) departments.

As in stroke, perception of sound and sight may precede recovery in expression by a considerable time. In theory, this information is widely known; in practice, it is frequently forgotten, and the patient can easily become the equivalent of a pillow in the bed to be talked over and around but never to. In patients who recover after a long time, this is commented on, often in terms of strongest resentment. In later stages of recovery, when speech content may be relatively normal, its articulation may be slow and confusing. It is of the utmost importance that staff and relatives should treat the patient as having a normal perception and comprehension, even if the evidence appears to the contrary. There is little to be lost by such a strategy, and everything to be gained.

Social workers

These staff are employed by the local authority, but ideally will work in hospitals or rehabilitation centres. Contact with relatives and counselling are an important part of their job. They will advise on benefits and aspects of guardianship, link with solicitors for the Court of Protection where necessary, and may act as the patient's advocate. They will be an integral part of the team and should attend all ward meetings. When the time comes for return of the patient into the community, they will have a particularly important role in preparing the care package at home. This will apply even if there is an intermediate stage after hospital in a residential rehabilitation unit. In some places, they may provide the continuity of care if there is no case manager. It should be borne in mind that 'care in the community' legislation will be in place, which will put the social services in the lead role of providing community care.

Nursing staff

Whilst the patient is in hospital, the nursing staff will have a 24-hour responsibility for the patient's care. This fact alone may make them the *de facto* leaders or managers of the rehabilitation team. To enable this to work well, some basic concepts of nursing care have to be examined. It is often quicker to help somebody to dress, shave or feed, but on a rehabilitation ward or unit it is important to be able to take longer and watch a patient attempt this for himself. In addition, specific techniques of movement, positioning and lifting patients may be recommended by the therapists and a consistency of approach within the unit is essential. There is nothing impossible about this, but it has to be consciously written into the operational policy of the unit to enable it to happen.

Where the patient has gone to a rehabilitation unit outside a hospital base, the relationships between these disciplines may change slightly. Provided the responsibilities of each group are clearly defined, preferably by interdisciplinary meetings, it is nearly always possible that a natural team leader will emerge.

Case managers

In the UK this concept started in a London teaching hospital. A therapist was appointed to act as a case manager for the entire rehabilitation process of any patient. Ideally the case manager is first introduced while the patient is on the intensive treatment unit. The manager follows the patient through the hospital system out into the community. It is extensively used in the US.

In Cornwall this has been undertaken by an occupational therapist, who has a shared commitment to the rehabilitation unit and the community. It is she who integrates the moves from hospital to home and, when possible, back to work. This post was initially part-funded by charity.

Carers and relatives

In the acute stage whilst consciousness is recovering, the presence of relatives can reassure the patient as to who he is and what has happened. Many brain-damaged survivors are said to have been able to recall, with considerable precision, information given them during the time when they appeared to be unconscious and uncommunicative. They recall this attention with deep gratitude and affection. Unfortunately, statistical proof of this statement is as yet impossible. On a completely common-sense basis, it appears a reasonable course of action, and in practical terms it is usually encouraged by all acute units where feasible.

A visitor's book may be used, where each relative or friend notes the date, the subject of any conversation that they may have had with the patient, and any observations made. It seems a simple and useful way of gathering information and involving the relatives from a very early stage in the programme of rehabilitation.

Relatives need to be included as part of the therapy team because they are the people most likely to be left with the major responsibilities and problems. A tremendous amount of co-operation and practical help must be given if they are to attempt this with any prospect of success.

Success will depend not only on the severity of the injury but on which relative has to look after the victim. The prospects of a satisfactory return home appear greatest when the injured person is young and where the parents are still able to care. If only one parent is available, then the chance of a successful return home is smaller. The impact on the family caused by TBI of a member has been carefully documented by Brooks et al. (1986). When the patients are middle-aged or elderly, a spouse may be the carer. It is difficult to resettle an elderly patient with brain damage with their children for a long time, as this is often unacceptable. Planned support, holiday relief and other forms of social and medical aid are necessary so that the problem for the caring relatives can be eased. These aids should be used as early as possible to help the whole family.

Disablement employment advisers (DEAs)

DROs are not members of the NHS in the UK but are responsible to the Department of Employment. If it appears that there is likely to be a problem of re-employment, then the earlier the DEA can be invoked the better. If it becomes apparent later that the patient is unable to get back to his/her original job, the DEA can arrange suitable assessment and retraining courses in UK government training centres (skill centres) or other suitable colleges or training institutions. If there is a case manager, occupational therapist or technical instructor attached to the unit, they may well be able to make contact with the DEA.

The advantage of recruiting the DRO early is that it will minimize the delay between the patient leaving hospital or rehabilitation centre and the time he/she starts work. A long period of delay before starting work is very destructive to morale for the vast majority of those for whom work has previously been part of their ethic.

Technical instructors

Technical instructors may either supervise retraining for an original job or assess and evaluate a suitable alternative. It is unlikely that these staff will be present in many hospitals, but they are represented in some rehabilitation centres. There needs to be close liaison between them and the occupational therapy department. In a few hospitals the instructors are actually part of such a department.

Although assessments carried out by technical instructors in hospitals and rehabilitation centres have no statutory significance in subsequent placement through employment rehabilitation centres and skill centres, they allow people to be presented to industrial rehabilitation with a higher chance of success than if they are presented from the hospital or home without such preparation. In addition, a technical instructor can supervise work, which may help to overcome resistance felt by some patients to the sort of craft or skill usually within the compass of occupational therapists.

Voluntary organizations

There are many organizations that may be involved in rehabilitation. Some, such as the League of Friends, may be able to provide some financial support or apparatus otherwise unobtainable, such as page-turners, reading aids and so forth. Headway has become established as the national charity with a particular interest in helping patients and their carers where there has been a head injury in the family. They are happy to be involved at an early stage. Local organizations differ widely in what they may offer, from advice and counselling through the acute stage to day support after discharge from hospital.

Discharge home

The decision to return a patient to the community should only be taken when there is a reasonable chance of success. There should be close liaison with the available community services. A gradual transition, possibly encouraging the carers to allow the patient home for short periods, should be attempted. These may be at first for a few hours only, then increasing to days and then overnight, either at weekends only or during the week. Successful trips home may encourage the relatives to take over completely. In many cases, it may have to be supervised by the social work department. They will also be responsible for ensuring that any statutory help is provided, and that the necessary adaptations to the home and work are undertaken and paid for.

Community rehabilitation teams

These started in Cornwall in 1985 so that there would be better co-operation between the field workers of social services and health authority. They started simply when a patient with severe head injury had been discharged into the community and there was no programme for him to follow and no single unit in which it could be undertaken. The speech therapist, occupational therapist, physiotherapist and social worker involved in his care used to meet regularly to plan ways to manage him.

This idea developed until there are now seven community rehabilitation teams in Cornwall, co-terminous with the social services boundaries. Members who attend do so unofficially but recognize that the time spent is well worth while in making contacts with their opposite numbers and saving time on the telephone and writing letters. It makes response to the patient's problems much quicker. The health authority representatives will include nursing staff from the community, medical staff from the hospitals and therapists from either. Social services will send occupational therapists, social workers and home care attendants. Officers from the housing, education and other council departments attend as necessary, and so do the disablement resettlement officer and clinical psychologist (Evans, 1987).

Long-stay care

The ideal outcome after TBI is for the patient to go home and take up his/her original job. When this is impossible, the patient may still be able to go home and be completely independent, despite being unable to do a job. The least satisfactory outcome is where, for whatever reason, the patient has to be admitted into long-stay care. This may happen for a variety of reasons. There may be nobody in the family to care for the patient at home or the physical or psychological consequences of the accident alienate potential carers so that they are unwilling to have the patient home. This causes conflict when the patient prefers to be at home, but has no insight that his/her behaviour is intolerable.

In theory, any patient, unless under Section, has a right to choose where he/she wants to live and with whom, and should be able to get support. This would be a needs-led service. In practice lack of facilities or money limits available options and most patients have to fit in to what is on offer, and this is a resource-led service. When this happens authorities, who act on his/her behalf do so but without the patient's agreement. A Court of Protection will look after the patient's financial interests, but their use is expensive and they have no control over anything other than finance. In the unlikely event of a patient being able to sign a valid power of attorney, administration of his long-term care is easier.

When there is a large insurance settlement, a choice can be made between buying residential care in a specialized unit (if such exists locally) and adapting and staffing a house or bungalow in the community. This offers an element of choice, but only about 10% of patients with TBI are in a position to make a claim. Settlements are always slow, usually not before 5 years after the accident. Structured settlement and interim payments are being sought more. Relatives should be advised to instruct a good solicitor specializing in this sort of claim as early as possible after the accident. It is expected that there will soon be a register of such specialists.

Most patients will not be able to sign a power of attorney. Social workers often work with solicitors to undo the legal tangles in this situation. Headway, a national charity, can advise relatives on all aspects of the effects of head injury. They will be able to put them in touch with the nearest branch. Many relatives comment on the feeling of isolation. Headway will help relatives to contact others who have been in the same situation. This can be of great comfort during a very stressful period. They run their own rehabilitation unit, for which costs currently are in the order of £1000 per week.

Long-stay units have proliferated but almost entirely in the private sector. Costs are high and in 1991 ranged between £750 a week for a nursing home specializing in head injury to £1700 a week for a hospital with an intensive rehabilitation programme or behaviour modification facility. In some cases, insurance companies will pay this cost. Other patients may be funded by health authorities, who find it less expensive to buy in this care when needed rather than provide it regularly in an NHS facility.

If there are no specialized unit and no funding, TBI survivors may be misplaced into geriatric units or unspecialized nursing homes and left without either satisfactory supervision or further rehabilitation. Some even remain in the acute hospital long after the hospital has a benefit to give because nowhere else is prepared to accept them.

Assessments

Quite often, assessments are merely displacement activities for staff; they often produce no valid information since no useful question was asked. If time used in assessment is to be well spent, then they need to be well designed and relevant. They will also be repeatable, recordable and retrievable.

Relevance

There are two widely separate reasons for initiating formal assessments, one being research and the other concerned with practical aspects of care. In the former it must be accepted that some information will be obtained which will be ultimately redundant. Provided this sort of assessment is not confused with the second group, which is much more practically orientated, then there is little problem. In any event, persuading therapists who are concerned with giving a service to do prolonged research-orientated assessments is difficult unless the project is thoroughly explained and there are enough staff to do them.

In units with no research staff, assessments need to be simpler and designed to produce the answers to important clinical management questions.

The two aims need not be incompatible, and a

well-designed research assessment does eventually help therapists to produce better service assessments with greater precision. Whiting & Lincoln (1980) designed assessments which established what point a patient had arrived at in the hierarchy of recovery. This gave the staff information about what the patient could do easily, what was impossible and what would be the next logical progression to make in treatment.

Repeatable

It should not matter which therapist has undertaken a particular assessment, provided they have been trained to do it. A study in which the observer error was minimized was undertaken at Oxford by Lincoln & Leadbetter (1979). This particular study was done on patients recovering from stroke, but the development of similar techniques is possible with patients who have suffered traumatic brain damage. They showed that recovery occurred in a hierarchy and, if this was graded accurately, it would identify the next level of activity to be retrained.

Recordable

Subjective narrative reports are misleading and time-consuming, though never entirely dispensable. If the luxury of such aids as videotape recording is unavailable, then the next best thing is either to devise or use available systems of scored assessments, where answers to the question of ability are done by a straight yes/no choice. Dozens of questionnaires have been produced for ADL which were reviewed by Donaldson (1973). She came to the conclusion that it was confusing to offer more than a five-point scale for any given activity, because as the precision required increased, so did observer error.

Retrievable

From the information observed, a huge stack of figures is easy to obtain, but to extract common sense is more difficult. However, with modern methods of information processing, data are storable on computer. Hamilton & Grainger (1989) and Evans (1991) have developed systems for scoring retrievable information.

Outcomes

Between 1973 and 1974 all the patients with a diagnosis of brain injury admitted to the Royal Air Force Rehabilitation Unit, Chessington, were examined carefully on arrival, their progress recorded in each department and their abilities measured with specially designed assessments. About 5 years later, most (more than 95%) were reviewed, mostly by interview and examination but some by questionnaire. In the 5-year review, five outcome measures were used. They were employability, financial status, accommodation, aids and adaptations needed for survival and dependency. The most useful of these were employability and financial status.

Employability

Most of the patients in the Chessington cohort were young and in employment at the time of their accident. They were followed up about 5 years after their injury. Most patients who sustain TBI are young so if they return to their original employment it is a good indicator of a successful programme of rehabilitation. The relative success or otherwise of the rehabilitation programme can then be measured, if needed, by the length of time off work.

If return to work is to a different job, the Registrar General's Classification of Employment can be used to compare the work undertaken after injury with that done before.

Five possible outcomes can be defined:
1 Return to original or equivalent job.
2 Unemployed.
3 Return to work, but at inferior job.
4 Still in training, or in sheltered work.
5 Unemployable.
It will be seen from Fig. 12.4 that over half this cohort of patients got back to full-time work. This compares with the estimate of 15% returning to work given in the MDS paper (McLellan *et al.*, 1988).

Figure 12.5 shows that, given this population and programme, no patient unconscious for less

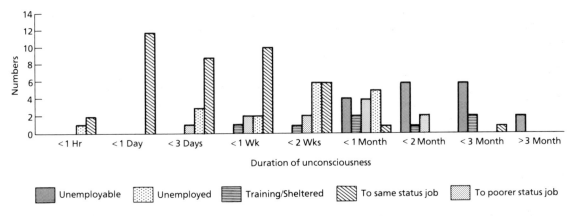

Fig. 12.4 Outcome in terms of employability.

than 2 weeks was unemployable. On the other hand, only 6.5% of those unconscious for more than 2 weeks were in any sort of work and only one was back in his original job (hence the description of 'disaster' for this group).

Financial status

During the follow-up interview and examination, the patient and relatives were asked about the family income and how it was derived. There were two basic categories: earned (by the patient) or from any other source.

Figure 12.6 shows the relationship between the duration of unconsciousness and the income of the patient (or his/her family) and whether it was earned or otherwise. The annual income recorded

represented the income (after tax) coming into the household. Earned income is obvious but the unearned income could come from pension, compensation or statutory allowances and benefits.

Where a patient was in a hospital or voluntary home, a figure of £12 000 p.a. was added, which was the contemporary cost of this care. All figures are at 1982 values.

To find equivalent 1991 values they should be multiplied by the increase in retail price index (RPI).

Accommodation

Despite the severity of the injuries, only five patients were in residential care at the time of review. They were all patients who had been un-

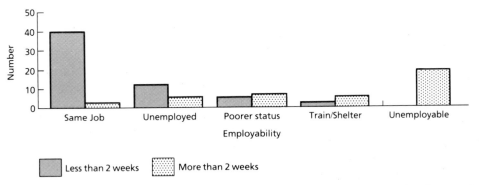

Fig. 12.5 Employability of survivors at 5 years. Only 6.5% were in work who had been unconscious for more than 2 weeks.

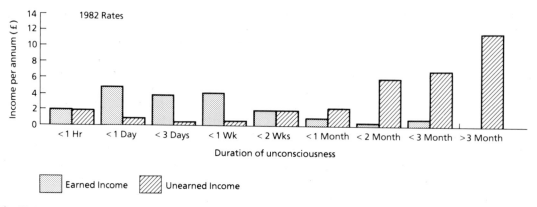

Fig. 12.6 Earned vs. unearned income of survivors.

conscious for 2 weeks or more. All the others were in their family homes and this says much for the level of family commitment. Community rehabilitation services were patchy and many relatives expressed their desolation at their lot, but could not see how to get help.

Aids and adaptations

These were divided into two categories: major and minor, the former being any equipment costing more than £100 and the latter that costing less. The same price bands were applied to mobility aids.

Dependency

This was measured by the amount of support needed each day and was broken down into four categories:

1 Total – needing constant attention.
2 Partial – attendants needed for some part of each day.
3 Relative independence – no attendant required but a major loss of job or social activity enforced.
4 Independent – this did not imply normality and might only be achieved by the use of an aid or appliance.

Specific problems

There are some specific problems which may require special attention. This list was compiled analysing the patients who could be said to have

failed. Failure is said to occur when the patient is unable to reintegrate in society. It may be because he/she cannot go home, is unemployable or depends on others for day-to-day needs, including financial support. In the group under discussion, four major factors emerged: epilepsy, behavioural change, impairment of memory and concentration, and the post-traumatic syndrome.

Epilepsy

Jennett (1985) found that four factors predisposed the incidence of late epilepsy after head injury. These were PTA of greater than 24 hours, focal signs, early incidence of an epileptic attack and a dural tear (or incision). Phenytoin is often given in the acute hospital, as it can be given intravenously. The MDS paper (McLellan *et al.*, 1988) recommends carbamazepine as the drug of choice, so this may be considered during rehabilitation as an alternative. It is said to cause fewer behavioural problems and to be less sedative. The biggest impact of epilepsy is on employment and driving, the two often being related. There is still no consensus in the use of anticonvulsants. However, the categorization given by Jennett does make a basis for a logical approach.

Behavioural problems

It is difficult to define behaviour problems, but in practice they are easy to recognize. Some patients who have suffered TBI display aggression or altered sexuality. Both cause much concern. Aggression may be verbal or physical, and, although the latter is more terrifying, neither is easy to live with.

Aggression may be due to misunderstanding and frustration on the patient's part. If aggressive behaviour has only been noticed in one department, it is unwise to assume that the patient is in the wrong. Staff or relatives may be the aggressors, often unwittingly. Some strategies which may help are to involve the patient in decisions that affect him, wherever possible to give him/her control over the situation and to keep him/her informed about what is taking place. It is most important to be consistent, as inconsistency of approach will produce insecurity and conflict. The staff must know how to respond to threats, either physical or verbal, and any sanctions that are threatened must be feasible.

Alteration of sexuality does not usually arise as an isolated problem. It is often associated with other changes in personality and behaviour, such as lack of caring and initiative, which corrode personal relationships. Sometimes altered sexuality is the outward manifestation of such degradation.

Increased sexuality may worry relatives and carers because it is indiscriminate and crude. It may range from lack of inhibition to promiscuity, with total disregard for the feelings of others. If it occurs, it should be remembered that this is often a transient phase during recovery, so need not cause panic. However, if it is not possible to control, consideration should be given to the risks of unwanted pregnancy. It may be possible to prevent this. If libido is decreased, the patient or partner may complain. Care needs to be taken not to assume a problem exists.

If ostentatious masturbation occurs, it causes concern to staff, relatives and carers. Fortunately, this is also normally transient. A consistent approach by which the patient is discouraged from masturbating in public may be sufficient. More draconian measures, such as the isolation of a patient or the administration of heavy sedatives, are rarely required. It may also be possible to anticipate problems.

When a problem presents, it is important to respond sympathetically. All members of staff need to be approachable and to listen for problems which may not be overtly stated. Many members of staff will feel inadequate to deal with problems of aggression or sexuality, but it is important that they know the members of staff who are prepared to listen and counsel. The clinical psychologist may take this role on, and may also offer advice to staff, relatives and other patients. They may also advise on behaviour modification programmes, such as the introduction of a token economy or other form of incentive which will provide positive responses for 'good' behaviour and a realistic negative one for 'bad'. It would seem preferable to adopt this approach before a pharmacological one, though some drugs are available.

Memory and concentration

Many patients who suffer mild or moderate brain damage make an excellent physical recovery. However, they may be unable to return to work and hold down a job, although in informal conversation there seems to be no major problem. Quite what qualities go to make up the ability to concentrate and to retain information is not yet known. Despite this, it is possible to try and clarify some aspects of memory for the sake of the relatives and friends. It may be possible that some help can be gained from the expertise of the clinical psychologist, but, unfortunately, in common with the medical profession, there is very considerable confusion as to what constitutes memory and how it may be defined.

Despite confusion, some definitions can be made. The first distinction to be drawn is between recall of information present before the accident, such as biographical details, work, family and general knowledge, and recall of information acquired after the head injury. It is the second aspect which causes confusion. It is agreed that there is a difference between short-term and long-term memory and that there are strategies for getting short-term information into a long-term store. It is not certain when long-term memory takes over from short-term; various definitions have placed this at anything from a few seconds to several minutes. It is possible that failure to acquire new information may be a failure to perceive new information.

Perhaps even more important than the actual aids is the willingness to recognize that a problem exists. Then these simple aids can help, and continued rehearsal may lead to the eventual abandonment of the aid. Barbara Wilson (1987) has highlighted possible ways of reducing the handicap of a poor memory.

Post-traumatic syndrome

Some patients whose injury seems trivial develop giddiness, headache and inability to concentrate where there seems to be no very good reason for it. This group is known variously as the post-traumatic or post-concussional syndrome. Whether it is organic or functional in origin has been extensively debated. The post-traumatic stress syndrome recently described has many of the features of the post-concussional syndrome, so it is possible that it is a general response to the stress of the injury. Even if there is no detectable lesion on X-ray, computerized tomography (CT) scan or clinical examination, some patients sustain damage which affects their future lives. In future, magnetic resonance imaging (MRI) scans soon after the injury may help.

There may be minor problems which remain undetected unless specifically sought. Such impairments may contribute to a vicious circle of poor concentration leading to difficulty in working.

Pre-injury personality

It is possible that patients who suffer injury come from specific sections of the population, even allowing for the already discussed age and sex differentials. It seems common sense that people who are aggressive are more likely to be involved in fights and accidents. Alcohol is thought to be a major factor. Information from the Road Research Laboratory confirms this.

In the Chessington study, time and care was taken to find out what the patient was like before the accident. If, before the accident, the patient was known to be a short-tempered, aggressive boor, or was a work-shy, alcoholic layabout, then the occurrence of severe head injury was unlikely to improve his personality. This could not always be assumed, since one particularly aggressive young man was welcomed home by his relatives with glee, for they found he was much less aggressive than before the accident. In general, it seemed that behaviour and motivation of a patient before the accident had an important bearing on his/her rehabilitation. Since some of these patients have no family support and a poor home environment, they often represent the biggest challenge.

Prognosis

A general prognosis can be given on the basis of statistics that are known about other patients. This assumes that the severity of the injury can be measured. At the moment, we can use duration of unconsciousness and PTA to do this. However, looking at even the small series from Chessington, it will be realized that while a prognosis can be given it will refer to a group rather than an individual. In the first stages after head injury, it is very difficult indeed to be accurate about the final outcome. If a firm prognosis is given at this stage and subsequently proved wrong, it causes greater stress for the family. The only basis upon which we can predict for the individual is that of the rate of recovery, and this has yet to be evaluated.

A young man who was involved in an aircraft accident sustained TBI and multiple injuries. He was unconscious for several weeks. The staff felt that he had no chance of survival and told his wife so. He did not die but by the time he recovered consciousness he had developed severe flexion contractures of knees, hips and elbows. The fractures were uniting in a poor position. His wife was now informed that he would never be able to walk, talk or go home. A year later, he was admitted to a rehabilitation centre, and continued to improve over the next 3 years. By that time, he was able to talk coherently, but needed operations on his eyes and on his limbs to relieve the contractures. His wife was then told that the patient might eventually be fit to go home.

By this time she had first become used to the idea that he would die, and then that would be in an institution of some sort as there was no prospect of his going home. Finally, she had to recognize that, though her husband would come home, he would have an altered personality. This sort of story is frequently heard. It emphasizes the extreme sensitivity needed when talking with relatives.

The need for research

Until quite recently it has been felt that recovery from head injury takes place during the first 6 months only. Any improvement observed later was believed to be adaptation but not neurological improvement. This view is now changing, and observations of workers over years suggest that recovery continues for longer than 6 months. In a conference in Bordeaux in April 1991, many of the issues were examined in considerable detail (Pelissier *et al.*, 1991). Speakers emphasized the underlying flexibility of the central nervous system to change, and this approach to the neurophysiology of recovery presents encouragement and an enormous challenge to those whose work is primarily concerned with neurological rehabilitation. The recognition of the plasticity of the nervous system, the presence of unused pathways capable of retraining and the recognition of the complexity of the synaptic system around the nerve cell give the encouragement to those concerned with rehabilitation that there may be a neurophysiological basis for recovery which is far better than mere adaptation.

Even though the mechanisms of recovery are becoming clearer, it has yet to be established that an intensive rehabilitation programme involving physiotherapy, occupational therapy and speech therapy, throughout the day and for several days a week, can be justified in terms of its ultimate effectiveness. Half the patients who went through Chessington went back to work, compared with 15% recorded in the MDS document (McLellan *et al.*, 1988). Even though this is not statistically sound, because there was no control population, it is suggestive. It is impossible to design controlled studies of rehabilitation, for ethical if no other reasons. It is likely to be more successfully made by repeated careful case studies.

This extract written 12 years ago for the first edition of this book serves as well today as then:

> The challenge consists in establishing that an intensive rehabilitation programme involving periods of physiotherapy, occupational therapy and speech therapy throughout the day for several days a week can be justified in terms of effectiveness. It is also necessary to establish whether one particular method of rehabilitation is better than another. There are many systems which have been devised and claims are made for each but there are no figures with which to support these arguments. This lack is due to the one fundamental deficiency in rehabilitation and that is of accurate measurements. Until these are available there is no scientific foundation for the belief that rehabilitation works. Inwardly, one may have the conviction that it does, but in the future, with increasing competition for funds, conviction alone will be inadequate.

References

Brooks D.N., Campsie L.M., Symington C., Beattie A., Bryden J. & McKinlay W. (1986) The five year outcome of severe blunt head injury: a relative's view. *Journal of Neurology, Neurosurgery and Psychiatry* **49**, 764–770.

Corkin S., Sullivan E. & Carr A. (1984) Prognostic factors for life expectancy after penetrating head injury. *Archives of Neurology* **41**, 975–977.

Donaldson S.W. (1973) A unified ADL form. *Archives of Physical Medicine and Rehabilitation* **54**, 175–179.

Evans C.D. (1987) Community rehabilitation. *Clinical Rehabilitation* **1**, 133–137.

Evans C.D. (1989) Long-term follow-up of head-injured patients. In Eames P. & Wood R.L. (eds) *Models of Brain Injury Rehabilitation*, pp. 184–203. Chapman & Hall, London.

Evans C.D., Gibson J., Jones T. & Williams M. (1993) A medical diagnostic index for rehabilitation. *Disability and Rehabilitation* **15**, 127–135.

Evans C.D. & Skidmore B. (1989) Rehabilitation in the community. In Eames P. & Wood R.L. (eds) *Models of Brain Injury Rehabilitation*, pp. 59–71. Chapman & Hall, London.

Field J.H. (1975) *A Study of the Epidemiology of Head Injury in England and Wales, with Particular Reference to Rehabilitation.* A report to the DHSS.

Hamilton B.B. & Grainger C.V. (1989) *A Uniform Data System for Rehabilitation: the Use of the International Classification of Impairments, Disabilities and Handicaps (ICIDH) in Rehabilitation*, pp. 42–45. Council of Europe, Strasburg.

Jennett B. (1985) Epilepsy (2) after head injury and craniotomy. In Raffle A. (ed.) *Medical Aspects of Fitness to Drive*. Medical Commission on Accident Prevention, London.

Kraus J.F., Black M.A., Hessol N. *et al.* (1984) The incidence of acute brain injury with severe impairment in

a defined population. *American Journal of Epidemiology*
119, 186–201.

Lincoln N.B. & Leadbetter D. (1979) Assessment of motor
function in stroke patients. *Physiotherapy* **65**, 48–51.

McLellan D. *et al.* (1988) *The Management of Traumatic
Brain Injury.* A report published by the Development
Trust for the Young Disabled, prepared by Working
Party of the Medical Disability Society, Royal College of
Physicians, London.

Pelissier J., Barat M. & Mazaus J.M. (1991) *Traumatisme
cranien grave et médecine de réeducation.* Masson, Paris.

Russell W.R. & Smith R. (1961) PTA in closed head injury.
Archives of Neurology **5**, 4.

Teasdale G. & Jennett B. (1974) Assessment of coma and
impaired consciousness: a practical scale. *Lancet* **ii**,
81–84.

Wade D. & Langton Hewer R. (1987) Epidemiology of
some neurological conditions with specific reference to
the work load on the NHS. *International Rehabilitation
Medicine* **8**, 129–137.

Whiting S.E. & Lincoln N.B. (1980) Assessment of activities of daily living in stroke patients. *British Journal of
Occupational Therapy* Feb., 44–46.

Wilson B. (1987) *Rehabilitation of Memory.* Guilford Press,
New York.

World Health Organization (1989) *Definitions from the Inter-
national Classification of Impairments, Disabilities and
Handicaps (ICIDH) in Rehabilitation.* Publications and
Documents Division, Council of Europe, Strasburg.

13: Rehabilitation after Stroke

R. LANGTON HEWER

Definitions, 157
Applied epidemiology, 158
   Incidence, 158
   Prevalence, 158
Assessment, 158
Recovery from stroke, 160
   Influence of 'therapy' on recovery, 160
   Intensity and timing of treatment, 160
   Activities of daily living, 161
   Walking, 161
   Arm recovery, 161
   Social and emotional recovery, 161
The stages of stroke, 162
Organization of stroke care, 162
   Care in hospital, 162
   In-patient rehabilitation units, 163
   Discharge into the community, 164
   Community support, 164
   The phase of residual disability, 164
Towards a model stroke service, 165
   Organization of services, 165
Final comments, 165

For many years stroke, and particularly its rehabilitation, was a Cinderella subject. Little attention had been devoted to it. There were few high-quality publications. There has, however, been a dramatic change during the last 10 years.

Stroke is now recognized as being a major cause of death and, even more importantly, of permanent disability. Managers have suddenly realized that the costs involved are enormous. There is now, also, the widespread view that the services offered to stroke patients are substandard (King's Fund Consensus Statement, 1988). A paradoxical situation has been reached, with large expenditure of money on the one hand and general dissatisfaction with the quality of service provision on the other. This chapter updates the previous contribution, written in 1982 (Langton Hewer, 1982). It is a pleasure to be able to document a number of different developments, together with a burgeoning interest in this previously neglected topic.

Definitions

The definition used in the Oxfordshire Community Stroke Project (1983), which embraces the WHO definition, is 'rapidly developing clinical symptoms and/or signs of focal, and at times global (applied to patients in deep coma and to those with subarachnoid haemorrhage), loss of cerebral function, with symptoms lasting more than 24 hours or leading to death, with no cause apparent other than of vascular origin'.

There have been many different attempts to define rehabilitation. For the purposes of this chapter, the one used by 26 neurological charities (Response to Health of the Nation, 1991) has been adopted: 'Rehabilitation for a disabled person involves all measures aimed at ensuring the highest possible quality of life, for the person concerned and his family, whatever the cause or severity of the disability.'

When faced with a person who is disabled as a result of a stroke (or, indeed, anything else), it may be useful to adopt the classification system suggested by the WHO (Aho *et al.*, 1980). Four terms are recognized as being important— pathology, impairment, disability and handicap. The example of a man of 50 who has suffered a left-hemisphere cerebral haemorrhage may be taken. The pathology is the haemorrhage. The impairment is the clinical reflection of the area of the brain that has been damaged. This may include dysphasia and paralysis of the right arm and leg. The term disability is used to describe the resultant disadvantage in terms of function—which might include difficulty with naming objects, inability to read, inability to write and inability to walk fast. The term handicap embraces the disadvantages faced by the disabled person in society, and may include loss of income, loss of friends and inability to do shopping unaided.

Medical rehabilitation involves a holistic approach, which involves a knowledge of all the four elements itemized above. It embraces, also, the prevention of functional deterioration, whether as a result of ageing, complications of the stroke or a further stroke.

Applied epidemiology

If there is to be a logical basis for stroke rehabilitation services, reliable information relating to the size and nature of the problem is required.

Incidence

The term 'incidence' refers to the number of new cases occurring within the general population per year. A number of studies have dealt with this topic. For instance, the Oxfordshire Community Stroke Project (1983) report an annual incidence of first stroke of 1.95 per 100 000 and a total incidence of 2.2 per 100 000, including recurrent cases. For both males and females, first-incidence rates increase with age and peak in the 75+ age-group. About 75% of strokes occur in persons aged 65 years of age or more. Such elderly people are liable to suffer with other disorders, including arthritis, coronary artery disease and general frailty.

An average health district of a quarter of a million persons will generate about 500 new strokes annually. At the end of 3 weeks, about 30% will have died and a further 30% will be fully independent. The core of the disability problem is the remaining 40%, comprising about 200 persons per quarter of a million population. The majority of disabled survivors will have initial weakness/paralysis of the arm and leg on one side of the body. About 20% of survivors will have some degree of dysphasia at 3 weeks. This latter figure falls rapidly to about 12% by 6 months (Wade *et al.*, 1986).

Prevalence

Studies of prevalence are notoriously difficult to undertake. In the field of stroke, there have been few. A survey of 14 225 persons in Copenhagen (Sorenson *et al.*, 1982) identified 115 stroke survivors, giving a prevalence of 518 per 100 000 population. Of these, 59% had residual neurological signs. However, most estimates of prevalence are based upon a combination of incidence and survival data. Kurtzke (1982) used an estimate of 600 per 100 000, 60% of whom would be disabled. Thus, in a population of a quarter of a million, there would be about 1500 stroke survivors, 900 of whom would be disabled. Most would be over the age of 65. Harris (1971) found that stroke was the cause of 24% of severe disablement in people living in the community.

Assessment

Assessment involves the identification, measurement and recording of deficits and problems. It is needed for both routine management and research.

Before a rehabilitation programme is commenced, it will be necessary to ascertain the precise nature and severity of any neurological, or other, deficits that exist. This will include such matters as cognitive state, language function, arm function and mobility. The use of assessment 'tools' enables problems to be identified and also quantified, so that the patient's progress can be monitored. In this way, a logical basis for treatment and management can be developed.

Research over the last 15 years has involved the measurement of recovery in large groups of patients, using formal assessments. This has enabled some of the rules of recovery to be defined, and has also started to make it possible for rehabilitation techniques to be evaluated. The subject of assessment has been discussed in detail elsewhere (Donaldson *et al.*, 1973; Wade *et al.*, 1985a). Any assessment technique used should, if used for research, have a number of characteristics, which would include the following:

1 Validity – i.e. it must measure what it is supposed to measure.

2 Repeatability – it should be possible for several observers to obtain the same result.

3 Sensitivity – the test must be sensitive enough to detect change in performance.

4 Communicability – the result of the test should

be able to be presented, if possible, in numerical terms so that it can be communicated to others.

5 Simplicity – the test should be easy for the patient and staff to understand and should be able to be undertaken reasonably quickly.

A considerable number of areas for potential assessment exist. Some of these are itemized below:

1 *Activities of daily living* (ADL). The patient's ability to look after himself and live independently is measured by scales that test the various ADL. There are many published scales. One of the scales most commonly used is the Barthel (Mahoney & Barthel, 1965), which has been found to satisfy the criteria listed above. The scale has been used in research and also in everyday clinical practice. For instance, a score of 15 out of 20 is usually reached before a patient can safely go home from hospital. This scoring system does not include information about communication or cognitive functioning. The functional independence measure (FIM) test is being increasingly used, particularly in the USA, as a general measure of functioning (Keith *et al.*, 1987).

2 *Quality of life after stroke.* So far, little attention has been paid to evaluating systematically the quality of life after stroke. Quality of life measures are useful not only in gaining a better understanding of patients' reactions to illness, but also for evaluating the efficacy of therapeutic interventions. A recent review (de Haan *et al.*, 1993) of 10 quality of life instruments has been undertaken. Most of these were generic quality of life measures but there was one stroke-specific instrument – the Frenchay activities index (Holbrook & Skilbeck, 1983).

3 *Orientation and intellect.* Most sophisticated tests can only be applied by a trained neuropsychologist. A variety of simple tests which can be used by medical clinicians and others are available. The most commonly used are the Hodkinson (1972) test and the minimental test battery (Folstein *et al.*, 1975).

4 *Perceptual function.* Many patients, particularly those with right-hemisphere damage, have disturbances of perception. A disorder of spatial orientation is one of the commonest problems identified. The Rivermead perceptual test (Bhavani & Cockburn, 1983) is probably the best for general use.

5 *Dysphasia.* Dysphasia is a disturbance of language function and is a common sequel of stroke. A formal assessment of speech and language is usually undertaken by speech therapists, and a large number of specialist tests exist. However, doctors need to be able to identify dysphasia and should be able to routinely test understanding of speech, naming and description of objects, reading and writing. A simple screening assessment technique exists – the Frenchay aphasia screening test (Enderby *et al.*, 1987). This produces a numerical score. The functional communication profile (FCP) (Sarno, 1969) is a test of functional speech and needs to be applied by a trained speech therapist. It has been found to be particularly useful in clinical work and for research.

6 *Arm function.* The arm is an extremely complex organ and has many functions, including manipulation of tools, writing, feeding, support, balance and gesture. A review of existing measures has recently been undertaken (Wade, 1989). It is suggested that the Frenchay arm test (Wade *et al.*, 1983) and the nine-hole peg test (Sharpless, 1982) are most suitable for routine use. The action arm test (Lyle, 1981), supplemented if necessary by dynamometric measurement of muscle strength (particularly grip), is probably the most appropriate for research purposes.

7 *Walking.* For routine purposes, it is necessary to know the following:

(a) How safely can the patient walk? Does he/she fall?

(b) How fast can the patient walk?

(c) How far can the patient walk?

It may also be helpful to have information about walking ability over different surfaces, e.g. carpet and rough ground. The ability to climb stairs is also important.

The component parts of gait, for example, stride length, step length and step frequency, can be measured (Robinson & Smidt, 1981). However, the speed of walking has been shown to correlate well with other indices of disturbed gait (Imms & Edholm, 1981). Chin *et al.* (1982) showed that, whilst controls walked at an average speed of 59 m per minute (i.e. approximately 1 m per second), stroke patients varied between 51 m per minute, for those who could walk without an aid, to 17 m per minute, for patients who walked with a zimmer frame. This technique has also been used to investigate the rate and extent of recovery (Wade et al., 1987a).

Recovery from stroke

The majority of patients who survive a stroke show significant functional recovery.

Adaptative recovery involves using alternative strategies – for example, using the unaffected hand for doing up buttons. Intrinsic recovery depends largely upon a return of neural control – for example, increase in the amount of voluntary movement in the paralysed hand. Adaptative and intrinsic recovery cannot be entirely separated. The mechanisms of intrinsic recovery are still largely speculative. It is important to note that both types of recovery can be hindered by complications such as severe depression or fractures. A number of detailed studies of recovery have been undertaken (Marquardsen, 1969; Andrews et al., 1981; Skilbeck et al., 1983; Partridge et al., 1987). The following general rules apply:

1 The amount of recovery depends largely upon the severity of the initial deficit. The more severe the initial deficit, the less the ultimate degree of recovery.

2 Recovery is fastest during the first 3 months and most recovery has occurred by the end of this time.

3 At most, 5–10% of recovery occurs between 6 months and 1 year.

4 It is highly exceptional for measurable recovery to occur beyond 1 year, although this has been recorded in sporadic cases.

5 All functions (for example, language, ADL, arm function and mobility) show the same general patterns of recovery.

Influence of 'therapy' on recovery

The term 'therapy' embraces the contribution of physiotherapists, occupational therapists and speech therapists. However, it is not possible to separate out the work done by therapists from that performed by other personnel, including doctors and nurses.

A principal objective of 'therapy' is to prevent complications. Thus, for example, fractures and contractures can almost certainly be prevented by avoiding premature attempts at walking and by frequent passive movements of the limbs. Attention to the psychological sequelae of stroke is important (see below). For example, the prevention and treatment of depression may be a significant way of influencing function.

A recent publication (Stroke Rehabilitation, 1992) summarized 17 of the main published controlled trials in rehabilitation effectiveness (Feldman et al., 1962; Meikle et al., 1979; Garraway et al., 1980a, b; Smith et al., 1981; David et al., 1982; Hamrin, 1982; Smith et al., 1982; Lincoln et al., 1984; Stevens et al., 1984; Sivenius et al., 1985; Strand et al., 1985, 1986; Wertz et al., 1986; Tallis, 1989; Indredavik et al., 1991; Sunderland et al., 1992). The evaluation of therapy is difficult and subject to major ethical constraints. The following observations can be made:

1 There have been very few randomized studies comparing no therapy with therapy.

2 The amount of formal therapy is small. One study (Wade et al., 1984) showed that physical therapy was given at an average amount of 46 minutes for each working day, which represented 3.4% of the patient's working day.

3 There appears to be a direct relationship between the severity of stroke and the amount of therapy actually given. Thus, the most severely disabled patients received the most therapy (Brocklehurst et al., 1978; Wade et al., 1984).

4 There have been a few trials which have compared different therapeutic techniques (Feldman et al., 1962; Inaba et al., 1973; Logigian et al., 1983). None have shown conclusively that any technique is superior to another. The effectiveness of routine speech therapy was compared in a randomized controlled design study with that given by volunteers (David et al., 1982). No difference between the two groups was found, although the amount of therapy given to the treatment group was only 2 hours per week.

Intensity and timing of treatment

Smith et al. (1982) conducted a randomized controlled trial on stroke patients discharged from hospital. There was evidence that intensive rehabilitation, defined as attendance at out-patients 4 full days per week, may benefit a 'middle band' (around 10%) of stroke patients who are healthy enough to tolerate an intensive therapy pro- gramme. However, the advantage beyond what would be expected from less intensive therapy (i.e. 3 half-days per week) was limited, and is not necessarily sustained. It is clear that any improve- ments that may occur must be considered alongside the personal costs associated with intensive re- habilitation regimes in terms of time and physical discomfort.

There have been a small number of uncontrolled studies of intensive therapy of aphasic patients (Vignolo, 1964; Hagen, 1973), but the results were not conclusive. An important study from the USA demonstrated an improved outcome from an average of 9 hours per week of speech therapy for aphasic patients (Wertz et al., 1986). A British study found no significant improvement in outcome for patients receiving only 2 hours of speech therapy per week (Lincoln et al., 1984). Several studies have suggested that early intensive therapy has a beneficial effect on the speed of early recovery, but the general finding is that the long-term status is not influenced (Garraway et al., 1980a; Hamrin, 1982).

Activities of daily living

There have been a considerable number of pub- lished studies on recovery of ADL function. Skilbeck et al. (1983) found that most improvement in the Barthel ADL score had occurred by 3 months. Sig- nificant late morbidity exists. The Bristol group found that, at 6 months, 31% of survivors needed help with dressing, and only 51% were inde- pendent for bathing (Wade & Langton Hewer, 1987).

Walking

It is generally agreed that 50–80% of stroke patients will be able to walk independently by 6 months. Wade et al. (1987a) assessed walking speed in a group of stroke survivors; only 22% could walk at a normal speed by 3 months. No infor- mation is available about the distance that patients can walk after a stroke. As far as is known, there have been no controlled studies that have demon- strated the effects of intervention, such as surgery or the use of a caliper, on walking speed and safety.

Arm recovery

The hemiplegic arm recovers less well than the leg. The Bristol study (Wade et al., 1983) found that only 14% of those who initially had a paralysed arm eventually regained normal arm function, and a further 25% made a partial recovery. The degree of recovery eventually achieved depended mainly upon the initial extent of loss. Severe sensory loss was a further adverse factor. A recent study (Sunderland et al., 1992) has shown that an in- tensively treated group do show improved function at 6 months as compared with a control group. Various techniques are currently being evaluated in an attempt to improve recovery, including the use of an arm suspension device to eliminate the effect of gravity, the use of computerized games which can be performed with the affected arm, and partial immobilization of the normal arm with the objec- tive of forcing the patient to use the affected limb (and thus, hopefully, avoiding the phenomenon of learned non-use).

Social and emotional recovery

Stroke causes considerable emotional and psy- chological distress, both to the patient and to the carer (Wade et al., 1985b). About one-third of survivors are depressed at any one time (Wade et al., 1987b). Sexual problems are common, and one study showed that only 36% of survivors main- tained their previous frequency of sexual inter- course (Fugl-Meyer & Jaasko, 1980). Of 50 spouses interviewed by Holbrook (1982), 38% found that stroke had an adverse effect on their sex life. Legh- Smith et al. (1986a) found that 58% of patients who had been driving before the stroke did not resume driving afterwards. Cessation of driving was associated with an increased frequency of de- pression, and with loss of social activities.

Many patients, even some with good physical recovery, are socially inactive and have high levels of psychological morbidity. The range of emotional disorders is wide and includes anxiety, agoraphobia and pathological emotionalism (House et al., 1991).

It appears that much of the psychological morbidity remains undetected and ignored. Few patients are prescribed antidepressant drugs. There therefore remains the possibility that some patients who have made a good physical recovery are seriously underperforming on account of the psychological and social problems.

The stages of stroke

Four arbitrary stages of stroke care can be recognized. The stages cannot be totally separated and it will quickly be realized, for instance, that rehabilitation and secondary prevention are closely linked.

1 *Prevention.* Clearly, prevention is better than cure. Preventive measures include the proper management of hypertension, transient ischaemic attacks, atrial fibrillation, major carotid stenosis, hyperlipidaemia, smoking and alcohol intake. A detailed discussion of preventive measures is clearly beyond the scope of this chapter, but the topic is of much importance – particularly for patients who have shown a reasonable degree of recovery from the first stroke.

2 *Acute phase.* The acute phase of stroke may be arbitrarily considered to occupy the first 7 days following the ictus. Proper rehabilitation starts from the first day. Important elements include the proper management of dysphagia, the prevention of pneumonia, the maintenance of proper hydration and correct positioning of paralysed limbs. In addition, it is important to take note of the profound psychological shock experienced by both patient and carers. An explanation of precisely what a stroke is will need to be given, and the relatives, particularly, must be given an idea of the prognosis.

3 *Recovery phase.* The recovery phase may be arbitrarily considered to cover the next 12 weeks. During this time, the majority of recovery will occur.

4 *Phase of long-term adjustment.* The phase of long-term adjustment stems from about 3 months post-stroke. Many stroke patients are left in a permanently disabled state, resulting in a profound change in lifestyle. An important objective at this point is to achieve the maximum physical function and the best possible psychological adaptation to residual disability.

Organization of stroke care

In the United Kingdom, between 50 and 70% of stroke patients are admitted to hospital (Wade &

Langton Hewer, 1985; Bamford *et al.*, 1986). The reasons for admission to hospital include the need to make an accurate diagnosis, the possibility of active medical treatment and, most importantly, social and nursing reasons. The Bristol study showed that about 25% of those not admitted to hospital are severely disabled (Wade & Langton Hewer, 1985). It might be expected that the proportion of people who remain at home would depend upon the quality and availability of domiciliary services (for example, home nursing, physiotherapy, etc.). However, a study of augmented domiciliary care (Wade *et al.*, 1985c) did not show any reduction in the hospital admission rate or in the duration of time spent in hospital.

Care in hospital

Carstairs (1976) found that 56% of stroke patients were discharged from general medical beds and 28% from geriatric beds. A more recent study, from Bristol (Wade *et al.*, 1985d), showed that stroke patients occupied 5.6% of all occupied beds in a general hospital and 20.6% of general medical beds. A recent Office of Health Economics (1988) study found that 42% of stroke patients were managed in general medical wards and 41% by geriatric medicine. About 7% were accommodated in neurological or neurosurgical wards, and 6% were admitted to beds under the care of general practitioners. A recent study of 91 000 discharges of stroke patients from hospital beds throughout England and Wales during 1989 showed that about 7% of patients were discharged from neurological beds (R. Langton-Hewer, unpublished data). It is clear, therefore, that an increasing number of inpatients, particularly those in the older age bracket, are looked after by geriatricians in the UK. Involvement of neurologists appears to be small.

The Bristol study (Wade *et al.*, 1985d) found that 42% of patients admitted to hospital died before discharge, 46% returned home or to the home of relatives and 12% were transferred to some form of institutional care. Those patients returning home stayed in hospital a median time of 16 days, although the mean time was 29.3 days. However, those patients who ultimately went to institutional care stayed in hospital for much longer – a median of 83 days (mean 131.5 days). It is clearly possible

Table 13.1 Major problems in the rehabilitation phase of stroke (King's Fund Consensus Statement, 1988)

---

1 Misunderstanding and rivalries between professionals
2 Breakdown of communication between professionals, patients and their carers
3 Insufficient appreciation of the impact of stroke on the patient's family
4 Ill-prepared and sometimes unplanned discharge home
5 Serious shortage of money
6 Long periods in which the patients are unoccupied
7 Ill-considered admission to hospital
8 Failure to recognize and respond to mood disturbance
9 Delegation of care to inadequately trained medical staff
10 Confusion caused by too many people being involved

---

that the time spent in an acute hospital could be reduced by an improvement in domiciliary care services, and possibly by earlier discharge to nursing homes or other residential care.

There has been much criticism, in the UK, of the care of stroke patients in general hospitals. These criticisms were voiced at a King's Fund Consensus Conference (1988). Details of some of the criticisms are given in Table 13.1. This conference appeared to identify major deficiencies in the provision of rehabilitation services, particularly in hospital. Because of the evident dissatisfaction with the present standards of provision within general hospitals, the establishment of stroke wards has been suggested. Several such wards have been set up in the UK and the majority are operated by geriatricians.

In-patient rehabilitation units

One of the first stroke units in the UK was that started by Professor Bernard Isaacs (1977). Since then, there have been several attempts to evaluate the effectiveness of such wards. Garraway *et al.* (1980b) conducted a randomized controlled trial comparing the management of the elderly in a special stroke unit with that in general medical wards of hospitals in Edinburgh. This study suggested that patients in the stroke unit made a more rapid recovery, but, at 1 year post-stroke, there

were no long-term benefits. The stroke unit patients occupied about 7% fewer beds during the first year than patients managed in general wards. A study in Dover (Stevens *et al.*, 1984) also showed little difference between outcome in the two groups. A third study (Strand *et al.*, 1985) compared 110 patients admitted to a six-bed special unit with 183 patients who were judged suitable for admission but could not be accepted into the stroke unit. The stroke unit patients in this trial did appear to do better than patients managed in general wards.

There is very little literature about essential elements of practice on a stroke ward. The following elements would need to be considered:

1 Assessment of neurological and disability status, using agreed assessment tools. These assessments would need to be repeated at regular intervals.
2 Evidence that short- and long-term goals have been set and modified as appropriate.
3 Complication rate on the ward – for example, fractures, pressure sores and stiff/painful shoulders.
4 Evidence that the patients were staying in hospital for an appropriate time – i.e. were not discharged prematurely and were not remaining in hospital unnecessarily.
5 Evidence that the psychological problems of stroke are recognized and catered for.
6 Evidence that the problem of boredom is specifically addressed. This is particularly important, bearing in mind that many patients are in hospital for 6 weeks or more.
7 Evidence that discharge into the community is properly planned and that all persons are fully informed.
8 Evidence that full records are kept in the hospital notes.
9 Evidence that specific problems have been addressed and that the elements of good practice are identified. These would include the following:
  (a) nutrition;
  (b) sleeping;
  (c) sitting/posture;
  (d) feeding;
  (e) leg swelling;
  (f) footwear;
  (g) management of the paralysed arm.
The principles of good practice in stroke wards need to be clearly identified and documented. So far, this has not been done.

Discharge into the community

The King's Fund Consensus Conference (1988) identified poor discharge planning as being a major problem. The following items are particularly important:

1 The need to carefully plan discharge into the community well in advance. In this way, the provision of community support can be organized.

2 Home alterations: certain alterations may need to be undertaken to the house before the patient goes home. If the patient cannot walk, it will be necessary to ensure that there is access to the house, toilet and garden.

3 The community staff must be informed in good time as to discharge plans.

4 A written summary of the patient's medical and disability status should be sent to the family doctor and community staff in advance of the patient's discharge.

5 It will be essential to ensure that the patient has been fully instructed in lifting and other techniques. The provision of written information about stroke, to both the carer and the patient, is likely to be important.

Community support

Once the patient leaves hospital, the family doctor will be in overall control of the medical situation relating to that particular patient. S/he will need to work in close collaboration with community staff, including remedial therapists and social workers. A variety of support services are available, including home aide and home care. For some severely disabled patients, there will be need for major community input, including some form of relief service, so that the carer can leave the house. Respite care, in a specially provided unit, may be appropriate.

The phase of residual disability

About 50% of stroke survivors will be left with a significant disability. Wade & Langton Hewer (1987) found that 47% of patients achieved 100% on the Barthel scale at 6 months, while 9% showed severe or very severe disability – scoring 45% or less on the Barthel scale. Of the total, 73% could walk alone, but only about one-third could walk at

a normal speed (Wade et al., 1987a). A study of services received by patients after discharge from hospital was undertaken by Legh-Smith et al. (1986b), who examined 436 survivors of the Bristol stroke study. Of the total, 38% were being visited by one or more community services (the major ones being district nursing, home help and meals on wheels), 10% were attending a day centre, and 19% of disabled patients were being looked after at home without any outside help. The number of patients who were seen in hospital out-patient clinics is unknown. In the Bristol series (Legh-Smith et al., 1986b), 56% of patients were in touch with their general practitioner.

There have been few studies investigating the value of long-term therapy and support. However, an important study by Smith et al. (1982) has been previously mentioned.

A recent study of long-term outcome of stroke showed that few patients or carers thought that more rehabilitation was necessary, but more than one-fifth identified a need for better support after discharge from hospital, counselling and more information about services for disabled people (Greveson & James, 1991).

Several studies have tried to improve the long-term physical, emotional and social function of patients with stroke. A small study evaluating the provision of booklets for patients and carers reported that many had found the booklets helpful, although there was no measurable effect on physical or social outcome (Pain & McLellan, 1990). The Leeds placement scheme prevented deterioration of physical function in a selected group of stroke patients, but had no impact on social activity (Geddes et al., 1989). The Bradford stroke trial showed that either attendance at a day hospital or physiotherapy at home maintained physical function up to 6 months after discharge from hospital, but many patients and carers remained emotionally distressed and socially restricted (Young & Forster, 1992).

Physiotherapy given at home may have a role, even 3 years after stroke, when a small improvement in mobility can be achieved. Social activities, however, remain unaffected (Wade et al., 1992).

Holbrook (1982) has postulated that patients with stroke experience four stages of adjustment to disability: crisis, treatment, realization and adjustment. It is possible that the treatment stage of recovery may currently be overemphasized in the medical model of care. New studies are needed to investigate ways of providing support, emphasizing the importance of psychosocial rehabilitation.

It is clear that the principal objective during the phase of long-term disability is to achieve the maximum possible quality of life at reasonable cost. Clearly, both the physical and the emotional sequelae of stroke must be considered.

Towards a model stroke service

When discussing the components of an ideal stroke service, some essential facts must be considered.

1 The high cost of stroke and the absence of evidence that good value is being obtained for the money spent. There is clearly the possibility that time in hospital could be reduced.

2 About 70% of patients are admitted to hospital, mainly for social, nursing and rehabilitative reasons. This is the principal identifiable expense to the NHS.

3 There is an increasing amount that can be done in the acute phase to ameliorate the effects of a stroke. A number of drugs are about to become available and there is preliminary evidence that some of these may be effective. At present, however, specific drug therapy is not available for most patients.

4 It is important to recognize that dysphagia occurs in nearly 50% of stroke patients and can lead to significant dehydration and malnutrition.

5 The prevalence of stroke disability is high. There is evidence that much distress and unhappiness are caused by stroke. In some instances, this may be preventable.

6 Stroke services, both in the community and in hospital, have up to now, been poorly organized and there are many deficiencies.

7 There is some evidence that segregation of patients into stroke units during the rehabilitation phase may be beneficial. Studies are needed to identify the important component features of a stroke rehabilitation programme, as delivered both in stroke units and elsewhere.

8 Many stroke patients remain permanently disabled. The psychological sequelae of stroke, for both the patient and the spouse, are profound. Many find adjustment difficult, and depression is common.

9 The value of comprehensive, long-term follow-up and support has not been fully evaluated.

10 The evidence that intrinsic recovery can be influenced by remedial therapy is, at the moment, inconclusive. However, therapy has an important role in the assessment of deficits, in the prevention of complications and in helping the patient and spouse to achieve his/her maximum potential.

11 The majority of recovery occurs in the first 3 months, but measurable recovery can occur in some patients up to 1 year post-stroke.

Organization of services

Stroke services require to be organized on a locality basis. Where possible, patients should be treated and rehabilitated as near as possible to their own home.

1 There should be a district policy for cerebrovascular disease and this should be updated from time to time.

2 The costs of stroke to the health authority should be identified annually.

3 There should be one, or possibly two, persons responsible for implementing the district stroke policy.

4 Consideration should be given to some form of segregation of patients into one place – i.e. a stroke ward.

5 There must be an effective community service. This must involve medical, nursing, social work and therapy elements.

6 There must be evidence of effective collaboration between the various elements of the district stroke service.

Final comments

Stroke rehabilitation is now recognized internationally as being an important and major topic for concern and research. There is an increasing interest in the subject by doctors, managers and organizations representing patients. The elements of a high-quality stroke service are now emerging, and there are an increasing number of high-quality publications on the subject. It is anticipated that, in the next 10 years, there will be further significant advances.

References

Aho K., Harmsen P., Hatano S., Marquardsen J., Smirnov V.E. & Strasser T. (1980) Cerebrovascular disease in the community: results of a WHO collaborative study. *Bulletin of World Health Organization* **58** (1), 133–130.

Andrews K., Brocklehurst J.C., Richards B. & Laycock P.J. (1981) The rate of recovery from stroke, and its measurement. *International Rehabilitation Medicine* **3**, 155–161.

Bamford J., Sandercock P., Warlow C. & Gray M. (1986) Why are patients with acute stroke admitted to hospital? *British Medical Journal* **1**, 1369–1372.

Bhavani G. & Cockburn J. (1983) The viability of the Rivermead perceptual assessment and implications for some commonly used assessments of perception. *British Journal of Occupational Therapy* **46**, 17–19.

Brocklehurst J.C., Andrews K., Richards B. & Laycock P. (1978) How much physical therapy for patients with stroke? *British Medical Journal* **1**, 1307–1310.

Carstairs V. (1976) Resource consumption and the cost to the community. In Gillingham F.J., Mawdsley C. & Williams A.E. (eds) *Stroke*, pp. 516–528. Churchill Livingstone, New York.

Chin P.L., Rosie A., Irving M. & Smith R. (1982) Studies in hemiplegic gait. In Clifford Rose F. (ed.) *Advances in Stroke Therapy*, pp. 197–211. Raven Press, New York.

David R., Enderby P. & Bainton D. (1982) Treatment of acquired aphasia: speech therapists and volunteers compared. *Journal of Neurology, Neurosurgery and Psychiatry* **45**, 957–961.

de Haan R., Aaronson N., Limburg M., Langton Hewer R. & van Crevel H. (1993) Measuring quality of life in stroke. *Stroke* **24** (2), 320–327.

Donaldson S.W., Wagner C.C. & Gresham G.E. (1973) A unified ADL evaluation form. *Archives of Physical and Medical Rehabilitation* **54**, 175–179.

Enderby P.M., Wood V.A., Wade D.T. & Langton Hewer R. (1987) The Frenchay aphasia screening test: a short, simple test for aphasia appropriate for non-specialists. *International Rehabilitation Medicine* **8**, 166–170.

Feldman D.J., Lee P.R., Unterecker J., Lloyd K., Rusk H.A. & Toole A. (1962) A comparison of functionally orientated medical care and formal rehabilitation in the management of patients with hemiplegia due to cerebrovascular disease. *Journal of Chronic Diseases* **15**, 297–310.

Folstein M.F., Folsten S.F. & McHugh P.R. (1975) Mini-mental state: a practical method for grading the cognitive state of patients for the clinician. *Journal of Psychiatric Research* **12**, 189–198.

Fugl-Meyer A.R. & Jaasko L. (1980) Post-stroke hemiplegia and sexual intercourse. *Scandinavian Journal of Rehabilitation Medicine* Suppl. 7, 158–166.

Garraway W.M., Akhtar A.J., Prescott R.J. & Hockey L. (1980a) Management of acute stroke in the elderly: preliminary results of a controlled trial. *British Medical Journal* **280**, 1040–1043.

Garraway W.M., Akhtar A.J., Hockey L. & Prescott R.J. (1980b) Management of acute stroke in the elderly: follow-up of a controlled trial. *British Medical Journal* **281**, 827–829.

Geddes J.M.L., Claydon A.D. & Chamberlain M.A. (1989) The Leeds family placement scheme: an evaluation of its use as a rehabilitation resource. *Clinical Rehabilitation* **3**, 189–197.

Greveson G. & James O. (1991) Improving long-term outcome after stroke – the views of patients and carers. *Health Trends* **23**, 161–162.

Hagen C. (1973) Communication abilities in hemiplegia: effect of speech therapy. *Archives of Physical and Medical Rehabilitation* **54**, 454–463.

Hamrin E. (1982) Early activation in stroke: does it make a difference? *Scandinavian Journal of Rehabilitation Medicine* **14**, 101–109.

Harris A.I. (1971) *Handicapped and Impaired in Great Britain. Part 1.* Office of Population, Censuses and Surveys, HMSO, London.

Hodkinson H.M. (1972) Evaluation of a mental test score for assessment of mental impairment in the elderly. *Age and Ageing* **1**, 233–238.

Holbrook M. (1982) Stroke: social and emotional outcome. *Journal of Royal College of Physicians* **16**, 100–104.

Holbrook M. & Skilbeck C.E. (1983) An activities index for use with stroke patients. *Age and Ageing* **12**, 166–170.

House A., Dennis M., Mogridge L., Warlow C., Hawton K. & Jones L. (1991) Mood disorders in the year after first stroke. *British Journal of Psychiatry* **158**, 83–92.

Imms F.J. & Edholm O.G. (1981) Studies of gait and mobility in the elderly. *Age and Ageing* **10**, 147–157.

Inaba M., Edberg E., Montgomery J. & Gillis M.K. (1973) Effectiveness of functional training, active exercise and resistive exercise for patients with hemiplegia. *Physical Therapy* **52**, 28–35.

Indredavik B., Bakke F., Solberg R., Rokseth R., Haaheim L. & Holme I. (1991) Benefit of a stroke unit: a randomised controlled trial. *Stroke* **22**, 1026–1031.

Isaacs B. (1977) Five years experience of a stroke unit. *Health Bulletin* **35**, 94–98.

Keith R.A., Granger C.V., Hamilton B.B. & Sherwin F.S. (1987) The functional independence measure: a new tool for rehabilitation. In Eisenberg M.G. & Greziak R.C. (eds) *Advances in Clinical Rehabilitation*, pp. 6–18. Springer Verlag, New York.

King's Fund Consensus Statement (1988) The treatment of stroke. *British Medical Journal* **297**, 126–128.

Kurtzke J.F. (1982) The current neurologic burden of

illness and injury in the United States. *Neurology* **32**, 1207–1214.

Langton Hewer R. (1982) Rehabilitation of stroke. In Illis L.S., Sedgwick E.M. & Glanville H.J. (eds) *Rehabilitation of the Neurological Patient*. Blackwell Scientific Publications, Oxford.

Legh-Smith J., Wade D.T. & Langton Hewer R. (1986a) Driving after a stroke. *Journal of Royal Society of Medicine* **79**, 200–203.

Legh-Smith J., Wade D.T. & Langton Hewer R. (1986b) Services for stroke patients one year after stroke. *Journal of Epidemiology and Community Health* **40**, 161–165.

Lincoln N.B., McGuirk E., Mulley G.P., Lendrem W., Jones A.C. & Mitchell J.R.A. (1984) Effectiveness of speech therapy for aphasic stroke patients. *Lancet* **i**, 1197–1200.

Logigian M.K., Samuels M.A., Falconer J. & Zagar R. (1983) Clinical exercise trial for stroke patients. *Archives of Physical and Medical Rehabilitation* **64**, 364–367.

Lyle R.C. (1981) A performance test for assessment of upper limb function in physical rehabilitation treatment and research. *International Journal of Rehabilitation Research* **4**, 483–492.

Mahoney F.I. & Barthel D.W. (1965) Functional evaluation: the Barthel index. *Maryland State Medical Journal* **14**, 61–65.

Marquardsen J. (1969) *The Natural History of Acute Cerebrovascular Disease: a Retrospective Study of 769 Patients*. Munksgaard, Copenhagen.

Meikle M., Wechsler E., Tupper A. *et al.* (1979) Comparative trial of volunteer and professional treatments of dysphasia after stroke. *British Medical Journal* **2**, 87–89.

Office of Health Economics (1988) *Stroke*.

Oxfordshire Community Stroke Project (1983) Incidence of stroke in Oxfordshire: first year's experience of a community stroke register. *British Medical Journal* **287**, 713–717.

Pain H.S.B. & McLellan D.L. (1990) The use of individualised booklets after a stroke. *Clinical Rehabilitation* **4**, 265–272.

Partridge C.J., Johnston M. & Edwards S. (1987) Recovery from physical disability after stroke: normal patterns as a basis for evaluation. *Lancet* **i**, 373–375.

Response to Health of the Nation, by 26 Neurological Charities (1991) *Neurological Provision: Key Areas and Targets*.

Robinson J.L. & Smidt G.L. (1981) Quantitative gait evaluation in the clinic. *Physical Therapy* **61**, 351–353.

Sarno M.T. (1969) *The Functional Communication Profile: Manual of Directions*. Rehabilitation Monograph 42. Institute of Rehabilitation Medicine, New York.

Sharpless J.W. (1982) The nine-hole peg test of finger–hand co-ordination for the hemiplegic patient. In Sharpless J.W. (ed.) *Mossman's A Problem-orientated Approach to Stroke Rehabilitation*, pp. 470–473. Charles C. Thomas, Springfield, Illinois.

Sivenius J., Pyorala K., Heinonen O.P., Salonen J.T. & Riekkinen P. (1985) The significance of intensity of rehabilitation after stroke – a controlled trial. *Stroke* **16**, 928–931.

Skilbeck C.E., Wade D.T., Langton Hewer R. & Wood V.A. (1983) Recovery after stroke. *Journal of Neurology, Neurosurgery and Psychiatry* **46**, 5–8.

Smith D.S., Goldenberg E., Ashburn A. *et al.* (1981) Remedial therapy after stroke: a randomised controlled trial. *British Medical Journal* **282**, 517–520.

Smith M.E., Garraway W.M., Smith D.L. & Akhtar A.J. (1982) Therapy impact on functional outcome in a controlled trial of stroke rehabilitation. *Archives of Physical and Medical Rehabilitation* **63**, 21–24.

Sorenson P.S., Boysen G., Jensen G. & Schnohr P. (1982) Prevalence of stroke in a district of Copenhagen. *Acta Neurologica Scandinavica* **66**, 68–81.

Stevens R.S., Ambler N.R. & Warren M.D. (1984) A randomised controlled trial of a stroke rehabilitation ward. *Age and Ageing* **13**, 65–75.

Strand T., Asplund K., Eriksson S., Hagg E., Lithner F. & Wester P.O. (1985) A non-intensive stroke unit reduces functional disability and the need for long-term hospitalisation. *Stroke* **16**, 29–34.

Strand T., Asplund K., Eriksson S., Hagg E., Lithner F. & Wester P.O. (1986) Stroke unit care – who benefits? Comparisons with general medical care in relation to prognostic indicators on admission. *Stroke* **17**, 377–381.

Sunderland A., Tinson D.J., Bradley E.L., Fletcher D., Langton Hewer R. & Wade D.T. (1992) Enhanced physical therapy improves recovery of arm function after a stroke: a randomised controlled trial. *Journal of Neurology, Neurosurgery and Psychiatry* **55** (7), 530–535.

Tallis R. (1989) Measurement and the future of rehabilitation. *Geriatric Medicine* **19**, 31–40.

University of Leeds (1992) Stroke rehabilitation. *Effective Health Care* **2**.

Vignolo L.A. (1964) Evolution of aphasia and language rehabilitation: a retrospective exploratory study. *Cortex* **1**, 344–367.

Wade D.T. (1989) Measuring arm impairment and disability after stroke. *International Disability Studies* **11**, 89–92.

Wade D.T. & Langton Hewer R. (1985) Hospital admission for acute stroke: who, for how long, and to what effect? *Journal of Epidemiology and Community Health* **39**, 347–352.

Wade D.T. & Langton Hewer R. (1987) Functional abilities after stroke: measurement, natural history and prognosis. *Journal of Neurology, Neurosurgery and Psychiatry* **50**, 177–182.

Wade D.T., Langton Hewer R., Wood V.A., Skilbeck C.E. & Ismail H.M. (1983) The hemiplegic arm after stroke: measurement and recovery. *Journal of Neurology, Neurosurgery and Psychiatry* **46**, 521–524.

Wade D.T., Skilbeck C.E., Langton Hewer R. & Wood V.A. (1984) Therapy after stroke: amounts, determinants and effects. *International Rehabilitation Medicine* **6**, 105–110.

Wade D.T., Langton Hewer R., Skilbeck C.E. & David R.M. (1985a) *Stroke – a Critical Approach to Diagnosis, Treatment and Management*. Chapman and Hall Medical, London.

Wade D.T., Legh-Smith J. & Langton Hewer R. (1985b) Social activities after stroke: measurement and natural history using the Frenchay activities index. *International Rehabilitation Medicine* **7**, 176–181.

Wade D.T., Langton Hewer R., Skilbeck C.E., Bainton D. & Burns-Cox C. (1985c) Controlled trial of a home-care service for acute stroke patients. *Lancet* **ii**, 323–326.

Wade D.T., Wood V.A. & Langton Hewer R. (1985d) Use of hospital resources by acute stroke patients. *Journal of Royal College of Physicians* **19**, 48–52.

Wade D.T., Langton R., David R.M. & Enderby P.M. (1986) Aphasia after stroke: natural history and as-sociated deficits. *Journal of Neurology, Neurosurgery and Psychiatry* **49**, 11–16.

Wade D.T., Wood V.A., Heller A., Maggs J. & Langton Hewer R. (1987a) Walking after stroke: measurement and recovery over the first 3 months. *Scandinavian Journal of Rehabilitation Medicine* **19**, 25–30.

Wade D.T., Legh-Smith J. & Langton Hewer R. (1987b) Depressed mood after a stroke – a community study of its frequency. *British Journal of Psychiatry* **151**, 200–205.

Wade D.T., Collen F.M., Robb G.F. & Warlow C.P. (1992) Physiotherapy intervention late after stroke. *British Medical Journal* **304**, 609–613.

Wertz R.T., Weiss D.G., Aten J. *et al.* (1986) Comparison of clinic, home, and deferred language treatment for aphasia: a Veterans Administrative Co-operative study. *Archives of Neurology* **43**, 653–658.

Young J.B. & Forster A. (1992) The Bradford stroke trial: results at six months. *British Medical Journal* **305**, 1085–1089.

14: Rehabilitation of Parkinson's Disease

D.E. BATEMAN

Importance of correct diagnosis, 169
  Case history, 169
Natural history, 170
Drug treatment, 170
  Introduction, 170
  L-Dopa and carboxylase inhibitor, 171
  Anticholinergics, 171
  Amantidine, 172
  Direct dopamine agonists, 172
  Bromocriptine, 172
  Lysuride, 172
  Pergolide, 172
  Apomorphine, 172
  Selegiline, 172
Approach to treatment, 173
  Management of fluctuations, 173
  Assessment of patients, 173
  Types of dyskinesia, 173
  Pain and dystonia, 174
  Neuropsychiatric problems, 174
  Constipation, urinary difficulties and sexual function, 175
  Sleep, 175
Non-drug treatment, 175
  Therapists, 175
  Parkinson's Disease Society, 175
Epidemiology and organization of services, 176

Importance of correct diagnosis

Effective rehabilitation requires accurate diagnosis. This is particularly true of Parkinson's disease, which can easily be confused with other akinetic rigid syndromes. Although the diagnosis of Parkinson's disease often seems and is easy, neurologists incorrectly diagnose it in about 20% of cases (Hughes *et al.*, 1992). Incorrect diagnosis leads to inappropriate medication with unnecessary side-effects; consequent mistaken prognosis increases the difficulty of management.

Case history

A 65-year-old woman was diagnosed as having Parkinson's disease by a specialist. Treatment was begun with L-dopa but was not realized to be ineffective due to failure of follow-up. The patient became increasingly disabled over the next 3 years with falls, eventually requiring nursing-home care. Further increase in L-dopa failed to improve the patient and the relatives were concerned by the rapid decline of a patient with apparent Parkinson's disease. A second opinion by a neurologist resulted in a diagnosis of multisystem atrophy (later confirmed at autopsy). Following correct diagnosis, the general practitioner and the relatives could cope and manage the problem successfully.

A number of conditions (see Table 14.1) are easily confused with Parkinson's disease, particularly multisystem atrophy and progressive supranuclear palsy; drug-induced Parkinson's disease is often forgotten or overlooked. The criteria for the diagnosis of Parkinson's disease are shown in Table 14.2.

Although many patients are now diagnosed as suffering from Parkinson's disease by their general practitioner and started on treatment, this has disadvantages. The true diagnosis may be obscured since some patients with multisystem atrophy have a mild short-lived response to L-dopa. The choice of drug treatment in Parkinson's disease is becoming more, rather than less, complicated and it is often useful to get specialist advice about the individual choice of drug treatment.

Initial referral to the neurologist is the first step in effective rehabilitation of a patient suspected of suffering from Parkinson's disease. The neurologist can confirm the diagnosis, communicate this to the

Table 14.1 Differential diagnosis of Parkinson's disease

Multiple system atrophy
Progressive supranuclear palsy
Drug-induced Parkinson's disease
Huntington's disease
Hydrocephalus
Dementias (e.g. Alzheimer's disease)
Corticobasal degeneration

Table 14.2 Diagnosis of Parkinson's disease

Positive features
Unilateral onset
Rest tremor
Excellent response to L-dopa

Negative features (reconsider diagnosis)
Symmetrical
Other signs
Early postural instability
Severe dysarthria/dysphagia
Irregular jerky tremor
L-Dopa intolerance
Eye movement disorder

patient and advise about best initial therapy. The patient should be reviewed once at this stage to ensure satisfactory response to the medication and to discuss any outstanding questions.

Natural history

Treatment with L-dopa has radically altered the natural history of Parkinson's disease. After a good initial response to treatment a number of new symptoms and problems emerge, not seen in untreated disease. By 5 years 50% of patients will have experienced these and by 10 years all (Lees, 1989). Failure to develop these should cast doubt on the diagnosis of idiopathic Parkinson's disease.

Patients start to notice that the effect of L-dopa wears off before the next dose. Instead of a contant relief of symptoms, stiffness, immobility and tremor return before the next tablet. Writhing movements — L-dopa-induced dyskinesias — develop, initially on the worst-affected side. Finally, patients experience fluctuations in their motor performance; abrupt changes in mobility occur and

doses fail to work, particularly in the afternoon — for reasons that are still unclear. These motor fluctuations are partly due to manipulations of the drug regime to overcome end-of-dose deterioration and dyskinesias, particularly the introduction of frequent small doses of L-dopa, and patients may be restored to cycles of predictable response if they are returned to three or four standard doses per day.

Understanding and managing these problems are a major challenge for patient and doctor alike. They can be simply understood by reference to Fig. 14.1. In early disease, disability is mild and the degree of dopaminergic stimulation is sufficient to keep the patient above the threshold for 'on' all day. Progression of the disease causes increasing 'off' disability so that, for the same amount of dopaminergic stimulation, there is less amount of 'on' above threshold and the amount of dopaminergic stimulation now falls below threshold before the next dose. If the dose is increased, dyskinesias appear, if they have not already done so, due to drop in the dyskinesia threshold with disease duration. The dose is often now reduced to avoid dyskinesias. A smaller dose, however, often fails to reach the threshold for 'on', causing failure of response or only brief duration of 'on' response. Referral to this model of the changes in response with disease duration should allow rational manipulation of the drug regime, so far as this is possible, to overcome the motor fluctuations.

Finally, as the disease progresses non-dopa-responsive symptoms appear, particularly postural instability.

It has been suggested that the natural history of Parkinson's disease in the young and old is different, with a smaller response to L-dopa in the elderly, less dyskinesia and a higher rate of dementia, but this has not been confirmed.

Drug treatment

Introduction

Drug treatment is the cornerstone of management and has transformed patients' lives. A series of fashionable changes in drug therapy have taken place, reflecting the pressure of the drug market and the difficulty in managing the long-term L-dopa syndrome. L-dopa/decarboxylase inhibitor is

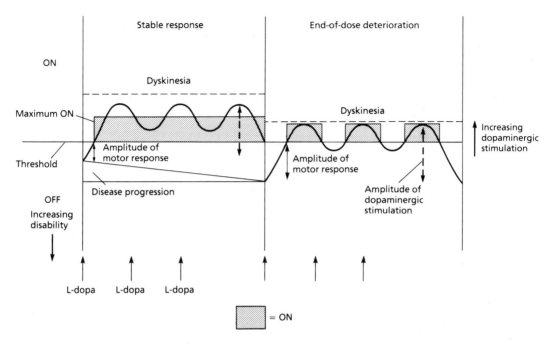

Fig. 14.1 The figure shows two clinical situations: stable response and end-of-dose deterioration. It is important to note that the degree of dopaminergic stimulation remains the same but the curve is shifted due to progression of the disease.

now used in smaller doses than previously because of fear of aggravating the motor fluctuations. Direct dopamine agonists are rarely used as single agents and tend to be used in combination with L-dopa.

L-Dopa with decarboxylase inhibitor

This is the most effective drug for idiopathic Parkinson's disease. It has a dramatic beneficial response and is well tolerated. Occasional nausea and vomiting occur, but idiosyncratic side-effects are rare. The major problem is the eventual development of the long-term L-dopa syndrome. The smallest necessary doses are given to provide symptomatic relief, rather than to restore the patient to normal.

Types of L-dopa preparation

Controlled-release L-dopa preparations were developed to combat the response fluctuations. Madopar CR is best used for early wearing off of drug effect. It is unhelpful in the management of motor fluctuations. Sinemet CR has different pharmokinetics

but has not been available long enough to determine its usefulness. The controlled-release preparations often have to be used with conventional L-dopa to provide a 'kick-start'.

Whether starting treatment with controlled-release preparations delays or prevents the development of the long-term L-dopa syndrome is not yet known and probably never will be.

A *dispersible* preparation of Madopar is available, which is useful for patients with swallowing difficulties or for those times when a more rapid onset of action is required, e.g. at night.

Anticholinergics

These improve tremor and rigidity but have no effect upon the most disabling akinesia. Side-effects are common, with dry mouth, blurred vision, urinary difficulties, poor memory and confusion. Because of these mental side-effects, it is unwise to use anticholinergics after the age of 60. Their place in treatment is for the young patient with disabling tremor.

Amantadine

This drug only produces mild benefit which is possibly of short duration, though patients often seem to deteriorate when it is stopped after many years. It is seldom used now. It has significant side-effects, causing livedo reticularis, oedema and confusion.

Direct dopamine agonists

The place of dopamine agonists (Lieberman et al., 1987) at present is in early add-on treatment to reduce the incidence of dyskinesias and motor fluctuations, a regime pioneered by Rinne (Rinne, 1987). Given alone, these drugs have only a small beneficial response and a high incidence of side-effects (nausea, vomiting, hypotension and neuropsychiatric problems), so that only 30% of patients continue with them. Starting these drugs with domperidone helps to avoid some of these.

They can also be given to patients when they develop motor fluctuations in an attempt to smooth out the response, due to their having a longer half-life than L-dopa. This is only partially successful, with mild benefit for about 6 months before the problems re-emerge (Lieberman et al., 1987).

Bromocriptine

This was the first semisynthetic ergot derivative to be regularly used in the treatment of Parkinson's disease. It has an interesting history. Originally used as first-line treatment, it was discarded because of lack of adequate benefit and because of side-effects. It was subsequently used in low dose as a single agent or as add-on treatment for motor fluctuations and finally seems to have found a place in early add-on therapy to reduce motor fluctuations and dyskinesias! It stimulates D2 receptors and there is some evidence that it requires intact presynaptic neurons for its antiparkinsonian effect. It has a longer duration of action than L-dopa, lasting for 3–5 hours.

Lysuride

This is a dopamimetic ergot derivative. It stimulates D2 receptors and also has strong 5-hydroxytryptamine agonist activity. Its action appears to be independent of presynaptic dopamine synthesis. Following intravenous injection, its duration of action is about 2–3 hours.

Pergolide

This is the most recently available (in the UK) postsynaptic dopamine agonist. Its pharmacological profile is different from those of bromocriptine and lysuride. Pergolide is an agonist at both D1 and D2 receptors. Its duration of action is about 4–8 hours.

Apomorphine

This drug is identical in effect to L-dopa. It is a direct D1 dopamine agonist. Given as a penject, it has a reliable and rapid onset of action after 15 minutes, lasting for about 45 minutes. Single injections can be used to rescue patients from failed responses or bad 'offs'. Alternatively it can be given as a subcutaneous infusion to smooth out the response. It is a valuable addition to the drug repertoire in appropriately selected patients (Stibe et al., 1988). The main disadvantage is the requirement for teaching and education of the patients in its use, which needs a nurse practitioner, who also has to be available to deal with problems. Side-effects are remarkably few, with nodules at the site of injection. Neuropsychiatric problems are infrequent. It may be superior to L-dopa in this respect and can be used to treat patients with a severe intractable neuropsychiatric syndrome due to L-dopa.

Selegiline

This drug was initially introduced to prolong the action of L-dopa, since it is a suicide inhibitor of monoamine oxidase inhibitor (MAO-B) – that is, it is metabolized by the MAO-B to form a product which combines irreversibly and lethally with the enzyme. The prescribing information indicated the need to reduce the dose of L-dopa by 10–20%. Subsequent studies have not confirmed that selegiline does prolong the action of L-dopa, showing how a drug can be licensed and used purely on the basis of a theory which proves incorrect in practice. History has repeated itself and the drug is now given to retard the progression of the disease without adequate proof of this. The impetus for this arose from the discovery of the mechanism of methylphenyltetrahydropyridine (MPTP) toxicity, which is prevented by selegiline. Despite the lack of evidence that idiopathic Parkinson's disease is caused in a similar way, a single study (Parkinson Study Group, 1989) showed that selegiline delayed the need for the introduction of L-dopa. This was interpreted as being due to an effect upon disease progression, but an acute symptomatic effect may have been the explanation. Further studies are awaited to clarify this. Selegiline is well tolerated, the main side-effects being confusion and insomnia, so that it should not be given after lunch.

Approach to treatment

This has to be tailored to the individual, with plans for the long term. Controversy over whether early or late L-dopa treatment should be started continues. If the patient's disability requires L-dopa, however, there is insufficient reason to withhold it. The aim is to provide adequate relief of symptoms and minimize disability, with least side-effects or long-term problems.

The best initial treatment is probably 400 mg of L-dopa in divided doses, with the addition of a direct dopamine agonist to minimize the development of long-term fluctuations. There is little to choose between the direct agonists. Bromocriptine is the most well known and so it is reasonable to start with this and to substitute lysuride or pergolide if and when problems occur. Current evidence is not strong enough to make addition of selegiline mandatory.

Management of fluctuations

This is the most difficult problem in management, with no simple solution. End-of-dose deterioration alone is simple to manage, with either more frequent doses of conventional L-dopa or a long-acting preparation. Motor fluctuations and dyskinesias are the real problem. Larger doses of L-dopa inevitably cause worse dyskinesias, which are often better tolerated by the patient than by the spouse, who usually complains of them. Smaller doses render the patient more parkinsonian and aggravate the fluctuations. For a short time, smaller, more frequent, doses of L-dopa will often help. The subsequent addition of a direct agonist can improve the

'on' time for a period of 6–12 months but is not a permanent solution.

The absorption of L-dopa is affected by large neutral amino acids (Nutt et al., 1984), so that taking the dose at least 30–60 minutes before the meal may help. Redistribution of the protein to the last meal of the day may be of some small benefit. Crushing or dissolving the tablets or capsules of L-dopa can improve speed of onset and benefit. Addition of selegiline at this stage sometimes seems to help. Subcutaneous apomorphine will rescue patients from afternoon 'offs' due to failure of response to L-dopa and, when given by infusion, can smooth out the response.

Patients need to understand their disease and the motor fluctuations, if possible, so that they can time their activities to the most predictable parts of the day, usually the mornings. Eventually, it has to be accepted by both patient and doctor that further adjustment of the drug regime is unlikely to help.

Assessment of patients

To enable adjustment of the medication, the following need to be determined:
1 % Time 'on'.
2 % Time 'off'.
3 Quality of 'on' and 'off'.
4 Severity and timing of involuntary movements.
It is often helpful to go through a day with the patient, discussing (i) the time to 'on', (ii) the duration and quality of 'on', and (iii) the severity and timing of involuntary movements, to see if further adjustments of the drug regime will be of help. If it is impossible to understand the pattern of dyskinesias and response to L-dopa, the patient must be admitted to hospital for observation. Alternatively, patients can fill in 'on' and 'off' charts, provided that they can clearly differentiate the two, which surprisingly many patients fail to do. Eventually, in severe and difficult cases, it has to be accepted that further manipulation of the drug regime is unlikely to be of help and to concentrate on helping the patient to manage his/her disability despite these limitations.

Types of dyskinesia

Dyskinesias are repetitive writhing and flailing movements of the limbs and body. Most often they occur at the peak of the dose and are present for the whole of the duration of the 'on'. In younger patients dyskinesias may occur at the onset of 'on' and as the patient goes 'off', called biphasic dyskinesia. This is a difficult situation to manage since increasing the dose initially stops the dyskinesias but the patient soon becomes dyskinetic continuously; reducing the dose aggravates them and produces less good 'on'. Controlled-release L-dopa or apomorphine can be of value here.

Pain and dystonia (Quinn et al., 1986)

Dystonic foot spasms may be an initial symptom of Parkinson's disease. Painful dystonic spasms of the foot and leg occur subsequently after treatment during the 'off' period, particularly in younger patients. Hence they are particularly troublesome in the morning, occurring when the patient puts his foot to the ground. A number of strategies can be tried to overcome them: night-time bromocriptine, baclofen, controlled-release L-dopa, first dose of L-dopa in bed, and, finally, lithium can be very effective in severe cases. Peak-dose and biphasic dystonia also occur. Pain is otherwise generally due to the 'off' state and relieved by turning 'on' if due to idiopathic Parkinson's disease. Other causes should be sought if this is not the case. Attempts should be made to relieve pain by modification of the drug regime, though in severe cases L-dopa may have to be stopped altogether. Beginning-of-dose pain can sometimes be relieved by overlapping the doses, or abbreviated by apomorphine.

Neuropsychiatric problems

Depression

Many patients with Parkinson's disease become depressed and disputes have arisen over whether this might be due to the disease or reactive to the disability. It is commonly characterized by dysphoria, pessimism and somatic complaints (Brown et al., 1988). If it is due to deterioration in motor function, it is important to try to reverse this if possible. Otherwise cognitive therapy and counselling are appropriate. If guilt and self-blame are features, treatment with antidepressants is appropriate.

Patients with long-standing Parkinson's disease may develop a fluctuating confusional state with paranoid delusions, sometimes of a sexual nature. This is probably due to a combination of the effects of the disease and drug treatment. The patient should be carefully examined to check that there is no intercurrent infection or medical disorder, with biochemistry screen, electrocardiogram (ECG), chest X-ray and urine culture. If these are negative, the most likely offending drugs should be reduced and withdrawn, i.e. anticholinergics and direct dopamine agonists. The dose of L-dopa should then be reduced to a minimum, with no L-dopa 1–2 days of the week if necessary. Clozapine (Wolters et al., 1990) can be used to treat some of the neuropsychiatric problems if they prove intractable, or occasionally apomorphine will prove less toxic than L-dopa. In principle, it is preferable to achieve mental clarity at the price of mobility.

Case history

A patient with a 36-year history of idiopathic Parkinson's disease became so deluded and confused that her husband could no longer manage her at home and she was admitted to a nursing home. Withdrawal of bromocriptine led to some improvement but she continued to be intermittently confused. Reduction in the dose of L-dopa to 400 mg daily resulted in mental clarity with no further episodes of confusion over 18 months' follow-up. She complains bitterly about lack of mobility. However, she is now back at home and her husband is able to look after her. Despite the lack of mobility, she is more independent, and able to converse with her husband. Her postural instability is so severe when mobile as to preclude walking, even if larger doses of L-dopa could be used.

Dementia

Among patients with Parkinson's disease, 10–15% develop dementia (Brown & Marsden, 1984). Onset of disease at an older age is a risk factor. Appropriate investigation is required and it is important to distinguish dementia from a fluctuating confusional state due to the medication. Additional support and respite care are likely to be needed.

Constipation, urinary difficulties and sexual function

Constipation is an early symptom and problem, best dealt with by dietary advice, or, if necessary, Celevac, Fybogel or lactulose. Urinary symptoms, such as frequency and urgency, occur, but incontinence is not a problem. Sexual difficulties (Brown et al., 1990), which are common and frequently overlooked, require advice and counselling.

Sleep

Sleep may be disturbed and is a difficult problem to resolve. This is often due to stiffness and rigidity causing discomfort and difficulty in turning over. Some patients find it easier, therefore, to sleep during the day, which further aggravates the problem. Long-acting preparations of L-dopa are of some benefit (Lees, 1987).

Non-drug treatment

Parkinson's disease is a chronic, progressive disorder. It is not purely a movement disorder, but affects mood and intellect as well. The difficulties in communication and the unpredictability of the motor disorder are further difficulties for the patients. Patients require considerable support, counselling and information about the disease. They need help to maintain their independence and dignity despite the disease.

Traditionally, no single person has been responsible for this aspect of care, information and support being gleaned from therapists, the social worker and the general practitioner, as well as the hospital consultant. This leads to confusion and inconsistency, if not omission. It is preferable if this is the major responsibility of one person, the key worker who counsels and organizes the necessary support. It is imperative to try to maintain independence, communication and self-reliance.

Consideration must be given to the following areas:
1 Communication of the diagnosis: patients complain that too often this is done in an uncaring, cold and inconsiderate way, without adequate back-up and support.
2 Further care and education.
3 Personal adjustment – job, relationships, sex.
4 Needs of the carers – particularly respite. The Parkinson's Disease Society has a holiday flat available.
5 Advice is required about employment, finances, retirement, benefits and allowances.

Therapists

The precise role of physiotherapy (Burford, 1988) and speech therapy (Johnson & Pring, 1990) is uncertain. Patients can certainly benefit from advice about trick movements to initiate walking, get out of the chair and turn over in bed and from group exercise classes to keep fit and maintain morale. Physiotherapy cannot correct bradykinesia or rigidity. Widely different treatment programmes are claimed to produce a favourable response, but it has been difficult to disentangle this from a nonspecific effect on mood and motivation. Research is needed to determine what sort of physiotherapy is effective, at what stage of the disease it should be given, and for how long.

Speech therapy can probably help with breath control to improve volume of speech and correct bad habits, but again cannot correct the basic deficit and has not always been shown to produce persistent and consistent benefit. Amplification aids and use of a metronome and pacing board can be useful. Again, more research is required to determine the precise use and benefit of speech therapy.

Both speech therapy and physiotherapy can be regarded like drugs, and proper trials are required to establish their place in treatment. Currently, they may be compared to a drug that may work while you take it but has no long lasting effect; for obvious practical reasons, it is impossible to take it all the time.

Occupational therapists are necessary to supply home and mobility aids. Alternative therapies should not be discouraged, and relaxation, aromatherapy, reflexology and music therapy may all be used to the patient's advantage, depending on personal preference.

Parkinson's Disease Society

This has played an enormous role in helping to develop welfare services and in basic research into the disorder. Local branches can be of enormous support to patients, providing education, counselling and social support.

Epidemiology and organization of services

Estimates suggest that a health district of 250 000 will have a total of 400 patients with idiopathic Parkinson's disease, three-quarters of whom will be disabled. In view of these large numbers, a comprehensive organized approach to their rehabilitation is required, involving consultant, general practitioner, therapists, counsellor and key worker. Services for Parkinson's disease patients need to be planned and properly organized. Fragmentation of the service causes extra work and makes it less effective. Few health districts have such a service and, though some are being developed, the best way of delivery of the rehabilitation is uncertain.

A Parkinson's disease clinic has the advantage that the resources and expertise can be concentrated, and specific physiotherapy, occupational therapy and speech therapy designed for the patients can be provided. A nurse practitioner/key worker is being evaluated in some areas. This person can potentially provide enormous help with advice, education and counselling, and referral at times of need to the appropriate services. For elderly patients, day-care facilities already available may be concentrated on specific groups, with the benefit of respite for the carer and associated physiotherapy and occupational therapy assessment. An education centre, which can also be used by the local Parkinson's Disease Society branch, could be useful.

References

Brown R.G. & Marsden C.D. (1984) How common is dementia in Parkinson's disease? *Lancet* **ii**, 1262–1265.

Brown R.G., Maccarthy B., Gotham A.M., Der G.J. & Marsden C.D. (1988) Depression and disability in Parkinson's disease: a follow-up of 132 cases. *Psychological Medicine* **18**, 49–55.

Brown R.G., Jahansi M., Quinn N. & Marsden C.D. (1990) Sexual function in patients with Parkinson's disease and their partners. *Journal of Neurology, Neurosurgery and Psychiatry* **53**, 480–486.

Burford K. (1988) The physiotherapist's role in Parkinson's disease. *Geriatric and Nursing Home Care* **8**, 14–16.

Hughes A.J., Daniel S.E., Kilford L. & Lees A.J. (1992) Accuracy of clinical diagnosis of idiopathic Parkinson's disease. *Journal of Neurology, Neurosurgery and Psychiatry* **55**, 181–184.

Johnson J.A. & Pring T.R. (1990) Speech therapy and Parkinson's disease. *British Journal of Disease and the Community* **25**, 183–194.

Lees A.J. (1987) A sustained release formulation of L-dopa in the treatment of nocturnal and early morning disabilities in Parkinson's disease. *European Neurology* **27**, 126–134.

Lees A.J. (1989) On-off fluctuations. *Journal of Neurology, Neurosurgery and Psychiatry*. Special Suppl.

Lieberman A.N., Goldatein M., Gopinthan G. & Neophytides A. (1987) D1 and D2 agonists in Parkinson's disease. *Canadian Journal of Neuroscience* **14**, 466–473.

Nutt J.G., Woodward W.R., Hammerstad J.P., Carter J.H. & Anderson J.L. (1984) The 'on-off' phenomenon in Parkinson's disease. *New England Journal of Medicine* **310**, 483–488.

Parkinson Study Group (1989) Effect of deprenyl on the progression of disability in early Parkinson's disease. *New England Journal of Medicine* **321**, 1364–1371.

Quinn N., Koller W.C., Lang A.E. & Marsden C.D. (1986) Painful Parkinson's disease. *Lancet* **i**, 1366–1369.

Rinne U.K. (1987) Early combination of bromocriptine and L-dopa in the treatment of Parkinson's disease. *Neurology* **37**, 826–828.

Stibe C.M.H., Kempster P.A., Lees A.J. & Sterm G.M. (1988) Subcutaneous apomorphine in Parkinsonian on–off oscillations. *Lancet* **i**, 403–406.

Wolters E., Hurwitz T.A., Mak E., Teal P., Peppard F.R., Renmick R., Calne R.N. & Calne D.B. (1990) Clozapine in the treatment of Parkinsonian patients with dopamimetic psychosis. *Neurology* **40**, 832–834.

15: Rehabilitation in Epilepsy

G.A. BAKER, D.W. CHADWICK
AND C.A. YOUNG

Epidemiology, 178
Remote symptomatic causes of epilepsy, 178
　Hypoxic–ischaemic cerebral insults, 178
　Head injury, 179
　Neurosurgical conditions and epilepsy, 180
　Cerebrovascular disease, 181
　Central nervous system infections and infestations, 181
　Other causes of symptomatic seizures and epilepsy, 181
Prognosis, 182
Medical and surgical management, 183
　Diagnosis, 183
　Pharmacological treatment, 184
　Surgical treatment, 192
Factors contributing to handicap, 195
　Seizures, 195
　Epilepsy as a psychosocial handicap, 197
　Epilepsy and psychiatric disorders, 198
　Epilepsy and employment, 199
　Epilepsy and education, 201
　Epilepsy and the family, 202
　Mobility, 203
Services for people with epilepsy, 205
　Service provision, 205
　Voluntary agencies, 206
Appendix, 206

The degree of social adaptation in work, school and recreation is the final criterion for health care delivery to the patient with epilepsy. (Porter, 1984)

For every person with epilepsy the first step in rehabilitation will always be the optimal control of seizures by appropriate medical or surgical treatment. Good evidence now exists to show that the psychosocial consequences of epilepsy decrease as the seizure-free period increases (Chaplin *et al.*, 1992; Jacoby *et al.*, 1992). It is not, however, an end in itself, but simply a step towards achieving the best possible quality of life for an individual. In targeting rehabilitation efforts, it must be recognized that the disability produced by epilepsy can be varied and derived from a wide variety of sources. The principal problem is the heterogeneity of epilepsy as a disorder. Epilepsy encompasses a wide variety of different seizure types and epilepsy syndromes. It is varied in its aetiology and may or may not be associated with the presence of other physical, intellectual and psychiatric handicaps. The prognosis also varies considerably, the majority of people with epilepsy achieving long-term seizure remission, either with or without continued treatment, the minority having a chronic lifelong epilepsy which results in considerable handicap. In addition to these overt problems, epilepsy is unusual in producing limitations that are more difficult to define. These derive from the unpredictability of seizures and the psychological problems associated with this, as well as the stigmatization that is still attached to the disorder, both by the community as a whole and because of perceived stigmatization by the sufferer (Scambler, 1989).

The complexity of disability in epilepsy means that for many people with epilepsy the clinician alone may possess neither the time nor the skills to address all the issues involved. For this reason optimal rehabilitation in epilepsy should involve a multidisciplinary team comprising clinicians, expert counsellors, nurses, social workers, clinical and educational psychologists and careers advisers. Optimizing the delivery of services needs efficient co-ordination between these agencies, which is most likely to be achieved within the context of an epilepsy clinic or a specialist assessment centre. The primary role of all the agencies involved is to offer the person with epilepsy the fullest and widest range of information. Ultimately, outcome will be determined by the individual's level of education

about his/her disorder and his/her adjustment to
the disorder.

Epidemiology

Despite problems with differing definitions of epilepsy and case ascertainment methods, there is
general agreement about the epidemiology of epilepsy in different populations (Sander & Shorvon,
1987). Incidence rates vary in an age-specific way
between approximately 20 and 70 per 100 000 per
year, whereas the prevalence for active epilepsy is
in the range of 4–10 per 1000. Age-specific incidence, prevalence and cumulative incidence are
described in Fig. 15.1 for a population in Rochester,
Minnesota. It can be seen that the incidence is
highest at the extremes of life but that there are
significant differences between the cumulative incidence and prevalence of epilepsy, indicating that
the majority of patients who develop epilepsy do
not suffer from a chronic disorder. The cumulative
incidence of epilepsy by the age of 70 may be as
high as 2–3% of the population.

Epilepsy can have a very varied aetiology, and
causes vary through life (Fig. 15.2). In the National
General Practice Study of Epilepsy, 60% of all patients had no identifiable cause for epilepsy (Sander

et al., 1990). A proportion of such patients may
have genetically determined epilepsy syndromes,
including childhood and juvenile absence epilepsy,
juvenile myoclonic epilepsy and epilepsy with tonic
−clonic seizures on awakening. These epilepsy syndromes are characterized by age-specific onset, the
presence of generalized spike-wave abnormalities
in the electroencephalogram (EEG) and the absence
of any associated neurological impairment (Commission on Classification and Terminology, 1989).
Symptomatic epilepsies present a much greater
challenge to rehabilitation because of the likelihood
of associated mental and physical handicap and
because of the poorer prognosis for seizure control.
It is therefore essential that rehabilitation efforts
take account of the cause of epilepsy.

Remote symptomatic causes of epilepsy

It is well recognized that a number of cerebral
insults predispose to the development of epilepsy.

Hypoxic−ischaemic cerebral insults

Mental and motor handicap present from birth
are commonly associated with seizure disorders.

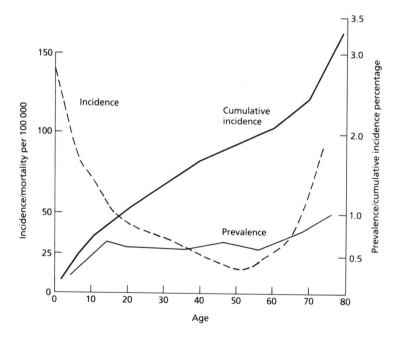

Fig. 15.1 Incidence, prevalence
and cumulative incidence rates for
epilepsy in Rochester, Minnesota,
1935–1974. (Reproduced from
Anderson *et al.* (1986) with
permission.)

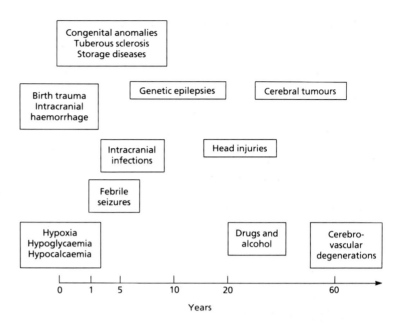

Fig. 15.2 Causes of seizures and epilepsy by age. (Reproduced from Chadwick D., Cartlidge N. & Bates D. (eds) (1989) *Medical Neurology*. Churchill Livingstone, Edinburgh.)

Zielinski (1974) found 20% of the epileptic population to be retarded or dull and Gudmundson (1966) found a similar proportion of mentally handicapped individuals to have epilepsy in Iceland. Cerebral palsy is also strongly associated with epilepsy and as many as 50% of individuals with both mental handicap and cerebral palsy have a seizure disorder (Hauser *et al.*, 1987). The more severe the mental and physical handicap the higher the risk of epilepsy (Gustavson *et al.*, 1977; Blomquist *et al.*, 1981; Edebol-Tysk, 1989). Pre- and perinatal hypoxia of one form or another seem to be the commonest single cause of mental handicap and cerebral palsy (Nelson & Ellenberg, 1986; Forsgren *et al.*, 1990).

The great majority of individuals with mental handicap and cerebral palsy develop seizures early in life, but up to 15% of patients may have a seizure disorder that starts after the age of 15 (Forsgren *et al.*, 1990). Whilst primary generalized seizures including myoclonus, tonic and atonic seizures and infantile spasms (as part of a symptomatic generalized epilepsy common in childhood), as individuals mature partial seizures and secondary generalized tonic–clonic seizures predominate (Forsgren *et al.*, 1990). In this population the outcome for epilepsy is poor, only 30% achieving seizure remissions of a year and a third having at least one seizure per month. Early brain damage is one of the most important factors predicting a poor outcome of epilepsy (Shafer *et al.*, 1988).

Hippocampal sclerosis is the most common pathological lesion in surgically treated patients with complex partial seizures (Babb & Brown, 1987) and a case-controlled study has suggested that complicated febrile seizures during childhood may be the aetiological factor in up to 20% of patients' complex partial seizures (Rocca *et al.*, 1987). Falconer (1971) suggested that prolonged febrile seizures produce such damage by leading to hypoxic–ischaemic cell loss in the hippocampus (Meldrum *et al.*, 1974). This hypothesis is now widely accepted, even though it is well recognized that simple febrile seizures do not seem to be associated with a high risk of late epilepsy (Nelson & Ellenberg, 1978).

Recognition of this aetiological factor is of particular importance in epilepsies in adolescents and young adults in view of the high prevalence of complex partial seizures, their poor response to antiepileptic drug treatment, and their excellent response to surgical treatment (see below).

Head injury

Of all concussive head injuries, 2% result in epilepsy (Annegers *et al.*, 1980) and head trauma was the cause of seizures in 3% of patients registered in the National General Practice Study of Epilepsy (Sander *et al.*, 1990). There can be no doubt that the more severe the head injury, the higher the risk of post-traumatic epilepsy (Jennett, 1975; Annegers *et al.*, 1980).

Missile injuries and epilepsy

Brain injuries caused by missiles provide a well-defined and relatively homogeneous group of injuries that fortunately are rare in civilian life. They have, however, been fully studied in cohorts of patients from the First World War through to the Vietnam War. In many, the localization and the extent of the injury are known to be anatomically precise and the relationship between the incidence of epilepsy and factors such as retention of foreign bodies, haematoma, brain infection and the extent of the cerebral injury can be determined. Overall, it would seem that 50% of patients with such injuries will eventually develop post-traumatic epilepsy and the relative risk of developing such epilepsy will initially be 580 times higher than a general age-matched population during the first year, falling to 25 times higher after 10 years (Salazar *et al.*, 1985).

Blunt injuries to the head

The most satisfactory unselected population of patients developing post-traumatic epilepsy has been studied by Annegers *et al.* (1980). This study utilized the records-linkage system of the Mayo Clinic to identify 2747 patients with head injuries between 1935 and 1974. The minimal clinical criteria for inclusion in the study was an injury resulting in loss of consciousness, post-traumatic amnesia or evidence of skull fracture. Patients were excluded if they died within 1 month of injury or had epilepsy predating the index head injury. The head injuries were classified as:
1 Severe – brain contusion, intracerebral or intracranial haematoma or 24 hours of unconsciousness or amnesia.
2 Moderate – skull fracture or 30 minutes to 24 hours of unconsciousness or post-traumatic amnesia.
3 Mild – briefer periods of unconsciousness or amnesia.

The overall risk of early seizures (within the first week) was 2.1%. This was greater in children (2.8%) than adults (1.8%). For severe head injuries the risk of early seizures rose to 30.5% in children and 10.3% in adults. For late seizures the risk in patients with severe injuries was 7.1% at 1 year and 11.5% at 5 years. For moderate injuries the corresponding figures were 0.7% and 1.6%, and for mild injuries 0.1% and 0.6%. The risk of seizures at any time is not significantly different from the general population for the group with mild head injuries. For all cases the risk of late seizures was 2.6 times greater than the expected risk. The relative risk was 12.7 in the first year, 4.4 in the next 4 years and thereafter 1.4.

The prognosis for post-traumatic epilepsy following blunt injuries is variable. In one series with prolonged follow-up for at least 15 years, approximately 50% of patients had no seizures for at least 5 years, 25% were experiencing between one and six seizures per year and the other 25% more than six seizures per year (Walker & Erculei, 1968).

Neurosurgical conditions and epilepsy

The overall incidence of seizures occurring after supratentorial craniotomy is 17% during a follow-up period of at least 5 years (Foy *et al.*, 1981a). The incidence varied from 3% to 92% depending on the condition for which the craniotomy was undertaken.

Approximately one-fifth of patients undergoing aneurysm surgery develop postoperative seizures (Cabral *et al.*, 1976; North *et al.*, 1983). The incidence varies according to the site of the aneurysm. Thus, approximate risks may be 7.5% from internal carotid aneurysm, 21% from anterior communicating aneurysm and 39% for a middle cerebral artery aneurysm (Cabral *et al.*, 1976; Foy *et al.*, 1981a). Additional factors influencing the incidence may be the presence of an intracerebral haematoma, cortical damage, splitting the Sylvian fissure, cerebral swelling and perioperative aneurysmal rupture, and the length of surgery (Foy *et al.*, 1981a, 1991). That at least part of the risk of epilepsy associated with aneurysm is associated with a surgical procedure is suggested by the 8.3% incidence in 261 conservatively managed survivors following aneurysmal subarachnoid haemorrhage reported by Storey (1967). Arteriovenous malformations and spontaneous intracerebral haematoma from other causes carry risks of epilepsy of 50% and 20% respectively, and surgical treatment does seem to be an additional risk factor for these conditions (Crawford et al., 1986).

The incidence of seizures commencing de novo following meningioma surgery is of the order of 20% (Foy et al., 1981a; North et al., 1983). The incidence is higher for parasagittal lesions than for convexity or basal tumours. Some 44% of patients who have preoperative seizures do not have any further seizures postoperatively. The incidence of seizures following frontal surgery for pituitary adenomas and craniopharyngiomas may be as high as 15% (Cast & Wilson, 1981; Foy et al., 1991).

Surgery for supratentorial abscess carries a very high risk. With sufficiently long follow-up, virtually all patients develop epilepsy (Legg et al., 1973; Foy et al., 1981b). Ventricular shunting procedures can be associated with a 24% risk of seizures (Copeland et al., 1982), and multiple shunt revisions and shunt infections significantly increase the risks.

The relationship between intracranial tumours and epilepsy is well recognized and results in a considerable pressure to investigate all patients presenting with epilepsy. In fact, brain tumours are responsible for late-onset epilepsy in only about 10% of cases from many series. The incidence of tumours rises steeply where seizures are clearly focal in nature (Raynor et al., 1959; Sumi & Teasdall, 1963). Tumours of the frontal, parietal and occipital lobes seem to carry the highest risk of epilepsy (Penfield & Jasper, 1954; Mauguiere & Courjon, 1978). The incidence of tumours causing complex partial seizures is lower (about 15%) (Currie et al., 1971). Gastaut found that 16% of 1702 epileptic patients with epilepsy beginning over the age of 20 had tumours on computerized tomography (CT) scanning (Gastaut & Gastaut, 1976).

The prognosis for tumour epilepsies is poor. Only 11 of 164 patients achieved a 1-year remission of epilepsy with antiepileptic drug treatment (Smith et al., 1992), and 50% of patients with tumour epilepsies in adult life die within 4 years. However, 20–30% show prolonged survival.

Whilst meningiomas should be treated surgically where this is practical and where the patient is not old or infirm, seizures will only be suppressed in about 40% of patients (Foy et al., 1981a).

Cerebrovascular disease

Cerebrovascular disease and stroke become an increasingly common cause of epilepsy in the later years of life (Loiseau et al., 1990; Sander et al., 1990). A community-based study of stroke showed an incidence of seizures by 1 year of 4% in patients with infarction (mainly for patients with total anterior circulation syndrome), 18% of patients with intracerebral haemorrhage and 28% of patients with subarachnoid haemorrhage (Burn et al., 1990). Other studies have emphasized that embolic or haemorrhagic stroke carries the highest risk (Lesser et al., 1985). However, asymptomatic carotid occlusion (Cocito et al., 1982) and cerebral infarction (Shorvon et al., 1984) may be found in patients presenting with epilepsy in later life, and seizures may also precede a stroke (Shinton et al., 1987; Burn et al., 1990). It has been estimated that cerebrovascular disease may account for 15% of new cases of epilepsy (Sander et al., 1990) and more than 50% of new cases in the elderly.

Central nervous system (CNS) infections and infestations

A wide range of viral, bacterial, opportunistic and parasitic infestations can be associated with seizures. Infections accounted for 3% of seizure disorders in the epidemiological study in Rochester, Minnesota (Hauser & Kurland, 1975). Annegers et al. (1988) examined the risks of unprovoked seizures following common CNS infections in 714 survivors of encephalitis and meningitis. Overall, the 20-year risk of developing unprovoked seizures was 6.8%, almost seven times the expected rate. Increased incidence of seizures was highest during the first 5 years after a CNS infection but continued to be elevated for as long as 15 years.

Other causes of symptomatic seizures and epilepsy

Neurodegenerative disorders can be associated with epilepsy. In Alzheimer's disease, seizures occur, usually late in the illness, in up to 15% of patients

(Romanelli *et al.*, 1990). Hauser *et al.* (1986) calculated a relative risk of 10 for autopsy-proven causes of Alzheimer's disease. Myoclonus is also evident, particularly in patients with familial Alzheimer's disease (Jacob, 1970) and with Alzheimer's change complicating Down's syndrome. In contrast, seizures appear rare in Pick's disease.

Several authors have noted an increased incidence of seizures in association with multiple sclerosis, the usual figure being quoted as around 5% of cases (Muller, 1949). It may be that seizures are particularly likely to occur as an acute symptomatic phenomenon related to plaque formation, and longer-term epilepsy seems to be uncommon (Kinnunen & Wikstrom, 1986).

Prognosis

The majority of studies of prognosis have been hospital-based, which has an adverse effect on outcome, patients with more severe and refractory epilepsy being more likely to be referred to specialist centres. In this respect, the study of Annegers *et al.* (1979) is of particular importance in being community- rather than hospital-based. In Rochester, 457 patients with a history of two or more nonfebrile seizures were followed for at least 5 years, and in the case of 141 for 20 years. The probability of being in a remission lasting for 5 years or more was 61% at 10 years, and as high as 70% at 20 years (Fig. 15.3). This large study is supported by a smaller one of 122 patients drawn from a general practice population (Goodridge & Shorvon, 1983). By 15 years after onset of seizures, 80% had achieved a 2-year remission, and only 38% were still taking antiepileptic drugs. Some further support for such high rates of remission is obtained from studies of patients followed prospectively from diagnosis and the commencement of therapy, which show that between 50% and 77% of such patients are 'controlled', depending on how control is defined (Turnbull *et al.*, 1985; Reynolds, 1987).

The age of onset of epilepsy is perhaps one of the most important factors influencing remission. There is general agreement that the commencement of seizures within the first year of life (when it is usually symptomatic of cerebral pathology) carries an adverse prognosis (Kiorobe, 1961; Sofijanov, 1982). Annegers *et al.* (1979) found that both par-

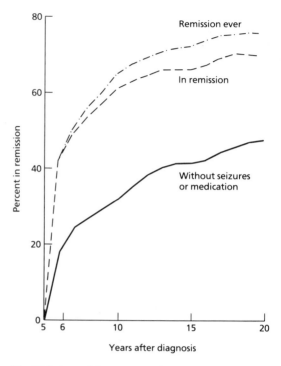

Fig. 15.3 Actuarial percentage of patients in remission following diagnosis of epilepsy. (Reproduced from Annegers *et al.* (1979), with permission.)

tial and generalized epilepsies had a better prognosis should they start before the age of 20.

The importance of the early course and treatment of epilepsy in its long-term outcome has been discussed in detail by Reynolds (1987). He has analysed data from a number of sources which show that the frequency of both partial and tonic–clonic seizures prior to treatment has an adverse effect on outcome and also that intervals between seizures may decrease progressively. As Hauser *et al.* (1982) have also shown that the risk of subsequent seizures increases from the first to the second and third seizures, it can be argued that these observations indicate that early and effective antiepileptic drug treatment may be capable of preventing the onset of chronic epilepsy.

Seizure classification is of importance in determining outcome. Remission rates range from approximately 60–80% for patients with only tonic–clonic seizures to between 20 and 60% in patients

Table 15.1 Factors affecting prognosis of epilepsy (Shafer *et al.*, 1988): univariate Cox regression estimate of relative risk from 298 patients

Factor	Relative risk (95% CL)	
	5 years seizure-free	5 years seizure-free and off medication
Age <16 at first fit	1.09 (0.82, 1.44)	1.96 (1.23, 2.8)
No early brain damage	2.15 (1.22, 3.78)	4.27 (1.35, 13.47)
No known aetiology	1.5 (1.05, 2.13)	2.64 (1.45, 2.84)
Never had a tonic–clonic fit	1.37 (1.03, 1.82)	2.19 (1.48, 3.24)
No generalized spike wave in third year EEG	3.47 (1.37, 8.8)	2.36 (0.56, 10.16)

with complex partial seizures (Juul-Jensen, 1964; Turnbull *et al.*, 1985). The combination of complex partial seizures with secondary generalized tonic–clonic seizures may have a particularly adverse prognosis (Rodin, 1968). In such patients it is common to find that, whilst tonic–clonic seizures come under good control with anticonvulsant therapy, partial seizures remain resistant to drug therapy (Rodin, 1968; Turnbull *et al.*, 1985). Other generalized epilepsies of childhood carry varying prognoses. Between 70% and 80% of patients with simple absences (*petit mal*) are likely to enter remission (Sofijanov, 1982). Complex absences show a lesser remission rate (33–65%), and in patients with the West or Lennox–Gastaut syndromes remission rates may be as low as 35–50%.

The evidence about the factors affecting the prognosis of epilepsy do not allow any very satisfactory quantification and assessment of the varying weights that prognostic factors carry. Some of these difficulties have recently been addressed by Shafer *et al.* (1988). This group examined the prognosis of 306 patients diagnosed between 1935 and 1978 and used Cox's proportional hazards model to investigate those factors determining the likelihood of achieving a 5-year seizure-free period and a 5-year seizure-free period off drugs. They calculated the relative risks and 95% confidence limits for a number of factors. Those of importance are presented in Table 15.1. It can be seen that no individual factor is very strongly predictive of remission but those that are include the absence of early brain damage, never having had a tonic–clonic seizure, and the absence of a generalized spike wave from a

number of EEGs. Similar factors were also predictive of 5-year seizure-free periods off antiepileptic drugs.

Medical and surgical management

The prime aim for any individual patient with epilepsy is to prevent the occurrence of further seizures by appropriate means involving the least harmful medical, or possibly surgical, treatment. The psychosocial outcome will be excellent in patients whose seizures can be well controlled (Jacoby *et al.*, 1992).

Diagnosis

An epileptic seizure is a brief, usually unprovoked, stereotyped disturbance of consciousness, behaviour, emotion, motor function or sensation which, on clinical grounds, results from cortical neuronal discharge. Epilepsy can only be diagnosed when seizures have recurred in an apparently spontaneous fashion on more than one occasion. (Rarely, individuals with epilepsy may have seizures provoked by reflex stimuli, e.g. visual.)

The diagnosis of epilepsy is clinical, based on a detailed description of events experienced by the patient before, during and after a seizure, and more importantly on an eye-witness account. In view of the social and economic implications, diagnostic errors need to be avoided. The first basic rule about the diagnosis of epilepsy, therefore, must be never to make a diagnosis unless the clinical evidence is wholly convincing and leaves no room for doubt. Where doubt does exist, no label should be attached and the clinician should rely on the passage of time and the further description of symptomatic events to allow a firm diagnosis. The chances of someone with epilepsy coming to harm from a delay in the diagnosis is minimal; the potential harm from a false positive diagnosis is certain and horrendous!

It is not enough, however, simply to decide that someone's attacks are epileptic in nature. Other questions must be answered. These include the following: (i) whether the seizures are related to an acute encephalopathy or whether they are due to epilepsy; (ii) where seizures are accepted as being part of an epilepsy, an adequate classification of the seizures and the epilepsy syndrome must be attempted, as this can have important prognostic, therapeutic and aetiological implications; and (iii) it may be necessary to determine whether there is an identifiable and independently treatable aetiology for an individual's epilepsy. Answering these questions has important consequences for rehabilitation (see above).

Pharmacological treatment

Starting therapy

Antiepileptic drug treatment has in the past been advocated before seizures occur. Such prophylactic treatment has been undertaken in patients with a high prospective risk of epilepsy after head injury (Jennett, 1975) and craniotomy for various neurosurgical conditions (Foy et al., 1981a). Because no clear evidence exists that antiepileptic treatment is effective in preventing late epilepsy (Temkin et al., 1990; Foy et al., 1992), it seems better to delay treatment until seizures have occurred rather than to adopt a policy of treatment of all potentially epileptic patients – particularly as there may be a relatively high incidence of side-effects with prophylactic treatment (Chadwick et al., 1984) and relatively poor compliance (McQueen et al., 1983).

Where two or more unprovoked seizures have occurred within a short interval, antiepileptic therapy is usually indicated. Problems do arise, however, in defining a short interval. Most would include periods of 6 months to 1 year within the definition, but difficulties arise in knowing whether seizures more widely separated in time demand therapy. Even where seizures occur in close temporal relationship, the identification of specific precipitating factors may make it more important to counsel patients than to commence drug therapy. The most common examples are febrile convulsions in children and alcohol-withdrawal seizures in adults. Less commonly, seizures may be precipitated in photosensitive subjects by television visual display units (VDUs) or other photic stimuli.

The choice of drug

There is now considerable evidence (Reynolds & Miska, 1981) that patients with newly diagnosed epilepsy should be commenced on treatment with a single drug. Up to 70–80% of patients quickly enter a prolonged remission of their seizures (Annegers et al., 1979; Turnbull et al., 1985). This raises the question of which of the available antiepileptic agents should be used as drugs of first choice for which patients. The major factors that influence the choice of antiepileptic drug are comparative efficacy and toxicity. The mode of action, spectrum of efficacy and toxicity are summarized in Table 15.2.

In practice, assumptions made about the comparative efficacy of antiepileptic drugs have been of major importance. While many clinicians have been persuaded that one is likely to be most effective against particular seizure types and epileptic syndromes, it is difficult to identify satisfactory clinical trials that support this contention (Chadwick & Turnbull, 1985). In children, the differences in efficacy between sodium valproate and ethosuximide, on the one hand, and phenytoin and carbamazepine, on the other, in the treatment of absence seizures seem too obvious to demand confirmation in a prospective clinical study. Studies do not, however, differentiate between the efficacy of sodium valproate and ethosuximide in absence epilepsy (Suzuki et al., 1972; Callaghan et al., 1982). Similarly, the preferential response of juvenile myoclonic epilepsy to sodium valproate seems to identify this as the drug of choice in this syndrome (Delgado-Escueta & Enrile-Bacsal, 1984). It is more doubtful whether there are major differences in efficacy between carbamazepine, phenytoin, barbiturates and sodium valproate in the treatment of partial epilepsies (Chadwick & Turnbull, 1985; Mattson et al., 1985).

Where differences in efficacy are marginal, the importance of comparative drug toxicity becomes

Table 15.2 Mode of action, spectrum of efficacy and toxicity of antiepileptic drugs (reproduced from Appleton *et al.*, 1991)

Carbamazepine

Trade name   Tegretol

Manufacturer   Ciba-Geigy

Structure

Mode of action   Limits repetitive firing of Na^+-dependent action potentials

Indications   Drug of choice: complex partial seizures (particularly if complicated by psychiatric disturbance), tonic–clonic and simple partial seizures

Dose
  Adults   300–1600 mg daily; initial dose low with slow increments (N.B. autoinduction of metabolism)
  Children   <1 year 100–200 mg; 1–5 years 200–400 mg; 5–10 years 400–600 mg; 10–15 years 0.6–1 g *or* commence on 10 mg/kg/day for 5–7 days; then 20–40 mg/kg/day thereafter

Optimal range   4–10 µg/ml (but little evidence to support this)

Side-effects
  Dose-related   Dizziness, double vision, unsteadiness nausea and vomiting
  Allergic   Rashes, reduced white cell count
  Chronic toxicity Few known: absence of major effects on intellectual function and behaviour is major benefit

Clobazam

Trade name   Frisium

Manufacturer   Hoechst

Structure

Mode of action   Allosteric enhancement of GABA-mediated inhibition

Indications   Occasional use: tonic–clonic and partial seizures, particularly perimenstrual (value is limited by development of tolerance)

Table 15.2 continued overleaf

Table 15.2 *Continued*

Clobazam *continued*

Dose
    Adults   Up to 30 mg daily in 2 or 3 doses
    Children   >3 years: half adult dose (maximum)

Optimal range   Not routinely measured

Side-effects
    Dose-related   Drowsiness and sedation
    Allergic
    Chronic toxicity

Clonazepam

Trade name   Rivotril

Manufacturer   Roche

Structure

Mode of action   Allosteric enhancement of GABA-mediated inhibition

Indications   Drug of choice: status epilepticus.
                Effective in: absence, myoclonus.
                Occasional use: tonic–clonic and partial seizures (value
                greatly limited by development of tolerance)

Dose
    Adults   Orally: 0.5–4 mg 3 times daily in slowly increasing doses
    Children   <1 year 0.5–1 mg/day; 1–5 years 1–3 mg/day; 6–12
                   years 3–6 mg/day *or* 0.1–0.2 mg/kg/day and usually
                   commence on 0.02 mg/kg/day

Optimal range   Not routinely measured

Side-effects
    Dose-related   Sedation and drowsiness
    Allergic
    IV   Inflammation of veins
    Chronic toxicity

Diazepam

Trade name   Valium Diazemuls Stesolid

Manufacturer   Roche KabiVitrum CP Pharmaceuticals

Structure

continued

Table 15.2 *Continued*

Diazepam *continued*

Mode of action	Allosteric enhancement of GABA-mediated inhibition
Indications	Drug of choice: status epilepticus. Occasional use: absence, myoclonus (value limited by development of tolerance)

Dose

Adults	Intravenous; rectal administration may be of value when venous access difficult. Little effect orally
Children	0.3−0.4 mg/kg (intravenous or rectal administration)

Optimal range	Not routinely measured

Side-effects

Dose-related	Sedation
Allergic	
Chronic toxicity	Habituation

Ethosuximide

Trade name	Zarontin Emeside
Manufacturer	Parke-Davis Laboratories for Applied Biology
Structure	

Mode of action	? Reduce low threshold calcium current in thalamus ? Enhancement of *non*-GABA-mediated inhibition
Indications	Drug of choice: simple absence

Dose

Adults	Up to 2 g/day in 2 or 3 doses
Children	<6 years 250 mg/day; >6 years 0.5−1 g/day *or* 20−40 mg/kg/day

Optimal range	40−10 µg/ml

Side-effects

Dose-related	Nausea, drowsiness, dizziness, unsteadiness, may exacerbate tonic−clonic seizures
Allergic	Rashes
Chronic toxicity	

Phenobarbitone

Trade name	Gardenal Luminal Prominal
Manufacture	May & Baker Winthrop Winthrop
Structure	

Table 15.2 continued overleaf

Table 15.2 *Continued*

Phenobarbitone *continued*

Mode of action	Enhancement of GABA-mediated inhibition
Indications	Effective in: tonic, clonic and partial seizures Occasional use: status epilepticus, absence, myoclonus
Dose	
Adults	Up to 200 mg/day in 2 or 3 doses
Children	Usually 4–5 mg/kg/day
Optimal range	15–35 µg/ml; both upper and lower limits modified by development of tolerance
Side-effects	
Dose-related	Drowsiness, unsteadiness
Allergic	Rashes
Chronic toxicity	Tolerance, habituation, withdrawal seizures. Adverse effects on intellectual function and behaviour

Phenytoin

Trade name	Epanutin
Manufacture	Parke-Davis
Structure	

Mode of action	Inhibits sustained repetitive firing effects on Na^+-dependent voltage channels
Indications	Drug of choice: tonic–clonic, simple and complex partial seizures
Dose	
Adults	200–600 mg/day in 1 or 2 doses
Children	5–8 mg/kg/day
Optimal range	10–20 µg/ml; the non-linear relationship between dose and serum concentration necessitates frequent blood-level monitoring
Side-effects	
Dose-related	Drowsiness, unsteadiness, slurred speech, occasionally abnormal movement disorders
Allergic	Rashes, swelling of lymph glands (pseudolymphoma), hepatitis
Chronic toxicity	Gingival hypertrophy, acne, coarsening of facial features, hirsutism, folate deficiency

---

continued

Table 15.2 *Continued*

Primidone

Trade name	Mysoline
Manufacturer	ICI
Structure	

Mode of action	As phenobarbitone
Indications	Occasional use: tonic–clonic and partial seizures

Dose
- Adults — 500–1500 mg/day in 2 or 3 doses
- Children — 10–30 mg/kg in 2 or 3 doses (rarely used)

Optimal range	As phenobarbitone – to which it is metabolized

Side-effects
- Dose-related — Drowsiness, unsteadiness; often tolerated poorly on initiation and a slow increase in dose advisable
- Allergic — See phenobarbitone
- Chronic toxicity — See phenobarbitone

Sodium valproate

Trade name	Epilim
Manufacturer	Sanofi
Structure	

Mode of action
- ? Enhancement of GABA-mediated inhibition
- ? Limits sustained repetitive firing
- ? Reduces effects of excitatory neurotransmitters

Indications	Drug of choice: idiopathic generalized epilepsies, partial and secondary generalized seizures

Dose
- Adults — 600–3000 mg in 2 or 3 doses
- Children — 20–60 mg/kg/day (usually 20–30 mg/kg/day)

Optimal range	Uncertain: blood levels vary considerably during the day and a single specimen is unreliable

Side-effects
- Dose-related — Tremor, irritability, restlessness; occasionally confusion
- Allergic — Gastric intolerance, hepatotoxicity (mainly children)
- Chronic toxicity — Weight gain; alopecia

Table 15.2 continued overleaf

Table 15.2 *Continued*

Vigabatrin

Trade name	Sabril
Manufacturer	Merrell Dow
Structure	$CH_2 = CH - CH - CH_2 - CH_2 - CO_2H$ with NH_2 branch
Mode of action	Enzyme-activated suicidal inhibitor of GABA aminotransferase
Indications	Treatment of partial epilepsy not satisfactorily controlled by other drugs
Dose	
Adults	2–4 g/day in 1 or 2 doses
Children	3–9 years 1 g/day; >9 years 2 g/day *or* 50–150 mg/ kg/day in 2 or 3 divided doses
Optimal range	Unrelated to known mode of action
Side-effects	The following have been reported but their relationship to the drug is not yet proven: drowsiness and fatigue, nervousness, irritability, depression, headache, confusion, psychosis, altered memory, mild gastrointestinal disturbance

a major consideration in the choice of antiepileptic agent. Antiepileptic drugs possess four distinct types of toxicity: acute dose-related toxicity, acute idiosyncratic toxicity, chronic toxicity and teratogenicity.

Acute dose-related toxicity

Most anticonvulsants, including phenytoin, carbamazepine, barbiturates and benzodiazepines, give rise to a non-specific encephalopathy associated with high blood concentrations. Patients exhibit sedation and nystagmus, and, with increasing blood levels, ataxia, dysarthria and ultimately confusion and drowsiness (Schmidt, 1982a). In some instances, seizure frequency may increase with high blood levels and occasionally involuntary movements are seen, particularly with phenytoin (Chadwick *et al.*, 1976). Phenytoin is especially likely to result in dose-related toxicity because of its unusual pharmacokinetics (see below). Carbamazepine may cause similar symptoms if the dose is not built up slowly. This is probably related to autoinduction of liver microsomal enzymes. Sodium valproate does

not appear to be associated with this typical syndrome of neurotoxicity, but some patients with high blood levels may exhibit restlessness and irritability (sometimes with a frank confusion state). Postural tremor is a common accompaniment (Turnbull *et al.*, 1983).

Undoubtedly, an important criterion influencing the choice of drug is the potential effects on cognitive function and behaviour. All antiepileptic drugs have adverse effects which can be detected at therapeutic concentrations and which become more apparent both with polytherapy and with increasing blood levels of individual drugs. The fact that newer agents such as carbamazepine and sodium valproate have fewer adverse effects on cognitive function and behaviour is perhaps one of the most powerful arguments for preferring these agents to longer-established antiepileptic drugs.

Acute idiosyncratic toxicity

Most antiepileptic drugs, particularly phenytoin and carbamazepine, may cause a maculopapular erythematous eruption, which in more severe cases may be associated with fever, lymphadenopathy and hepatitis (Schmidt, 1982a). The incidence of allergic skin reaction with phenytoin may be as high as 10% and with carbamazepine up to 15% (Chadwick *et al.*, 1984). It may be possible to avoid such reactions with a cautious build-up of initial doses. Rarer, but potentially more serious, idiosyncratic reactions can occur, although these are unpredictable and less likely to influence the choice of drug. Marrow aplasia seems to be extremely rare and fears concerning carbamazepine appear largely unfounded. Concern has arisen because of reports of fatal cases of liver failure in association with sodium valproate therapy. These largely concern children under the age of 2 years who are often multiply handicapped and receiving many different antiepileptic drugs. It may be that they have an underlying error of metabolism that predisposes them to liver failure (Dreifuss *et al.*, 1987). Vigabatrin has been associated with confusion and psychosis, particularly in patients with a previous psychiatric history.

Chronic toxicity

Antiepileptic drugs are unusual in that they may be administered to patients over long periods as treatment for chronic epilepsy. This may lead to the development of a wide variety of syndromes of chronic toxicity (summarized in Table 15.3). A number of factors seem to predispose to the development of these disorders, i.e. the use of polypharmacy, the dosage and the length of therapy. While it appears that sodium valproate and carbamazepine may have fewer chronic toxic effects than barbiturates and phenytoin, the length of time that elapsed before quite common chronic toxic effects were recognized with the older agents should warn us that continued vigilance is needed in the use of the new antiepileptic drugs (Reynolds, 1975).

Teratogenicity

All antiepileptic drugs must be regarded as potentially teratogenic. Phenytoin and probably barbiturate antiepileptic drugs seem to increase the risk of major fetal malformation by two to three times; the most common malformations are harelip and cleft palate and cardiovascular anomalies. The

Table 15.3 Chronic toxicity of anticonvulsants

Nervous system
Memory and cognitive impairment
Hyperactivity and behavioural disturbance
Pseudodementia
Cerebellar atrophy
Peripheral neuropathy

Skin
Acne
Hirsutism
Alopecia
Chloasma

Liver
Enzyme induction

Blood
Megaloblastic anaemia
Thrombocytopenia
Lymphoma

Immune system
IgA deficiency
Drug-induced SLE

Endocrine system
Decreased thyroxine levels
Increased cortisol and sex hormone metabolism

Bone
Osteomalacia

Connective tissue
Gum hypertrophy
Coarsened facial features
Dupuytren's contracture

Pregnancy
Obstetric complications
Teratogenicity
Fetal hydantoin syndrome

risks are higher with polytherapy than with monotherapy. This teratogenicity, together with the unpleasant cosmetic side-effects of these drugs, should limit their use in women. There appears to be an association between neural tube defects and exposure to sodium valproate. Estimates of this risk suggest it is 1–2%, i.e. 10 times the expected rate (Lindhout & Schmidt, 1986). Early screening with ultrasound, alpha-fetoprotein and amniocentesis for neural tube defects therefore seems to be indicated in women becoming pregnant while taking sodium valproate. However, screening should also be undertaken in patients receiving carbamazepine, as this drug may be associated with up to a 1% risk of neural tube defects (Rosa, 1990).

With increasing study of the problem of teratogenicity in women with epilepsy, the higher risk of neural tube defects with more than one drug might argue a genetic link between some forms of epilepsy and this malformation.

Long-term management of drug therapy

Patients with chronic epilepsy have in the past been exposed to increasing doses of multiple drugs, with frequent changes of drugs and dosages. Such a policy needs to be questioned. In patients receiving, and complying with, optimal doses of a single antiepileptic drug, the addition of further agents is likely to result in a significant (>75%) improvement in seizure control in only approximately 10% of patients (Schmidt, 1982b; Crawford & Chadwick, 1986). Such a policy, however, inevitably increases the risks of dose-related, idiosyncratic and chronic toxicity. In essence, a law of diminishing returns applies. Thus, for this group of patients an appropriate aim may be not complete remission of seizures but a compromise of reduced seizure frequency with less severe seizures, to be achieved with one or, at most, two drugs.

Some patients may continue to have seizures but are not disabled by them; they may have very infrequent seizures or seizures that are minor in their symptomatology or confined to sleep. In such patients, assuming that a single drug has been used appropriate to the seizure type and epilepsy syndrome, there is usually little to be gained from alternative drugs or addition of drugs.

Patients who continue to be disabled by the occurrence of seizures despite treatment with a single drug in optimal dosage demand further careful consideration. In particular, it is important to consider whether there are factors that would explain an unsatisfactory response to therapy, e.g. known structural pathology, the presence of complex partial seizures or poor compliance. If this is not the case, then it is important to review the diagnosis. A common reason for failure of therapy

is that the patient does not have epilepsy. Furthermore, it must be remembered that some patients have both true epileptic seizures and pseudoseizures. Has the drug that has been used been an appropriate one? In particular, it is important to differentiate clearly between generalized absence seizures and partial seizures, which may in some instances be similar in their symptomatology.

Where none of these conditions apply, it may be reasonable to try alternative drugs as monotherapy, and in some instances to undertake a trial of the addition of a second drug. However, this demands careful discussion with the patient and the understanding that the second drug will be withdrawn in the absence of satisfactory sustained response.

Finally, patients with intractable partial seizures in spite of adequate drug therapy may benefit from surgical treatment.

Surgical treatment

Whilst the surgical treatment of epilepsy was pioneered in the UK over 100 years ago, it has never been made widely available to patients with epilepsy. The increasing sophistication of EEG investigation, neurological imaging and neuropsychology, however, means that this form of treatment can be highly successful in large numbers of patients. It has been estimated that at least 75 000 patients in the USA may be suitable for surgical treatment (Dreifuss, 1987) and in the UK there may be well over 2000 patients who would benefit.

The philosophy of surgical treatment requires either the accurate identification of a localized site of seizure onset (by neurophysiological with or without neuroradiological techniques) or the disconnection of epileptogenic zones so as to interrupt seizure spread in a palliative procedure (callosotomy or multiple pial resections). Inevitably, excisions of epileptogenic lesions and zones will also involve, to some degree, interruption of their connections.

Engel (1987) reviewed the varying procedures undertaken at centres world-wide. Some form of temporal lobe surgery was involved in 68% of operations, whilst extratemporal cortical excisions accounted for 24% of operations, hemispherectomies for 2% and corpus callosotomy for 6%. To be considered for any of these procedures, patients will need to demonstrate a history of medically refractory epilepsy. There may be some controversy about a precise definition of refractory epilepsy, but this will usually be established within 2 years of onset if appropriate antiepileptic drugs have been administered singly or in combination in optimal doses. Thereafter, there can be little optimism that the manipulation of drug therapy is likely to radically alter the outcome of epilepsy in such a patient. Patients will be sufficiently disabled by their epilepsy to warrant the risks of surgical treatment and the necessary presurgical evaluation. There should be a high probability that an improvement in seizure control will be expected to lead to a significant improvement in the individual's quality of life. Other factors determining suitability of treatment will relate to the type of procedure to be performed, but the above criteria may be relaxed where neurological imaging shows the presence of a lesion that may be a low-grade tumour, which would demand surgical treatment in its own right.

Temporal lobe surgery

There is no doubt that patients with mesiotemporal lesions experience the best results from temporal lobe surgery (Engel, 1987). The ideal candidate for temporal lobe surgery will have a history of seizures typical of a medial temporal onset, an initial epigastric aura being the most common mode of onset (Duncan & Sagar, 1987). The two pathologies with the best outcome are those of mesial temporal sclerosis (Ammon's horn sclerosis) or an indolent glioma of the medial temporal region (Oxbury & Adams, 1989). In the former, a history of a prolonged febrile seizure before the age of 4 or 5 is a particularly strong clinical indicator. Patients should usually be between the ages of 12 and 30, as psychosocial adjustment may be more difficult in patients having resective surgery after the age of 30 (Crandall *et al.*, 1987). Patients will show a unilateral, anterior temporal, interictal spike, and sphenoidal or other ictal recordings may confirm a temporal onset to seizures.

Having defined the ideal patient, it must be recognized that many patients who do not conform to these criteria will, nevertheless, have a significant chance of benefiting from temporal lobe surgery, though they may require more detailed presurgical evaluation.

Presurgical evaluation

A detailed clinical history is essential to describe the clinical features of seizures and past medical history. Developmental and educational histories are particularly important.

Neuropsychological assessment is essential. An overall intelligence quotient (IQ) of <70 would tend to indicate diffuse cerebral damage, which reduces the likelihood of a good outcome of surgery. Particular evaluation of verbal and visual memory can be important in defining deficits affecting each of the temporal lobes. Neuropsychological testing after intracarotid Amytal is helpful in further defining memory deficits related to each temporal lobe. Where there is agreement between the side of interictal temporal spiking and a lateralized memory deficit on Amytal testing, the likelihood of a good outcome is high. Amytal testing is also important in ensuring that memory function in the temporal lobe contralateral to that on which surgery is being considered is adequate to sustain memory postoperatively.

Brain imaging has become increasingly important. Modern generations of CT scanners may detect small structural lesions such as gliomas and arteriovenous malformations that previously would have been missed. Magnetic resonance imaging (MRI) seems to possess ever greater sensitivity, particularly for atrophic and gliotic lesions. In specialist centres, functional imaging using positron emission tomography (PET) or single-photon emission computerized tomography (SPECT) may also be of some value. Epileptogenic zones are characteristically hypometabolic and hypoperfused during the interictal state, but may become hypermetabolic and hyperperfused ictally or immediately postictally (Engel *et al.*, 1982; Fish, 1989).

Perhaps the most controversial element of preoperative assessment is the extent of neurophysiological investigation. There is no doubt that some patients with typical histories of febrile seizures, unilateral memory deficit and purely unilateral anterior temporal spiking interictally can reasonably be offered temporal lobectomy without further investigation (Polkey, 1987). Sphenoidal recordings have frequently been used in the past but it can be questioned how much extra information such recordings give compared with an electrode placed

Table 15.4 Survey results: outcome with respect to epileptic seizures (reproduced from Engel, 1987)

Classification	Hemispherectomy	Anteriotemporal lobectomy	Extratemporal resection	Corpus callosum section
Total patients	88	2336	825	197
Total centres	17	40	32	16
No. seizure-free	68	1296	356	10
Percentage	77.3	55.5	43.2	5.0
Range	0–100	26–80	0–73	0–13
No. improved	16	648	229	140
Percentage	18.2	27.7	27.8	71.0
No. not improved	4	392	240	47
Percentage	4.5	16.8	29.1	23.9
Range	0–33	6–29	17–89	10–38

on the surface where such a wire would be inserted. In less typical patients, some form of long-term recording will usually be necessary. The technique of foramen ovale recording is probably subject to few complications and has proved invaluable in several centres (Wieser *et al.*, 1985). More sophisticated recordings can be obtained following the insertion of subdural electrodes and stereotactically implanted depth electrodes or a combination of the two (Hahn & Luders, 1987).

The outcome of temporal lobe surgery and other operations is summarized in Table 15.4. The most common surgical procedure is the *en bloc* anteriotemporal lobectomy pioneered by Falconer *et al.* (1955). More recently, amygdalohippocampectomy

Table 15.5 Complications of temporal lobectomy (reproduced from Oxbury & Adams, 1989)

Complication	Incidence
Visual field defect	
Asymptomatic homonymous upper quarter	Most cases
Symptomatic homonymous upper + partial lower quarter	15%
Transient diplopia	Common with *en bloc* resection
Persistent hemiplegia	2%
Psychiatric disorder	2%
Persistent dysphasia	1%

has been pioneered for patients in whom it can be shown that there is a definite medial temporal onset to seizures (Yasargil & Wieser, 1987). This procedure may potentially offer results as good as classical *en bloc* resection with hopefully a reduced morbidity. The complications of temporal lobe surgery are summarized in Table 15.5.

Extratemporal cortical excisions

The outcome of such procedures is somewhat less satisfactory than temporal lobe surgery, but extratemporal resections can reasonably be considered in patients with localized extratemporal lesions defined by imaging techniques and in patients where neurophysiological investigation reveals a consistent focal onset to seizures outside the temporal lobe. Complex partial seizures arising from frontal–orbital areas may be particularly helped by surgery (Quesney, 1986).

Hemispherectomy

This procedure may be suitable for patients with intractable epilepsy and an infantile hemiplegia with a useless hand. Overall, 70–80% of patients become seizure-free following this operation, and behavioural abnormalities can also improve. The operation, however, fell into disrepute, as up to 25% of those undergoing hemispherectomy developed delayed complications (Oppenheimer, 1966). Most suffered from recurrent subdural haemorrhage from the subdural membrane lining the hemispherectomy cavity. Adams (1983) modified the hemispherectomy procedure to eliminate the large extradural space and to insulate the ventricular system from the subdural cavity. Hemispherectomy should probably now be restored to its previous position in children with infantile hemiplegia and epilepsy, and also in those rare children with chronic progressive focal encephalitis (Rasmussen's syndrome; Rasmussen *et al.*, 1958). Recently, the operation has also been used in the treatment of infants with infantile spasm syndrome where EEGs and functional imaging techniques indicate a unilateral onset to seizures.

Callosotomy

Section of the corpus callosum and hippocampal commissure is an accepted palliative procedure for uncontrolled, secondarily generalized seizures (Spencer *et al.*, 1987). The procedure seeks to prevent the generalization of seizures, particularly those that generalize rapidly, resulting in falls (tonic and atonic seizures). Early procedures were often complicated by ventriculitis, meningitis and hydrocephalus, by more severe and frequent focal seizures immediately postoperatively and by a characteristic disconnection syndrome of mutism, apraxia of the non-dominant limbs, agnosia, apathy, confusion and infantile behaviour. Refinements of the surgical procedure and the introduction of anterior and two-stage operations have reduced the morbidity. In some series, up to 80% of patients have had a complete cessation of generalized seizures with falls, although about 25% may have more intense partial seizures than previously. It also seems that a callosotomy may reduce the incidence of status epilepticus.

The selection criteria for corpus callosotomy are more poorly defined than for other surgical procedures. The operation will be most commonly considered in children and adolescents with very severe epilepsy with multifocal origin to seizures or with seizures of sudden onset resulting in falls.

Factors contributing to handicap

Despite the best medical and surgical endeavours, many patients do face life with a chronic epilepsy.

In planning rehabilitation for an individual with persisting epilepsy, the impairments contributing to the disability and handicap must be carefully assessed. These will include:
1 Seizures.
2 Associated handicaps.
3 Psychological and psychiatric handicap.
4 Social and legal handicap.

Seizures

Because seizures are varied in the clinical phenomena that they produce, they can cause very variable degrees of disability and handicap.

The Commission on Classification of Seizures (1989) contrasts seizures which have a generalized onset and those that begin locally (partial seizures). Seizures with a generalized onset are not associated with a warning or aura and therefore frequently cause a greater impairment, particularly when such seizures are associated with significant motor phenomena. In particular, sudden tonic, atonic or tonic−clonic seizures frequently result in injury. Tonic−clonic seizures are also associated with prolonged postictal confusion, which also adds to handicap. However, even brief absence seizures can themselves represent a problem when they occur extremely frequently and have an adverse impact on concentration and learning.

Partial seizures are usually but not always associated with an aura. This may be beneficial to patients in that it allows them to take sensible precautions prior to loss of consciousness or may allow them to utilize a variety of methods to reduce the impact of their seizures. One important role of antiepileptic drugs is to prevent the spread of seizure activity during partial seizures, and they therefore reduce seizure duration and severity. Thus, the patient who presents with complex partial seizures may continue to experience the auras to his/her seizures on treatment but is not in other ways handicapped. This can be a satisfactory outcome.

Seizures occurring at different times of the day may similarly produce variable degrees of disability. In particular, seizures that occur during sleep, most commonly partial seizures, produce less handicap than do those that occur during the day. Similarly, generalized seizures with a predisposition to occur shortly after waking may not have significant consequences for employment.

Seizures contribute to disability by interrupting normal activity and by producing forms of behaviour that may be hazardous or be misinterpreted by observers. Of greater concern to patients and their families is the risk of accidental injury or even death (Mittan & Locke, 1982) because of seizures. Rehabilitation needs to include sensible counselling to reduce the risks to people with epilepsy from accidental injury from seizures during everyday life.

Mortality from epilepsy

All available studies show an increased mortality ratio for epilepsy of between two and three times the expected (Hauser & Hesdorffer, 1990). A number of factors appear to contribute to this excess mortality. The greatest excess seems to occur in the early years of life (Hauser et al., 1980) and to be more obvious in men. The risk of mortality is greatest in the early years following diagnosis, and is highest for patients with tonic–clonic seizures and seizures that recur frequently.

Much of the excess mortality seems to be associated with the underlying aetiology of an epilepsy rather than the occurrence of seizures themselves. The risk is higher for patients with a symptomatic epilepsy than for those with idiopathic epilepsy (Hauser et al., 1980). The association of epilepsy with cerebrovascular disease in later life probably accounts for the excess mortality associated with the diagnosis of epilepsy in the elderly. The association with mental handicap and cerebral palsy in younger age-groups seems of considerable importance (Satishchandra et al., 1988). Both neoplasms and arteriovenous malformations contribute to the excess mortality from symptomatic epilepsies.

Considerable controversy surrounds the role of sudden unexpected death in people with epilepsy. A number of studies have highlighted cases in which people with epilepsy are found dead, usually in bed (Leestma et al., 1984; Neuspiel & Kuller, 1985). It is usually assumed that deaths are related to seizures and possibly to associated cardiac dysrhythmias. However, the only study to compare risks of sudden death in people with epilepsy with those of the rest of the community failed to find any excess mortality for those with epilepsy (Annegers et al., 1984). Accidental death is more common in

epilepsy than would be expected, drowning being the commonest cause. While status epilepticus continues to be associated with mortality, its rarity means that it does not contribute significantly to the excess mortality associated with epilepsy.

Accidental injury

Injuries due to falling are not uncommon in people with epilepsy but most injuries are not severe. The Rochester study (Hauser et al., 1980) demonstrated a standardized mortality ratio (SMR) of 2.3 for fatal accidents. However, non-fatal accidents (head injury, burns, fractures, dental injuries, near-drowning) are much more common. Intuitively, these are more likely to occur in patients whose epilepsy involves frequent loss of consciousness with or without falls. Unfortunately, very few systematic analyses have been performed and, indeed, no prospective study of incidence of these events has been undertaken.

Hauser et al. (1983) have shown that patients with epilepsy are over-represented in a study of non-fatal head trauma. These patients account for 7.4% of admissions to five New York hospitals, which was three times expected incidence for a population of similar age distributions. Accidents in those with epilepsy were significantly more likely to be due to falls and less likely to be sustained in a road traffic accident than non-epileptic trauma victims. There was a greater chance of alcohol use in relation to head injury in the epileptic group, but even when these cases were excluded the increased risk persisted.

Rusell-Jones & Shorvon (1989) found that 2.7% of seizures at the Chalfont Centre for Epilepsy resulted in a clinically significant head injury, but only one in over 9000 seizures was complicated by skull fracture or intracranial haematoma.

There have been no studies of the incidence of burns in unselected populations of patients with epilepsy. However, it is agreed that epilepsy is a cause of burns in approximately 10% of cases (Maisels, 1964; Tempest, 1970). Bhatnagar et al. (1977), in a retrospective review of presentations on an Indian burns unit, identified epilepsy as the cause of 2.6% of all burns, but 8.4% of those requiring admission. In a study of patients attending an epilepsy clinic (Hampton et al., 1988), 38% of patients had a history of any burn with 13% seeking hospital treatment, 4% requiring admission and 1% needing skin grafting. Those who sustained burns were older, had a longer history of epilepsy and were more likely to have complex partial seizures than those who had no history of burns. Spitz (1992) presents 10 patients with severe burns, of whom eight had more than two seizures per month and six of whom were alone at the time of the injury. A consistent feature of these reports is that patients do not recall being warned by their physicians about the risk of burns or particular risk activities.

Other injuries are common. Hampton *et al.* (1988) report 58% of patients with a history of injury, with 13% sustaining a fracture or dislocation, 10% dental trauma and 13% multiple injuries.

Interventions

What approach should be taken in counselling patients about the risk of accidental injury? There is an obvious dilemma in that strategies which reduce risk may cause considerable limitation of quality of life. It is an area in which compromises must be made.

It must be clear (see above) that patients can be identified who are at particular risk. For others, reassurance about the low risks of serious accident injury appears appropriate, perhaps with advice to avoid climbing to significant heights, to use microwave cooking in preference to gas or electric hobs, and to ensure that fires are adequately guarded. Showers are preferred to baths, and swimming in open water best avoided. For most people a full range of leisure activities should be possible, though perhaps with some accompanying supervision where appropriate (e.g. swimming in a pool, cycling on a busy road).

For patients with frequent seizures complicated by falls, more supervision and attendance may be necessary, and occasionally protective helmets may be worn, although these may be regarded as unduly stigmatizing by some.

Epilepsy as a psychosocial handicap

The social, psychological and emotional problems encountered with epilepsy have been extensively reviewed in terms of the frequency of seizures and the additional effects of associated neurological handicaps, including the effects of anticonvulsant therapy and societal attitudes towards people with epilepsy (Dodrill *et al.*, 1980; Betts, 1981; Masland, 1988). High rates of psychosocial problems among individuals with epilepsy have been reported, and these may be the result of the unpredictability and the severity of seizures, rather than their frequency. No matter how well controlled a person's seizures are, the fear of seizures may always be present, for epilepsy is more often a threat than an active condition (Lechtenberg, 1984). The fear evoked by the unpredictable nature of the seizures may lead to social withdrawal, with loss of existing friendships and an inability to form new relationships. Loss of employment or inability to compete in the job market may lead to loss of self-esteem and to financial hardship. These factors not infrequently result in anxiety, depression and a loss of sense of control. This loss of control may have serious psychological consequences, including feelings of helplessness and low self-esteem (Garber & Seligman, 1980; Betts, 1981).

Dealing with these various psychological and social factors is crucial to making a positive adjustment to epilepsy. Even those persons who appear to adjust successfully must continually cope with the fears and uncertainties imposed by epilepsy. Emotional factors may become the most important determinants of the motivation to carry out a medical regime and adapt to an altered life situation (Laaksonen, 1983).

The process of adjusting to epilepsy is complex, with patients having to make changes in the way they think, feel and act as a result of the diagnosis. Scambler (1992) distinguishes five dimensions contributing to the adjustment process: accommodation, rationalization, concept of self, sociability and fulfilment. According to Scambler, accommodation refers to the reaction to the physical properties of seizures, for example many people fear that seizures may lead to serious injury or death (see above). The process of rationalization refers to making sense of one's medical history and attempting to understand its cause. In patients with epilepsy where no explanations are forthcoming, patients may generate their own theories. Epilepsy may also have the effect of diminishing patients' perception of their own self-worth. There is also evidence that epilepsy may negatively affect the extent and quality of relationship that patients may have with family friends and work colleagues. This may result in some patients attempting to conceal their condition from others. Epilepsy may also constitute an obstacle to patients' individual sense of achievement in a number of social roles and contexts.

Interventions

It is important to help patients and their families gain a greater understanding about their epilepsy and in doing so demystify any beliefs they have about their condition. It is also important for clinicians to be aware of the importance and timing of communicating the diagnosis of epilepsy, as often a diagnosis marks the beginning of a protracted, and sometimes lifelong, process of adjustment to having epilepsy. Physicians can exercise considerable influence on the accommodation of the diagnosis by the patient and their family. According to Scambler (1992), successful accommodation is likely to be facilitated by medical intervention to reduce seizure frequency with minimal treatment, combined with therapy for possible psychological or psychiatric sequelae of epilepsy or medication or psychosocial factors (Hermann et al., 1990).

Perhaps even more importantly, successful accommodation may be influenced significantly by good communication between physician and patient. A number of the concerns that patients have about their epilepsy could be substantially resolved if acknowledged and discussed.

Physicians also have an important role in helping patients adapt to their epilepsy. Physicians can take care to maximize the time taken to communicate the diagnosis. They can provide much more information about medication, aetiology and the psychosocial consequences of epilepsy. Schneider & Conrad (1983) have also argued that patients and their families should be incorporated into a shared care philosophy in the management of the epilepsy with the physician. This would entail good two-way communications between the patient and the physician and allow the opportunity for the patient to discuss issues important to them.

Physicians, through what they say and what they do, undoubtedly influence how people cope with

their epilepsy. By rethinking the patient–physician consultation, physicians might better facilitate the coping process.

Families also play an important role in relation to how well patients adjust to their epilepsy. In some families parents perceive epilepsy as something unwelcome or bad, and are motivated by a desire to protect their offspring. They unwittingly coach their children to perceive epilepsy in the same way. Overprotection is a major source of anger and resentment in people with epilepsy (Hoare, 1984) and has been associated with behavioural and emotional problems in children. The long-term effect of overprotection is likely to impede normal development and impair the capacity to establish peer relationships (Fenton, 1983). Successful management of patients with epilepsy should not merely rely on the reduction of seizure frequency but on a holistic assessment of the physical, social and psychological well-being of the individual, their general perception of their quality of life and confidence in their ability to adapt to living with epilepsy. This will normally require a multidisciplinary team approach, with specialists from neurology, psychology, psychiatry, social work and, where possible, counsellors and advisers from the Epilepsy Association. The provision of such a team will increase the likelihood of addressing all the needs of the patient with epilepsy (see below).

Epilepsy and psychiatric disorders

The relationship between epilepsy and psychiatric disorders has evoked much discussion. A number of studies on unselected populations of patients have demonstrated an increased incidence of psychiatric illness in patients with epilepsy (Pond & Bidwell, 1959; Gudmundson, 1966). These studies provide evidence that the increased incidence occurs in both adults and children and that having epilepsy rather than other chronic conditions is associated with increased psychopathology. Several studies support the view that the incidence of psychiatric illness was greater in people with temporal lobe epilepsy. These studies, however, have been criticized on methodological grounds, particularly the ascertainment of psychiatric illness and the categorizations of seizure types. A recent general practice survey (Edeh & Toone, 1987), using an accurate measure of psychiatric disorder and a detailed examination of seizure type, has shown that psychiatric morbidity (especially anxiety and non-psychiatric depression) occurs more commonly in people with epilepsy than would be expected by chance and is particularly common in patients with focal epilepsy as opposed to primary generalized epilepsy.

There have been a number of conflicting studies investigating the incidence and prevalence of psychosis in patients with epilepsy. Pond & Bidwell (1959), in a study of 14 general practices, found 29% of their sample had a history of psychiatric illness but none had been, or were, psychotic. In contrast, a number of out-patient studies (Currie et al., 1971; Bruens, 1974) have reported an incidence of between 2 and 5%. In an earlier study of 69 patients with schizophrenia-like psychosis, 80% were found to have focal temporal lobe EEG abnormalities (Slater et al., 1963), leading the authors to conclude that the characteristics of the psychoses accompanying epilepsy were distinct from functional psychosis. This finding has not, however, been confirmed in subsequent prospective studies (Perez et al., 1980, 1985).

Because of a number of methodological problems, including selection bias and a lack of homogeneity in the psychosis syndrome (Toone, 1986), the relationship between epilepsy and psychosis remains unclear. This has undoubtedly led to an overestimation of the incidence and prevalence of psychosis in epilepsy (Hauser & Hesdorffer, 1990). Further controlled population-based research is clearly necessary to overcome such pitfalls and clarify the relationship between psychosis and epilepsy. It is clear that a small proportion of patients with epilepsy will present with either chronic or short-lived psychosis. In such cases, hospital admission may be needed from time to time, particularly for an acute crisis, especially where overt psychiatric illnesses develop. Particularly difficult cases may benefit from an admission to a specialized epilepsy clinic assessment centre.

Epilepsy has also been linked to a higher incidence of self-harm and suicide. Exact figures for incidence of suicide and self-harm among individuals with epilepsy, however, are difficult to acquire. A review of diverse studies on mortality and suicide in epilepsy (Barraclough, 1980) confirmed that there was an increased risk of suicide in individuals with epilepsy. Barraclough estimated the incidence as five times higher than expected in those with temporal lobe epilepsy. It has been suggested that feelings of helplessness, lack of control, low self-esteem and anxiety were important risk factors in the aetiology of suicide.

If seizures can be controlled by medication and if patients are provided with adequate information about the extent to which their lives may or may not be restricted, then they may be capable of developing effective coping strategies and avoid such extreme measures as suicide.

Epilepsy and employment

The importance of work for patients with epilepsy has been well established (Scambler, 1989). The Reid report on *People with Epilepsy* highlighted the importance of work in determining social and financial status, role in society, aspects of personal satisfaction, social companionship, self-esteem, discipline and purpose (Central Health Services Council, 1969).

The vocational difficulties experienced by individuals with epilepsy (unemployment and underemployment, limitations in vocational choice) have been well documented (Fraser & Clemmons, 1989). It is estimated that there are approximately 200 000 people of working age with epilepsy in the UK, and that between 50 000 and 100 000 of these may experience moderate or severe problems with epilepsy (Floyd, 1986).

Some studies have shown that unemployment rates among epileptic patients do not appear to differ greatly from those of the general population (Scambler & Hopkins, 1980). Certainly, in populations of people with a remote history of epilepsy, employment rates may approach the norm (Jacoby, 1992). In times of greater unemployment, these findings may be no longer valid. A recent study in an area of high unemployment by Elwes et al. (1991) found that patients with epilepsy had much greater difficulty in finding work. Patients with epilepsy were less likely to leave school with qualifications or undergo subsequent training apprenticeships. They were more likely to be single, live in rented accommodation and be unskilled manual workers.

In some countries, apart from legislative barriers to employing patients with epilepsy (Table 15.6), there is also evidence of deliberate discrimination. This commonly arises through misinformation and misunderstanding of the nature of epilepsy, rather than the requirements of many occupations. In addition, people with epilepsy may perceive potential employers as hostile, fearful and indifferent,

Table 15.6 Some occupations affected by statutory barriers (UK)

Occupation	Regulations	Effect
Aircraft pilot	Manual of Civil Aviation Medicine produced by International Civil Aviation Organization	Applicants shall have no established medical history or clinical diagnosis of epilepsy
Ambulance driver	Follow PSV regulations (see below)	Barrier if fit occurred since age of 5 for drivers or crew. Clerical work available for those who develop epilepsy in employment
Armed services:		
Army	Army Act 1955; Manual of Military Law	Applicants are rejected on grounds of epilepsy and likely to be discharged if they develop epilepsy during employment. If they have had no fits since childhood, each case is considered individually
Navy		Medical regulations state any attacks at any age would debar from entry
RAF	Recruiting regulations in Air Force Act 1955 as amended in Army and Air Force Act 1961 and the Armed Forces Acts of 1966, 1971 and 1976	Proven epilepsy with a few exceptions is bar to recruitment. People developing epilepsy during service are given a medical employment standard which limits their employment
Coastguard	Civil Service Medical Advisory Service policy based on individual merit	Coastguards come into a category which requires special physical qualifications, therefore medical examination is arranged in all cases to determine fitness to undertake the full range of duties
Diver	Health and Safety at Work Act 1974. Diving Operations at Work Regs. 1981 (SI 1981/399)	Any history of fits (apart from febrile convulsions) will preclude granting a Certificate of Medical Fitness to Dive, which must be renewed every 12 months
Fire brigade	Fire Service Act 1947: Fire Services Appointments (and Promotion) Regs. 1965	A history of epilepsy renders a man unsuitable for operational fire duties
HSV, PSV and taxi-driver	Statutory Instrument 1309 HGV (Drivers' Licences) Regs. 1977. Amendment 429, 1982 — consolidated in 1984, 1925 Reg. 4 Section 22 Public Passenger Vehicle Act 1981 PSV 1985, Statutory Instrument 214 Reg. 5a	The amending regulations for Group II entitlement 'an epileptic attack since attaining the age of 5 years' amended to 'a liability to epileptic seizures'. This liability to be assessed by the ability to meet all of the following criteria: (i) free of epileptic attack for at least the last 10 years; (ii) no anti-epileptic medication taken during this 10-year period; (iii) no continuing liability to epileptic seizure. The last requirement would exclude persons who have some structural intracranial lesion thus increasing the risk of seizure

continued

Table 15.6 *Continued*

Occupation	Regulations	Effect
Merchant seaman	DoT Merchant Shipping (Med. Exam) Regs. 1983 Statutory Instrument 1983 No. 808, Merchant Shipping Notice M1144	Absolute barrier on applicants with history of fits since age 5. Serving seamen who develop epilepsy may be employed after 2 years free of seizures on a ship carrying a medical officer and provided they are not involved in the safety of ship or passengers
Nurse and midwife	Nurses, Midwives and Health Visitors Act 1979 SI 1983/873 – midwives only	Epilepsy is not mentioned specifically. Nurses: each training authority sets own standards. Midwives: prospective trainees must provide evidence that they are not knowingly suffering from any disabilities which might preclude them from carrying out the duties of a midwife
Police	Statutory qualifications contained in Police Regulations 1979. Regulation 14(1) (C) relates to general health criteria for entry – not specific to epilepsy	Applicants currently having fits not recruited. Those with past history dealt with on individual basis. Also applies to traffic wardens, drivers, etc.
Prison service	No Statutory Instrument regarding health standards for prison service	Recent history of epilepsy debars an applicant on grounds of security for posts at prison officer grade. Applicants to other grades of prison service are considered individually
Teacher in state school	Education (Teachers) Regulations, 1982	Applicants must be 3 years free of seizures. Teachers in post may be barred from teaching PE, craft, science and home economics
Train driver	No statutory requirements for medical fitness	Absolute barrier if fit ever occurred (London Regional Transport) or if fit occurred since age 5 (British Rail). Also applies to LRT guards and track operatives

HSV: heavy goods vehicle; PSV: public service vehicle; LRT: London regional transport.

even where there is no evidence for this (Scambler, 1987).

The findings from the above studies clearly indicate the need for individual vocational counselling from professionals with an understanding of patients with epilepsy. In Great Britain such a service can be obtained through the Health and Safety Executive's Employment Medical Advisory Service, which is open to employers, employees and job applicants alike. The Department of Employment also produces good written information about employment and epilepsy and this is in addition to the information provided by the voluntary epilepsy associations. Local information about employment prospects can be obtained through disability re-

settlement officers, who are normally contacted through job centres.

Ideally, patients with epilepsy should be offered employment or training based on their skills, experience and qualifications, but one commonly expressed problem is when and how epilepsy should be declared to a prospective employer. Codes of good practice do exist but seem rarely observed. Many application forms contain a request for medical information with no guarantee that it will be assessed by anyone with medical or occupational health expertise. Whilst employers should be informed of a previous diagnosis of epilepsy before employment begins, it seems inappropriate to elicit information at such an early stage.

The Civil Service will only make health enquiries after interview, assessment of qualifications and experience, and a job offer. At this stage, a specialist's report may be requested and suitability assessed by a specialist in occupational health.

It is not unreasonable to advise patients faced with requests for medical information on a first application to leave these sections of the form blank, but to declare epilepsy at the time when a job offer might be made.

Epilepsy and education

In the UK, the 1981 Education Act stressed that children with special needs should be educated, whenever practical, in mainstream schools. It is estimated that, of the 60 000 children with epilepsy, only a small number will be attending special schools (Radley, 1987). Despite this, there is potential for discrimination inherent in formulating policies for school activities based on generalizations about children with epilepsy (Thompson & Oxley, 1993). Amongst those children with epilepsy in mainstream schooling, there is considerable evidence of a significant number of children underachieving, particularly in the areas of reading, spelling and arithmetic (Aldenkamp, 1987). This has been attributed to a number of factors, including the occurrence of nocturnal attacks, brief epileptic discharges which can result in transient cognitive impairment, and high levels of medication and polypharmacy (Cull & Trimble, 1989). In addition, other psychological variables have been implicated, including parental and teacher expectations, misconceptions about epilepsy, absence from school, low self-esteem and anxiety due to stress at home (Thompson & Oxley, 1993).

Where a child is considered to have special education needs, the 1981 Education Act requires those to be specified in a process known as statementing. The educational needs of the child are assessed by a multidisciplinary team and include the views of the parents. On the basis of the statement, the local education authority is required to meet those special needs. The Advisory Centre for Education (ACE) publishes a wide range of information relating to education law and provision. ACE also offers free telephone advice.

Interventions

The importance of good communication between parents and school authorities cannot be overestimated. Parents deciding not to disclose their child's epilepsy remain a problem, with the unfortunate consequences of a child being mislabelled as a daydreamer or having behavioural problems. A number of reports have endorsed the need for frank and open discussion between parents, teachers and primary health care services. Parents and teachers may also hold inaccurate beliefs about epilepsy and have differing expectations about levels of achievement. Information packages are readily available for both teachers and parents which provide valuable information about epilepsy and managing different seizure types (Rogan, 1992).

The education of the child about his or her epilepsy is also an important factor in the child's adjustment at school and in the home. The effect of keeping the child uninformed is to increase the probability of social and emotional maladjustment. Making a child feel different can have adverse consequences for self-esteem and lead to social withdrawal, reduced motivation and school phobia (Kato et al., 1979). It is important, therefore, to maintain the child's self-image in order to maximize adjustment to school. Finally, there is a continuing need to monitor the child's educational and social development. Continuous unobtrusive monitoring by teachers and parents enhances the likelihood of pre-empting difficulties in school performance. Information from the school and home can be useful to the physician in prescribing medication.

Epilepsy and the family

With early onset of epilepsy, it appears reasonable to assume that particular parenting styles may affect some aspects of the personality of the patient. This may take the form of overprotection: parents, fearful of the risks involved when seizures cannot be completely controlled, often dominate and prevent the child from gaining normal independence. Conversely, it may lead to rejection of the child. The same attitudes may prevail in the school environment, and may exercise a major impact on the child's academic, emotional and social development. Emotional maladjustment has been shown to be more common in children with epilepsy than in those with non-neurological handicaps (Hoare, 1984), as has educational underachievement (Britten *et al.*, 1986).

Coming to terms with the diagnosis of epilepsy affects not only the individual but also his or her family. There is a growing body of evidence that having epilepsy can have an adverse effect on relationships within the family and within the individual's peer group. It is not uncommon to observe high levels of anxiety and resentment in families where epilepsy is prominent and seizures are frequent and uncontrolled (Taylor, 1989).

In some families with epilepsy, inappropriate coping styles develop, including overprotection and parental overinvolvement. This may lead to emotional, cognitive and social underdevelopment in the child with epilepsy. Children may also learn to use their condition to manipulate other family members. Parents are often in the difficult position of balancing the safety of the child against allowing him or her to engage in normal activities with their associated risks. In some families, a preoccupation with the child's epilepsy may be detrimental to the well-being of other family members, leading to deep-seated resentment. Parents may also have lowered expectations of the child with epilepsy, compared with his/her siblings. In a recent study, negative parental reactions to epilepsy were associated with high levels of psychosocial maladjustment in children with epilepsy and their siblings (Hoare, 1984).

Epilepsy is the commonest neurological problem in adolescence, a time when young people are considering their own identity, sexuality and independence. The effects of epilepsy can severely disrupt this natural period of development. Parental overprotection and restrictions on social activities may result in social isolation. Inability to form friendships may have a detrimental effect on psychological health, resulting in anxiety, depression and non-compliance with medication (Clement & Wallace, 1990; Thompson & Oxley, 1993). Young people may have fears about sexual problems and sexual performance (Betts, 1988). Thompson & Oxley (1993) argue that young people with problematic epilepsy have a very poor understanding of sexual development and this is a direct consequence of overprotection. Research has also shown that people with epilepsy are less likely to marry or have children. This may be due partly to poor social skills

as a result of low levels of confidence, self-esteem and the overprotectiveness of families. It may also be due to social isolation as a result of fear of seizures and the subsequent restrictions on social activities (Lechtenberg, 1984; Hoare, 1988).

Interventions

It is clear from research that many families with epilepsy not only require clear factual information but may also need emotional support. This information should be regularly repeated and updated when and where necessary. The general practitioner will have an important role in counselling the family and directing them to appropriate support groups. Recent evidence has suggested that rehabilitation courses for children and their families can be successful in helping patients and their families adjust to epilepsy. Families with a member with chronic epilepsy may also benefit from respite care, home help and holiday opportunities. Some assistance with these areas may be available through charitable epilepsy support agencies.

Some adolescents will need assistance in achieving independence, and this may only be possible through the intervention of an agency outside the family. A social rehabilitation programme, including working with other family members, may be an appropriate method for helping an individual make progress towards personal development. Unfortunately, such programmes are not readily available and only centres with an expertise in epilepsy and a strong multidisciplinary team are likely to provide them (Thompson & Shorvon, 1991). In terms of sexual development, a proportion of young people with epilepsy will require clear information and careful counselling.

Mobility

People with epilepsy have restricted mobility, because of legal restrictions on driving and difficulty using public transport when seizures are not well controlled. This contributes to feelings of social isolation and to reduced employment prospects.

Driving

The Road Traffic Act 1982 (UK) states that a person who suffers from epilepsy must have been free from attacks for a period of 2 years to become eligible to hold an ordinary driving licence. If attacks continue during sleep, there must be a history of attacks only during sleep for a minimum of 3 years. These rules apply whether or not the person is on antiepileptic medication. Licences for people with a history of epilepsy are issued for a limited period and made subject to periodic review.

In the UK anyone who holds a driving licence and has a seizure is obliged to inform the Driver and Vehicle Licensing Authority (DVLA) at Swansea and may expect his/her licence to be revoked until he can fulfil the above regulation. Seizures include auras and myoclonic jerks, as well as all types of more major seizures. Doctors and other health professionals should give unambiguous explanation of current regulations, and advise patients not to drive in the intervening period before the DVLA informs them of the decision regarding their licence. Patients who seem unwilling to comply with the regulations should be reminded that their insurance cover will be invalid and that there are legal penalties, as well as potential risks to themselves and others. It is advisable to record such advice in the case notes. Only under the most exceptional circumstances should any health professional consider contacting the DVLA him/herself about an individual patient. They must be persuaded that an individual's continued driving offers a significant risk to society as a whole and they would be well advised to consult their medical defence organization.

Under present regulations, a seizure which follows a change or attempted withdrawal of anticonvulsant medication must be declared and would result in application of the above regulations, even if the original medication was immediately resumed. This should be explained to patients who hold a driving licence and who are contemplating drug withdrawal.

Vocational licences

Recent amendments to the Road Traffic Act have allowed drivers requesting a HGV or PSV licence who have had a seizure of any type after their fifth birthday to be reassessed. Drivers must meet the following requirements:

1 have been free of epileptic attack for at least the last 10 years;

2 have not taken anti-epileptic medication during this 10-year period;

3 do not have a continuing liability to epileptic seizure.

Single seizures or other unexplained loss of consciousness

Patients with a single seizure or other unexplained loss of consciousness may be banned from driving for 1 year. However, patients with cerebral pathology, such as head injury or stroke, who have had a single seizure may be banned for 2 years. Patients are obliged to inform the DVLA even if epilepsy has not been diagnosed, as the regulations require the licence-holder to notify the DVLA if they have had any disability which affects their fitness to drive. Epilepsy, a seizure or an unexplained loss of consciousness would all constitute such a disability.

The regulations governing fitness to drive vary between countries (Parsonage, 1992).

Fare concessions

Concessions are available for people with epilepsy but availability and regulations vary between local authorities. Schemes include free travel, reduced fares and a system of tokens, which may be usable towards taxi fares. Details of local schemes can be obtained through local council transport offices, passenger transport executives, bus operators, local authority officers and public libraries.

The disabled person's railcard is available to permanently and severely disabled people who are entitled to attendance allowance, mobility allowance (under revision) or special disablement allowance. Valid for a year, it provides fare reductions. Further details are found in the leaflets *Disabled Person's Railcard* and *BR and Disabled Travellers*.

Travel abroad

1 People with epilepsy intending to travel, particularly abroad, require adequate medical cover, including a 24-hour emergency service.

2 Most standard travel insurance policies do not cover claims arising from a pre-existing condition.

3 Special travel policies exist, but many would not cover people with active epilepsy, as they exclude

those who are under out-patient care at a hospital or clinic, or who have received medical treatment in a variable time period before the journey (3–12 months). One policy which provides travel insurance extended to cover people with epilepsy demands a medical report supporting fitness to travel, excludes claims arising from swimming and requires the patient to carry an adequate supply of medication. All policies significantly restrict the total medical expenses claim they will allow, and charge additional premiums.

Services for people with epilepsy

Service provision

The DHSS (1986) recommends that all patients with seizures should be referred for 'diagnosis, initial assessment and recommendation for management' to a neurologist or other consultant with a special interest in epilepsy. Children should be seen by a paediatric neurologist or paediatrician (DHSS, 1986).

The accessibility of consultant referrals is limited by the low ratio of experienced clinicians to population. In the UK there is estimated to be one full-time consultant neurologist per 373 000 persons, one consultant paediatrician per 14 000 children and one paediatric neurologist per 738 000 children (DHSS Medical Manpower and Education Division, 1988; OPCS, 1990). These shortfalls mean that many people with epilepsy are assessed by general physicians and geriatricians, not all of whom have a special interest or expertise in epilepsy.

After initial assessment and recommendation for management, patients who have good seizure control can be managed by their general practitioners. While this applies to 70–80% of people developing epilepsy, the remainder pose greater problems. This includes patients with intractable epilepsy, resistant to medical treatment. Some may have associated disabling conditions, leading to complex disability and handicap.

Such patients require co-ordinated input from a number of sources, ranging from neurosurgery to neuropsychology. Unfortunately, the accessibility is again limited. There is one neurosurgeon per 512 000 population (DHSS Medical Manpower and Education Division, 1988; OPCS, 1990), only a

minority of whom perform surgery for relief of epilepsy (Hart & Shorvon, 1990). There are approximately 50–60 clinical neuropsychologists in the UK.

The DHSS (1986) recommend that the facilities available for the investigation of epilepsy should include routine EEG, CT, MRI, routine X-ray, electrocardiography, serum drug level monitoring, haematology and clinical chemistry services. Access to such services is far from uniform (Langton Hewer & Wood, 1990).

Assessment of patients with epilepsy resistant to medical treatment, who may have underlying structural disease or whom may benefit from surgery, requires more sophisticated investigations. These include ambulatory and invasive EEG monitoring, clinical neurophysiology, neuropsychology, cerebral angiography and neuropathology, and are available only in specialist centres.

The lack of qualified and experienced professionals and of appropriate facilities means that few patients with epilepsy can be offered the full range of services which may benefit them.

Epilepsy clinics

The management of patients with seizures continuing despite drug treatment merits a dedicated specialist clinic. A number of government-sponsored reports supported the concept of such clinics, to be run in close association with a neurology department. The Reid report recommended that such clinics take a multidisciplinary approach (Central Health Services Council, 1969), but there has been some resistance to this being necessary for all patients (Morgan & Kurtz, 1987), and the DHSS report concluded that the majority of patients can be managed by a neurologist or other specialist (DHSS, 1986). A minority will have multiple problems – physical disability, mental handicap, psychiatric or learning difficulties – in conjunction with epilepsy, and for these patients a multidisciplinary approach is imperative. The concentration of limited experience and equipment means that such clinics are likely to be organized at regional specialist centres.

The benefits of epilepsy clinics were shown by a prospective randomized study comparing care in a neurology clinic and in an epilepsy clinic. Patients attending the epilepsy clinic had fewer drug side-effects, and were better informed and more satisfied (Morrow, 1990). Audit of an epilepsy clinic showed that the proportion of patients on monotherapy increased and a third of referrals had >50% reduction of seizure frequency following attendance (Crawford & Wilson, 1990).

Assessment centres

There are four epilepsy centres which provide detailed medical evaluation, including psychosocial assessment, rehabilitation, research and teaching. Currently, the number of specialist centre places is less than 60 for adults and 30 for children. The DHSS (1986) suggested an expansion of such facilities and recommended that the funding should be on a supraregional level direct from the DHSS. The emphasis of care has shifted from residential placement to rehabilitation and return to the community.

Residential care

The provision of residential places for people with epilepsy has fallen, with improved medical management and a move from institutionally based to community care. However, a minority of people with intractable epilepsy and other difficulties, such as physical or psychological disability, may be very difficult to maintain in a community setting. After detailed evaluation, including assessment of the domestic circumstances, some form of residential care may be felt to offer a more supportive environment.

In the UK there are five centres providing long-term residential care. Collectively, these institutions account for about 1000 beds. In addition, about 30% of people with mental handicap who live in institutions have epilepsy.

Voluntary agencies

Voluntary agencies serve several important functions for people with chronic conditions: support and counselling groups for patients and relatives, formation of pressure groups to lobby for improved services, fund-raising for research, and education of patients, professionals and the public. Their role is particularly important for chronic conditions such as epilepsy, where patients may feel socially isolated and have wider needs than conventional medical care can address (Keller, 1990).

In the UK, the National Society for Epilepsy and the British Epilepsy Association produce health education material and assist local support groups. Counselling is also provided by societies in Merseyside, Wales and Scotland (see Appendix). Government reports have recommended close liaison between such local agencies and the medical profession, who might work together in settings such as epilepsy clinics.

Appendix

Assessment centres for epilepsy (UK)

Bootham Park Hospital
Bootham
York YO3 7BY
Tel: 0904 54664

National Society for Epilepsy
Chalfont Centre for Epilepsy
Chalfont St Peter
Buckinghamshire SL9 0RJ
Tel: 024 07 3991

David Lewis Centre*
Alderley Edge
Mobberley
Cheshire SK9 7 UD
Tel: 056 587 2613

Maudsley Hospital – Epilepsy Unit*
Denmark Hill
London SE5 8AZ
Tel: 071 703 6333

National voluntary organizations (UK)

British Epilepsy Association
Anstey House
40 Hanover Square
Leeds LS3 1BE

*Not designated special assessment centres, but provide an assessment facility for people with epilepsy.

For membership enquiries
Tel: 0532 439393
For general information
Tel: 0345 089599
Regional offices:
London Tel: 071 929 4069
Belfast Tel: 0232 248414

Epilepsy Association of Scotland (Glasgow)
48 Gowan Road
Glasgow G5 11JR
Tel: 041 427 4911

Epilepsy Association for Scotland (Edinburgh)
13 Guthrie Street
Edinburgh EH1 1JG
Tel: 031 226 5458

Irish Epilepsy Association
249 Crumlin Road
Dublin W12
Tel: 01 557500

Mersey Regional Epilepsy Association
Walton Hospital
Liverpool, L9 1AE
Tel: 051 525 3069

References

Adams C.B.T. (1983) Hemispherectomy – a modification. *Journal of Neurology, Neurosurgery and Psychiatry* **46**, 617.

Aldenkamp A.P. (1987) Learning disabilities in children with epilepsy. In Aldenkamp A.P., Alpherts W.C.J., Meinardi H. & Stores G. (eds) *Education and Epilepsy*, pp. 21–37. Swets and Zeitlinger, Lisse.

Annegers J.F., Hauser W.A. & Elverback L.R. (1979) Remission of seizures and relapse in patients with epilepsy. *Epilepsia* **20**, 729.

Annegers J.F., Grabow J.D., Groover R.V. *et al.* (1980) Seizures after head trauma: a population study. *Neurology* **30**, 683.

Annegers J.F., Hauser W.A. & Shirts S.B. (1984) Heart disease mortality and morbidity in patients with epilepsy. *Epilepsia* **25**, 699.

Annegers J.F., Hauser W.A., Beghi E. *et al.* (1988) The risk of unprovoked seizures after encephalitis and meningitis. *Neurology* **38**, 1407.

Appleton R., Baker G.A., Chadwick D. & Smith D. (1991) *Epilepsy*. Martin Dunitz, London.

Babb T.L. & Brown W.J. (1987) Pathological findings in epilepsy. In Engel J., Jr (ed.) *Surgical Treatment of the Epilepsies*, pp. 511–540. Raven Press, New York.

Barraclough B. (1981) Suicide and epilepsy. In Reynolds E. & Trimble M. (eds) *Epilepsy and Psychiatry*, pp. 72–76. Churchill Livingstone, Edinburgh.

Betts T.A. (1981) Depression, anxiety and epilepsy. In Reynolds E.H. & Trimble M.R. (eds) *Epilepsy and Psychiatry*, pp. 60–71. Churchill Livingstone, Edinburgh.

Betts T.A. (1988) People with epilepsy as parents. In Hoare P. (ed.) *Epilepsy and the Family*, pp. 49–52. C.C. Williams, Manchester.

Bhatnagar S.K., Srivastava J.L. & Gupta J.L. (1977) Burns: a complication of epilepsy. *Burns* **3**, 93–95.

Blomquist H.K., Gustavson K.H. & Holmgren G. (1981) Mild mental retardation in children in a northern Swedish county. *Journal of Mental Deficiency Research* **25**, 169.

Britten N., Morgan K., Fenwick P.B.C. & Britten H. (1986) Epilepsy and handicap from birth to age thirty-six. *Developmental Medicine and Child Neurology* **28**, 719–728.

Bruens J.H. (1974) Psychoses in epilepsy. In Vinken P.L. & Bruyn L.W. (eds) *Handbook of Clinical Neurology*, Vol. 15, pp. 593–610. North Holland, Amsterdam.

Burn J.P.S., Sandercock P.A.G., Bamford J. *et al.* (1990) The incidence of epileptic seizures after a first ever stroke. *Journal of Neurology, Neurosurgery and Psychiatry* **53**, 810.

Cabral R.J., King T.T. & Scott D.F. (1976) Epilepsy after two different neurological approaches to the treatment of ruptured intracranial aneurysm. *Journal of Neurology, Neurosurgery and Psychiatry* **39**, 1052.

Callaghan N., O'Hare J., O'Driscol D. *et al.* (1982) Comparative study of ethosuximide and sodium valproate in the treatment of typical absence seizures (petit mal). *Developmental Medicine and Child Neurology* **24**, 830.

Cast I.P. & Wilson P.J.E. (1981) Pituitary tumours. *Journal of Neurology, Neurosurgery and Psychiatry* **44**, 371.

Central Health Services Council (1969) *People with Epilepsy: Report of a Joint Sub-committee of the Standing Medical Advisory Committee and the Advisory Committee of the Health and Welfare of Handicapped Persons.* HMSO, London.

Chadwick D. & Turnbull D.M. (1985) The comparative efficacy of antiepileptic drugs for partial and tonic–clonic seizures. *Journal of Neurology, Neurosurgery and Psychiatry* **48**, 1073–1077.

Chadwick D., Reynolds E.H. & Marsden C.D. (1976) Anticonvulsant-induced dyskinesias: a comparison with dyskinesias induced by neuroleptics. *Journal of Neurology, Neurosurgery and Psychiatry* **39**, 1210.

Chadwick D., Shaw M.D.M., Foy P. *et al.* (1984) Serum anticonvulsant concentrations and the risk of drug induced skin eruptions. *Journal of Neurology, Neurosurgery and Psychiatry* **47**, 642.

Chaplin J.E., Yepez Lasso R., Shorvon S.D. & Floyd M. (1992) National general practice study of epilepsy: the social and psychological effects of a recent diagnosis of epilepsy. *British Medical Journal* **304**, 1416–1418.

Clement M.J. & Wallace S.J. (1990) A survey of adolescents with epilepsy. *Developmental Medicine and Child Neurology* **32**, 849–857.

Cocito L., Favle E. & Reni L. (1982) Epileptic seizures in cerebral arterial occlusive disease. *Stroke* **13**, 189.

Commission on Classification and Terminology of the International League Against Epilepsy (1989) Proposal for revised classification of epilepsies and epileptic syndromes. *Epilepsia* **30**, 389–399.

Copeland G.P., Foy P. & Shaw M.D.M. (1982) The incidence of epilepsy after ventricular shunting operations. *Surgical Neurology* **17**, 279.

Crandall P.H. (1987) Cortical resections. In Engel J. (ed.) *Surgical Treatment of Epilepsies*, p. 377. Raven, New York.

Crawford P. & Wilson S. (1990) Epilepsy clinics: do they improve epilepsy management? *Acta Neurologica Scandinavica* **82** (Suppl. 133), 32.

Crawford P.M. & Chadwick D. (1986) A comparative study of progabide, valproate, and placebo as add-on therapy in patients with refractory epilepsy. *Journal of Neurology, Neurosurgery and Psychiatry* **49**, 1251.

Crawford P.M., West C.R., Chadwick D.W. & Shaw M.D.M. (1986) Cerebral arteriovenous malformations and epilepsy: factors in the development of epilepsy. *Epilepsia* **27**, 270.

Cull C.A. & Trimble M.R. (1989) Effects of anticonvulsant medications on cognitive functioning in children with epilepsy. In Hermann B. & Seidenberg M. (eds) *Childhood Epilepsies: Neuropsychological, Psychosocial and Intervention Aspects*, pp. 83–103. John Wiley, Chichester.

Currie S., Heathfield K.W.G., Henson R.A. & Scott D.F. (1971) Clinical course and prognosis of temporal lobe epilepsy: a survey of 666 patients. *Brain* **94**, 173–190.

Delgado-Escueta A.V. & Enrile-Bacsal F. (1984) Juvenile myoclonic epilepsy of Janz. *Neurology* **34**, 285–294.

Department of Health and Social Security (DHSS) (1986) *Report of the Working Group on Services for People with Epilepsy: a Report to the Department of Health and Social Security, the Department of Education and Science and the Welsh Office.* HMSO, London.

Department of Health and Social Security (DHSS) Medical Manpower and Education Division (1988) *Health Trends* **20**, 101–109.

Dodrill C.B., Batzel L., Queisser H.R. & Temkin N.R. (1980) An objective method for the assessment of psychological and social problems among epileptics. *Epilepsia* **21**, 123–135.

Dreifuss F.E. (1987) Goals of surgery for epilepsy. In Engel J. (ed.) *Surgical Treatment of the Epilepsies*, p. 31. Raven Press, New York.

Dreifuss F.E., Santilli N., Langer D.H. *et al.* (1987) Valproic acid fatalities: a retrospective review. *Neurology* **37**, 379.

Duncan J.S. & Sagar H.J. (1987) Characteristics, pathology and outcome after temporal lobectomy. *Neurology* **37**, 405.

Edebol-Tysk K. (1989) Epidemiology of spastic tetraplegic cerebral palsy in Sweden. I. Impairments and disabilities. *Neuropediatrics* **20**, 41.

Edeh J. & Toone B. (1987) Relationship between interictal psychopathology and type of epilepsy: results of a survey in general practice. *British Journal of Psychiatry* **151**, 95–101.

Elwes R.D.C., Marshal J., Beattie A. & Newman P.K. (1991) Epilepsy and employment. A community based survey in an area of high unemployment. *Journal of Neurology, Neurosurgery and Psychiatry* **54**, 200–203.

Engel J. (1987) Outcome with respect to epileptic seizures. In Engel J. (ed.) *Surgical Treatment of the Epilepsies*, p. 553. Raven Press, New York.

Engel J., Kuhl D.E., Phelps M.E. & Crandall P.H. (1982) Comparative localization of epileptic foci in partial epilepsy by PET and EEG. *Annals of Neurology* **12**, 529.

Falconer M.A. (1971) Genetic and related aetiological factors in temporal lobe epilepsy: a review. *Epilepsia* **12**, 13.

Falconer M.A., Hill D., Meyer A. *et al.* (1955) Treatment of temporal-lobe epilepsy by temporal lobectomy: a survey of findings and results. *Lancet* **i**, 827.

Fenton G. (1983) Epilepsy. In Lader M. (ed.) *Handbook of Psychiatry 2: Mental Disorder and Somatic Illness.* Cambridge University Press, Cambridge.

Fish D. (1989) CT and PET in drug-resistant epilepsy. In Trimble M.R. (ed.) *Chronic Epilepsy, Its Progress and Management*, p. 59. Wiley, Chichester.

Floyd M. (1986) A review of published studies on epilepsy and employment. In Edwards F., Espir M.L.E. & Oxley J. (eds) *Epilepsy and Employment – a Medical Symposium on Current Problems and Best Practices*, pp. 3–8. ICSS no. 86. Royal Society of Medicine, London.

Forsgren L., Edvinsson S.-O., Blomquist H.K. *et al.* (1990) Epilepsy in a population of mentally retarded children and adults. *Epilepsy Research* **6**, 234.

Foy P.M., Copeland G.P. & Shaw M.D.M. (1981a) The incidence of postoperative seizures. *Acta Neurochirurgica* **55**, 253.

Foy P.M., Copeland G.P. & Shaw M.D.M. (1981b) The natural history of postoperative seizures. *Acta Neurochirurgica* **57**, 15.

Foy P.M., Chadwick D.W., Rajgopalan N. *et al.* (1992) Do prophylactic anticonvulsant drugs alter the pattern of seizures following craniotomy? *Journal of Neurology, Neurosurgery and Psychiatry* **55**(9), 753–757.

Fraser R.T. & Clemmons D.C. (1989) Vocational and psychosocial interventions for youths with seizure disorders. In Hermann B. & Seidenberg M. (eds) *Childhood Epilepsies: Neuropsychological, Psychosocial and Intervention Aspects*, pp. 201–219. John Wiley, Chichester.

Garber J. & Seligman M. (eds) (1980) *Human Helplessness: Theory and Applications.* Academic Press, New York.

Gastaut H. & Gastaut J.L. (1976) Computerised transverse axial tomography in epilepsy. *Epilepsia* **17**, 325–331.

Goodridge D.M.G. & Shorvon S.D. (1983) Epileptic seiz-ures in a population of 6000. II: treatment and prog-nosis: *British Medical Journal* **287**, 645–647.

Gudmundson G. (1966) Epilepsy in Iceland. *Epilepsia* **43** (Suppl. 25), 1–124.

Gustavson K.H., Holmgren G., Jonsell R. & Blomquist H.K. (1977) Severe mental retardation in children in a northern Swedish county. *Journal of Mental Deficiency Research* **21**, 161.

Hahn J.F. & Luders H. (1987) Placement of subdural grid electrodes at the Cleveland Clinic. In Engel J. (ed.) *Surgical Treatment of the Epilepsies*, p. 621. Raven, New York.

Hampton K.K., Peatfield R.C., Pullar T., Bodansky H.J., Walton C. & Feely M. (1988) Burns because of epilepsy. *British Medical Journal* **296**, 1659–1660.

Hart Y.M. & Shorvon S. (1990) Surgery for epilepsy in the United Kingdom. *Acta Neurologica Scandinavica* **82** (Suppl. 133), 21.

Hauser W.A. & Hesdorffer D.C. (1990) *Epilepsy: Frequency, Causes and Consequences*. Demos Publications, New York.

Hauser W.A. & Kurland L.T. (1975) The epidemiology of epilepsy in Rochester, Minnesota, 1935 through 1967. *Epilepsia* **16**, 1.

Hauser W.A., Annegers J.F. & Elveback L.R. (1980) Mor-tality in patients with epilepsy. *Epilepsia* **21**, 339.

Hauser W.A., Anderson V.E., Loewenston R.B. & McRo-berts S.M. (1982) Seizure recurrence after a first un-provoked seizure. *New England Journal of Medicine* **307**, 522.

Hauser W.A., Rich S.S., Jacobs M.P. & Anderson V.E. (1983) Patterns of seizure occurrence and recurrent risks in patients with newly diagnosed epilepsy. *Abstracts of the 15th Epilepsy International Symposium*, p. 16. American Epilepsy Society, Hartford, Connecticut.

Hauser W.A., Morris M.L., Heston L.L. & Anderson V.E. (1986) Seizures and myoclonus in patients with Alzheimer's disease. *Neurology* **36**, 1226.

Hauser W.A., Shinnar S., Cohen H. *et al.* (1987) Clinical predictors of epilepsy among children with cerebral palsy and/or mental retardation. *Neurology* **37** (Suppl. 1), 150.

Hermann B.P., Whitman S., Wyler A., Anton M. & Van-derzwagg R. (1990) Psychosocial predictors of psycho-pathology in epilepsy. *British Journal of Psychiatry* **156**, 98–105.

Hoare P. (1984) Does illness foster dependency? A study of epileptic and diabetic children. *Development and Medical Child Neurology* **26**, 20–24.

Hoare P. (1988) The development of psychiatric disorders among school children with epilepsy. *Developmental Medicine and Child Neurology* **26**, 3–13.

Jacob H. (1970) Muscular twitchings in Alzheimer's dis-ease. In Wolsteholme G.E.W. & O'Connor M. (eds) *Alzheimer's Disease and Related Conditions*, p. 75. J & A Churchill, London.

Jacoby A., Johnson A.L. & Chadwick D. (1992) The psychosocial outcomes of antiepileptic drug withdrawal. *Epilepsia* **33**, 1123–1131.

Jennett W.B. (1975) *Epilepsy After Non-missile Head Injuries*, 2nd edn. Heinemann Medical Books, London.

Juul-Jensen P. (1964) Epilepsy: a clinical and social analysis of 1020 adult patients with epileptic seizures. *Acta Neurologica Scandinavica* **40** (Suppl. 5), 1.

Kato H., Mori T., Moriuchi T. & Kaiyak K. (1979) Psy-chosocial aspects of schoolchildren with epilepsy: schoolchildren who fell into school phobia. *Folia Psy-chiatrica and Neurologica Japonica* **33**, 437–439.

Keller D.J. (1990) Do self-help groups help? *International Disability Studies* **12**, 66–69.

Kinnunen E. & Wikstrom J. (1986) Prevalence and prog-nosis of epilepsy in patients with multiple sclerosis. *Epilepsia* **27**, 729.

Kiorobe E. (1961) The prognosis of epilepsy. *Acta Psy-chiatrica Scandinavica* **36** (Suppl. 150), 166.

Laaksonen R. (1983) The patient with recently diagnosed epilepsy psychological and sociological aspects. *Acta Neurologica Scandinavica* **67** (Suppl. 93), 52–59.

Langton Hewer R. & Wood V.A. (1990) *Neurology Services in the United Kingdom. A Report of the Association of British Neurologists*. Association of British Neurologists, London.

Lechtenberg R. (1984) *Epilepsy and the Family*. Harvard University Press, Cambridge, Mass.

Leestma J.E., Kalelkar M.B., Teas S.S. *et al.* (1984) Sudden unexpected death associated with seizures: analysis of 66 cases. *Epilepsia* **25**, 84.

Legg N.J., Gupta P.C. & Scott D.F. (1973) Epilepsy fol-lowing cerebral abscess: a clinical and EEG study of 70 patients. *Brain* **96**, 259.

Lesser R.P., Luders H., Dinner D.S. & Morris H.H. (1985) Epileptic seizures due to thrombotic and embolic cere-brovascular disease in older patients. *Epilepsia* **26**, 622.

Lindhout D. & Schmidt D. (1986) In-utero exposure to valproate and neural tube defects. *Lancet* **i**, 1392–1393.

Loiseau J., Loiseau P., Duche B. *et al.* (1990) A survey of epileptic disorders in southwest France: seizures in elderly patients. *Annals of Neurology* **27**, 232.

McQueen J.K., Blackwood D.H., Harris P. *et al.* (1983) Low risk of late post-traumatic seizures following severe head injury: implications for clinical trials of prophy-laxis. *Journal of Neurology, Neurosurgery and Psychiatry* **46**, 899.

Maisels D.O. & Corps B.V.M. (1964) Burned epileptics. *Lancet* **i**, 1298–1301.

Masland R.L. (1988) Psychosocial aspects of epilepsy. In Porter E.J. & Morselli P.L. (eds) *The Epilepsies*, pp. 356–377. Butterworths, London.

Mattson R.H., Cramer J.A., Collins J.F. *et al.* (1985) Comparison of carbamazepine, phenobarbital, pheny-toin and primidone in partial and secondary generalised tonic–clonic seizures. *New England Journal of Medicine* **313**, 145–151.

Mauguiere F. & Courjon J. (1978) Somatosensory epilepsy: a review of 127 cases. *Brain* **101**, 307.

Meldrum B.S., Horton R.W. & Brierley J.B. (1974) Epileptic brain damage in adolescent baboons following seizures induced by allylglycine. *Brain* **97**, 407.

Mittan R. & Locke G. (1982) Fear of seizures: epilepsy's forgotten problem. *Urban Health* Jan./Feb. 40–41.

Morgan J.D. & Kurtz Z. (1987) *Special Services for People with Epilepsy in the 1970s*. HMSO, London.

Morrow J. (1990) An assessment of an epilepsy clinic. In Chadwick D.W. (ed.) *Quality of Life and Quality of Care in Epilepsy*, pp. 96–105. Royal Society of Medicine, London.

Muller R. (1949) Studies on disseminated sclerosis with special reference to symptomatology, course and prognosis. *Acta Medica Scandinavica* **133** (Suppl. 222), 1.

Nelson K.B. & Ellenberg J.H. (1978) Prognosis in children with febrile seizures. *Paediatrics* **61**, 720.

Nelson K.B. & Ellenberg J.H. (1986) Antecedents of cerebral palsy, multivariate analysis of risk. *New England Journal of Medicine* **315**, 81.

Neuspiel D.R. & Kuller L.H. (1985) Sudden and unexpected natural death in childhood and adolescence. *Journal of American Medical Association* **254**, 1321.

North J.B., Penhall R.K., Hanieh A. *et al.* (1983) Phenytoin and postoperative epilepsy: a double blind study. *Journal of Neurosurgery* **58**, 672.

Office of Population Censuses and Surveys (OPCS) (1990) *Population Trends* **62**, 2.

Oppenheimer H.B. (1966) Persistent intracranial bleeding as a complication of hemispherectomy. *Journal of Neurology, Neurosurgery and Psychiatry* **29**, 229.

Oxbury J.M. & Adams C.B.T. (1989) Neurosurgery for epilepsy. *British Journal of Hospital Medicine* **41**, 372.

Parsonage M. (1992) *Epilepsy and Driving Licence Regulation*. Report by the ILEA/IBE Commission on Drivers' Licensing.

Penfield W. & Jasper H. (1954) *Epilepsy and the Functional Anatomy of the Human Brain*. Little, Brown, Boston.

Perez M.M. & Trimble M.R. (1980) Epileptic psychosis — diagnostic comparison with process schizophrenia. *British Journal of Psychiatry* **137**, 245–249.

Perez M.M., Trimble M.R., Murray N.M.S. & Reider I. (1985) Epileptic psychosis: an evaluation of PSE profiles. *British Journal of Psychiatry* **146**, 155–164.

Polkey C.E. (1987) Anterior temporal lobectomy at the Maudsley Hospital, London. In Engel J. (ed.) *Surgical Treatment of the Epilepsies*, p. 641. Raven, New York.

Pond D.A. & Bidwell B.H. (1959) A survey of epilepsy in fourteen general practices. *Epilepsia* **1**, 285–299.

Porter R.J. (1984) Epilepsy: 100 elementary principles. In Walton J.N. (ed.) *Major Problems in Neurology*, Vol. 12. W.B. Saunders, London.

Quesney L.F. (1986) Seizures of frontal lobe origin. In Pedley T.A. & Meldrum B.S. (eds) *Recent Advances in Epilepsy*, Vol. 3, p. 81. Churchill-Livingstone, Edinburgh.

Radley R. (1987) The educational needs of children with epilepsy. In Oxley J. & Stores G. (eds) *Epilepsy and Education*, pp. 9–14. Medical Tribune Group.

Rasmussen T., Olszewski J. & Lloyd-Smith D. (1958) Focal seizures due to localized chronic encephalitis. *Neurology* **8**, 435.

Raynor R.B., Paine R.S. & Carmichael E.A. (1959) Epilepsy of late onset. *Neurology* **9**, 111.

Reynolds E.H. (1975) Chronic antiepileptic toxicity: a review. *Epilepsia* **16**, 319.

Reynolds E.H. (1987) Early treatment and prognosis of epilepsy. *Epilepsia* **28**, 97.

Reynolds N.C. & Miska R.M. (1981) Safety of anticonvulsants in hepatic porphyrias. *Neurology* **31**, 480.

Rocca W.A., Sharbrough F.W., Hauser W.A. *et al.* (1987) Risk factors for complex partial seizures: a population-based case-control study. *Annals of Neurology* **21**, 22.

Rodin E.A. (1968) *The Prognosis of Patients with Epilepsy*. Charles C. Thomas, Springfield, Illinois.

Rogan P.J. (1992) *Epilepsy: a Teacher's Handbook*. Roby Education Ltd., Merseyside.

Romanelli M.F., Morris J.C., Ashkin K. & Coben L.A. (1990) Advanced Alzheimer's disease is a risk factor for late-onset seizures. *Archives of Neurology* **47**, 847.

Rosa F.H. (1990) Spina bifida in maternal carbamazepine exposure cohort data. *Teratology* **41**, 587.

Rusell-Jones D.L. & Shorvon S.D. (1989) The frequency and consequences of head injury in epileptic seizures. *Journal of Neurology, Neurosurgery and Psychiatry* **52**, 659–662.

Salazar A.M., Jabbari B., Vance S.C. *et al.* (1985) Epilepsy after penetrating head injury. I. Clinical correlates. *Neurology* **35**, 1406.

Sander J.W.A.S. & Shorvon S.D. (1987) Incidence and prevalence studies in epilepsy and their methodological problems: a review. *Journal of Neurology, Neurosurgery and Psychiatry* **50**, 829.

Sander J.W.A.S., Hart Y.M., Johnson A.L. & Shorvon S.D. (1990) National General Practice Study of Epilepsy: newly diagnosed epileptic seizures in a general population. *Lancet* **336**, 1267.

Satishchandra P., Chandra V. & Schoenberg B.S. (1988) Case-control study of associated conditions at the time of death in patients with epilepsy. *Neuroepidemiology* **7**, 109.

Scambler G. (1987) Sociological aspects of epilepsy. In Hopkins A. (ed.) *Epilepsy*, pp. 497–510. Chapman and Hall, London.

Scambler G. (1989) *Epilepsy*. Tavistock, London.

Scambler G. (1992) Coping with epilepsy. In Laidlaw J., Richens A. & Chadwick D.W. (eds) *A Textbook of Epilepsy*, 4th edn. Churchill Livingstone, Edinburgh, New York.

Scambler G. & Hopkins A. (1980) Social class, epileptic activity and disadvantage at work. *Journal of Epidemiology and Community Health* **34** (2), 129–133.

Schmidt D. (1982a) *Adverse Effects of Antiepileptic Drugs*.

Raven Press, New York.

Schmidt D. (1982b) Two antiepileptic drugs for intractable epilepsy with complex-partial seizures. *Journal of Neurology, Neurosurgery and Psychiatry* **45**, 1119.

Schneider J. & Conrad P. (1983) *Having Epilepsy: the Experience and Control of Illness*. Temple University Press, Philadelphia.

Shafer S.Q., Hauser W.A., Annegers J.F. & Klass D.W. (1988) EEG and other early predictors of epilepsy remission: a community study. *Epilepsia* **29**, 590.

Shinton R.A., Zezulka A.V., Gill J.S. & Beevers D.G. (1987) The frequency of epilepsy preceding stroke. *Lancet* **i**, 11.

Shorvon S.D., Gilliat R.W., Cox T.C.S. & Yu Y.L. (1984) Evidence of vascular disease from CT scanning in late onset epilepsy. *Journal of Neurology, Neurosurgery and Psychiatry* **47**, 225.

Slater E., Beard A.W. & Glithero E. (1963) The schizophrenia-like psychoses of epilepsy. *British Journal of Psychiatry* **109**, 95−150.

Smith D.F., Hutton J.L., Sandemann P.M. *et al.* (1992) The prognosis of primary intracerebral tumours presenting with epilepsy: the outcome of medical and surgical management. *Journal of Neurology, Neurosurgery and Psychiatry* **54**, 915−920.

Sofijanov N.G. (1982) Clinical evolution and prognosis of childhood epilepsies. *Epilepsia* **23**, 61.

Spencer S.S., Gates J.R., Reeves A.R. *et al.* (1987) Corpus callosum section. In Engel J. (ed.) *Surgical Treatment of the Epilepsies*, p. 425. Raven, New York.

Spitz M.C. (1992) Severe burns as a consequence of seizures in patients with epilepsy. *Epilepsia* **33**, 103−107.

Storey P.B. (1967) Psychiatric sequelae of subarachnoid haemorrhage. *British Medical Journal* **3**, 261−266.

Sumi S.M. & Teasdall R.D. (1963) Focal seizures: a review of 150 cases. *Neurology* **13**, 582.

Suzuki M., Maruyama H., Ishibashi Y. *et al.* (1972) *A Double-blind Comparative Trial of Sodium Dipropylacetate and Ethosuximide in Epilepsy in Children with Special Emphasis on Pure Petit Mal Seizures* (Japanese). *Medical Progress* **82**, 470−488.

Taylor D. (1989) Psychosocial components of childhood epilepsy. In Hermann B. & Seidenberg M. (eds) *Childhood Epilepsies: Neuropsychological, Psychosocial and Inter-vention Aspects*, pp. 119−142. John Wiley, Chichester.

Temkin N.R., Dikmen S.S., Wilensky A.J. *et al.* (1990) A randomized, double-blind study of phenytoin for the prevention of post-traumatic seizures. *New England Journal of Medicine* **323**, 497.

Tempest M. (1970) Burns and epileptic patients: a survey of admissions to original burns centre over a period of 20 years. In Malles P., Barkely T.L. & Konckova Z. (eds) *Research in Burns: Transaction of Third International Conference on Research in Burns*, pp. 54−57. Hans Huber, Berne.

Thompson P. & Oxley J. (1993) Social aspects of epilepsy. In Laidlow J., Richens A. & Chadwick D. (eds) *A Textbook of Epilepsy*, pp. 661−704. Churchill Livingstone, Edinburgh.

Thompson P.J. & Shorvon S.D. (1991) The epilepsies. In Greenwood R.J., Barnes M.P., McMillan T.M. & Ward C.D. (eds) *Neurological Rehabilitation*. Churchill Livingstone, Edinburgh.

Toone B. (1986) Epilepsy with mental illness: interrelationships. In Trimble M.R. & Reynolds E.H. (eds) *What is Epilepsy? The Clinical and Scientific Basis of Epilepsy*. Churchill Livingstone, Edinburgh.

Turnbull D.M., Rawlins M.D., Weightman D. & Chadwick D.W. (1983) Plasma concentrations of sodium valproate: their clinical value. *Annals of Neurology* **14**, 38.

Turnbull D.M., Howell D., Rawlins M.D. & Chadwick D. (1985) Which drug for the adult epileptic patient: phenytoin or valproate? *British Medical Journal* **290**, 815−819.

Walker A.E. & Erculei F. (1968) *Head-injured Men 15 Years Later*. Charles C. Thomas, Springfield Illinois.

Wieser H.G., Elger C.E. & Stodieck S.R.G. (1985) The 'foramen ovale electrode': a new recording method for the preoperative evaluation of patients suffering from mediobasal temporal lobe epilepsy. *Electroencephalography and Clinical Neurophysiology* **61**, 314−322.

Yasargil M.G. & Wieser H.G. (1987) Selective amygdalo-hippocampectomy at the University Hospital, Zurich. In Engel J. (ed.) *Surgical Treatment of the Epilepsies*, p. 653. Raven, New York.

Zielinski J.J. (1974) *Epidemiology and Medicosocial Problems of Epilepsy in Warsaw*. Final report on research program No. 19-P-58325-F-01. Psychoneurological Institute, Warsaw.

16: The Rehabilitation of Multiple Sclerosis

L.C. SCHEINBERG AND C.R. SMITH

The disease, 212
Evaluating the patient, 212
Symptoms of multiple sclerosis, 213
Primary symptoms and treatment, 213
   Gait disturbance, 213
   Bladder, bowel and sexual dysfunction, 216
   Upper extremity involvement, 217
   Fatigue, 217
   Dysarthria, 218
   Dysphagia, 218
Secondary symptoms and treatment, 218
   Decubitus ulcers, 218
   Fibrous contractures, 219
Tertiary symptoms and treatment, 219
Conclusion, 219

The disease

Multiple sclerosis is a chronic disease of the central nervous system in which the myelin is damaged for unknown reasons and the axons are relatively spared. The aetiology and pathogenesis are unknown, although a combination of viral and autoimmune factors are suspected. Clinically, it is often manifested as an unpredictable gait disorder due to ataxia, paresis and/or spasticity associated with fatigue, urinary, bowel, sexual and sensory findings. The usual onset is in the second or third decade of life, with a predilection to affect women. The course varies from benign, with a few sensory findings and minimal disabilities after many years, to unfavourable, with serious disabilities from motor impairments in a short period after onset. Among all disabilities at all ages, it ranks first as the one requiring the patient to seek help for basic life activities; after trauma and rheumatological disorders, it is the next leading cause of severe disability.

Because of its tendency to produce motor findings, e.g. weakness, incoordination, spasticity and bladder and bowel dysfunction, and the failure of any pharmacological intervention to modify its course, it is a major challenge to the field of rehabilitation.

Evaluating the patient

When first seen, the average patient is often young and sometimes frightened by the diagnosis.

The initial evaluation of the patient includes a complete history of the illness, with the demographic, occupational, social and psychological aspects meticulously detailed. The *Minimal Record of Disability for Multiple Sclerosis* (MRD), developed by the International Federation of Multiple Sclerosis Societies (1985), is an excellent guide for the clinical evaluation of patients with multiple sclerosis (see Appendices). The impairment portion is based on the Kurtzke disability status scale (Kurtzke *et al.,* 1977), which evaluates the patient in a number of functional systems: pyramidal, cerebellar, brain stem, sensory, bowel and bladder, visual and cerebral (or mental). The scale ranges from 0 = normal to 5 = severe loss of this function. Coupled with a scale heavily weighted for ambulation, wherein, for example, 0 represents normal neurological examination and 1.5 represents normal functions but the presence of certain signs, e.g. Babinski or vibratory decrease; 6.0 represents unilateral assistance (cane, crutch or brace); 7.5 essentially represents restricted to wheelchair but able to enter and leave chair alone; 9.0 represents the bedbound patient but able to communicate and eat and 10 represents death due to multiple sclerosis; this enables the examiner to give an expanded disability status scale score (EDSS) (Kurtzke, 1983). It allows the examiner to designate a single EDSS score to each patient and follow his/her course in therapy or clinical trials.

One should attempt to evaluate the patient's disabilities using the activities of daily living methods and scales of the occupational therapist. The MRD has this in a reasonably quantitative manner. The handicap scale is less objective but important.

In the initial evaluation of the patient, the physician should attempt to determine the major problems as the patient sees them and tailor the therapy to these problems initially. For the sake of gaining the patient's confidence, it is always useful to begin with a problem in which the outcome is favourable, e.g. spasticity, urinary findings or fatigue, and not to begin with a more hopeless situation, such as ataxic gait or advanced cognitive changes.

Symptoms of multiple sclerosis

The symptoms of multiple sclerosis can be conveniently categorized as primary, secondary or tertiary. *Primary* symptoms reflect the strategic effects of a discrete plaque of demyelination on neurological function, e.g. monocular visual loss due to optic neuritis, incontinence of urine due to myelopathy, and intention tremor due to demyelination of the cerebellar outflow tracts. *Secondary* symptoms are non-neurological complications that are a direct consequence of primary symptoms and include urinary tract infection (UTI) due to urinary retention, pressure sores due to immobility and aspiration pneumonia due to dysphagia. Finally, *tertiary* symptoms are the psychological, social and vocational consequences of the disease on the patient, family and community.

The needs of patients, especially those most severely affected, are best served in a comprehensive care setting where a team approach can be coordinated. Team members include neurologists, specialized nurses, occupational medicine and physical therapists, social workers and psychologists. There must be an established working relationship with other medical practitioners, such as specialists in internal medicine and physical medicine, urologists, orthopaedists and psychiatrists, to assist when special needs arise. The MS comprehensive care centre must coordinate care so that the patient's needs are satisfied by those most familiar with the ramifications of the disease.

Primary symptoms and treatment

Primary symptoms include gait disturbances; bladder, bowel and sexual dysfunction; disorders of the upper extremities; fatigue; dysarthria; and dysphagia. These symptoms must be addressed first; however, attention to all symptoms is necessary to provide optimal rehabilitation and prevent complications.

Gait disturbance

Walking is often a major problem for patients with multiple sclerosis. A disturbance in gait may be the result of spasticity, weakness, ataxia or any combination of these findings.

In the earliest phases of gait impairment, patients may complain of easy fatiguability or difficulty in running. If the symptoms progress, they may note dragging of one or both legs after prolonged exercise. The symptoms may fluctuate throughout the day and become worse in high ambient temperatures. Equilibrium may be defective, and the patient will frequently fall. Patients become more dependent on the banisters of staircases and must stop and rest when walking any distance. If the disease is progressive, independent gait may become hazardous, and gait aids are required. Unfortunately, for some patients, even with aids, walking becomes impossible and the use of a wheelchair is inevitable.

Careful evaluation of the history and physical examination is necessary to identify the precise mechanism of abnormal gait. Patients with symptomatic spasticity, for example, may also report spasms of the lower limbs, which may be painful, occur at night and interfere with sleep. Weakness and spasticity can produce complaints of 'heaviness' or 'dragging', but patients suffering from spasticity may describe their lower limbs as being 'stiff'. The physical examination detects which of these causes are present and provides an estimate of the relative contribution of each to the complaint.

Cerebellar disturbances are among the most common symptoms of multiple sclerosis, and cerebellar ataxia is probably the most frequent finding responsible for gait complaints. Patients describe losing their balance, especially when turning. They may weave from side to side or lean toward the side of the lesion. On examination, most patients will have at least some difficulty with tandem gait. Although patients often have findings that suggest abnormal dorsal column function in the lower limbs, such as impaired vibratory or position sense, sensory ataxia is rarely a primary cause of imbalance or gait impairment.

Depending on the cause of gait disturbance, various treatment regimens are available. When the primary cause of gait disturbance is spasm, an antispastic agent is usually effective. Of the currently available antispastic drugs, baclofen is the most beneficial in relieving stiffness and spasms. A small dose should be used initially and slowly increased until a positive response is noted. For some patients, large doses may be necessary for optimal response, with surprisingly few side-effects (Smith *et al.*, 1991). The drug should be taken with meals to avoid the side-effects of drowsiness and nausea. Careful titration is important. Diazepam is also an effective antispastic agent, but it is not tolerated as well as baclofen and should be used only in patients who do not respond to or cannot tolerate baclofen.

Passive stretching through the full range of movement is beneficial in patients suffering spasms (Delisa & DeLateur, 1983). All extremities suffering from spasms should be stretched several times a day to relieve the spasms and prevent fibrous contracture of muscles and joint ankylosis. Most patients may require the assistance of a physical therapist until they learn the techniques. Various other types of exercise are beneficial, e.g. swimming.

When spasticity does not respond to medical management, chemical neurectomy with phenol (5%) may be necessary (Moore, 1971). Recent reports indicate that intrathecal baclofen, given through an indwelling pump and catheter, may be effective and well tolerated (Penn *et al.*, 1989). See also Chapter 24 for management of spasticity. As a last resort in patients with severe, long-standing urinary retention, severe sensory loss in the lower extremities and paraplegia who do not respond to any other forms of treatment, intrathecal administration of alcohol may be beneficial.

When weakness is the cause of gait disturbances,

management depends on distribution, severity and acuteness of onset. Exercise is the mainstay of therapy for these patients. The exercise programme should be tailored to the patient's physical capabilities and be either passive or active.

In active-range-of-motion exercises, the patient actively moves the joint through as wide a range as possible (with gravity eliminated when weakness is severe) and then progresses as strength permits to moving the joint in the antigravity position. The assistance of a therapist or the use of weights or pulleys may be required to counterbalance the joint when the patient is too weak to move the joint actively. The two types of active–restrictive exercises currently employed are isometric and isotonic (Delisa & DeLateur, 1983). In passive exercises, the patient moves the joint through its full range of motion as resistance, either by a therapist or by equipment, is applied in the opposite direction. A complete exercise programme must include cardiovascular exercises, such as swimming, running and cycling.

When weakness interferes with gait, orthotics may be necessary. A thorough understanding of the pathological anatomy and the patient's requirements is necessary for the proper prescription of an orthosis. The patient must understand the purpose and benefit of the device; it must be comfortable, relatively easy to take off and put on and reasonably attractive (Redford, 1985).

Patients with upper motor neuron lesions often experience foot drop during the swing phase of gait, mediolateral ankle instability and insufficient push-off while standing (Lehman, 1985). This is caused by weakness of the foot dorsiflexors and evertors, which may be aggravated by spasticity. Therefore, the orthosis should provide resistance against plantar flexion during the swing phase, increase ankle stability at the time of heel strike, and be relatively rigid during push-offs (Lehman *et al.*, 1983). The polypropylene ankle–foot orthosis (PAFO) meets many of these requirements.

There are several types of polypropylene ankle–foot orthosis. All are worn inside the patient's shoe and secured by a strap around the calf. They differ in degree of rigidity and ankle support, and are generally made to provide a slight degree of dorsiflexion (5°–10°) to minimize toe drag. However, this may lessen knee stability (Lehman *et al.*, 1970).

Rather than letting the foot down slowly from heel strike to foot flat by contracting the foot dorsiflexors, the patient rocks over the posterior portion of the heel; this causes a bending movement at the knee, which must be overcome by the knee extensors. Therefore, the degree of dorsiflexion should be only as much as needed. Alternatively, part of the heel can be cut off at a 45° angle or a cushion wedge can be inserted into the heel (Simons et al., 1967); this will move the ground-reactive force forward.

Once fitted, the orthosis should be checked to ensure that the calf band does not impinge on the peroneal nerve, that it does not place undue pressure on any part of the skin (especially in patients with impaired sensation or spasticity), that the axis of the ankle joint for plantar and dorsiflexion closely approximates the location of the anatomical joint axis during movement, and that the patient exhibits good function during ambulation (Lehman, 1985). When the patient is standing, the sole and heel of the shoe should be flat on the floor. The entire gait cycle should be observed. If the orthosis exceeds the length required for toe clearance, the patient's knee may buckle while walking. Hyperextension of the knee will occur if there is too much plantar flexion or the sole plate extends too far forward (Lehman, 1985).

One common alignment problem involving the knee is genu recurvatum, resulting from muscle imbalance, in which the patient stabilizes the knee by extending it. Usually, this is limited by the posterior joint capsule and extension-limiting knee ligaments. However, these may gradually yield. Patients with this problem who wear a PAFO can limit this tendency by placing the ankle in dorsiflexion and forcing the knee to bend during the first part of stance (Lehman et al., 1983).

If genu recurvatum is severe, it can be managed by a knee–ankle foot orthosis (KAFO) designed to keep the knee in slight flexion. Alternatively, some patients do best with knee supports, such as the Swedish knee cage.

When ataxia is responsible for gait interference, Frenkel's exercises are recommended (Frenkel, 1929). These exercises are done in four positions (lying, sitting, standing and walking) and incorporate total patterns, righting reflexes and stabilization mechanisms, while stressing prime movements.

When walking becomes dangerous, an assistive device may be necessary. Gait aids should provide as much assistance as is needed but no more. The more complicated the gait aid, the more cumbersome the gait. The patient should be trained to use the aid in a way that will closely mimic his/her normal gait pattern.

Canes provide the least support. A cane provides weight-bearing relief in the range of 20–25% of body-weight (Jebson, 1967). Because there is only a single point of contact with the body, there is limited support. Usually, a cane is held in the hand opposite the involved side; this provides a more physiological gait as the opposite arm and leg move together. When the dysfunction is unilateral, this shifts weight away from the involved limb (Varghese, 1986). The length of the cane should be adjusted so that the highest point is at the level of the greater trochanter (Hoberman & Basmajian, 1984).

Crutches, either axillary or non-axillary, provide two points of contact with the body, resulting in more support. Axillary crutches can transfer as much as 80% of body-weight away from the lower extremities; non-axillary crutches can transfer 40–50% (Jebson, 1967). Non-axillary crutches, the most commonly prescribed for patients with multiple sclerosis with paraparesis, require adequate axial balance.

Walkers provide maximal support but at a slow and awkward pace. They are useful in patients with poor balance. Walkers with wheels are appealing to patients with weak or dysmetric upper extremities; however, they cause a measure of instability that can be dangerous (Varghese, 1986). A walker should be placed 25–30 cm in front of the patient, and the patient should stand erect with elbows flexed 15°–20° (Burgess & Alexander, 1975).

Before using any type of gait-assistance device, the patient must be instructed in its proper usage. An experienced physiotherapist should work with the patient until the patient feels secure standing and walking. S/he must be able to demonstrate the ability to negotiate stairs, inclines and curbs, and should feel comfortable with the prescribed aid.

When walking with an assistive device becomes unsafe or impossible, a wheelchair may be necessary. It often serves as a supplementary means of transportation and provides a degree of independence that might not be possible otherwise. However, some patients depend too heavily on a wheelchair. Therefore, it is important to stress that the wheelchair is to be used as an alternative means of transportation and that walking, even with an aid, is preferred.

The patient should be fully clothed and wearing any braces normally worn when fitted for a wheelchair. The hips and knees should be at 90° flexion and the ankles in a neutral position. It is important to note the distance from the soles of the shoes to the upper horizontal level of the seat (add 5 cm to compensate for elevation of the footrests); the distance between the outer borders of the thighs; the distance from the back of the seat to within four finger-breadths from the back of the knee, taken along the midline; the height of the armrest (the forearm should be at right angles to the arms with the palms down, plus 2.5 cm); and the distance between the chair and the lower angle of the scapula.

Normally, the footrest should be adjusted so that two finger-breadths can be placed under the thigh at the forward end of the seat. This extra lift for the thighs is not advisable in patients predisposed to ischial pressure sores. The legs should not dangle over the end of the seat because of the danger of sciatic nerve compression.

Once provided with a wheelchair, the patient should be trained to propel the chair backward and forward, to turn it and to know how and when to use the brakes. In addition, the patient must be taught how to transfer properly from the wheelchair. An unassisted standing transfer requires adequate balance while sitting, strong voluntary control of hip and knee extensors or adequate extensor spasticity of the lower extremities, and reasonably strong upper extremities. Physical therapists teach the techniques for transferring into and out of bed, or to other surfaces, into and out of the bath and on to and off the toilet (Ellwood, 1982).

Bladder, bowel and sexual dysfunctions

Urinary symptoms occur in the majority of patients with multiple sclerosis and are typically conjoined with bowel and sexual complaints. 'Irritative' urinary symptoms that indicate uninhibited detrusor contractions include urgency, frequency, nocturia and urgency incontinence; complaints

suggestive of urinary retention include a weak urinary stream, incomplete emptying, with 'double voiding', and spontaneous interruptions of the urinary stream. These symptoms may also occur in combination. Therefore, attempting to detect the nature of the disturbance based on history alone frequently yields inaccurate conclusions and errors in treatment (Blaivas et al., 1984).

Urinary symptoms directly resulting from the neurological lesions of multiple sclerosis can be categorized as failure to store urine, failure to empty the bladder or a combination of the two (Blaivas, 1979). Patients with failure to store urine have a small-capacity bladder with involuntary detrusor contractions. Patients with failure to empty urine may have either detrusor paralysis (rare in multiple sclerosis) or outlet obstruction due to detrusor–external sphincter dyssynergia (DESD) (Blaivas et al., 1981a). DESD occurs due to failure to co-ordinate detrusor contraction with external urinary sphincter relaxation. It results from lesions above the sacral segments of the spinal cord but below the pontine reticular formation – the site of an important facilitatory centre for bladder reflexes (Blaivas et al., 1981b). DESD causes obstruction of urinary flow and an elevated residual urine, predisposing to UTI.

When urinary complaints are present, the goals of intervention include: identify complicating UTI, prevent further complications and control neurological symptoms. A microscopic urinalysis and culture of urine should be obtained on the first evaluation or if there is any subsequent change in symptoms. If infection is present, it should be treated with appropriate antibiotics. A postvoiding residual urine (PRU) should be determined on all patients with urinary symptoms before initiating treatment to ensure proper therapy. All patients with a significant PRU should be treated with urinary antiseptics.

Anticholinergics or smooth-muscle relaxants are usually effective in patients whose bladders fail to store urine.

Some patients with hyper-reflexic bladders can be taught to induce voiding by triggering detrusor contractions. These triggers may include suprapubic tapping, stroking the glans penis, rubbing the thigh or pulling on pubic hair. Patients with DESD should not void by reflex triggering because it may cause ureteral reflux. Patients with DESD should not use Crede's method to reduce residual urine.

Clean, intermittent self-catheterization, a simple and safe technique proved to reduce the frequency of UTI and relieve symptoms, is recommended in patients with high PRUs (Blaivas *et al.*, 1984). Patients who are obese, who have impaired vision, sensation, manual co-ordination or intellect, or who suffer from spasticity of the adductors of the thighs will require assistance in performing this technique.

If a patient is not able to perform intermittent self-catheterization, an indwelling catheter may be necessary as a last resort. A suprapubic vesicostomy with continuous catheterization is preferable to uretheral catheterization because it is easier to keep clean and avoids acute epididymitis in men.

Bowel complaints are at least as common as urinary symptoms, with the most frequent complaint being constipation (Glick *et al.*, 1982). Although this may be attributed directly to the effects of the neurological lesions on bowel motility, there are other important contributing factors, e.g. diet, fluid intake and medication. Constipation is usually treated conservatively by instructing the patient to increase his/her intake of fluid to six to eight glasses of liquid daily and to eat high-fibre foods. If constipation persists, a laxative or enema may be necessary. Diarrhoea is not a symptom of multiple sclerosis and should suggest another problem, such as spurious diarrhoea because of faecal impaction (Levine, 1985).

Sexual complaints occur as frequently as bladder and bowel symptoms, which is not surprising because all three functions are probably subserved by similar spinal pathways. The most frequent complaint in men is impotence; for women, decreased libido is the most frequent complaint (Barrett, 1977). Sexual problems may relate to the psychological ramifications of the disease as well as to the effects of the neurological lesions (Kalb *et al.*, 1987). Also, many medications interfere with sexual responses and may contribute to the problem.

Treatment depends on the cause. Psychological problems are treated with individual, group or couple counselling. Intracavernous papaverine has proved beneficial in cases of impotence. See also the management of sexual disability in Chapter 28.

Upper extremity involvement

Many patients have symptoms referable to the upper limbs, such as weakness, clumsiness, tremor or numbness. Initially, difficulty with tasks requiring fine motor control, such as buttoning a shirt or writing, is described. Corticospinal, dorsal column or cerebellar involvement may be responsible for impaired digital dexterity. When severe, involvement of the upper limbs may cause the patient to become totally dependent on others for all activities of daily living, thereby robbing him/her of his/her self-esteem.

Treatment includes the use of various adaptative devices, such as long straws to aid with drinking and devices that spread pants, turn pages, hold cards and extend the patient's reach. Upper extremity orthotics are not usually recommended because they may hinder the performance of activities impaired by multiple sclerosis. However, static forearm splints and hand rolls may be beneficial. Although motor-point phenol blocks may be effective for unremitting upper extremity spasticity, their benefit is often short-lived and repeat blocks are often needed.

Fatigue

Most patients who complain of fatigue find it to be among the most disabling of symptoms (Freal *et al.*, 1984). Descriptions include a 'washed-out', 'exhausted' or 'lacking in energy' sensation. It is usually most prominent in the mid- to late afternoon and increases in severity with physical exercise and high ambient temperature and humidity. Rest, but not necessarily sleep, is usually restorative. The pathophysiological basis for multiple sclerosis-related fatigue is unknown, but conduction failure through partially demyelinated regions is suspected. Because many depressed patients complain of fatigue and fatigue is frequent in multiple sclerosis, depression is a major differential. Various historical features distinguish multiple sclerosis-related fatigue from fatigue associated with depression. Patients with depression usually wake in the morning feeling tired; patients with multiple sclerosis-related fatigue are at their best in the morning. Although patients may describe considerable frustration with this symptom, the typical vegetative signs of depression are notably lacking. Also, many medications used to treat some of the other symptoms of multiple sclerosis are associated with fatigue as an adverse effect.

To help alleviate fatigue, patients should organize their day around the times when fatigue is worse to permit rest periods when needed. High-fatigue activities should be scheduled for times when fatigue is less likely. Patients should learn to sit, slide and toss rather than stand, lift and carry.

Dysarthria

Many patients with dysarthria have cerebellar causes for speech impairment, although pseudobulbar palsy from bilateral corticobulbar involvement also occurs. Patients with cerebellar speech disturbances may have nystagmus and intention tremor of the limbs. The severity of speech disturbance generally parallels the severity of neurological impairment.

Because most clinically significant disorders of motor speech are partly amenable to treatment, a speech pathologist should be consulted. Patients with defective articulation should be instructed to slow their rate of speech to allow more time for the tongue to compensate for the loss of control. With severe articulatory failure, exercises utilizing specific speech muscles may be required.

Patients with severe motor speech disturbance sometimes do not benefit from direct exercise of articulators or contextual speech therapy. For these patients, alternatives to speech, e.g. picture, word, phrase and alphabet boards, may assist them in attempts at communication. Also, voice synthesis computers are available, but they are quite costly.

Dysphagia

Although rarely severe, dysphagia is a potentially serious complication of multiple sclerosis because it can lead to aspiration. A thorough history and clinical evaluation are necessary to detect dysphagia. The history should include questions regarding the onset, course, effects of various food consistencies, results of swallowing and presence of coughing or choking. The evaluation should include range, rate and accuracy of lip, tongue and soft palate movement during speech; reflex activity; and swallowing. Coughing and choking generally indicate aspiration into the airway. The presence or absence of the gag reflex is not by itself an indication of the patient's ability to swallow (DeJong, 1979). Radiography is the only accurate means of determining the cause of aspiration (Logemann, 1986).

Poor tongue control can result from cerebellar dysfunction or from pseudotumour palsy. Treatment for the loss of tongue control includes compensatory positional changes or exercises to increase the tongue's range of motion, strength and control (Logemann, 1986).

To alleviate delayed or absent triggering of the swallowing reflex, the patient may flex his head in preparation for the swallow and eat thicker foods in smaller amounts. Thermal stimulation of the anterior faucial arches, soft palate or posterior tongue has also proved effective.

If the larynx fails to close while swallowing, the patient should inhale, hold his breath at the height of inspiration, swallow, and then cough while exhaling. Whenever residue remains in the pharynx or upper airway, the patient should cough and clear any residue before inhaling after swallowing (Logemann, 1986).

If dysphagia is severe, a percutaneous gastrostomy may be necessary.

Secondary symptoms and treatment

Secondary symptoms are those that occur as a direct result of the neurological disturbances. They include decubitus ulcers, fibrous contractures, aspiration pneumonia and urinary tract infections (the latter two have been discussed). Although they are a large cause of morbidity in patients with multiple sclerosis, these symptoms are preventable. Prevention is achieved by supervision of patients at risk.

Decubitus ulcers

Decubitus ulcers (pressure sores) are caused by sustained pressure of the tissues under bony prominences. In addition to postural abnormalities, alterations of the mental status, significant sensory impairment and urinary incontinence accelerate their development. Without proper care, superficial skin lesions can quickly develop into deep ulcerations, which may extend, by sinus tracts, into adjacent joints or bones.

Patients at risk for developing decubitus ulcers are those with weakness of the legs severe enough to preclude ambulation and those who suffer from significant loss of sensation, intellectual impairment, bladder or bowel incontinence or poor nutrition.

Superficial sores can be managed conservatively with the use of antiseptic washes and saline dressings. The primary approach is to prevent further pressure until the initial reddened area is healed entirely. Deeper sores often require operative management, resulting in prolonged hospitalization.

To prevent decubitus ulcers, the patient should examine his/her skin regularly for signs of tissue compromise. Patients in wheelchairs should sit in a way that evenly distributes pressure over the buttocks and posterior thighs. They should also do pressure-relieving exercises every 15 minutes and be provided with wheelchair cushions designed to fit their body contours.

If capable, patients who are bedridden must learn to turn themselves by using side-rails and overhead trapezes. If the patient is not able to turn him/herself, s/he must be turned every 2 hours. Customized mattresses filled with air, water, hydrophilic gels or fluidized silicone beads are beneficial.

Fibrous contractures

Unremitting spasticity can lead to irreversible shortening of muscles which, especially in the lower limbs, can severely compromise the patient's position in a wheelchair or bed. Once fibrous contractures occur, the only form of treatment is tenotomy of the involved muscles. Fibrous contractures can also lead to ankylosis of adjacent joints, further complicating management. The extent of these complications may be difficult to appreciate because of coincidental spasticity. Occasionally, it is necessary to examine the affected limbs under anaesthesia, which relieves spasticity, to determine the precise mechanism of severely altered posture. It is important that patients with severely altered posture, especially those who have flexion deformities of the lower limbs, be considered for surgical correction. Otherwise, many individuals will develop pressure sores due to the inability to be positioned properly.

Tertiary symptoms and treatment

Tertiary symptoms are the psychosocial and vocational issues that complicate the lives of many patients with multiple sclerosis. Multiple sclerosis is a disease that causes considerable stress (LaRocca et al., 1987) and coping with this stress depends on the adequacy of premorbid coping strategies and the ability to mobilize support from internal and external sources. External sources of support include relationships with family and friends, occupational affiliations and medical interventions. Attitudes toward health and societal role, as well as pre-existing stress-reducing strategies, constitute some of the internal support mechanisms and also provide them with the necessary assistance to re-establish control. Individual and family counselling and vocational rehabilitation, as well as referral to support groups such as the local branches of the National Multiple Sclerosis Society, are ways that the health-care provider can favourably influence outcome.

Conclusion

Although there is no cure for multiple sclerosis, the physician can provide the patient with symptomatic treatment and rehabilitation. Treatment is all-encompassing and includes a careful assessment of the patient's neurological and associated symptoms; knowledge of the patient's intellectual, emotional and social skills and demands; and an understanding of the patient's support network. To provide optimal treatment, the physician must work closely with speech, physical and occupational therapists, social workers and rehabilitation specialists, and with the patient and his family.

The physician treating patients with multiple sclerosis faces a complex challenge but reaps his/her rewards in the patient's small victories in his/her battle against this disease.

Acknowledgements

This work was supported by NIDRR Grant No. H133B80018-92 and the Schmulka Aronson Charitable Trust Funds. The authors are grateful to Roxane Baer for editorial assistance and Eileen Blight for her secretarial skills in typing this manuscript.

References

Barrett M. (1977) *Sexuality and Multiple Sclerosis.* Multiple Sclerosis Society of Canada, Toronto.

Blaivas J.G. (1979) Management of bladder dysfunction in multiple sclerosis. *Neurology* **30**, 12–18.

Blaivas J.G., Sinha H.P., Zayed A.A.H. & Labib K.B. (1981a) Detrusor external sphincter dyssynergia. *Journal of Urology* **125**, 542–544.

Blaivas J.G., Sinha H.P., Zayed A.A.H. & Labib K.B. (1981b) Detrusor external sphincter dyssynergia: a detailed electromyographic study. *Journal of Urology* **125**, 545–548.

Blaivas J.G., Holland N.J., Giesser B., LaRocca N., Madonna M. & Scheinberg L. (1984) Multiple sclerosis bladder: studies and care. *Annals of the New York Academy of Science* **436**, 328–345.

Burgess E. & Alexander A. (1975) Mobility aids. In *Atlas of Orthopedics.* Mosby, St Louis.

DeJong R. (1979) *The Neurologic Examination,* 4th edn. Harper & Row, New York.

Delisa J.A. & DeLateur B.J. (1983) Therapeutic exercise: types and indications. *American Family Physician* **28**, 227–233.

Ellwood P.M. (1982) Transfers: method, equipment and preparation. In Kottke F.J., Stillwell G.K. & Lehman J.F. (eds) *Krusen's Handbook of Physical Medicine and Rehabilitation,* 3rd edn, pp. 473–491. W.B. Saunders, Philadelphia.

Freal J.E., Kraft G.H. & Coryell S.K. (1984) Symptomatic fatigue in multiple sclerosis. *Archives of Physical Medicine and Rehabilitation* **65**, 135–138.

Frenkel H.S. (1929) In Granger F.B. (ed.) *Physical Therapeutic Technique.* W.B. Saunders, Philadelphia.

Glick M.E., Meshkinpoor H. & Haldeman S. (1982) Colonic dysfunction in multiple sclerosis. *Gastroenterology* **83**, 1002–1007.

Hoberman M. & Basmajian J.V. (1984) Crutch and cane exercises and use. In Basmajian J.V. (ed.) *Therapeutic Exercise,* 4th edn, pp. 267–284. Williams and Wilkins, Baltimore.

International Federation of Multiple Sclerosis Societies (1985) *Minimal Record of Disability for Multiple Sclerosis.* International Federation of Multiple Sclerosis Societies, New York.

Jebsan R. (1967) Use and abuse of ambulation aids. *Journal of American Medical Association* **199**, 63–68.

Kalb R.C., LaRocca N.G. & Kaplan S.R. (1987) Sexuality. In Scheinberg L.C. & Holland N.J. (eds) *Multiple Sclerosis: a Guide for Patients and Their Families,* 2nd edn, pp. 177–196. Raven Press, New York.

Kurtzke J.F. (1983) Rating neurologic impairment in multiple sclerosis: an expanded disability status scale (EDSS). *Neurology (Cleveland)* **33**, 1444–1452.

Kurtzke J.F., Beebe G.W., Nagler B., Kurland L.T. & Auth T.L. (1977) Studies on the natural history of multiple sclerosis and early prognostic features of the later course of the illness. *Journal of Chronic Diseases* **30**, 819–830.

LaRocca N.G., Kalb R.C. & Kaplan S.R. (1987) Psychological issues. In Scheinberg L.C. & Holland N.J. (eds) *Multiple Sclerosis: a Guide for Patients and Their Families,* 2nd edn, pp. 197–213. Raven Press, New York.

Lehman J.F. (1985) Lower limb orthotics. In Redford J.B. (ed.) *Orthotics Etcetera,* pp. 278–351. Williams and Wilkins, Baltimore.

Lehman J.F., Warren C.G. & deLateur B.J. (1970) Biomechanical evaluation of knee stability in below knee braces. *Archives of Physical and Medical Rehabilitation* **51**, 688–695.

Lehman J.F., Esselman P.C., Ko M.J., Smith J.C., deLateur B.J. & Dralle A.J. (1983) Plastic ankle–foot orthoses: evaluation of function. *Archives of Physical and Medical Rehabilitation* **64**, 402–407.

Levine J.S. (1985) Bowel dysfunction in multiple sclerosis. In Maloney F.P., Burks J.S. & Ringel S.P. (eds) *Interdisciplinary Rehabilitation of Multiple Sclerosis and Neuromuscular Disorders,* pp. 62–64. J.B. Lippincott, Philadelphia.

Logemann J.A. (1986) Treatment for aspiration related to dysphagia: an overview. *Dysphagia* **1**, 34–38.

Moore C.D. (1971) *Regional Block: a Handbook for Use in the Clinical Practice of Medicine and Surgery,* 4th edn. Charles C. Thomas, Springfield.

Penn R.D., Savoy S.M., Corcos D. *et al.* (1989) Intrathecal baclofen for severe spinal spasticity. *New England Journal of Medicine* **320**, 1517–1521.

Redford J.B. (1985) Principles of orthotic devices. In Redford J.B. (ed.) *Orthotics Etcetera,* pp. 1–20. Williams and Wilkins, Baltimore.

Simons B.C., Jebsen R.H. & Wildman L.E. (1967) Plastic short leg brace fabrication. *Orthopedic and Prosthetic Appliance Journal* **21**, 215–218.

Smith C.R., LaRocca N.G., Giesser B.S. & Scheinberg L.C. (1991) High-dose oral baclofen: Experience in patients with multiple sclerosis. *Neurology* **41**, 1829–1831.

Varghese G. (1986) Crutches, canes and walkers. In Redford J.B. (ed.) *Orthotics Etcetera,* 3rd edn, pp. 453–463. Williams and Wilkins, Baltimore.

17: Natural History and Rehabilitation in Spinal Cord Damage

H.L. FRANKEL

Terminology, 221
Causes of spinal cord lesion, 222
Natural history, 223
  Motor function, 223
  Sensory function, 223
  Bladder function, 223
  Bowel function, 224
  Sexual function, 224
  Vascular changes, 224
  Natural history in completely untreated patients, 224
Prognosis of spinal cord function, 224
Management and rehabilitation: early stages, 227
  Position, 227
  Care of joints and soft tissues, 227
  Period of mobilization, 228
The active phase of rehabilitation, 228
  Skin care, 230
  Bladder care, 231
  Bowel training, 233
Skeletal complications, 234
  Para-articular ossification, 234
  Pathological fractures, 234
  Charcot joints, 234
Spasticity, 234
  Positioning and physiotherapy, 235
  Drug treatment, 235
  Peripheral surgical procedures, 235
  Injections, 235
Pain, 235
  Phantoms, 236
  Root pains, 236
  Hyperpathic pains, 236
Autonomic dysreflexia, 236
Special equipment, 237
  Electric chairs, 237
  Cars, 237
  Calipers, 237
Sport, 237

Terminology

The term 'paraplegia' indicates motor and sensory paralysis of the lower limbs with involvement of bladder, bowel and male sexual function. The word 'tetraplegia' (quadriplegia) implies a higher spinal cord lesion causing partial or complete paralysis of the upper limbs in addition to paralysis of the chest, trunk, abdomen and lower limbs as well as impairment of the bladder and bowel and male sexual function. When applied to the description of an individual patient the word 'complete' implies total loss of all motor and sensory function. The word 'incomplete' implies any lesser degree. For assessment of prognosis and follow-up, the classification introduced by Frankel *et al.* (1969) is used:

1 *Complete* (A). This means that the lesion is found to be complete, both motor and sensory, below the segmental level named.

2 *Sensory incompleteness only* (B). This implies that there is some sensation present below the level of the lesion but that the motor paralysis is complete below that level. This applies to sensory sparing as well as sacral sparing.

3 *Motor useless* (C). This implies that there is some motor power present below the lesion but it is of no practical use to the patient.

4 *Motor useful* (D). This implies that there is useful motor power below the level of the lesion. Patients in this group can move the lower limbs and many can walk with or without aids.

5 *Recovery* (E). This implies that the patient is free of neurological symptoms, i.e. no weakness, no sensory loss, no sphincter disturbance. Abnormal reflexes may be present.

To indicate the exact level of a lesion, the last normal segment is used, i.e. tetraplegia complete below C6 segment means that C6 segment is intact and C7 and the distal spinal cord are not in connection with the brain.

This chapter is confined to spinal cord lesions of acute onset and of a non-progressive nature. It is based on experience at the National Spinal Injuries Centre, Stoke Mandeville Hospital, and does not include multiple sclerosis, malignant tumours involving the spinal cord, or other progressive neurological diseases.

Causes of spinal cord lesion

In the UK the majority of non-progressive acute spinal cord lesions are due to trauma, the main causes being road accidents, industrial accidents, domestic accidents and sporting accidents. Most of these are due to fracture dislocations or severe fractures of the vertebral column and the major cause in relationship to the level of bony injury is shown in Table 17.1, which is the result of an analysis of 682 such patients admitted to Stoke Mandeville Hospital within 14 days of injury. The

Table 17.1 The level of bone injury to the spine in 682 patients

Vertebral injury	Cervical	T1–10	T11, 12; L1	Lumbar	Total
Road accidents					
Car (and lorry):					
Driver	46	20	24	3	93
Passenger	42	23	21	3	89
Motor cycle:					
Driver	36	50	12	1	99
Pillion	1	6	5	2	14
Bicycle	12	5	7	0	24
Pedestrian	11	2	8	0	21
					340
Aeroplane	1	1	6	0	8
Work					
Fall down	16	31	62	4	113
Dropped upon	2	8	12	3	25
Crushed	2	3	19	2	26
Hit	4	0	12	0	16
Other	1	0	0	0	1
					181
Domestic					
Fall	28	18	15	1	62
Dropped upon	0	1	0	0	1
Crushed	0	1	1	0	2
Hit	1	1	1	0	3
Other	1	2	1	0	4
					72
Sport					
Diving	41	0	1	0	42
Riding	0	4	3	1	8
Rugby football	5	0	0	0	5
Gymnastics	5	0	0	0	5
Other	4	1	4	2	11
					71
Assault	0	1	1	0	2
Attempted suicide	0	4	3	1	8
					10
Total	259	182	218	23	682

cause of the accident in different countries varies. In certain parts of Africa the commonest cause is falling from coconut trees. Penetrating injuries are much more common in other countries. In North and South America gunshot wounds are much more common and in South Africa stab wounds are frequent.

Stoke Mandeville Hospital also treats patients with non-traumatic spinal cord lesions whose onset and stability mimic those of traumatic causes, the commonest being transverse myelitis, benign tumours, vascular disturbances of the spinal cord (anterior spinal artery thrombosis, spinal strokes, arteriovenous malformation and decompression sickness) and abscesses – either pyogenic or tuberculous – compressing the spinal cord.

Natural history

Following a physical transection of the spinal cord there is complete and permanent paralysis of voluntary motor power below the affected segment with complete and permanent loss of somatic sensory function and there is severe impairment of bladder, bowel and male sexual function as well as visceral and autonomic function. The evolution in time of each of these functions is briefly described below.

Motor function

Although there can be no recovery from a complete transection, the initial paralysis is usually somewhat higher than the final paralysis. On the second or third day after an acute transection, the level of paralysis commonly rises by one segment. Over the next weeks this returns to the original level and then finally may end up one segment lower than the original physiological lesion; this pattern of events is of significance if the lesion is in the cervical region. Paralysis is at first of the flaccid type. Tendon reflexes and plantar responses may be present in the first hours after injury; then there is a period of spinal shock during which these reflexes are apparently abolished. The period of spinal shock varies from days to weeks and is usually shorter in younger patients and those with higher spinal cord transections. In general the period of spinal shock as assessed by the tone of the paralysed muscles and the absence of tendon reflexes and plantar

responses is roughly related to the period of spinal shock as assessed by the evolution of bladder, bowel and vascular functions, but this correlation is not accurate in individual patients. Following the period of spinal shock, tone in the paralysed muscles returns and subsequently becomes abnormally high and varying degrees of 'spasticity' develop.

In cases where distal spinal cord is destroyed by the trauma or where all the spinal roots are destroyed, particularly in fracture dislocations of the lumbar spine, there is a permanent flaccid paralysis.

Sensory function

Following complete transection of the spinal cord the changes in level by a segment or so described for motor function are also seen in the sensory level.

Bladder function

Following spinal cord injury there is usually a period of severe disturbance of bladder function, which may be classified as follows:

1 *Complete retention.* This is almost invariable in adult Europeans, but West Indians and European children may not have a period of complete retention.

2 *Passive incontinence* due to overflow from the distended bladder.

3 *Periodic micturition*
  (a) by reflex activity of the automatic bladder, or
  (b) by expressing the urine by using the muscles of the abdominal wall or pressing on the lower abdomen with the hand.

The time-scale for the development of an automatic bladder or an expressive bladder is extremely variable and tends to be shorter in patients with high spinal cord lesions and in younger people, particularly in children. The average time for starting periodic micturition was found to be 4.3 weeks and the average time until catheterization could be stopped was 8.8 weeks (Frankel, 1974).

If the bladder was left entirely to itself, it is possible that many patients would die of renal failure in the first weeks. Some form of catheterization is almost invariably used in patients with complete spinal cord lesions and the various methods are described later in this chapter.

Bowel function

The small intestine

Immediately following a high spinal cord transection there may be a period of ileus, particularly on the second or third day. This can give rise to gross abdominal distension and dilated stomach, particularly if the patient is given excessive fluids early on or allowed to eat solid food in the first few days. It is particularly dangerous in patients with tetraplegia, as their ventilation may already be seriously impaired. Following these early days, small-intestinal function appears to return to normal, as judged by normal absorption of food and the normal transit time of a barium meal. The ileus is likely to recur throughout the patient's subsequent life if he is given an anaesthetic, even for relatively minor procedures such as dental extraction.

Large-intestinal and rectal function

Immediately following a complete spinal cord transection, rectal tone is low and faeces tend to accumulate in the sigmoid colon. During this period laxatives and digital evacuations are required. Subsequently, patients with upper motoneuron lesions tend to develop reflex defaecation while those with lower motoneuron lesions do not. In both cases there is permanent loss of bowel sensation and control.

Sexual function

Patients with high spinal cord lesions tend to have an initial priapism. Subsequently patients with complete spinal cord lesions above T12 often have reflex erections and no psychically induced erections; most such patients are incapable of having seminal emissions. Patients with complete cauda equina lesions below T12 segment may be capable of having psychically induced erections and/or having seminal emissions.

Vascular changes

The resting blood-pressure in patients with high spinal cord lesions is low. Problems of postural hypotension and autonomic dysreflexia are dealt with subsequently. The degree of 'hypotension' is related to the level of the spinal cord transection, as shown in Figs 17.1(a) and 17.1(b).

Natural history in completely untreated patients

Tetraplegics

A tetraplegic patient is breathing entirely with his/her diaphragm and accessory muscles of respiration and is therefore unable to cough effectively. It is, therefore, usual for such a patient to drown in his/her own secretions within the first 12 days after injury. If, as is likely, he/she also develops an ileus and dilated stomach, he/she may die sooner of inhalation of vomit.

Paraplegics

Paraplegics and any surviving tetraplegics are likely to develop severe penetrating pressure sores, contractures and severe urinary tract complications. If they are given no prophylaxis against these and no treatment when they develop, they are likely to die of the pressure sores within a few months, usually due to osteomyelitis and septicaemia; if for any reason they survive longer than this, they are likely to die of severe urinary tract complications within 2 years. The full natural history of this disorder is of course only rarely seen in civilized countries; however, as soon as the level of care and supervision of a paraplegic patient falls below an excellent standard, various aspects of this natural history manifest themselves remorselessly.

The alterations in human physiology and their natural consequences, as described above, are the background against which these patients must be rehabilitated. As there is at present no 'treatment' for the spinal cord lesion itself, our rehabilitation must be based on utilizing all remaining intact functions and on a detailed understanding of the altered physiology of the patient.

Prognosis of spinal cord function

The prognosis varies with the type of injury and my experience is limited to closed spinal cord injuries.

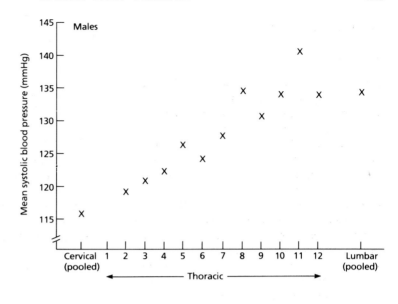

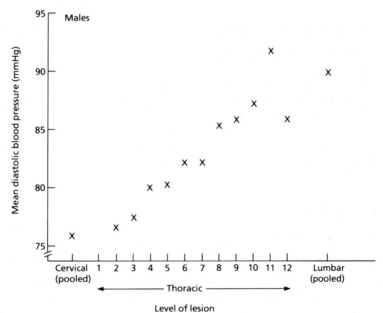

Fig. 17.1 (a) Mean systolic blood
pressure/level of spinal cord lesion.
(b) Mean diastolic blood
pressure/level of spinal cord lesion.

Where the initial spinal cord lesion is physiologically incomplete, the prognosis for some improvement or recovery is good. Even where the initial examination reveals a physiologically complete lesion, a certain number of patients make a partial or substantial recovery. Figure 17.2 shows a change in neurological status in 218 patients with tetraplegia (from Frankel *et al.*, 1969). The first letter in each square, for grade, shows each patient's status on admission to Stoke Mandeville Hospital and the second letter shows his/her status on discharge. This indicates that even when there is a complete lesion initially there is a small chance of some or substantial recovery. If the lesion remains physio-

Cervical injuries

A/A 81	AB 21	AC 10	AD 11	AE 0
BA 3	BB 9	BC 2	BD 14	BE 5
CA 0	CB 1	CC 4	CD 11	CE 5
DA 0	DB 0	DC 0	DD 30	DE 11
EA 0	EB 0	EC 0	ED 0	EE 0

Fig. 17.2 In each square of the grid are two letters of the alphabet, the first related to the neurological lesion on admission and the second to the neurological lesion on discharge. The numbers of patients are indicated. (Reproduced by permission of the editor of *Paraplegia*.)

logically complete for 14 days, then the prospect of any significant recovery is extremely slight. In patients who do eventually make a substantial recovery, the onset of useful motor function in the lower limbs may be delayed for many weeks. I have seen several patients who, though they had sensory sparing, had complete motor paralysis at 6 weeks, but who subsequently made a substantial recovery, sometimes good enough to walk without the aid of sticks. For the rest of this chapter I describe the management and expected course for patients with complete permanent lesions. For most purposes, management of patients with incomplete lesions is easier and the complications are less severe. The only exception to this is that patients with slightly incomplete lesions may have a far greater spasticity than those with complete lesions, and patients with substantially incomplete lesions often have greater difficulty in adjusting psychologically to their residual disability than those who are far more severely and completely paralysed.

There is no evidence that any surgical procedures can enhance recovery of spinal cord function. There is recent evidence that drugs such as high-dose methylprednisolone (Bracken *et al.*, 1990) and

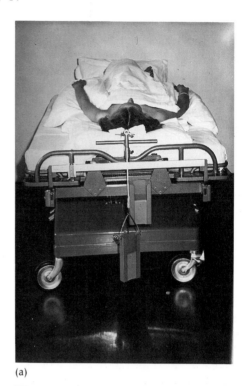

(a)

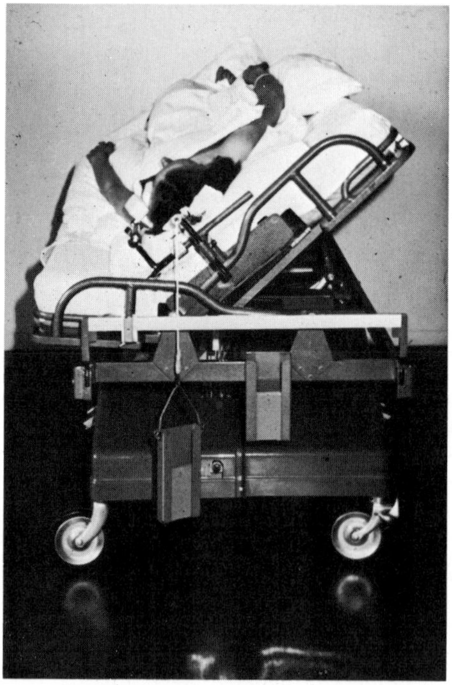

(b)

Fig. 17.3 Stoke Mandeville turning bed.

GM-1 ganglioside (Geisler *et al.*, 1991) may have a marginally beneficial effect on outcome if given soon after injury.

Management and rehabilitation: early stages

This phase of management covers the period that the patient spends in bed during the stabilization of the fracture or fracture dislocation. It usually varies from 6 to 12 weeks, although some patients may require more than 12 weeks in bed and some patients who have no substantial skeletal problems may be mobilized within a few days of the onset of their paralysis. Patients who have had a surgical stabilization of their vertebral injury may be mobilized within days or weeks, depending on the type of stabilizing procedure.

The phase of bedrest consists of postural management of the spinal column injury, which at Stoke Mandeville is achieved by posturing the patient on a Stoke Mandeville/Egerton turning bed in a position appropriate to the injury (Fig. 17.3). The patient is turned on this turning bed 3-hourly to prevent pressure sores and, in addition, there is a daily inspection of all his/her pressure points. As long as the patient is admitted to a spinal injuries centre in the early stages, pressure sores are totally avoidable.

Position

If a paralysed or partly paralysed muscle is overstretched for long periods of time, recovery will be impaired; the patient must therefore be nursed in a posture which keeps muscles in a neutral position. This is particularly important where the opposing muscle is unparalysed or less paralysed. For example, a patient with traumatic tetraplegia complete below the C6 segment will have active power in his/her deltoids, biceps and extensor carpi radialis longus and will tend to adopt a posture of abduction and internal rotation of the shoulders, flexion of the elbows, and extension, with radial deviation, at the wrists. Not only will this cause contractures, but any partial recovery which might be hoped for in the triceps will be prevented. In such cases, where opposing muscles are unparalysed, the patient's position may have to be corrected frequently because he/she is able to flex the elbows actively but cannot extend them again.

Care of joints and soft tissues

When paralysed limbs and joints are allowed to remain in the same position for prolonged periods, soft-tissue contractures will develop extremely rapidly unless specific measures are taken to prevent them. The tendency to form contractures is most pronounced in the early weeks after the onset of paralysis, and during that time a full range of passive movement must be given to every joint at least twice daily, 7 days a week. As long as such care is started on the first day of the paralysis, it is possible to perform a complete range of movements gently without the use of any undue force. Use of powerful passive movements may be necessary in a previously neglected patient but should be avoided whenever possible as it may cause damage to the soft tissues and overvigorous physiotherapy may play some part in the production of para-articular ossification.

During the period of bedrest, rehabilitation of the bladder and bowel will have started but not yet be under the patient's own management. During this period the patient will learn of the prognosis of his/her lesion. If the lesion is still complete after 2 weeks, the physician will be virtually certain of the prognosis. The exact timing of when the patient is told this prognosis varies with different physicians and of course with different patients. It is the author's practice to wait until the patient asks for his/her prognosis for at least the first few weeks. Very often the patient refrains from asking and then the subject must be carefully approached. If the patient is being treated in a spinal injuries centre, he/she will already be aware of the presence of wheelchair-bound patients around him/her and is very likely to make his/her own enquiries from other patients or trained or untrained staff before wanting to discuss it with the doctor. The majority of patients with complete lesions do understand and to some degree accept the permanence of their lesion by the time 10 weeks have passed. The amount of professional help, support and counselling that is given to patients on this aspect varies from centre to centre, and doubtless the patient community is itself the main source of information and support. It is common to see severe reactive depression or denial of permanence of the injury. These are usually temporary phases, but if they become prolonged they interfere with the process of physical and social rehabilitation and drug treatment seems to be useless. It has not been established whether any form of psychotherapy or sophisticated counselling has any beneficial effect. The presence of a trained psychologist and counsellors in a spinal injuries team certainly speeds up the identification of those patients with the greatest problems.

During the acute phases and during the period of bedrest, it is of course natural that the patient's relatives and friends visit as frequently as possible. The staff at the centre take this opportunity of getting to know them and enlisting their co-operation in future planning.

Towards the end of the period of bedrest, strict immobilization of the spine is stopped and a period of mobilization and back- or neck-strengthening exercises in bed is started. In most cases normally innervated muscles traverse the spinal fracture site; during the period of immobilization there is relative atrophy of these muscles and they can be strengthened by systematic exercises with the patient lying down so that his/her spinal fracture is more adequately stabilized when he/she starts to sit up.

Period of mobilization

Sitting up

In patients with high spinal cord lesions the normal reflex arc controlling the blood pressure in the sitting or standing position is largely abolished when the spinal cord lesion is above the level of the sympathetic outflow. By an arbitrary method of training, described below, it is usually possible to maintain an adequate blood pressure in these patients:

1 Sit the patient up very slowly in a winding bed.
2 When the patient can tolerate the sitting position, repeat the process several times each day.
3 All patients should eventually tolerate the sitting position for prolonged periods without any loss of consciousness.

The mechanisms by which this training is successful are due in part to the activation of the renin–angiotensin system and also the subsequent rise in plasma aldosterone (Mathias & Frankel, 1988) and the secretion of arginine vasopressin (Poole et al., 1987) and the ability of the patient to perfuse his/her brain adequately with a low blood pressure. The use of abdominal binders and elastic stockings and the administration of ephedrine 15 mg before raising the patient from the horizontal may help to achieve circulatory readjustment in this phase.

In the early stages in the wheelchair, pitting oedema of the ankles is relatively common. This should be managed by limiting the number of hours which the patient spends sitting up, by elevating the legs while in bed and occasionally by the use of well-fitting elastic stockings.

The active phase of rehabilitation

Once the patient can tolerate the sitting position in a wheelchair, the more active phase of his/her rehabilitation starts. This is a combined operation between the physician, nurses, physiotherapists, occupational therapists and social workers. Different members of this team are relatively more important at certain phases and for certain activities; thus the nurses will lead in training the patient in the prevention of pressure sores and management of bladder and bowels and in some centres they also teach patients in dressing. Physiotherapists are responsible for the care of the joints and teach transfers, standing and ambulation. The occupational therapist will largely concentrate on training of the upper limbs and on dressing for tetraplegics, as well as advising on adaptations and rehousing.

The actual techniques of physiotherapy and occupational therapy are unremarkable and are deployed as appropriate to the condition of the patient. An excellent account of the different techniques is available in Bromley (1985).

The general principle on which our physical rehabilitation is based is to both strengthen and increase the skill of the remaining intact musculature.

By the time the patient is ready to leave the spinal injuries centre, he/she should be approaching the optimum level of independence for his/her particular cord transection. Obviously the degree of independence achieved and the length of time taken also depend on the patient's age and moti-

Table 17.2 C3. Lowest muscles: sternomastoid; trapezius − part; diaphragm − part

Independent	Assisted	Dependent
Talking Swallowing	Breathing − *ventilator*, part- or full-time Coughing ⎫ Writing ⎬ *mouth stick* or *POSSUM* Typing ⎪ Telephoning ⎭ Environmental controls − *POSSUM* *Electric wheelchair*	Drinking Feeding Turning Lifting Washing Shaving Dressing Bowels Urinal Transfers − sometimes *hoist* Car − *special safety belt*

Table 17.3 C4. Lowest muscles: trapezius; rhomboid; diaphragm − part

Independent	Assisted	Dependent

Talking
Swallowing
Breathing
	Coughing
	Writing − *mouth stick*
	Typing − *electric continuous paper*
	Telephoning − *POSSUM and other*
	  adaptation
	Environmental controls − *POSSUM*
	Shaving − *electric razor on stand*
	  Electric wheelchair
	Drinking
		Feeding
		Turning
		Lifting
		Washing
		Dressing
		Bowels
		Urinal
		Transfers − sometimes *hoist*
		Car − *special safety belt*

Table 17.4 C5. Lowest muscles: deltoids; biceps; diaphragm

Independent	Assisted	Dependent
Talking	Coughing	Bowels
Drinking − *thermos mug*	Feeding	Urinal
Teeth cleaning − *strap to hold brush*		
Swallowing		
Hair brushing − *strap to hold brush*	Transfers	Car
Breathing	Turning	
Make-up − some	Lifting	
Push self-propelled *wheelchair* on flat surface	Washing	
Writing − *pen holder*		
Typing − *electric typewriter*	Dressing	
Telephoning − *POSSUM* or *adaptation*	Transfers −	
Shaving − *electric shaver*	sometimes *hoist*	

Table 17.5 C6. Lowest muscles: branchioradialis; extensor carpi radialis longus; triceps – sometimes

Independent	Assisted	Dependent
As C5 plus:		
Typing – *standard typewriter*	Coughing	Bowels
Feeding	Turning	Urinal
Teeth cleaning		
Hair brushing		
Hair washing		
Washing		
Lifting		Car – *most*
Dressing – some	Dressing – some	
Cooking		
Kitchen work		
Writing – some – no aid		
Transfers – some using *sliding board*	Transfers – some, *hoist* or manual	
Push *wheelchair* up incline 1 in 12	Standing – in *standing frame*	
Car – some, *hand-controlled car, automatic gearbox*		

Table 17.6 C7. Lowest muscles: triceps; wrist flexors

Independent	Assisted	Dependent
As C6 plus:		
Turning (most)	Coughing	Bowels (most)
Washing (some)	Turning (few)	Urinal (most)
Dressing (most)	Washing (some)	Car (some)
Wheelchair – 'back wheel balance' (some)	Dressing (few)	
Bowels (few) – *suppository inserter*	Transfers (few) – *hoist* or manual	
Urinal (few) apply and empty	Standing – in *standing frame*	
Transfers (most) – some use *sliding board*		
Family shopping – assisted		
Car (some) – *hand-controlled, automatic gearbox*		

vation. The expected goals that can be achieved by typical representative cord lesions are shown in the tables for patients with complete lesions below C3, C4, C5, C6, C7, C8, T7, T10, T12, L3 and L4 (Tables 17.2–17.9). These tables also show any special personal equipment that the patients may use.

Skin care

It is most important that patients fully understand the mechanisms by which their lack of sensation can cause pressure sores. If they do not have a full understanding of this subject, they may take inappropriate action when something goes wrong. They are taught to lift themselves at 10-minute intervals while in the wheelchair and to turn themselves at 3-hourly intervals while in bed. Patients with high tetraplegia are unable to lift themselves and they either have to be lifted by someone else (at hourly or 2-hourly intervals) or sit on a gel cushion or a ripple cushion. The Roho cushion is very expensive but is the most effective means of pressure equali-

Table 17.7 C8. Lowest muscles: finger extensor; finger flexors

Independent	Assisted	Dependent
As C7 plus:		
Turning	Coughing with respiratory infection	
Washing	Ambulate with *calipers* in parallel bars (not usually attempted)	
Dressing		
Transfers		
Full control of *wheelchair* – can mount 15 cm kerb		
Car – *hand controls, automatic gearbox*		
Bowels		
Urinal		
Standing – in *standing frame*		

Table 17.8 T7. Lowest muscles: intercostals

Fully independent for all personal needs in a suitable environment
Never stand (some), may develop more severe demineralization of bones and fracture easily
Stand in *frame* (some)
Ambulate with *long calipers* in *bars* (some), with *rollator* (some), with *elbow crutches* (some). Negotiate stairs (few). Most patients spend all day in a *wheelchair* and ambulate for exercise or special occasions

Table 17.9 T12, L3 and L4

T12. Lowest muscles: abdominals
As T7 but more patients ambulate with *elbow crutches*; however, the majority spend most of the day in a *wheelchair*

L3. Lowest muscles: quadriceps; adductors
Walk with *long calipers* and *elbow crutches*, occasional *wheelchair* use

L4. Lowest muscles: quadriceps; hamstrings
Walk with *short calipers* and *sticks*

zation that we have tried. Its use should be reserved for those with very high spinal cord lesions and those who have had recurrent problems with their ischial regions.

The patients and attendants are taught to inspect all their pressure areas daily and if there is the slightest redness or bruising they must keep off that point entirely until the condition has resolved.

Although the patients are taught to lift themselves at 10-minute intervals, certain patients, by trial and error, can extend this period gradually to once every half an hour. Likewise, for safety we prefer 3-hourly turning while the patient is in bed. Certain patients can lie in one position for longer than this, particularly if a large-cell ripple mattress is used. It is often possible for the patient to lie on his/her side for 3 hours then turn on to his/her back and remain there for the rest of the night – approximately another 6 hours. If the patient becomes ill for any reason and has a fever, he/she is taught that more frequent turning is temporarily necessary under those conditions.

The patient's entire future is dependent upon his/her ability to prevent pressure sores. The importance of prophylaxis and the inevitability of pressure sores in the absence of adequate prophylaxis is repeatedly pointed out to the patient and the vast majority of patients absorb this information and act accordingly. A small proportion of patients (approximately 5%) develop recurrent pressure sores after their discharge from hospital, and this small proportion of patients makes up a substantial part of the workload of our readmission wards.

Bladder care

The natural history of the untreated bladder in patients with spinal cord lesions was described earlier in this chapter. The major problem in the early stages of rehabilitation is protecting the patient's urinary tract from damage and chronic infection during the phase of complete or partial retention of urine. In European adults this almost invariably means some form of catheterization, either urethral or suprapubic. Nowadays urethral catheterization, either with an indwelling catheter or by intermittent catheterization, is almost always practised.

Foley catheters are the most commonly used indwelling catheters. These should be of small size (16 French gauge (Fg)) and should be inserted aseptically, and in male patients the penis must lie in an upwards direction. If the penis is allowed to lie between the legs with an indwelling catheter in position, there is severe pressure on the urethral wall at the penoscrotal junction and the urethral diverticulum, and sometimes a fistula at that site will occur. While the urine remains sterile, continuous closed drainage is recommended. Once the urine becomes infected (usually within a few days), the patients should have daily bladder wash-outs.

A Gibbon catheter may be used in the first instance and, with a small Gibbon catheter size 10 Fg or 12 Fg, the urine may remain sterile for several weeks, particularly if the patient has a high fluid output. Once the urine does become infected, these small catheters almost invariably block and it is necessary to change to a Foley catheter.

Whether a Foley catheter or a Gibbon catheter is used, eventually a period of bladder training must be undertaken and this is usually attempted between 8 and 10 weeks after the injury. In recent years the early use of a small-bore suprapubic catheter has been introduced. It is particularly useful in female patients and in tetraplegic men.

Intermittent catheterization

At Stoke Mandeville Hospital the favoured method of management in the early weeks is by intermittent catheterization, using a non-touch technique. This has been fully described elsewhere (Guttmann & Frankel, 1966; Frankel, 1974). Basically, the patients are catheterized three times in every 24 hours. Catheterization is performed with a soft flexible Jacques-type catheter. Each catheterization is performed by a doctor assisted by a nurse or an orderly. It is essential for this method of management that the fluid intake is controlled so

that at each catheterization not more than 600 ml of urine is in the bladder. It is also essential that all the urine is removed from the bladder on each occasion and, as the bladder is atonic in the early stages, this needs suprapubic pressure while the catheter is slowly withdrawn. If during this period a subclinical urinary infection occurs, it is promptly treated with systemic antibiotic. If a severe urinary infection supervenes with rigors and high fever, then the method is temporarily abandoned and an indwelling catheter is used until the acute infection is over (usually in 3–4 days).

Catheterization three times a day is continued until the patients are passing urine reliably between catheterization; then the midday catheterization is omitted and fluid intake increased. As soon as the residual urine is less than 200 ml, catheterization is reduced to once daily. When the residual urine is less than 100 ml, catheterization is finished. It is soon after catheterization is stopped that any residual infection which may have been acquired during the period of catheterization is likely to be troublesome, and at this stage careful bacteriological control and the appropriate antibiotic treatment are very important. The majority of patients have sterile urine at the end of their treatment, but in many cases subclinical or clinical infections may recur in the later stages. Some patients require bladder neck or extensive sphincter surgery.

After such treatment at Stoke Mandeville Hospital, most male patients leave hospital catheter-free. If they have a complete spinal cord lesion, they will almost certainly be using a urinal device and we favour the condom-type urinal, where the condom is glued to the penis with condom glue. These condoms are satisfactory for the majority of patients except those who have a retracting penis and those who are allergic to either the condom or the glue. These allergy problems have been well described by Bransbury (1979). A few patients are now managed by long-term intermittent self-catheterization. A few have long-term indwelling suprapubic catheters, a few have long-term indwelling urethral catheters and occasionally a sacral anterior root stimulator is used.

Many of our female patients leave hospital catheter-free and attempt to keep dry by regular visits to the lavatory where they stimulate their bladder by whatever method works for them.

Unfortunately, most female patients with complete cord lesions are sometimes wet in between such times and have to wear absorbent pads and waterproof pants. The management of the female's urinary incontinence, which was for years the weakest point in the rehabilitation of paraplegics, has been improved in recent years. Patients with good use of their hands can often use long-term intermittent self-catheterization, sometimes with the help of anticholinergic bladder relaxants. Patients with high lesions, who cannot catheterize themselves, may be managed with the use of a long-term, indwelling, suprapubic catheter; again, they will usually use anticholinergic bladder relaxants. Patients with upper motor neuron lesions who are able to transfer to a toilet may obtain very good continence by the use of a sacral anterior root stimulator, combined with section of the posterior roots of S2, 3 and 4. The use of long-term, indwelling, urethral catheters should be avoided as it eventually leads to the destruction of the female urethra. Once this has occurred, the only way for the patient to be dry is to divert her ureters into an ileal conduit.

Bowel training

During the first few weeks after injury, laxatives and digital evacuations will almost certainly be required; these digital evacuations should be preceded by glycerin suppositories and should be performed carefully and gently; if undue violence or stretching occurs during the phase of spinal shock the anus may be overstretched and the onset of 'automatic defaecation' may be delayed or prevented.

After the stage of spinal shock, attempts are made to teach the patient 'planned defaecation'. The reservoir for faeces is the sigmoid colon and not the rectum. The rectum should be empty except immediately before defaecation. The ability of the sigmoid colon to act as a reservoir seems to be unimpaired in the paraplegic; it is the awareness of faeces passing into the rectum and the ability to assist or prevent their further passage which is lacking. As the last line of defence against faecal incontinence is permanently lost, our efforts must be directed to preserving the remaining function, i.e. the holding function of the colon. This can be

done by completely emptying the sigmoid colon by appropriate stimulation at regular intervals and by ensuring that the rectum is also completely emptied.

At a later stage a mild laxative is taken on alternate evenings – senna is as good as anything. The smallest dose which has been found to be effective is used; the best time to take the laxative is determined in each case by trial and error. The laxative should 'load the gun and take off the safety catch, but should not pull the trigger'. The final stimulus should be one which can be accurately timed and in most cases glycerin suppositories are suitable – they stimulate and lubricate; the time between insertion and evacuation of the colon is usually 10–20 minutes. Dulcolax (bisacodyl) suppositories are sometimes more effective but may take 1–2 hours to act. Other accessory methods of stimulation may also be used, the most important being the utilization of the gastrocolic reflex, abdominal straining or abdominal massage and rectal stimulation with the finger.

In patients with upper motoneuron lesions, when the rectum is filled from above it usually empties itself reflexly and completely, and in such patients digital evacuations are rarely required if the patient waits long enough.

In patients with lower motoneuron lesions, the sigmoid colon will still empty itself into the rectum when stimulated. Although the patient may be able to expel some faeces from his/her rectum by straining, in most cases some faeces are left in the rectum. As the anal sphincters are lax, there is then faecal leakage, so most of these patients need to remove some faeces digitally.

Having emptied the colon and rectum completely, the rectum should remain empty until the colon is stimulated again 2 days later. This is only a general plan. Every patient needs individual advice and much depends on previous bowel habit, neurological lesion and degree of motility. There are a number of things which can disturb this method of management, the most important of which is constipation. The method I have described depends on the delivery of a moderate amount of formed stool – neither too hard nor too soft – to the rectum. If a considerable length of colon is loaded with hard faeces, liquid faeces may be forced past the stale faeces and cause spurious diarrhoea. In such cases a faecal softener such as dioctyl can be given, followed by larger doses of laxatives and by enemas.

The second cause of failure may be due to a change of diet or activity. Patients confined to bed may need larger doses of laxative. This is probably due to inactivity rather than inability to sit on the lavatory. We attempt to teach most patients to have their bowels open on a lavatory with a padded seat, but this is largely for social convenience. I do not think that the sitting position is of great importance to the act of defaecation: lying on the side with legs flexed is also effective.

The results of adequate bowel training are most gratifying. It prevents ill health due to constipation and avoids social embarrassment. The success of the method is shown by the fact that, although the necessity to interfere with his/her own bowel function is at first distasteful and embarrassing to a new patient, very few patients who attend for check-up report any serious difficulty, and the colleagues and friends of most paraplegics are unaware that these patients have any dysfunction of their bowels.

Skeletal complications

In the early stages paraplegics are prone to develop contractures (described earlier) and para-articular ossification. In later stages they are prone to suffer from pathological fractures and Charcot joints.

Para-articular ossification

A small proportion (approximately 5% in our experience) of paralysed patients develop para-articular ossification. This starts as a hard swelling, usually within a muscle, and gradually develops into ectopic new bone. It occurs most commonly around the hip joint, but may develop in the lower end of the quadriceps or around the elbow or shoulder joint. If it is allowed to progress, it may form a complete extra-articular ankylosis. The joint itself is never directly involved.

While this condition may undoubtedly start at the site of a haematoma, the majority of paraplegics who develop haematomas do not develop para-articular ossification, and why it occurs in some patients is unexplained. Once the condition is suspected, an X-ray should be taken. Although in the first week or two it may show only a soft-tissue swelling, it then becomes radio-opaque over the next few weeks. Gentle passive movements usually prevent the development of a complete extra-articular ankylosis. These movements must be continued twice a day, 7 days a week, until the disease process becomes inactive. The degree of activity can be judged on clinical and radiological grounds and by the alkaline phosphatase, which is substantially raised during the active phase. Patients who have had para-articular ossification at one site are liable to develop it at other sites, either spontaneously or in response to soft-tissue injuries.

Pathological fractures

All paralysed patients develop substantial demineralization of their lower limbs and this process continues for 1–2 years after the onset of their paralysis. Subsequently the patients may fracture their lower limbs, either by falling from their wheelchair, or from some relatively minor trauma, for example when attempting to put on their socks. The fractures usually heal rapidly. We attempt to reduce the demineralization of the skeleton by regular weight-bearing. In patients with low lesions this is done by standing and walking with the aid of calipers; in patients with higher lesions regular use of a standing frame is recommended. We have not yet been able to prove conclusively that regular standing lessens demineralization or lessens the frequency of pathological fractures.

Charcot joints

These are liable to occur over a number of years whenever there is a discrepancy between motor and sensory function around a particular joint. The knee joint and ankle joint of patients with cauda equina lesions are particularly vulnerable if the patients walk with inadequate calipers. Charcot joints of the spine below the original fracture are quite common as a radiological phenomenon, but are usually of little clinical significance.

Spasticity

Some degree of spasticity is expected to develop in all patients where there is some remaining viable isolated spinal cord. Patients with complete lesions do not usually have such intense spasticity as those who have incomplete lesions. However, in some patients with complete lesions the spasticity is disabling in that it prevents certain activities being carried out without assistance. Spasticity as such should only be treated if it is inhibiting the patient's independence; a certain degree of spasticity and spontaneous movement is helpful to the patient's circulation and skin and, if the patients are taught to understand this effect, they will learn to accept spasticity as being beneficial and not evil or frightening.

If the spasticity is disabling, the following techniques may be used in attempts to treat it.

Positioning and physiotherapy

Careful positioning, as described above, will tend to cause a balanced and acceptable form of spasticity. Physiotherapy, in the form of regular passive movements, and standing are beneficial. Hydrotherapy in a warm pool (33°C) for periods of up to half an hour often causes temporary relief of spasticity, which enables the patient to become more active. Cooling a muscle with ice or cold water can also give temporary localized relief of spasticity, but this cannot be used for the whole of the lower part of the body as it would induce hypothermia.

Drug treatment

In general, drugs are only to be used on a temporary basis until other measures can produce some improvement.

Diazepam in doses ranging from 6 mg to 40 mg per day in divided doses has a definite effect on spasticity (Corbett *et al.*, 1972) but, unfortunately, it causes marked drowsiness and is unsuitable for patients who wish to drive cars.

Baclofen, 15–45 mg in divided doses, has also been used for spasticity, but the author has had less success with this drug. It also causes drowsiness and on occasions mental disturbance and hallucinations, both during its administration and when it is stopped.

Dantrolene sodium, starting with doses of 25 mg t.d.s. and gradually working up to 100 mg q.d.s., very often has an effect on spasticity; this drug works directly on the muscle fibres and in effective doses may increase the patient's weakness. However, many patients find they can compensate for greater weakness and gain benefit from the drug. The drug sometimes gives rise to a feeling of drunkenness, probably due to an effect on the muscles of speech, but most patients can overcome this side-effect with time.

Peripheral surgical procedures

Peripheral operations on tendons, in particular division of contracted hamstring tendons and lengthening of the Achilles tendons, may be beneficial. Obturator neurectomy is a relatively simple method of permanently abolishing adductor spasticity in the legs. Tenotomy of the adductors is often followed by wound infections, as is any operation in the groins of paraplegics. Division of the iliopsoas, either below the inguinal ligament or intraabdominally, is sometimes beneficial.

Surgical anterior rhizotomy gives permanent relief of spasticity, but because of the number of roots that require treatment it is a major procedure and is rarely carried out. Posterior rhizotomy is now rarely used but has been reintroduced by means of percutaneous radio-frequency rhizotomy. Intrathecal baclofen from an automated, implanted reservoir can give spectacularly good results in selected patients. This is an invasive procedure with a high risk of serious complications but can be justified in cases of intractable spasticity.

Injections

Injections of 6% phenol in water into motor points is successful in the right hands. Intrathecal alcohol abolishes spasticity completely but unfortunately causes further impairment of bladder and bowel function and increases the patient's liability to develop pressure sores. Intrathecal phenol can be given in a more controlled and localized manner, but the beneficial effects are rarely permanent.

Pain

The majority of paraplegic patients are pain-free. However, up to 10% of patients with closed injuries may suffer chronically disabling pains and the proportion is much higher when the spinal cord injury is due to a gunshot wound. Although the pains are of many different types they can be broadly divided into three categories: phantoms, root pains and hyperpathic pains.

Phantoms

These are analogous with the phantoms of amputees. The phantom sensations are not necessarily painful but are usually described as unpleasant. They usually manifest themselves well below the level of the cord transection, often in the feet, rectum or genitalia. Within a closed community like a spinal injuries centre, there are occasionally epidemics of particular types of phantom pain. There have been occasions when in one ward there were four patients with penile phantoms. They usually respond to explanation of the nature of the phenomenon. Very often the patient can be persuaded to think of the phantom as pleasant rather than unpleasant. Drug treatment with large doses of Tegretol and an antidepressant is sometimes successful.

Root pains

These are severe pains occurring in the segmental distribution, within anaesthetic segments one or two segments below the last intact segment. In patients with gunshot wounds they may start very soon after the injury; in patients with closed injuries they rarely start less than 2 months after injury. Patients who have complications such as pressure sores, which delay their mobilization for many months, are much more prone to these pains. We do not know the cause of the pains, or whether there is any abnormal 'electrical' activity in the stump of the cord. They are extremely difficult to manage and sometimes even major procedures, such as cordectomy a segment or two above the lesion or surgical or chemical division of the spinothalamic tract, may produce no improvement. Dorsal root entry zone (DREZ) lesions may be successful in certain patients. The most helpful measures are of a general nature, i.e. early, active mobilization and a full programme of rehabilitation, including physiotherapy, occupational therapy and sport. Mild analgesics are usually useless and strong analgesics are addictive. Tegretol and an antidepressant may give partial relief. The majority of patients can learn to tolerate the pains if they are well settled at home and in full-time employment. In a very small proportion of cases the rest of their life is a misery because of the pains. These patients typically provoke hostility and resentment in the medical and nursing staff as well as the other patients. The reason for this is not clear; possibly it is because we cannot stand the repetition of details and symptoms that we are powerless to alter, possibly some of these patients do have a different personality, and often in their preparaplegic history there is evidence of them having suffered from chronic painful conditions. I have no personal experience of electrical stimulation of the spinal cord to control these pains, but it is probably no more helpful than any other powerful placebo.

Hyperpathic pains

Some patients, particularly cervical patients, have hyperpathia or hyperalgesia in partially innervated segments of the border of their lesions. This is not usually a permanent phenomenon, but it can be very distressing, so the patient cannot bear to be touched, even by the lightest bedclothes, on that part. Occasionally regular freezing of the affected part with an iced spray or crushed ice gives relief.

Autonomic dysreflexia

The phenomenon has been extensively studied in recent years and has been reviewed by Frankel & Mathias (1976) and Mathias & Frankel (1988). It is a most interesting phenomenon which occurs in patients with high spinal cord lesions. In response to certain stimuli, the most important of which are bladder contraction, rectal contraction, ejaculation and skeletal muscle spasms, there is an intense vasoconstriction below the level of the spinal cord lesion. This results in a rapid marked degree of hypertension with compensatory bradycardia (the vagus nerves are intact in these cases). Associated with this, there is usually sweating of the face and neck, a mottled erythema of the trunk to just above the groin, dilatation of the pupils and, in severe cases, a throbbing headache. Blood pressure can rise to extreme heights – for example from 100/60 to 260/150 mmHg (13.5/8 – 35/20 kPa) within a few heartbeats of the onset of the stimulus – and very occasionally these acute episodes of hypertension cause cerebral haemorrhage. Autonomic dysreflexia is a non-specific warning of what would normally be a painful condition below the level of the lesion. The best treatment is to remove the cause, e.g. emptying a full bladder. In an emergency, the blood pressure may be reduced by the use of ganglion-blocking agents or with glyceryl trinitrate or nifedipine.

Special equipment

Almost all paraplegics require a wheelchair and at Stoke Mandeville Hospital we favour folding, self-propelling wheelchairs of the Carters/Everest and Jennings type. The vast majority of adult patients can be suited by either a standard wheelchair or a junior wheelchair, and a small number by a slim adult chair. For the majority of patients we recommend a 4-inch Sorbo cushion; only those who cannot lift themselves are provided with a gel, ripple or Roho cushion. A small number of patients who have used them for many years prefer to have the driving wheels at the front of their chair, but the vast majority have 24-inch driving wheels at the back with 7- or 8-inch castors at the front.

As a development of sports wheelchairs, new types of lightweight wheelchairs have been developed. These are not only lighter in weight but have a different 'geometry' which makes them inherently less stable but much easier to propel and control. As long as the patient has a good sitting position, these new wheelchairs are an immense improvement on previous models and are now favoured by almost all patients who can afford their considerable expense.

Electric chairs

Patients who are unable to push a wheelchair can be provided with an electrically propelled one. There is an immense range of commercially available wheelchairs, most of which are very expensive.

Cars

Most paraplegics can get in and out of a car unaided, fold up their wheelchair and pull it into the car behind them or next to them. They can drive a hand-controlled car, preferably with an automatic gearbox. Many of our young male patients enjoy changing gear, although the number of actions involved in declutching and changing gear is considerable. Surprisingly many tetraplegics, even those with complete C6 lesions, have learnt to drive cars and some have even passed the test of the Institute of Advanced Motorists!

The wheelchair and the hand-controlled car form the basis of the paraplegic's independence.

Calipers

For patients with lesions above L3, long calipers (not ischial-bearing), with lockable knee joints and built-in foot-raising device (usually backstops), are used. For patients with good strength in their quadriceps and no power in their hamstrings we prescribe a long caliper with an open knee joint but with a posterior sling to prevent hyperextension.

Sport

Sport for paraplegics was introduced by Sir Ludwig Guttmann at Stoke Mandeville soon after the Second World War. At that time darts, table tennis, archery, swimming and wheelchair polo were played, although the last sport was too dangerous and was replaced by wheelchair basketball. Many other sports have since been added, in particular wheelchair racing, fencing, weight-lifting, bowls and various field events.

It is our present practice to try to interest all new paraplegics and tetraplegics in some of the sports that are within their capacity. Not only is this beneficial for the physical exercise, but it is sometimes the first 'fun' for newly paralysed patients. It also aids their self-confidence and their reintegration into society.

Most patients do not continue with active sport at a later stage, but a few of them become interested in competitive sports and become extremely proficient, participating in regional, national, international and Olympic competitions. Apart from giving those chosen few some very enjoyable international trips, the International Stoke Mandeville Games and Olympics have had a profound influence on the attitude of society towards the disabled throughout the world. Indeed, when the

Para-Olympics were held in Japan in 1964, the Japanese set up a spinal injuries centre 2 years in advance of these games so that they would have some paraplegics who could compete! The Guttmann Sports Centre at Stoke Mandeville, together with the Olympic Village there, were named in memory of the late Sir Ludwig Guttmann, the Founder of the National Spinal Injuries Centre.

References

Bracken M.B., Shepard M.J., Collins W.F., Holford T.R., Young W., Baskin D.S., Eisenberg H.M., Flamm E., Leo-Summers L., Maroon J., Marshall L.F., Perot P.L., Piepmeier J., Sonntag V.K.H., Wagner F.C., Wilberger J.E. & Winn H.R. (1990) A randomized, controlled trial of methylprednisolone or naloxone in the treatment of acute spinal cord injury. *New England Journal of Medicine* **322** (20), 1405–1411.

Bransbury A.J. (1979) Allergy to rubber condom urinals and medical adhesives in male spinal injury patients. *Contact Dermatitis* **5**, 317–323.

Bromley I. (1985) *Tetraplegia and Paraplegia.* Churchill Livingstone, Edinburgh.

Corbett M., Frankel H.L. & Michaelis L. (1972) A double blind, cross-over trial of Valium in the treatment of spasticity. *Paraplegia* **10**, 19–22.

Frankel H.L. (1974) Intermittent catheterization. *Urologic Clinics of North America* **1**, 115–124.

Frankel H.L. & Mathias C.J. (1976) The cardiovascular system in tetraplegia and paraplegia. *Handbook of Clinical Neurology* **26**, 313–333.

Frankel H.L., Hancock D.O., Hyslop G., Melzak J., Michaelis L.S., Ungar G.H., Vernon J.D.S. & Walsh J.J. (1969) The value of postural reduction in the initial management of closed injuries of the spine with paraplegia and tetraplegia, part one. *Paraplegia* **7**, 179–192.

Geisler F.H., Dorsey F.C. & Coleman W.P. (1991) Recovery of motor function after spinal cord injury – a randomized placebo-controlled trial with GM-1 ganglioside. *New England Journal of Medicine* **324** (26), 1829–1838.

Guttmann Sir L. & Frankel H.L. (1966) The value of intermittent catheterization in the early management of traumatic paraplegia and tetraplegia. *Paraplegia* **4**, 63–83.

Mathias C.J. & Frankel H.L. (1988) Cardiovascular control in spinal man. *Annual Reviews of Physiology* **50**, 577–592.

Poole C.J.M., Williams T.D.M., Lightman S.L. & Frankel H.L. (1987) Neuroendocrine control of vasopressin secretion and its effect on blood pressure in subjects with spinal cord transection. *Brain* **110**, 727–735.

18: Rehabilitation of Progressive Neuromuscular Diseases

M. DE VISSER

Epidemiology, 240
Assessment, 240
Muscular dystrophies, 241
    Duchenne muscular dystrophy (DMD), 241
    Facioscapulohumeral muscular dystropy (FSHD), 242
Hereditary motor and sensory neuropathies (HMSN), 243
    Treatment, 243
    Prevention, 243
Spinal muscular atrophies (SMA), 243
    Natural history, 243
    Treatment, 244
    Prevention, 245
Motor neuron diseases, 245
    Treatment, 246
Post-polio syndrome, 246
    Treatment, 246

Neuromuscular disorders encompass all diseases of the anterior horn cell, peripheral nerve, neuromuscular junction and muscle. By far the majority of neuromuscular diseases are hereditary, manifest with progressive muscle weakness and are incurable. Only in a few neuromuscular diseases, such as myasthenia gravis, polymyositis and dermatomyositis, which are responsive, at least in part, to treatment, weakness may be reversible. After establishing the diagnosis, which is of great importance with regard to prediction of outcome and genetic counselling, treatment of the patient with a progressive neuromuscular disease should be initiated, preferably early in the course of the disease. In the absence of any effective drug treatment, physical methods of management are still the mainstay of treatment. Since neuromuscular diseases are relatively rare, the setting up of randomized control trials of methods of management is severely hampered. Brooke *et al.* (1989) advocated the use of natural history-controlled trials, which require fewer patients and proceed more quickly than randomized trials. So far, few aspects of supportive treatment, such as prevention of disabling contractures by stretching exercises, the use of leg braces and the optimal treatment of spinal deformity, have been adequately investigated, with the exception of patients with Duchenne muscular dystrophy (DMD) and spinal muscular atrophy (SMA). It is a common experience that therapeutic manoeuvres employed by physiotherapists to treat secondary disabilities, e.g. muscular pain or joint stiffness, are often beneficial. However, other special procedures, such as range of motion manoeuvres and muscle strength exercise, which are designed to improve strength and mobility, are poorly investigated. Nevertheless, physiotherapy and occupational therapy are always integrated in the overall management of the patient with a chronic neuromuscular disease. Many patients derive great psychological benefit from the close interaction with their therapist, not least because they are taught new ways of coping with disability. The rehabilitation approach may vary considerably from disease to disease and depends not only on the clinical appearance and the natural course of the disease but also on the pathogenesis.

Rehabilitation in a child with a severe neuromuscular disorder is based on the premise that, despite the briefness of the child's life, the life must approximate to normal as much as possible and be free of severe discomfort (Binder, 1989; Eng, 1989). *Mutatis mutandis*, the same holds true for adult sufferers from a neuromuscular disease. Counsel and support for the patient or the parents in understanding the diagnosis, and also its genetic implications, are of great importance. Organizations which are specifically concerned with the patients' interests may play an important role in helping the patients cope with their chronic disease.

Counselling is a continuous process. In diseases

with a poor prognosis, such as the severe form of SMA, DMD or amyotrophic lateral sclerosis (ALS), the problem of 'resuscitate' or 'not to resuscitate' has to be settled a long time before respiratory failure is imminent. In the same context, the patient or his/her family should be helped in choosing between the options of staying at home rather than being transferred to the hospital at the final stage of the disease.

This chapter will first deal with some general aspects of chronic neuromuscular diseases which are of importance for the overall management, followed by a discussion in detail of a few specific diseases: the common forms of muscular dystrophy (DMD and facioscapulohumeral dystrophy (FSHD)) and SMA (the autosomal recessive proximal form), hereditary polyneuropathies, ALS and post-polio syndrome.

Epidemiology

In considering the epidemiology of neuromuscular diseases, considerable variations in prevalences and incidences are often found in different studies. These variations in disease frequencies are not only the result of the use of different diagnostic criteria, but are also due to incomplete case ascertainment. A survey of the world literature on the population frequencies of various inherited neuromuscular diseases affecting children and adults has been carried out by Emery (1991). Such information may be valuable with regard to genetic counselling and also to the planning of strategies for the welfare needs of the handicapped people in the population.

Hereditary motor and sensory neuropathies (HMSN) are the most frequently occurring group of diseases among neuromuscular disorders (Table 18.1).

Assessment

Neuromuscular diseases are predominantly characterized by muscle weakness, which may result in difficulties with mobility and decreased functional capacity of the upper limbs but also, dependent on the distribution of weakness, difficulties with swallowing, chewing, speaking or breathing. In some diseases, involvement of extraocular muscles and, in particular, ptosis is so severe that the patient is functionally blind. Secondary complications may develop, e.g. contractures and scoliosis, which in themselves further incapacitate the patient. Other neurological deficits, such as sensory disturbances (e.g. in neuropathies), impairment of the autonomic nervous system (e.g. in Guillain–Barré syndrome and some neuropathies) and mental retardation (e.g. in DMD and myotonic dystrophy), may also contribute to the patient's disability.

Reliable neuromuscular assessment is needed to document the natural history of a disease and subsequently to determine the results of therapeutic interventions. Therefore, an evaluation system must be disease-specific. Traditional methods, such as the manual muscle test, clinical neurological examination and various rating scales, often include subjective elements and lack sensitivity and reproducibility. Functional testing uses daily activities to monitor disease progression and appeals to the patient, who appreciates improvement in function more readily than improvement in strength. However, limitations of functional testing are its lack of sensitivity and inability to detect a subtle change in muscle strength and the difficulty of applying standard statistical methods for analysis. Furthermore, a single test is often not appropriate throughout all stages of the disease. The same holds true for measurements such as manual muscle test and quantitative myometry, which become technically difficult to perform at some stage in the

Table 18.1 Prevalences and incidences ($\times 10^{-6}$) of the commoner neuromuscular diseases in the general population

	Prevalence	Incidence
Muscular dystrophies		
Duchenne	19.5–95.0*	97–311†
Facioscapulohumeral	2.2–66.9	3.8–26.0
Myotonic dystrophy	9.1–96.2	28.9–44.6
Spinal muscular atrophies‡	7.3–41.8	56.4–59.7
Hereditary motor and sensory neuropathies	14–282	—
ALS	10–70	4–18

* Prevalence in total male population.
† Incidence in total male population.
‡ Type I: severe Werdnig–Hoffmann disease; type II: intermediate; type III: benign Kugelberg–Welander disease.

course of DMD, ALS and SMA (Moxley, 1990).

Muscular dystrophies

Duchenne muscular dystrophy (DMD)

Natural history

Weakness is first evident in the muscles of the pelvic girdle and is noted when the child starts walking. In many cases, the first attempts to walk are delayed. Subsequently all skeletal muscles become involved, but weakness of the facial musculature, the sternomastoids, the intercostals and the diaphragm are relatively late developments in the disease. Brooke *et al.* (1989) have carefully documented the natural history of DMD in 283 boys who have been followed up to 10 years, using a protocol that accurately measured their function, strength, contractures and back curvature. A relatively rapid decline in function begins at the age of 6 or 7 years, ending in loss of (braced) ambulation at about 12 or 13 years. Scoliosis is a major problem in the clinical management of DMD. The development of a significant scoliosis before the age of 11 appeared to be rare. After the age of 11, approximately 75% of the patients developed a scoliosis, which rapidly deteriorated after the age of 13.

Analysis of the causes of death suggested that there were two different groups. There were some patients who had evidence of cardiomyopathy whose respiratory function was adequate, but the majority had evidence of respiratory failure in the months prior to death, with little evidence of impaired cardiac function. The mean ages of death were 14.7 and 16.7 years respectively.

Treatment

Numerous drugs have been initially thought to be beneficial but had to be discarded as worthless after careful evaluation. However, in a natural history-controlled study, Griggs *et al.* (1991) showed that administration of prednisone was associated with definite improvement in strength, pulmonary function and functional ability. The therapeutic efficiency of a novel approach, i.e. potential replacement of dystrophin by injecting normal myoblasts into the muscles of patients, was poor (Karpati *et al.*, 1993).

The effects of supportive therapy (i.e. bracing, physical therapy and back stabilization) were also assessed in the study of Brooke *et al.* (1989). Stretching exercises together with bracing are commonly recommended (Dubowitz & Heckmatt, 1980; Kingston & Moxley, 1989). However, no positive correlation could be detected between the use of passive joint-stretching exercises and the prevention of contractures. Yet there was a significant correlation between the use of lightweight leg braces or night splints and the prevention of contractures. Comparison with a study published by DeSilva *et al.* (1987), showing that without using braces loss of ambulation occurs at approximately 9 years of age, suggests that bracing is an effective form of treatment. The additional time of 3 years prevents the development of severe contractures (Dubowitz & Heckmatt, 1980; Brooke *et al.*, 1989) and scoliosis (Rodillo *et al.*, 1988; Brooke *et al.*, 1989). Apart from this benefit, the use of orthoses enhances the child's mobility and independence (Dubowitz & Heckmatt, 1980), although it has also been argued that the wheelchair often provides much better mobility (Gardner-Medwin, 1977).

Tenotomy for release of contractures in DMD is of practical value in the context of fitting orthoses. However, Rideau *et al.* (1983) claimed a 2-year extension of independent braced ambulation in DMD by the use of radical surgery, including correction of Achilles tendon contractures and pes cavus, transfer of the tibialis posterior muscle to the dorsum of the foot, extensive tenotomies of contracted muscles around the hip and occasional transplant of the iliopsoas muscle to correct the forward pelvic tilt. These authors also claimed that early surgery in DMD patients between the ages of 4 and 6 years gave the children a normal gait and either stabilized or improved their function. In this context, the introduction of percutaneous tenotomies, requiring a short postoperative period (Siegel *et al.*, 1968), is considered an important step forwards since it is well known that in DMD immobility leads to loss of strength. Recently, Manzur *et al.* (1992) performed a randomized controlled trial of early surgical treatment in DMD. Although surgery corrected the tendo Achilles contractures there was no beneficial effect on strength or function.

Once the child becomes chair-bound, there is a

rapid acceleration of the contractures. Particular attention should be paid to maintaining a good posture of the ankles at 90° in the wheelchair. If the back cannot be kept straight by posture alone, a lightweight spinal brace can be fitted, although patient compliance is often poor (Brooke et al., 1989). Obesity can become a major problem in chair-bound patients and cause respiratory compromise, and therefore dietary management is needed.

In the study carried out by Brooke et al. (1989), the effect of back surgery (i.e. Luque procedure), which was usually performed in patients with a curve exceeding 35°, was assessed. In the majority, pulmonary function either improved or stabilized and only a few patients who had a low forced vital capacity of 1 litre or less showed a further decline and died. In contrast, Miller et al. (1991) demonstrated that segmental spine fusion had no beneficial effect upon decline of respiratory function. However, their operated group was somewhat more affected in terms of both respiratory function and spine curve. The advantages of spine fusion included improved sitting comfort and/or appearance, and resolution of previous back pain.

Respiratory muscle training in patients with DMD showed no benefit and may even be potentially hazardous, since the weak respiratory muscles may already be close to their fatiguing threshold (Smith et al., 1988; Rodillo et al., 1989).

Management of end-stage respiratory failure is still a matter of debate. Prolonging life with assisted ventilation has not been thought justified by some (Miller & Kakulas, 1986) and has been advocated by others (Bach et al., 1987; Kingston & Moxley, 1989; Heckmatt et al., 1990). Night-time intermittent positive-pressure ventilation via a nasal mask has proved to be very effective in the management of chronic respiratory failure (Heckmatt et al., 1990).

Among DMD patients, their parents and professionals, surveys have been conducted in order to explore the need and availability of life expectancy information and counselling. The majority of the patients and parents indicated that, in the overall management of the DMD patient, focusing on these aspects, particularly with regard to extending life by means of ventilator support, is of paramount importance, but that they seldom received it. Remarkably, most of the professionals stated that

the opposite was true, in the sense that they provided either short-term or long-term counselling (Madorsky et al., 1984; Miller et al., 1988).

Prevention

Since the Duchenne gene has been isolated at Xp21, deletions or, rarely, duplications have been found in over 65% of DMD and Becker muscular dystrophy (BMD) patients (Den Dunnen et al., 1989). The use of this molecular genetic technique and of restriction fragment length polymorphism linkage analysis and the application of immunocytochemical analysis to the gene product dystrophin in muscle greatly improved the accurate assessment of carrier status and made antenatal diagnosis possible (Ginjaar et al., 1991).

The clinical definitions of DMD (wheelchair-bound at the age of 12 or 13 years) and BMD (still ambulatory at the age of 16 years) are arbitrary, but genetic studies are beginning to yield new prognostic information. The nature of the mutation and the amount and size of dystrophin appear to be prognostic indicators for DMD and BMD patients (Bulman et al., 1991).

Facioscapulohumeral muscular dystrophy (FSHD)

The main features of FSHD are early asymmetrical weakness and atrophy of the shoulder girdle muscles, often preceded by facial weakness. Early in the course of the disease, the muscles of the upper arms and the foot extensors are affected. Subsequently, weakness spreads to the abdominal, pelvic girdle and thigh muscles, and to the wrist and finger extensors. FSHD runs a benign course, with only a minority of the patients becoming wheelchair-bound. Contractures and skeletal deformities are rare (Padberg, 1982).

Treatment

Although active exercise programmes are recommended and have been conducted in anecdotal cases (McCartney et al., 1988), there is no evidence for benefit in terms of improvement in function.

Operations to improve the function of the arm and the cosmetic handicap by stabilization of the shoulder have been designed for the FSHD patient with severe weakness of the scapular fixators but relatively strong deltoid muscles (Girolami *et al.*, 1990).

Prevention

FSHD is an autosomal dominantly inherited disease. Autosomal recessive cases have been reported but are poorly documented. Sporadic cases should always prompt the physician to make a careful examination of the parents, and one should consider the possibility of non-paternity. In the case of non-affected parents, the sporadic case may be a *de novo* mutant.

In 1990 the FSHD gene was mapped to chromosome 4q (Wijmenga *et al.*, 1990). Subsequent detection of *de novo* deletions in new FSHD patients has proved to be useful for diagnostic purposes (Wijmenga *et al.*, 1992).

Hereditary motor and sensory neuropathies (HMSN)

HMSN are characterized by slowly progressive weakness and wasting and mild sensory loss, predominantly in the distal muscles of the legs and the feet, and, only at a later stage, also in the lower arms and the hands. Foot deformities, e.g. pes cavus, are a hallmark of the disease. Specific foot complaints include pain under the metatarsal heads, claw toes, foot fatigue and difficulty in fitting regular shoes.

Onset is mostly in (early) childhood or adolescence. There are seven different types of HMSN divided on the basis of pathology, pattern of inheritance or associated features (Dyck *et al.*, 1993). The most common types are HMSN I and II.

Treatment

In patients with mild foot involvement, properly fitting shoes or boots or orthotic aids can be effective (Alexander & Johnson, 1989). The efficacy of stretching exercises for flexible deformities has never been proved.

If conservative treatment is insufficient, surgical management of the cavus foot, tailored to the individual patient, should be considered. Various surgical techniques, such as tendon lengthening, transfer or occasionally tenotomy, but often also

osteotomies and arthrodeses, are carried out in an attempt to correct alignment and alleviate symptoms. Evaluation of long-term results of various surgical procedures showed variable results. A satisfactory outcome following soft-tissue procedures which can postpone the need for triple arthrodesis has been reported (Roper & Tibrewal, 1989). Analysis of the results of triple arthrodesis were controversial. Wetmore & Drennan (1989) observed an unsatisfactory outcome in nearly half of their patients, whereas Wukich & Bowen (1989) claimed that 86% of their patients were satisfied with their result. However, these reviews were retrospective and consequently have their limitations. Prospective natural history-controlled trials have not yet been conducted.

Prevention

HMSN types I and II usually follow an autosomal dominant trait. There is marked variability of expression of the gene and therefore, in the case of genetic counselling, individuals at risk with dubious clinical abnormalities should also be examined electrophysiologically.

In the autosomal dominant demyelinating form of HMSN, type I, a duplication is found on chromosome 17 which is considered to be the mutation responsible for the disease (Raeymaekers *et al.*, 1991). The presence of the duplication in an individual establishes the diagnosis. However, its absence does not necessarily indicate that the individual is not a heterozygote, since linkage to chromosome 1 has been found in certain autosomal dominant HMSN I families. Furthermore, there are forms of HMSN with another mode of inheritance which have a similar phenotype.

Spinal muscular atrophies (SMA)

Natural history

SMA is characterized by muscle weakness caused by degeneration of anterior horn cells. Although there are many different forms of SMA, the most common condition is the autosomal recessive proximal form of SMA. The distribution of weakness tends to be symmetrical and to affect the proximal muscles of the limbs more than the distal and the lower limbs more than the upper. Depending on severity, the bulbar, axial and intercostal muscles can also be affected, whereas the facial muscles, the extraocular muscles and the diaphragm tend to be spared. Classification has been a matter of debate for decades and will only be settled when the gene(s) involved have been identified. A simple classification based on clinical severity has been proposed by Dubowitz (1978):

1 *Severe SMA*. Infant unable to sit unsupported.

2 *Intermediate SMA*. Infant achieves ability to sit unaided, but is unable to stand or walk unaided.

3 *Mild SMA*. Child achieves ability to stand and walk unaided.

Studies on linkage analysis (Brzustowicz *et al.*, 1990; Gilliam *et al.*, 1990; Melki *et al.*, 1990a,b) have revealed that it seems likely that all the cases of classical autosomal recessive proximal SMA of infancy and childhood, of varying severity, conform to a single gene at locus 5q, comparable with the dystrophin gene responsible for both DMD and BMD. Thus, it is suggested that there might be a continuum between the severe infantile form at the one end and the mild juvenile form at the other end. However, the important issue of intrafamilial heterogeneity remains to be clarified. Therefore, from the point of view of prognosis and management, clinical classification is still important.

The severe form (also called Werdnig–Hoffmann disease), which usually has its onset *in utero* or in the first months after birth, is characterized by severe weakness of the legs and arms, marked trunk and intercostal weakness, hypotonia and poor head control. Swallowing dysfunction becomes more obvious as the weakness progresses. The prognosis is poor and the majority of these infants will die within the first year of life as a result of pneumonia.

The intermediate type has its onset within the period of 6 to 12 months of age. Initially, the child may appear normal, but the child never acquires the ability to stand or walk unsupported. The prognosis is variable and depends on the degree of respiratory deficit.

The mild type (Kugelberg–Welander disease) has its onset after the age of 18 months following a period of normal walking. The prognosis is relatively good, and many will survive well into adult life.

Associated characteristic clinical features include fasciculations, particularly visible in the tongue,

and tremor of the fingers in the intermediate and mild forms. All children with the intermediate form of SMA and the patients with the mild form who have stopped walking develop progressive kyphoscoliotic deformity, which further impairs their functional ability, respiratory function and cosmetic appearance.

Respiratory problems either are restrictive or arise from bronchopulmonary congestion with obstruction (Rideau *et al.*, 1989). The severity of the restrictive syndrome is highly variable and probably related to the spinal deformity. Once the initial phase of the disease is complete, there is often a prolonged stable phase (plateau phase) in the curve of the total vital capacity, which can be explained by a stable diaphragmatic function (Rideau & Delaubier, 1988). This is in sharp contrast with DMD, in which the plateau phase is brief. Bronchopulmonary congestion with obstruction can be explained by the absence of effective coughs, which is, at least partially, related to weakness of the abdominal muscles.

Dubowitz (1989) stresses that the apparent nonprogressive nature of the condition following the initial onset is a striking feature of, especially, the intermediate and mild form. This is at variance with the results of a retrospective analysis of 56 patients with SMA, showing that there was progression in all patients (Russman *et al.*, 1983). Since retrospective reviews are fraught with potential errors, a co-operative study has been initiated to study the natural history in SMA. Although manual muscle testing and functional testing were very useful in delineating the natural history in DMD, it appeared not to be very sensitive for testing strength in very weak, non-ambulatory patients with chronic SMA. Quantitative muscle testing, using a fixed myometric system, provided greater sensitivity (Dallas–Cincinnati–Newington Spinal Muscular Atrophy Study Group, 1990a,b). A recent prospective, collaborative study by Russman *et al.* (1992) in which 37 patients with SMA were evaluated over an 18 months period showed that none had lost strength, but four had lost function.

Treatment

Therapeutic trials are only useful after the natural history of the disease has been defined.

Rehabilitation of the child with a severe form of SMA is mainly directed to encouragement of the parents to develop a level of comfort in nurturing, feeding and providing mobility for an otherwise immobile child (Eng, 1989). Proper feeding, sometimes with supplemental nasogastric drip, is needed to maintain an adequate nutritional status. Suctioning prior to feeding or postural drainage in case of increased secretions may be helpful. The child should be placed lying on his/her side in the midst of family activity and passive range-of-motion exercises should be executed on all extremities in order to prevent painful joint stiffness.

From a rehabilitation point of view, most of the efforts have been concentrated on the patients with the intermediate form. With adequate orthotic help in terms of early fitting of lightweight knee–ankle–foot orthoses with ischial support and releasing knee joint, unsupported standing or even independent ambulation may be achieved (Granata et al., 1989). Furthermore, orthoses have also proved to be effective in preventing contractures and scoliosis. For children who have achieved independent standing posture but not walking, the swivel walker is a good device. The best age to fit a child with orthoses is under 2 years since the prerequisite for fitting is the absence of contractures (Granata et al., 1989). When children with intermediate SMA begin to sit, their backs become kyphotic and subsequently a scoliotic curve develops, usually between 2 and 4 years of age. In spite of the continuous daily use of a spinal brace, the spinal deformity progresses (Lonstein, 1989). Scoliosis shows the same progression in patients with the Kugelberg–Welander type of SMA who stopped walking because of progressive muscle weakness of the lower limbs. Since non-operative treatment does not arrest the progression of scoliosis, surgical stabilization has to be the definitive treatment. After a careful preoperative assessment, including an extensive pulmonary work-up, spinal fusion is performed at the onset of the adolescent growth spurt. The aims of surgical treatment are to prevent progression of the deformity, rebalancing the head and the trunk on the pelvis and making a sitting position possible, and to slow down the deterioration of respiratory function related to progression of the deformity. The Luque method is considered to be the method of choice, as satisfac-

tory correction is obtained without requiring postoperative immobilization (Cervellati et al., 1989).

Prevention

There are now several microsatellite markers on either side of the SMA gene enabling the pre-natal diagnosis of the disease in most families with 79% accuracy (Morrison et al., 1993). However, the question of clinical heterogeneity remains to be solved, not only in terms of prognosis, but also because the mode of inheritance may not always be purely autosomal recessive (Müller & Clerget-Darpoux, 1991).

Motor neuron diseases

Motor neuron diseases (MND) are characterized by progressive loss of upper and/or lower motor neurons, leading to deficits in voluntary motor function. MND encompass several different syndromes, depending on clinical signs. SMA is designated by signs of lower MND only and manifested by limb weakness and wasting, regardless of whether cranial muscles are affected. Progressive bulbar palsy is dominated by weakness of cranial muscles of the lower motor neuron type. ALS is characterized by both upper and lower motor neuron signs. Primary lateral sclerosis designates a syndrome manifest by pyramidal features alone. There are still debates about terminology. SMA and ALS may actually be different diseases but, on the one hand, patients may never show upper motor neuron signs clinically and none the less at autopsy the corticospinal tracts appear to be affected, whereas, on the other hand, in post-mortem series cases of pure motor neuron degeneration are equally rare. In most series ALS is the most common form of MND, followed by SMA and bulbar palsy. We will confine ourselves to ALS in this section.

The major symptoms of ALS are due to weakness. Limb weakness and wasting may first be evident in the arms, in the legs or in all limbs simultaneously. Weakness may be asymmetric at first, but ultimately all limbs are involved. Involvement of cranial muscles is essentially restricted to dysphagia and dysarthria and may be due to bulbar or pseudo-bulbar palsy or both; facial weakness may be

present but is rarely symptomatic. Mastication is
affected late, and oculomotor weakness only occurs
in long survivors who have been on a respirator
(Mizutani *et al.*, 1990). Respiratory muscles are
usually affected late in the disease, although some
patients may present with acute respiratory insufficiency (Norris *et al.*, 1987). Fasciculations may not
be seen clinically or may be (very) active. The
disease is inexorably progressive, and the mean
duration is about 3 years. Death is almost always
due to pulmonary complications of respiratory
muscle weakness and/or bulbar paralysis.

Using a reliable and valid testing protocol, the
Tuft quantitative neuromuscular examination,
which investigates the pulmonary function, oro-
pharyngeal function, timed functional activities and
isometric strength, the natural history of ALS was
defined (Munsat *et al.*, 1988). It was observed that
the rate of motoneuron loss was linear. Bulbar
function deteriorated more slowly than respiratory,
arm and leg function. The loss of leg strength was
slower than in the arm. There was no correlation
between age at onset and rate of deterioration or
different regions of onset. Considerable variance in
deterioration rate was found between individuals.

Treatment

Various drug trials have been carried out but most
of these studies showed no significant efficacy.

Despite the lack of curative therapy, great progress has been made in the development of technologies to assist patients with ALS. Elaborate
devices for communication, orthotic aids, wheelchairs with various modifications and refinement
of surgical procedures such as percutaneous gastrostomy can do a great deal to enhance the patient's
autonomy and increase his quality of life (Norris *et
al.*, 1987; Sinaki, 1987). Occupational therapists
can be of great help to these patients by assisting
them to learn the use and application of various
assistive devices for independence in self-care.

In considering any form of symptomatic treatment, one should always keep in mind that there
has to be an equilibrium between improvement in
the quality of life and the unnecessary prolongation
of suffering.

Respiratory support with a cuirass and negative-
pressure ventilation may provide considerable

subjective improvement in sleep and exercise tolerance and relief of daytime fatigue, orthopnoea and
morning headache in patients with symptoms
due to respiratory muscle weakness in the absence of severe bulbar impairment (Howard *et al.*,
1989). Invasive respiratory support will frequently
lead to ventilator dependence and is therefore
controversial.

Post-polio syndrome

The post-polio syndrome becomes symptomatic at
least 15 years after the original attack of poliomyelitis anterior acuta. After a variable degree of
recovery, there is a period of stabilization during
which patients are fully active. Then, insidiously,
they begin to experience new difficulties, such as
weakness, loss of muscle bulk, fatigue, decreased
functional ability or pain. These symptoms are
usually observed in muscles that had been previously affected. The post-polio syndrome runs a
slowly progressive course, but, in patients who
have been left with a considerable handicap
after the original attack, minor changes in muscle
strength may markedly decrease their functional
abilities. However, an evaluation of a proportion of
a cohort of subjects who had well-documented
paralytic polio in Olmsted County, Minnesota,
revealed that the number of individuals requiring
major lifestyle changes is small (Windebank *et al.*,
1991).

The pathogenesis has not yet been elucidated,
but clinical, morphological and electrophysiological
data support the hypothesis that the syndrome
is caused by deterioration of an overworked and
enlarged motor unit. A retrospective study on the
potential risk factors for the development of new
muscle weakness revealed a significant relationship
between functional recovery from poliomyelitis
and the risk of subsequently developing post-polio
syndrome (Klingman *et al.*, 1988).

Epidemiological data about the frequency of the
post-polio syndrome are as yet based on estimates
in the US and vary from 22 to 87% (Halstead &
Rossi, 1985; Cosgrove *et al.*, 1987).

Treatment

The role of exercise is controversial. On the one
hand, believers in the 'overworked motor unit'

theory are of the opinion that muscles that are already being used extensively in normal activities of daily living should not be stressed further (Maynard, 1985). On the other hand, it was demonstrated that training programmes were capable of producing an increase in strength in previously affected muscles (Einarsson, 1991). Patients experiencing the late sequelae of polio usually feel better when they reduce their daily activities in terms of modifying work or home environments. In some patients, increasing weakness forces them to use assistive devices such as a cane, orthotic aids, or even a wheelchair in order to continue to perform their most valued daily activities. The key to successful lifestyle modification is education of the patient in energy conservation.

References

Alexander I.J. & Johnson K.A. (1989) Assessment and management of pes cavus in Charcot–Marie–Tooth disease. *Clinical Orthopaedics and Related Research* **246**, 273–281.

Bach J.R., O'Brien J., Krotenberg R. & Alba A.S. (1987) Management of end stage respiratory failure in Duchenne muscular dystrophy. *Muscle and Nerve* **10**, 177–182.

Binder H. (1989) New ideas in the rehabilitation of children with spinal muscular atrophy. In Merlini L., Granata C. & Dubowitz V. (eds) *Current Concepts in Childhood Spinal Muscular Atrophy*, pp. 117–125. Springer-Verlag, Vienna.

Brooke M.H., Fenichel G.M., Griggs R.C. *et al.* (1989) Duchenne muscular dystrophy: patterns of clinical progression and effects of supportive therapy. *Neurology* **39**, 475–481.

Brzustowicz L.M., Lehner T., Castilla L.H. *et al.* (1990) Genetic mapping of chronic childhood-onset spinal muscular atrophy to chromosome 5q11.2–13.3. *Nature* **344**, 540–541.

Bulman D.E., Murphy E.G., Zubrzycka-Gaarn E.E., Worton R.G. & Ray P.N. (1991) Differentiation of Duchenne and Becker muscular dystrophy phenotypes with amino- and carboxy-terminal antisera specific for dystrophin. *American Journal of Human Genetics* **48**, 295–304.

Cervellati S., Palmisani M., Bonfigliolo S. & Savini R. (1989) Surgical treatment of scoliosis in spinal muscular atrophy. In Merlini L., Granata C. & Dubowitz V. (eds) *Current Concepts in Childhood Spinal Muscular Atrophy*, pp. 175–192. Springer-Verlag, Vienna.

Cosgrove J.L., Alexander M.A., Kitts E.L., Swan B.E., Klein M.J. & Bauer R.E. (1987) Late effects of polio-myelitis. *Archives of Physical Medicine and Rehabilitation* **68**, 5–7.

Dallas–Cincinnati–Newington Spinal Muscular Atrophy (DCN-SMA) Study Group (1990a) A methodology to measure the strength of SMA patients. *Muscle and Nerve* Suppl. 13, S7–S10.

Dallas–Cincinnati–Newington Spinal Muscular Atrophy (DCN-SMA) Study Group (1990b) Sensitivity of the DCN-SMA Study Group methodology. *Muscle and Nerve* Suppl. 13, S13–S15.

Den Dunnen J.T., Grootscholten P.M., Bakker E. *et al.* (1989) Topography of the Duchenne muscular dystrophy (DMD) gene: FIGE and cDNA analysis of 194 cases reveals 115 deletions and 13 duplications. *American Journal of Human Genetics* **45**, 835–847.

DeSilva S., Drachman D.B., Mellits D. & Kuncl R.W. (1987) Prednisone treatment in Duchenne muscular dystrophy: long term benefit. *Archives of Neurology* **44**, 818–822.

Dubowitz V. (1978) *Muscle Disorders in Childhood*, pp. 149–156. W.B. Saunders, Philadelphia.

Dubowitz V. (1989) The clinical picture of spinal muscular atrophy. In Merlini L., Granata C. & Dubowitz V. (eds) *Current Concepts in Childhood Spinal Muscular Atrophy*, pp. 13–19. Springer-Verlag, Vienna.

Dubowitz V. & Heckmatt J. (1980) Management of muscular dystrophy: pharmacological and physical aspects. *British Medical Bulletin* **36**, 139–144.

Dyck P.J., Chance P., Lebo R. & Carney J.A. (1993) Hereditary motor and sensory neuropathies. In Dyck P.J. *et al.* (eds) *Peripheral Neuropathy*, pp. 1094–1136. W.B. Saunders, Philadelphia.

Einarsson G. (1991) Muscle conditioning in late poliomyelitis. *Archives of Physical Medicine and Rehabilitation* **72**, 11–14.

Emery A.E.H. (1991) Population frequencies of inherited neuromuscular disorders – a world survey. *Neuromuscular Disorders* **1**, 19–29.

Eng G.D. (1989) Rehabilitation of the child with a severe form of spinal muscular atrophy (type I, infantile or Werdnig–Hoffmann disease). In Merlini L., Granata C. & Dubowitz V. (eds) *Current Concepts in Childhood Spinal Muscular Atrophy*, pp. 113–115. Springer-Verlag, Vienna.

Gardner-Medwin D. (1977) Objectives in the management of Duchenne muscular dystrophy. *Israel Journal of Medical Sciences* **13**, 229–234.

Gilliam T.C., Brzustowicz L.M., Castilla L.H. *et al.* (1990) Genetic homogeneity between acute and chronic forms of spinal muscular atrophy. *Nature* **345**, 823–825.

Ginjaar I.B., Soffers S., Moorman A.F.M. *et al.* (1991) Fetal dystrophin to diagnose carrier status. *Lancet* **ii**, 258–259.

Girolami M., Merlini L., Ballestrazzi A., Granata C. & Giannini S. (1990) New technique of fixation of the scapula in facioscapulohumeral muscular dystrophy

(FSH). *Journal of the Neurological Sciences* **98** (Suppl.), 428.

Granata C., Magni E., Sabattini L., Colombo C. & Merlini L. (1989) Promotion of ambulation in intermediate spinal muscular atrophy. In Merlini L., Granata C. & Dubowitz V. (eds) *Current Concepts in Childhood Spinal Muscular Atrophy*, pp. 127–132. Springer-Verlag, Vienna.

Griggs R.C., Moxley R.T. III, Mendell J.R., Fenichel G.M., Brooke M.H., Pestronk A., Miller J.P. and the Clinical Investigation of Duchenne Dystrophy Group (1991) Prednisone in Duchenne dystrophy: a randomized, controlled trial defining the time course and dose response. *Archives of Neurology* **48**, 383–388.

Halstead L.S. & Rossi C.D. (1985) New problems in old polio patients: result of a survey of 539 polio survivors. *Orthopaedics* **8**, 845–850.

Heckmatt J.Z., Loh L. & Dubowitz V. (1990) Night-time nasal ventilation in neuromuscular disease. *Lancet* **i**, 579–582.

Howard R.S., Wiles C.M. & Loh L. (1989) Respiratory complications and their management in motor neuron disease. *Brain* **112**, 1155–1170.

Karpati G., Ajdukovic D., Arnold D. *et al.* (1993) Myoblast transfer in Duchenne muscular dystrophy. *Annals of Neurology* **34**, 8–17.

Kingston W.J. & Moxley R.T. (1989) Treatment of muscular dystrophies. *General Pharmacology* **20**, 263–268.

Klingman J., Chui H., Corgiat M. & Perry J. (1988) Functional recovery: a major risk for the development of postpoliomyelitis muscular atrophy. *Archives of Neurology* **45**, 645–647.

Lonstein J.E. (1989) Management of spinal deformity in spinal muscular atrophy. In Merlini L., Granata C. & Dubowitz V. (eds) *Current Concepts in Childhood Spinal Muscular Atrophy*, pp. 165–173. Springer-Verlag, Vienna.

McCartney N., Moroz D., Garner S.H. & McComas A.J. (1988) The effects of strength training in patients with selected neuromuscular disorders. *Medicine and Science in Sports and Exercise* **20**, 362–368.

Madorsky J.G.B., Radford L.M. & Neumann E.M. (1984) Psychosocial aspects of death and dying in Duchenne muscular dystrophy. *Archives of Physical Medicine and Rehabilitation* **65**, 79–82.

Maynard F. (1985) Post-polio sequelae – differential diagnosis and management. *Journal of Orthopedics* **8**, 857–861.

Melki J., Abdelhak S., Sheth P. *et al.* (1990a) Gene for chronic spinal muscular atrophies map to chromosome 5q. *Nature* **344**, 767–768.

Melki J., Sheth P., Abdelhak S. *et al.* and the French Spinal Muscular Atrophy Investigators (1990b) Mapping of acute (type I) spinal muscular atrophy to chromosome 5q12–14. *Lancet* **ii**, 271–273.

Miller G. & Kakulas B.A. (1986) Management of

Duchenne muscular dystrophy in Western Australia. In Dimitrijević M., Kakulas B. & Vrbová C. (eds) *Recent Achievements in Restorative Neurology. 2. Progressive Neuromuscular Diseases*, pp. 15–27. Karger, Basle.

Miller J.R., Colbert A.P. & Schock N.C. (1988) Ventilator use in progressive neuromuscular disease: impact on patients and their families. *Development Medicine and Child Neurology* **30**, 200–207.

Miller, R.G., Chalmers A.C., Dao H., Filler-Katz A., Holman D. & Bost F. (1991) The effect of spine fusion on respiratory function in Duchenne muscular dystrophy. *Neurology* **41**, 38–40.

Mizutani T., Aki M., Unakami M. *et al.* (1990) Development of ophthalmoplegia in amyotrophic lateral sclerosis during long-term use of respirators. *Journal of the Neurological Sciences* **99**, 311–319.

Morrison K.E., Daniels T.J., Suthers G.K. *et al.* (1993) Two novel microsatellite markers for prenatal prediction of spinal muscular atrophy (SMA). *Human Genetics* **92**, 133–138.

Moxley R.T. III (1990) Functional testing. *Muscle and Nerve* Suppl. 13, S26–S29.

Müller B. & Clerget-Darpoux F. (1991) Becker's model and prenatal diagnosis in proximal spinal muscular atrophy (SMA): a note of caution. *American Journal of Human Genetics* **49**, 238–240.

Munsat T.L., Andres P.L., Finison L., Conlon T. & Thibodeau L. (1988) The natural history of motoneuron loss in amyotrophic lateral sclerosis. *Neurology* **38**, 409–413.

Norris F.H., Smith R.A. & Denijs E.H. (1987) The treatment of amyotrophic lateral sclerosis. In Cosi V., Kato A.C., Parlette W., Pinelli P. & Poloni M. (eds) *Amyotrophic Lateral Sclerosis: Therapeutic, Psychological, and Research Aspects*, pp. 175–182. Plenum Press, New York.

Padberg G.W.A.M. (1982) Facioscapulohumeral disease. Thesis, Intercontinental Graphics, Hendrik Ido Ambacht.

Raeymaekers P., Timmerman V., Nelis E. *et al.* (1991) Charcot–Marie–Tooth neuropathy type 1a (CMT Ia) is most likely caused by a duplication in chromosome 17p11.2. *Neuromuscular Disorders* **1**, 93–97.

Rideau Y., Glorion B. & Duport G. (1983) Prolongation of ambulation in the muscular dystrophies. *Acta Neurologica (Napoli)* **5**, 390–397.

Rideau Y. & Delaubier A. (1988) Management of respiratory neuromuscular weakness. *Muscle and Nerve* **11**, 407.

Rideau Y., Delaubier A., Guillou C. & Mettey R. (1989) Respiratory rehabilitation in spinal muscular atrophy. In Merlini L., Granata C. & Dubowitz V. (eds) *Current Concepts in Childhood Spinal Muscular Atrophy*, pp. 133–152. Springer-Verlag, Vienna.

Rodillo E.B., Fernandez-Bermejo E., Heckmatt J.Z. & Dubowitz V. (1988) Prevention of rapidly progressive scoliosis in Duchenne muscular dystrophy by prolongation of walking with orthoses. *Journal of Child Neurology* **3**, 269–274.

Rodillo E.B., Noble-Jamieson C.M., Aber V., Heckmatt J.Z., Muntoni F. & Dubowitz V. (1989) Respiratory muscle training in Duchenne muscular dystrophy. *Archives of Diseases in Childhood* **64**, 736–738.

Roper B.A. & Tibrewal S.B. (1989) Soft tissue surgery in Charcot–Marie–Tooth disease. *Journal of Bone and Joint Surgery* **71B**, 17–20.

Russman B.S., Melchreit R. & Drennan J.C. (1983) Spinal muscular atrophy: the natural course of disease. *Muscle and Nerve* **6**, 179–181.

Russman B.S., Iannacone S.T., Buncher C.R. *et al.* (1992) Spinal muscular atrophy: new thoughts on the pathogenesis and classification scheme. *Journal of Child Neurology* **7**, 347–353.

Siegel I.M., Miller J.E. & Ray R.D. (1968) Subcutaneous lower limb tenotomy in the treatment of pseudohypertrophic muscular dystrophy. *Journal of Bone and Joint Surgery* **50A**, 1437–1443.

Sinaki M. (1987) Physical therapy and rehabilitation techniques for patients with amyotrophic lateral sclerosis. In Cosi V., Kato A.C., Parlette W., Pinelli P. & Poloni M. (eds) *Amyotrophic Lateral Sclerosis: Therapeutic, Psycho-logical, and Research Aspects*, pp. 239–252. Plenum Press, New York.

Smith P.E.M., Coakley J.H. & Edwards R.H.T. (1988) Respiratory muscle training in Duchenne muscular dystrophy. *Muscle and Nerve* **11**, 784–785.

Wetmore R.S. & Drennan J.C. (1989) Long-term results of triple arthrodesis in Charcot–Marie–Tooth disease. *Journal of Bone and Joint Surgery* **17A**, 417–422.

Wijmenga C., Frants R.R., Brouwer O.F., Moerer P., Weber J.L. & Padberg G.W. (1990) Location of facioscapulohumeral muscular dystrophy gene on chromosome 4. *Lancet* **ii**, 651–653.

Wijmenga C., Hewitt J.E., Sandkuyl L.A. *et al.* (1992) Chromosome 4q DNA rearrangements associated with facio-scapulo-humeral muscular dystrophy. *Nature Genetics* **2**, 26–30.

Windebank A.J., Litchy W.J., Daube J.R., Kurland L.T., Codd M.B. & Iverson R. (1991) Late effects of paralytic poliomyelitis in Olmsted County, Minnesota. *Neurology* **41**, 501–507.

Wukich D.K. & Bowen J.R. (1989) A long-term study of triple arthrodesis for correction of pes cavovarus in Charcot–Marie–Tooth disease. *Journal of Pediatric Orthopaedics* **9**, 433–437.

19: Rehabilitation of Peripheral Nerve Disorders

C.B. WYNN-PARRY AND J. COWAN

Neuropraxia, 250
Axonotmesis, 250
Neurotmesis, 251
Treatment, 252
Trick movements, 252
  Shoulder, 252
  Elbow, 252
  Hand, 253
  Leg, 253
Splintage, 253
  Median nerve, 253
  Ulnar nerve, 253
  Radial nerve, 254
  Leg, 255
Reconstructive surgery, 255
  Shoulder, 256
  Paralysis of wrist extension, 256
  Paralysis of opposition, 256
  Claw hand, 256
  Leg, 257
Brachial plexus lesions, 257
  Clinical picture, 257
  Treatment, 258
  Pain in brachial plexus lesions, 259
Re-education, 261
  Motor re-education, 261
  Sensory re-education, 261
Pain, 263
  Causalgia, 264
Electrodiagnostic techniques, 264
  Brachial plexus lesions, 266
  Root lesions, 266
  Facial nerve, 267
The future, 267

Peripheral nerves can be affected by a wide variety of diseases – infective, metabolic, immunological, toxic, malignant and heredofamilial.

This chapter deals with injuries to peripheral nerves. The classic work of Seddon (1972) describes three major types of disorder – neuropraxia, axonotmesis and neurotmesis.

Neuropraxia

Neuropraxia is defined as a temporary block to conduction, commonly due to pressure; electrical impulses, both natural and externally evoked, fail to traverse the damaged area, but there is no Wallerian degeneration. Electrical excitability is retained proximally and distally to the site of the block. If there is stimulation distally, there will be a motor response but little or no sensation. If stimulation is proximal to the block, there will be sensation but little or no motor response. There is no wasting and trophic lesions do not develop. It used to be thought that neuropraxia always recovered within 6 weeks, but now it is recognized that such blocks can be very prolonged. We have seen patients with compression of the ulnar nerve at the elbow with virtually complete sensory and motor paralysis which has lasted 18 months, but who have recovered almost full function within a few days of decompression.

Ochoa *et al.* (1977) have shown that compression blocks are associated with mechanical changes in the nerve such that a node of Ranvier is invaginated into the myelin sheath. Metabolic changes occur under the block and it is possible that ischaemia also plays a part.

Electromyographic (EMG) studies will help to demonstrate the block; the amplitude to supramaximal stimulation recording over a muscle supplied by the nerve will be markedly reduced above the point of compression compared with that below, and the mixed nerve action potential will be similarly reduced.

Axonotmesis

In axonotmesis, damage is more severe. The nerve sheath is intact, the axon cylinder disintegrates,

Wallerian degeneration occurs and regeneration takes place at a rate of about 1 mm a day in adults and 2 mm in children. As the internal architecture is maintained intact, little or no misrouteing of axons occurs and the functional result is nearly perfect.

However, in traction lesions of nerves, particularly the brachial plexus, there may be a considerable degree of torsion, with disorganization of the architecture of the nerve; cross-innervation and disordered function are then inevitable.

Axonotmesis usually follows a severe closed injury in which the nerve is crushed, e.g. paralysis of the radial nerve in a fracture of the midshaft of the humerus.

Neurotmesis

In neurotmesis the whole nerve is divided, including the sheath. Recovery is impossible without surgical suture. Each peripheral nerve has a special vulnerability to particular types of damage. Some common types are listed below.

1 *Median nerve.* At the wrist, such as a laceration due to a fall on glass, putting the hand through a window, suicide attempts, compression of the carpal tunnel by malunited or badly reduced Colles fracture, myxoedema, rheumatoid flexor tenosynovitis or idiopathic thickening of the transverse carpal ligament.

2 *Ulnar nerve.* Vulnerability at the wrist in falls on glass or putting the hand through a window. Prolonged pressure in the palm in carpentry, in dispatch-riders or in lorry drivers crashing their gears can damage the deep branch. It is liable to damage in fractures and dislocations around the elbow joint, either immediately or as the result of late deformity stretching the nerve in the cubital tunnel (tardy palsy), pressure by Osborne's band, occupational palsy due to prolonged leaning on the elbows, pressure of osteophytes in osteoarthritis and joint effusions or destructive change in rheumatoid disease.

3 *Radial nerve.* Temporary block is common when compressed over the arm of a chair – 'Saturday night palsy'. Axonotmesis is seen in midshaft fractures of the humerus when the nerve is compressed as it travels around the spiral groove and in dislocations of the shoulder, and also after too vigorous attempts to reduce them.

4 *Musculocutaneous nerve.* A rare lesion, but occurring in humeral fractures and in some cases of shoulder dislocation. It may coexist with traction lesions of the upper trunks of the brachial plexus and is thus difficult to diagnose.

5 *Axillary nerve.* This nerve is still sometimes referred to by the old name of circumflex nerve. The nerve is commonly involved in dislocations of the shoulder and in neuralgic amyotrophy (acute brachial neuritis). Owing to inadequate clinical examination, axillary nerve palsies can be diagnosed when the true disorder is a traction of the fifth cervical nerve root. It is surprising how often the wasting of the spinati is missed, although this should be confirmed with EMG if possible, because, if there is shoulder pain, there may be a reduction in bulk of these muscles as a result of disuse rather than denervation. Abduction and elevation are often possible in pure deltoid paralysis using trick movements (see below), whereas it is never possible if the external rotators are paralysed.

6 *Brachial plexus* palsies are considered in a separate section (see below).

7 *Femoral nerve.* This can be damaged in fractures of the femur or in organizing haematomas after direct violence injuries.

8 *Common peroneal nerve.* This is sometimes referred to by the old name of lateral popliteal nerve. The nerve is commonly involved in direct violence injuries to the knee, in dislocations of the knee and in too tight plasters in the treatment of fractures of the lower limb.

9 *Sciatic nerve.* This is easily damaged in dislocations and fracture dislocations of the hip. It is occasionally damaged during total hip replacement operations. For some reason, the lateral part of this nerve is particularly vulnerable. This results in a clinical picture that is identical to that seen in common peroneal nerve lesions at the head of the fibula.

All peripheral nerves are liable to damage by gunshot wounds, either by direct violence or by the cavitation effect of a high-velocity missile passing close by. Regeneration always takes longer and is often incomplete, owing to the considerable degree of intraneural fibrosis. Nerves are liable to pressure by intrinsic tumours (neurofibroma, schwannoma) or extrinsic factors (ganglia, lipoma) or tight bands. A whole group of entrapment neuropathies are now known, such as compression of the median in the carpal tunnel, the ulnar nerve in Guyan's canal at the wrist and by Osborne's band at the elbow, or the median nerve by the anomalous ligament of Struther's at the elbow or between the two heads of pronator teres. There are other such syndromes. A full review is given in Staal (1970). Some are so rare that their very existence can be questioned.

Treatment

If a nerve is divided, it must of course be repaired. In closed injuries, it may not always be necessary; for example, 70% of radial nerve palsies associated with fractures of the midshaft of the humerus recover spontaneously.

The decision to explore depends on a sound knowledge of the natural history of injuries associated with nerve lesions (Seddon, 1972). If a nerve is compressed, it usually requires release. The decision will depend on the degree of clinical involvement: sensory loss or wasting is almost an absolute indication for surgery. The aim is to prevent such a degree of damage, which may well be irrecoverable, by early surgery. Nerve conduction testing has shown that, if on stimulating the median nerve at the wrist and recording at the abductor pollicis brevis muscle the distal motor latency is more than 7 ms, surgery is indicated, as it is known that spontaneous recovery will not occur (Goodman & Gilliatt, 1961).

In many situations the EMG studies indicate a much more profound degree of nerve involvement than appears clinically. Serial studies will show if the lesion is progressive and if it will require urgent surgical treatment.

There are many principles governing the timing of surgical treatment and the type of operation that should be performed in an individual case. The subject is well discussed by Sir Sydney Sunderland (1991). Only a few points will be mentioned here. The sooner that a repair is made the better, given that the surgeon is competent and has the time to do a proper job, that the patient is in good general condition and that any complicating wounding of the tissues around the nerve lesion has had a chance to heal and that the risk of infection has passed. If the delay between injury and repair becomes greater than six months, the chance of a good result begins to lessen. On the other hand, good results

have occasionally been claimed for lesions repaired years after injury, so it may be worth operating late. The type of operation performed depends on individual circumstances. When the condition of the nerve ends is good, and where the ends can be opposed both without tension and without greatly flexing adjacent joints, end-to-end repair should be performed. Otherwise, nerve grafting should be considered.

Trick movements

In certain cases of muscle paralysis, other muscles can perform the movements normally carried out by those paralysed. They are worth careful study, for if one is ignorant of them one may be deceived into thinking the muscles are working when they are not. Moreover, absence of the typical trick movements in a presumed nerve lesion raises serious doubt as to the diagnosis. Finally, patients can often be taught to use trick movements for function.

Shoulder

In paralysis of the deltoid, the external rotators, in particular the infraspinatus, will rotate the humerus, allowing the clavicular head of pectoralis major to act as an abductor. The long heads of biceps and triceps, as they cross the joint, assist in the movement. It is very unusual not to be able to teach patients with deltoid paralysis in axillary nerve lesions to gain full elevation against considerable resistance. If the infraspinatus is paralysed (C5 root lesion, combined suprascapular and axillary nerve lesions), this action is not possible.

Elbow

Elbow flexion is still possible in paralysis of muscles innervated by the musculocutaneous nerve by using brachioradialis (radial nerve supply), and this can be a very strong movement.

In a C5, C6 palsy, all the usual elbow flexors are paralysed, but slight elbow flexion can sometimes be obtained by strong pronation, wrist extension and finger flexion. The long flexors and extensors and the pronator teres arise from the lower part of the humerus and, by contracting from their insertion to their origin, can flex the elbow joint. Just occasionally, this movement is strong enough to allow limited function. Its importance lies in realizing that the ability to bend the elbow does not mean that the biceps and brachialis (or brachioradialis) are necessarily working. The muscles must always be palpated in order to judge if there is a contraction.

Hand

In complete paralysis of radial or posterior interosseous nerves, it is always possible to extend the interphalangeal (IP) joint of the thumb, provided that the patient is allowed to abduct the thumb in the plane of the palm. This is because the abductor pollicis brevis and the flexor pollicis brevis both insert into the extensor expansion of the thumb. By applying a little resistance to the radial border of the thumb, the immediate attempt to abduct the thumb can be appreciated.

Sometimes powerful wrist flexion followed by relaxation can result in wrist extension and fool the examiner into thinking that the wrist extensors are working when they are not. It is a sure sign of a trick movement when the patient produces the opposite movement to that desired in an effort to obtain a rebound. Again, attempted finger extension results in flexion of the metacarpophalangeal (MP) joints, due to the action of the interossei pulling down on the extensor hood.

Ulnar nerve

When the patient attempts to abduct the thumb, the flexor pollicis longus substitutes for the paralysed adductor and the IP joint of the thumb flexes (Froment's sign). The long extensors can imitate finger abduction and the long flexors imitate finger adduction. If the patient puts his/her hand on the table palm down, raises his/her middle or ring finger and tries to abduct it, he/she will be unable to do so as the extensor is now fully occupied by keeping the finger in the air. Instead the whole wrist and hand move on the immobile finger – a very characteristic sign.

Median nerve

When the patient attempts opposition, the IP joint of the thumb is hyperflexed in an attempt to approximate the tip of the thumb to the finger tips by the action of flexor pollicis longus, which is spared in a lesion at the wrist.

When the patient attempts abduction in the plane of the palm away from the index finger, the thumb goes into radial abduction by the action of the abductor pollicis longus.

Leg

The knee can be extended in the presence of paralysis of the quadriceps (femoral nerve) by snap action of the gastrocnemius. We have seen a patient with poliomyelitis whose glutei and quadriceps were paralysed on one side who was still able to walk without sticks and only a slight limp by gastrocnemius action and strong contraction of quadratus lumborum raising up the pelvis.

In complete common peroneal nerve palsy it may appear as if the extensors are working when the patient makes a strong flexion movement in the toes and relaxes them – this is the rebound phenomenon.

Splintage

Paralysed muscles are liable to shorten due to overaction of the unopposed antagonists, and splintage may be necessary if deformity threatens. Much the most important reason for splinting is to provide function, and lively splints can harness some of the trick movements described to allow function.

Median nerve

Here one must splint the thumb so that it is held away from the index finger in palmar abduction. This can be either by a static opponens splint or by a lively splint in which a spring is placed at the MP joint of the thumb. This helps the flexor pollicis longus to oppose the thumb to the fingers. It also prevents the thumb from being held adducted against the index finger.

Ulnar nerve

Not all patients need splinting, but, if there is a marked hyperextension deformity of the little and ring fingers at the MP joints, then some device to

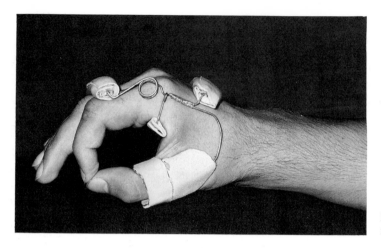

Fig. 19.1 Splint for combined median and ulnar nerve lesion.

prevent this is required. We use a splint which both prevents this hyperextension and allows active movements at the MP joints by a spring coil. As only a small palmar bar is used in this splint, the fingers are free for function. We prefer this lively splint to the static knuckleduster, which is too cumbersome and less effective.

In a combined median and ulnar nerve lesion, two splints are combined (Fig. 19.1). These lively splints are easy to make and are made in some centres by occupational therapists. They are cheap, easy to clean, comfortable, light and unobtrusive and patients really do wear them for work or hobbies.

Radial nerve

The dropped wrist is a serious bar to hand function, for the grip is weak in palmar flexion of the wrist. A lively cock-up splint is valuable, for this supports the wrist in dorsiflexion and by virtue of the spring at the wrist allows active movements. A spider attachment for the thumb and the fingers is used by a few patients in an attempt to provide some release of finger flexion into extension. Some patients find their function is perfectly satisfactory wearing a simple wrist support like the Futura splint.

There is no indication to splint the shoulder in abduction in deltoid paralysis. There is no danger of deformity and no one has yet devised a lively splint to offer active abduction that does not prove to be a gross encumbrance.

In paralysis of elbow flexion (musculocutaneous nerve lesion, C6 root palsy) when there is no trick action to provide functional movements, such as brachioradialis or a strong Steindler effect, a splint can be provided to allow the patient to fix his/her elbow in one of the four desired positions of flexion. It comprises an upper arm and forearm trough, joined by an elbow hinge with a ratchet which the patient locks him/herself. This splint thus puts the hand in the position of function. The splints can be provided in standard sizes which are altered to suit the individual patient and, within a few hours of fitting, the patient has mastered its use with the help of the occupational therapist or orthotist.

In C6 or C7 palsies where, in addition, there is paralysis of wrist extension, a cock-up piece is attached to the forearm trough. In total paralysis, a flail arm splint over the paralysed upper limb offers some function. It consists of the elbow splint already described to give variable fixed elbow flexion, which is attached to the upper limb by a shoulder support. On the distal end of the volar surface of the forearm piece is a platform into which are slotted the standard devices for an artificial arm. These include: split hook; pliers; dividers; and driving attachment. Operation of the device is by a harness around the opposite shoulder. The patient can then put objects into the attachments and use the splint as a support, leaving the other arm free.

Whether the patient has had reconstructive surgery to the plexus, such as grafting or neurotization, or whether spontaneous recovery is expected, any improvement will be slow. It will take months before even proximal muscle function can be expected. Recovery of nerve function can continue for 2 years. If the patient is not encouraged to keep the paralysed arm as part of his/her body image, he/she may become so one-armed that, when recovery does occur, he/she will not use it. The use of the splint does allow body image to be maintained and 70% of 61 patients splinted used their splints for work, hobbies or both. All found the support given to the shoulder to be valuable. It was cosmetically more acceptable than a flail arm (Wynn Parry, 1981).

Most patients whose arm has been amputated never use any supplied prosthesis. Few young men or women relish the loss of their arm and they dislike being seen with a stump on the beach or by the pool. We feel that the flail arm splint allows both function and retention of the natural limb.

If, in the future, giant strides in the design of artificial limbs are made, the above policy may be changed. In the meantime, we believe that amputation should only be offered if recurrent trophic lesions are a serious nuisance (and this is rare), or in some of the cases in whom there is great difficulty in learning to use the uninjured, non-dominant arm.

Leg

In a few patients with permanent paralysis of the quadriceps, it may be necessary to prescribe a calliper. The Stanmore cosmetic calliper is light, easy to apply and well tolerated (Fig. 19.2).

In sciatic or common peroneal nerve palsies, the dropped foot needs support. It is worth trying an ortholene (high-density polypropylene) orthosis which fits into the shoe. Often this will give enough stability to the ankle to allow normal function. Well-fitting boots may give extra support. If the ankle still gives way, a traditional iron calliper, fixed through the heel of the shoe, should be tried.

Reconstructive surgery

When paralysis is permanent, there are a number of surgical procedures which can offer excellent function. These are indicated, for example, when so much nerve tissue has been lost in an injury that nerve grafting is impossible, or when regeneration

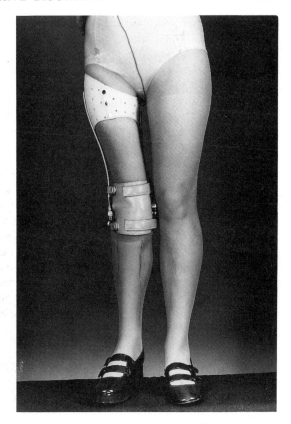

Fig. 19.2 Stanmore caliper for quadriceps paralysis.

has not occurred because of intraneural fibrosis or the lesion is known to be irrecoverable, as, for example, in avulsion of one or more roots of the brachial plexus.

The timing of these procedures is important. If it is known that recovery is impossible, the sooner the surgery, the quicker the patient can return to normal life. When recovery is possible, the time during which it may occur depends on the length of the damaged path. One day (and perhaps a fraction more) should be given for each millimetre, measured from the site of the lesion to the distal point of the normal nerve, before failure of recovery is diagnosed. During the period of waiting, functional splintage will allow the patient to return to work so that nothing is lost.

Surgical procedures can offer either stabilization of a flail joint (arthrodesis) or tendon transfer, which can be used to regain movement. The transfer of a tendon means that some of the original function of the tendon will be lost. Before embarking on such a procedure, a very careful assessment is made by physiotherapist and occupational therapist. This is made over sufficient time and in a realistic environment so that it can be established that the planned procedure will improve function and that the loss of transferred tendon function will not obviate any resulting benefit. These decisions cannot and must not be made in the clinic. Usually we admit our patients to our rehabilitation ward and spend 3 days on comprehensive assessment. Often a spell of intensive therapy, including time in the workshop, will build up more power in the muscles whose tendons are to be transferred, thus making the procedure more successful. No tendon whose power is less than 4− on the Medical Research Council (MRC) scale should be transferred. This is because a muscle will lose one grade of strength on transfer.

The effect of an arthrodesis can be imitated by applying a plaster of Paris and observing the patient's function. Both s/he and the medical team can then be convinced of the value of the planned operation.

Shoulder

Arthrodesis of the shoulder is sometimes useful. It is always necessary if elbow flexion is to be provided by transfer of pectoralis to biceps.

To restore elbow flexion, several procedures are available. If both the long and the short extensors are spared and strong, then the Steindler procedure is used. The origins of the long flexors and extensors are mobilized and reinserted higher up the humerus. If these muscles are unavailable, then the Clark–Brooks transfer is used, in which the pectoralis major is inserted into the biceps. The drawback here is that elbow flexion is accompanied by adduction, both because of the action of the pectorals as adductors and also because in brachial plexus lesions, which are the commonest indication for this operation, the external rotators are paralysed. In this event, if adduction is a bar to function, external rotation osteotomy of the humerus allows a more natural arc of flexion.

Whole-muscle transfer with its neurovascular pedicle has been used successfully, the latissimus dorsi being the most effective. The biceps is usually removed to allow room for the transfer.

Operations to restore shoulder abduction are disappointing, but occasionally the Zachary transfer can be valuable. The tendons of latissimus dorsi and teres major are inserted into the tendon of infraspinatus, thus converting internal rotators into external rotators. A full passive range of movement, an intelligent patient and an intensive rehabilitation programme are all essential if this operation is to succeed. Many patients feel that they can dispense with abduction, managing well with the normal arm, but just occasionally this procedure may make all the difference to a particular person with a particular problem.

Paralysis of wrist extension

In the pure radial nerve palsy with all other upper limb muscles spared, the standard procedure is flexor carpi ulnaris to extensors of fingers and thumb, pronator teres to extend wrist and palmaris longus to abductor pollicis longus.

If at least one of these tendons is unavailable for transfer, as happens in plexus lesions, then an arthrodesis of the wrist gives stability and releases a tendon for transfer to give active finger extension to release grasp.

Paralysis of opposition

In pure median nerve lesions, transfer is usually only indicated if the patient has some functional sensation in the median distribution. Otherwise, s/he is unlikely to use the transfer.

The best transfer is flexor sublimis of the ring finger. The tendon is taken round the tendon of flexor carpi ulnaris as a pulley and is inserted into the extensor expansion of the thumb. If flexor digitorum sublimis is unavailable, extensor pollicis brevis or extensor indicis can be used.

In a high median nerve lesion, when the flexors to the index and middle fingers are paralysed, these tendons are connected to the flexor profundus of the ulnar two fingers (supplied by the ulnar nerve) and produce a mass flexor action.

Claw hand

Dynamic transfers to correct hyperextension at the MP joints and to provide active flexion at those joints are disappointing – they usually act as a tenodesis. Zancolli's procedure is the simplest and in most cases the most effective. The volar plate is plicated, thus bringing the MP joints into slight flexion.

Leg

The most satisfactory reconstructive procedures are around the ankle. Arthrodesis of the hip or knee certainly offers stability in paralysis of these joints, but is a very major decision and may seriously impair the patient's comfort in daily life.

Transfer of tibialis posterior or peroneus longus to the insertion of tibialis anterior will correct the tendency to inversion or eversion and allow active dorsiflexion. A flail ankle can be made stable by arthrodesis.

Brachial plexus lesions

Trauma to the brachial plexus is an excellent example of a serious peripheral nerve lesion. It deserves special consideration.

By far the commonest causes of lesions of the brachial plexus are road traffic accidents, with motorcycle accidents forming the majority. Goldie & Coates (1992) found 254 cases in Britain in 1987, as a result of a postal survey. Using this information, Birch (1992) estimates that there are probably 300–350 severe cases a year.

Most are traction lesions, the plexus being stretched between its two points of attachment at the transverse processes of the vertebrae proximally and the clavipectoral fascia distally. If the lesion is very violent, there may be actual ruptures of one or more of the C5, 6 or 7 roots. Very violent injuries cause avulsion of the roots from the cord, and this is commonest in C8 and T1 roots, whose ligamentous attachments of the transverse processes of the vertebrae are much looser or even non-existent.

In most cases the traction is caused by sudden distraction of the neck on the arm as the body is thrown off the machine, while the arm tends for a fraction of a second to retain its hold on the handlebars. Pressure lesions can occur; drunk or comatose patients have been seen who have lain for many hours on their arm and suffered diverse degenerative lesions, but almost always these re-

cover nearly completely for there is no distracting force to cause intraneural fibrosis and the lesion is in continuity. Stab wounds and surgical errors cause clean division of the roots or trunks and should be repaired as a primary procedure and usually do well. It is traction lesions that cause the greatest problems in diagnosis and management.

The clinical patterns commonly seen in practice are:
1 Complete C5, 6 in continuity.
2 Complete C5, 6, 7 in continuity.
3 Rupture C5, 6; C7, 8, T1 in continuity.
4 Rupture C5, 6; avulsion C7, 8, T1.
5 Avulsion of all five roots.
However, all combinations are seen and two- or even three-level lesions occur – for example, rupture of C5, 6, avulsion of C7, 8, T1, and rupture of median and musculocutaneous nerves in the axilla.

The fact that the infraspinatus rarely recovers in plexus lesions may be due to damage to the suprascapular nerve round the suprascapular notch. In many instances, there are two, three or even four separate accidents. The patient is thrown off his/her motor cycle on impact and stretches the plexus. Next he/she hits the oncoming car and may further damage nerves or roots. Then he/she strikes the road, suffering further injury, and well-meaning bystanders may then inflict a fourth injury when moving the patient from the road.

Clinical picture

1 *C5 lesion*. Inability to abduct, externally rotate or elevate the arm.
2 *C5, 6 lesion*. In addition, inability to flex the elbow or to adduct the humerus.
3 *C5, 6, 7 lesion*. In addition, inability to extend the elbow, wrist, fingers or thumb.
4 *C8 lesion*. Paralysis of the finger flexors, some wrist flexors and sometimes the thenar muscles.
5 *T1 lesion*. Paralysis of all the intrinsic hand muscles.

Over 30 years ago exploration of the plexus for possible repair was given up. So much fibrosis was found that it was impossible to recognize nerve tissue from fibrosis, ruptures were rarely found and yet, despite these gloomy operative findings, reasonable recovery did occur in the upper roots. The work of Narakas (1977) has shown that ruptures are now much more common, occurring in up to one-third of cases – possibly because now that crash helmets are obligatory many patients with injuries so severe that they would have been killed without wearing a helmet are now surviving and we are seeing much more damage to the plexus.

This is important, for ruptures are susceptible to nerve repair, and return of function to at least those muscles supplied by C5, 6 and 7 can be expected. Repairs of C8 and T1 have a less certain prognosis as the time for regeneration is so long (up to 3 years) that muscle fibrosis occurs before reinnervation. It is significant that, in the series of one of the authors (Wynn Parry, 1974) of 134 cases treated without operation, one-third of upper trunk lesions did not recover and these may well have been ruptures.

The diagnosis is therefore important. We suspect rupture if the accident has been particularly violent (high speed with multiple injuries), if the lesion of that root is complete and if there is a strongly positive neuroma sign at the root of the neck referred to that root's dermatome. By this we mean that tapping causes painful tinglings, much more violent than the standard Tinel and definitely unpleasant. If the roots are avulsed from the cord, then the prognosis is hopeless and it is important to establish this early on. The diagnosis depends on the fact that in such avulsion injuries the posterior root ganglion remains intact and, although the patient has complete sensory loss in the distribution of that root, both the root and the nerve will still conduct an impulse. Therefore sensory conduction studies will show a response. If there is associated nerve damage more distally, as is quite common, the amplitude of the sensory action potentials will be lower than normal, but the detection of a measurable response in the presence of anaesthesia indicates a preganglionic component. These studies have replaced the histamine test, which relied on the axon reflex to produce a flare in a preganglionic lesion. If there is a complete lesion both proximal and distal to the ganglion, the electrical findings will be those of a postganglionic lesion and, taken on their own, underestimate the severity of the injury.

A Horner's syndrome indicates involvement of the sympathetic supply at T1 and therefore a lesion proximal to the ganglion. Myelography and mag-netic resonance imaging (MRI) scans show filling of root pouches due to tearing of the dura away from the cord. They are not completely reliable. In some cases they underestimate the severity of damage and, in other cases, recovery has been seen despite a positive myelogram. If the patient suffers intense, burning, crushing pain, this strongly suggests a preganglionic lesion.

If the lesion is a traction lesion in continuity (where there is neither rupture nor avulsion), then spontaneous recovery is likely and there may be less of a need for surgical exploration. Much depends on the experience of the surgeon. When expertise is less, the risk of damage to nerves and blood vessels as a result of the operation becomes important. When expertise is great, then the fact that the true state of affairs cannot be learned without exploration becomes a compelling argument. During an operation, a skilled individual can use direct stimulation of nerves to further assess the severity of a lesion.

In summary, the three types of lesion can often be distinguished as follows:

1 *Avulsion*. Very violent injuries; multiple injuries; severe burning crushing pain; Horner's syndrome (T1); complete lesion; retention of sensory conduction; positive myelogram.

2 *Rupture*. Violent injury; complete lesion; negative myelogram; absent sensory conduction; no Horner's syndrome; no pain; positive neuroma sign.

3 *Traction in continuity*. Mild or no violence; may be complete lesion – if surviving units are found on EMG or contraction is detected clinically, this indicates an incomplete lesion with an excellent prognosis (Wynn Parry, 1974); absent sensory conduction; negative myelogram; no Horner's syndrome; no pain; progressive, painless Tinel's sign.

Treatment

When there is to be an operation, accurate diagnosis will help in the planning of the procedure. The terminology used below follows that of Sunderland (1991).

If the lesion is in continuity, it is left alone. If ruptures are found, they are repaired directly or with nerve grafts. If nerve has been avulsed from muscle, neurotization (direct reimplantation of nerve into muscle) can be performed. If there is extensive loss of nerve tissue or a two-level lesion (C5, C6 roots and musculocutaneous nerve, for example), then grafting may be impossible. Nerve cross-grafting may then be indicated. In this, intercostal nerves and the spinal accessory nerves can be joined to the upper trunk, the lateral cord or the musculocutaneous nerve, using additional grafts when necessary.

If nerve repair is performed, recovery will be incomplete. One can hope for reasonable elbow flexion, shoulder adduction and perhaps wrist or even finger flexion. It is possible that repair decreases troublesome pain. The limited objectives of such operations must be explained carefully. The long time between operation and any functional improvement must be appreciated. Patients may fail to take advantage of a useful return of function because their outlook is dominated by a feeling of disappointment that recovery is incomplete and a determination to wait until there is further improvement before using the limb.

Birch (1992) has produced an excellent review of the results of different forms of surgery, based on his own extensive experience.

It is important to keep the limb in good condition, so that advantage can be taken of any recovery that occurs. The patient should be taught how to put the insensitive joints through a full range of passive movement, to prevent contracture. The care of anaesthetic skin must be learned. This can all be achieved during a short hospital stay. Out-patient follow-up is important to check that the patient is following the necessary routine and to reinforce morale.

When recovery begins, therapy is again prescribed, preferably in short intensive courses. Patients are given activities to continue with at home and goals to achieve.

Recovery may continue for 3 years for proximal and even longer for distal ones. Once this period is over, the situation should be discussed with the patient. There may be a place for reconstructive surgery. Stabilization of joints or tendon transfer can be considered. If these measures either are unlikely to help or are of limited success, a permanent splint may be the solution. If so, it is justified to make a special splint and incorporate refinements that would be unjustifiable as a temporary measure. A good example is a C5, 6, 7 palsy which shows only limited recovery with weak elbow flexion, no rotation or elevation of the shoulder, no recovery of wrist or finger extension and weakness of wrist flexion due to either C7 supply or partial involvement of C8. Neither a Steindler procedure nor tendon transfers for wrist or finger extension are feasible. A splint with a rotation element to allow positioning of the arm in variable rotation, elbow lock and a wrist dorsiflexion piece can be worn as a permanent orthosis. These splints are more expensive than the ready-made variety, requiring time and skill to produce, but are amply justified in such circumstances.

It used to be recommended that patients with flail arms due to avulsion of the plexus were best treated with amputation of the arm, arthrodesis of the shoulder and fitting of a prosthesis. Such a procedure was urged at an early stage before the patient became totally one-armed regarding function. This approach is no longer followed. Most patients with prostheses for brachial plexus palsy do not actually wear their arm (Ransford & Hughes, 1977), almost all becoming fully one-armed within 2 months, and such early amputation is unjustifiable as it is usually impossible to assess the exact nature of the lesion and the prognosis so soon after injury.

Pain in brachial plexus lesions

Avulsion of the nerve roots usually results in pain. It can be accompanied by one of the most distressing pains imaginable. The pain may begin almost immediately, but more usually 2–3 weeks after the injury. It is consistently described as burning, gnawing or gripping, and there are often severe tinglings like electric shocks. There may be stabbing pains. Often there is more than one kind of pain. In such situations, it is useful to ask the patient to describe which pain is the worst. The pain is usually consistently present, as a background. Many patients also experience periodic paroxysms of pain building up to a crescendo over many seconds, until they feel as if they are about to burst. During these paroxysms, they cannot continue conversations or activities. Some have paroxysms lasting minutes at a time and may have to retire to be alone. In some there is a regular pattern of crescendos, paroxysms and periods of increased pain, such that they can learn their particular pattern and adjust their activities to it. Strangely enough, pain does not usually waken them, although many use hypnotics to induce sleep.

Some patients have some sensation in a shoulder whose muscles are denervated. The resultant subluxation can be very uncomfortable. A sling may be of great help here.

In general, outside influences have little effect on the pain – quite unlike causalgia. An occasional patient does report that jostling of the whole limb can start off a cycle of pain. Few patients gain any relief from analgesics. Often such patients have been started on opiates in an attempt to help. The patient may become habituated to these drugs and, while realizing that the pain is no better, appreciates that he/she feels bad if the drug is rapidly withdrawn. Some patients do claim benefit from opiates, but close questioning often reveals that the drugs are probably working by inducing sleep – a form of oblivion.

When there is a stabbing component to the pain, carbamazepine may well be of value. This must be introduced at a low dose and should be increased gradually to a maximum tolerated level before giving up, otherwise an important opportunity may be missed.

Keeping busy in work, conversation, hobbies and sport seems to diminish the pain. An early return to work or training may be the only way to help the pain. Conversely, it is when the patient wishes to relax, at the end of a hard day that the pain is most troublesome.

Transcutaneous electrical (nerve) stimulation (TNS) helped pain in 50% of 52 patients. In all, there was some afferent impulse to modulate. The best example may well be one patient with total avulsion of C6–T1 with sparing of some of C5. Three months later, he was admitted to our rehabilitation ward where TNS was tried. Stimulating over the back of the neck at C3–C7 and the root of the neck, pain was substantially relieved after two treatments, and relief for most of the day followed regular use for 2 hours twice daily. In general, however, TNS is of greater value in patients with pain due to postganglionic lesions.

It is known that total deafferentation of a section of the cord causes the release of spontaneous discharges in the cells of laminae I and V in the dorsal horn some 10–30 days after section (Loeser et al., 1968) and it is presumably this mechanism that is at work. This fits with the central nature of the pain, unrelieved by external events, and the timing after injury.

Patients are demoralized and disturbed by this pain; they cannot understand how a totally anaesthetic and flail arm can be painful. Some ask for amputation, but this, of course, never relieves the pain. The pain is a result of the central nervous system damage that occurs when the roots are avulsed from the spinal cord. Patients are helped by a careful explanation of the cause of the pain, and by realizing that the pain is acknowledged and taken seriously.

Pain can be so distressing to the patient and his/her family and so worrying to the doctor that operative lesions to the central nervous system are considered. Thermocoagulation of the dorsal root entry zone (DREZ) of the spinal cord can be performed. This was modified and popularized by Nashold (Nashold & Ostdahl, 1979). Thomas (1988) found that about two-thirds of patients treated had useful pain relief. In many, the benefit is permanent, but we have seen patients in whom the benefit has faded at least 1 year after the procedure. Permanent side-effects, attributable to the DREZ lesion, occur in about 10% of patients.

Most patients either lose their pain after variable intervals or become so adapted to it that it no longer seriously affects their activities. It usually lasts at least a year; thereafter the proportion each year with severe pain lessens. Pain has ceased to be a problem in about 60% of patients with preganglionic lesions 3 years after the injury (Wynn Parry et al., 1987). A significant proportion of the rest find that pain has ceased to be an issue by 5 years post-injury, leaving perhaps 10% with permanent severe pain. Within these numbers, the term 'ceased to be an issue' is meant to include both those who no longer feel significant pain and those who are able to cope despite feeling significant pain. When patients with postganglionic lesions are included, then about 15% have severe pain 2 years after injury (Bonnard & Narakas, 1985). Birch (1992) believes that cross-grafting with intercostal nerves may result in a great reduction in pain.

Re-education

Motor re-education

During the stage of paralysis, while awaiting reinnervation, the patient is taught daily passive movements to keep a full range and given appropriate lively splintage to encourage maximum function. Apart from periodic review to ensure that joints are supple, splints satisfactory and the patient at work, no formal physiotherapy is required. We are not impressed by the case for daily electrical stimulation of denervated muscle to prevent atrophy and it has never been shown to affect the work output of muscle in man. All experiments have been either on animals or have used plethysmography as a judge of muscle bulk, and there are objections to this as a criterion of muscle function. One can have significant wasting with excellent power; bulk represents tissue fluid and fat among other ingredients. We have treated over 800 nerve lesions and have found that, when reinnervation occurs, muscle power and bulk return without the need for stimulation. When recovery is detected clinically, the patient should be encouraged to attend for a short period of intensive exercise to relearn the use of muscles that may have been paralysed for many months. He/she can continue these at home. Review should be frequent (2- to 3-monthly) and periodic short spells of physiotherapy and occupational therapy instituted to capitalize on recovery. Splints can be discarded as soon as function allows and once muscle power has returned to MRC grade 3. The best form of treatment is realistic occupational therapy chosen with a mind to the patient's work or hobbies. Carpentry, metal-work, gardening and printing with adapted handles are all popular with men and indeed with many women, but most women prefer household activities, typing, sewing and craft-work. For lower limb injuries, lathes and fretsaws can be adapted to provide progressive resistance. All types of games, both hand games such as blow football, weighted draughts, car race games (Wynn Parry, 1981) and gymnasium activities, can be encouraged. For nerve injuries in

the leg, progressive cycle rides, walking, circuit training and later football are useful.

Regular muscle strength charting on the MRC scale and measurement of maximum strength and stamina using spring balances or strain gauges are valuable as a check on progress both for patient and doctor. The more objective measures that can be recorded the better.

Sensory re-education

During the paralysed stage there will be anaesthesia in the distribution of the nerve. Quite soon after injury, there is ingrowth of adjacent normal nerves into the denervated area and this can be quite extensive. The radial nerve has been seen to take over the pulp of the thumb and half the pulp of the index finger in median nerve lesions. Trophic lesions may occur in the anaesthetic area, particularly in median nerve and sciatic lesions. The patient must be carefully and repeatedly instructed by the therapist on avoiding these lesions: care in smoking, avoiding putting the hand on a radiator or hot stove, equal care in cold weather and when using the refrigerator. Gloves should always be worn in cold weather in nerve lesions involving the hand and thick woollen socks in sciatic or medial popliteal nerve lesions.

Functionally, the most important sensory nerve is the median. It used to be thought that stereognosis never recovered after median nerve lesions; only protective sensation could be expected. It was believed that misrouteing of axons was inevitable as they crossed the suture line and a high proportion would innervate the wrong receptors. Moreover, it was believed that there was sensory specificity: special receptors and tracts with no overlap subserving the various modalities such as touch, pain, pressure, heat and cold.

The most widely used index of sensory recovery is two-point discrimination (2PD). As Onne pointed out in 1962, 2PD is invariably poor, being over 20 mm in adults in the fingertips after median nerve sutures. In children, however, values of 2PD can approach normal. There was thus an entrenched belief that the results of median nerve sutures might be satisfactory for motor recovery, but would always be poor for sensation.

Working in a military environment with highly

skilled technicians, we found (Wynn Parry & Salter, 1976; Wynn Parry 1981) that co-operative patients who needed their hands for skilled work could be re-educated to a level of stereognosis not far short of normal and that this was functionally most valuable.

As soon as some sensation returns to the finger-tips, training is started. The patient is blindfolded and the unaffected part of the hand covered with gauze fingerstalls. He/she is then presented with a number of wooden blocks of various shapes — square, rectangular, oval, etc. — and asked to feel around them and identify their shape. This is a good introduction to the patient in his/her first essay into learning again how to build up an image in the mind by tactile stimuli. If s/he fails to identify the object, s/he is asked to look at it and relate what s/he sees to what s/he feels. The process is then repeated with the blindfold on and continued until s/he has learned all the shapes. Next, different textures such as felt, wool, canvas, sheepskin and rubber are presented to the blindfolded patient and s/he tries to recognize these, describing out loud his/her impressions and building up a progressive image. She/he attempts recognition again and if s/he fails s/he looks at the texture and feels it, relating visual to tactile impressions. When successful with most textures s/he graduates to objects, thus summating texture, shape, temperature and density. Large objects are used first, then smaller ones. It is important to use objects with which the patient is familiar. Tables 19.1 and 19.2 show our regime.

Training sessions are short to avoid fatigue, 15 minutes twice a day, and a relative is taught the technique so that the training can be continued at home. Quite quickly, with training, patients become more aware of their hand and begin to use it for everyday activities which they had avoided previously. At regular intervals, usually 3-weekly, tests are carried out using different textures and objects. The patient is not told the results so that there will not be a training effect from the tests. Most patients regain satisfactory stereognosis and some have been able to return to intricate skilled work requiring 'blind' finger activities and to play keyboard instruments.

In 23 patients, after median nerve sutures, the average time for recognition of textures at the start of training was 34 seconds, most patients being able to recognize four textures. After an average of 9 weeks' training, seven textures could be recognized in an average time of 19 seconds. Similarly, the average time for recognition of objects was 23 seconds and after 9 weeks' training this fell to 11 seconds, the patient being able to recognize seven more objects (Wynn Parry & Salter, 1976).

We have confirmed Onne's work that 2PD is grossly abnormal in such patients and Tables 19.1 and 19.2 show that 2PD can be poor and yet sensory function excellent. Two-point discrimination most probably measures nerve fibre density and as such is useful as an academic test to gauge proportion of fibres reaching the periphery, but it is no use as a test of *function*. We believe that clinical sensory testing should include the recognition of objects and textures. Finally, it must be appreciated that when one attempts to feel an object to recognize it, one automatically moves it between fingers and thumb. Attempts to identify (correctly) something laid statically on the fingertip, as in the 2PD test, always fail.

This gives the clue as to how retraining may work. Clearly the ability to regain stereognosis is incompatible with the specificity theory of sensation, for it is well recognized that there is con-

Table 19.1 Recognition times of objects 19 months after median and ulnar nerve suture at the wrist

	Seconds
String	17
Pencil	3
Small bottle	8
Nailbrush	4
Match	7
Shuttlecock	2

Table 19.2 Two-point discrimination in mm 19 months after suture of the median nerve (figures in parentheses are 2PD on equivalent site on normal hand)

	Index	Middle	Ring	Little	Thumb
Proximal	9 (2)	10 (3)	9 (3)	10 (3)	9 (1)
Middle	10	8	11	11	
Distal	8 (2)	9 (2)	15 (2)	13 (2)	12 (1)

siderable misrouteing of axons. It is now believed that although there is certainly some degree of end-organ specificity, many fibres respond to several different types of stimuli, and it is the pattern of activity both spatially and temporally that determines the nature of sensation. The pattern of impulses reaching the cord will depend on a large number of variables, including the frequency, interval between discharges and sequential firing of fibres.

In retraining, one is attempting to train the patient to learn a new code, for the pattern of firing will be abnormal due to a smaller number of fibres firing with a slower conduction speed. Central remodelling certainly occurs and sensory re-education is eminently worth trying in all patients with median nerve lesions who need that sensation in daily life. Sometimes hyperaesthesia is a serious problem for stereognosis, and we have found that transcutaneous electrical stimulation proximal to the nerve applied for periods of 1 hour or more regularly several times daily can inhibit the hyper-aesthesia and allow much improved stereognosis.

Localization is an important parameter of sensation and is always disordered after nerve sutures in adults. This too can be easily trained. The patient is blindfolded, touched in various places and asked to locate the touch. If wrong, s/he opens his/her eyes and relates what s/he sees to where s/he feels it; re-education usually only takes 3 weeks of training.

Pain

A number of peripheral nerve disorders are associated with pain. These include painful neuromata, causalgia, irritative neuritis, painful amputation stumps and plexus avulsion. Even the most skilled suture of nerve does not prevent a number of fibres escaping from the sheath and forming a neuroma; this is usually painless, although many patients have a persistent strongly positive Tinel's sign at the suture line. In some cases, this may be very painful and cause severe painful paraesthesiae when knocked or rubbed and permanent tinglings in the distribution of the affected nerve. This may be so distressing as to exclude all use of the hand. Often resuture and even two attempts at resuture are tried, and we have seen patients in whom, even

after the highest class of surgery with interfascicular grafting under microscope cover, the pain returns, often more severely than before.

If the neuroma is only painful on pressure or touch, then a wristband with a hole around the neuroma and a cover on top of it may be enough. But if there are spontaneous pain and paraesthesiae then other measures must be sought. It is possible that there are two mechanisms to this pain – one peripheral and one central. Wall & Gutnick (1974) showed that the terminal neuroma after cutting the sciatic nerve in a rat produces spontaneous discharges which can be suppressed by proximal electrical stimulation of the nerve.

Some deafferentation occurs with nerve lesions and the balance between large- and small-diameter afferent activity in the dorsal horn is changed so that there is excessive activity in laminae I and V and pain is felt. As Cevero et al. (1976) showed, electrical stimulation of the large-diameter afferent fibres can suppress this activity. We have found TNS most helpful in these patients.

We apply our electrodes just proximal to (never over) the painful area and adjust the parameters of pulse width, amplitude and repetition rate according to the patient's reaction. We stimulate for many hours at a time and feel sure that the reports of disappointment with this technique are due to inadequate stimulation time. Most patients are stimulated twice a day and are encouraged both during and between stimulation to use their hand normally. There is thus a big advantage in admitting such patients to a rehabilitation ward so they may have a full programme of stimulation and activity in physiotherapy and occupational therapy departments. It is believed that this allows normal movement patterns to replace the abnormal ones set up by the neuroma. Many patients are provided with their own stimulator, and wear it all day if necessary. Some patients need to use the stimulator for many weeks or even indefinitely; a few gain immediate and permanent relief after two or three sessions. Some 'escape' from the effect, and the treatment becomes gradually less useful, so prolonged follow-up is necessary.

We find that about 65% of patients with painful neuromas or irritative neuritis, e.g. ulnar neuritis at the elbow, respond satisfactorily. Vibration, massage and acupuncture are all believed to work in a similar way, but in our hands TNS is pre-eminent, and only if it fails do we attempt other peripheral modulating techniques.

Painful paraesthesiae in the sole of the foot are common and very distressing after sciatic nerve lesions. Some patients prefer total anaesthesia to this spontaneous sensation and ask for nerve section. TNS can be helpful and is best used permanently, for the firm pressure of walking on the sole modifies the pain, presumably by increasing afferent input. Repeated nerve blocks with long-acting anaesthetics are sometimes dramatically successful and can be used in combination with TNS. A firm ortholene anklet pressing on neuromas of the sural nerve have been helpful also. But these painful peripheral nerve conditions have, in our hands, proved much more intransigent than in the upper limb.

Hand surgeons are all too familiar with the painful amputation stump – often of a tip of a finger – leading to successive amputations at higher levels, only for the pain to return and even to spread to other unaffected fingers. In the same way as in painful neuromas, multiple operations must be avoided. Once pain has been present for any length of time, it becomes central, and peripheral destructive surgery only adds to the deafferentation and compounds the issue. TNS and vibration are often dramatically successful in these cases and should always be given an extended trial.

We have seen extraordinary results from TNS in patients with painful phantom limbs, even when treated many years after amputation. One patient whose pain had been present for 18 years was treated thus. First she felt the fingers of the phantom unclench, then straighten, then the elbow straightened and she then lost her pain completely after a week's stimulation, 2 hours twice daily. She now uses the stimulator a few times a week to keep the pain at bay. Similar spectacular results in avulsion injuries are, alas, rare, possibly because the avulsion produces much more severe central damage and sets off more reverberating circuits than a traumatic amputation.

Causalgia

This extraordinary condition follows partial nerve lesions and is commonly seen after missile wounds near the median and sciatic nerves. The term should be reserved for such cases and not used for pain in plexus avulsion – the nature and reaction to treatment are entirely different.

The patient feels a constant burning in the hand or foot, which is slightly relieved by applying moisture – some patients go around with the part wrapped in moist towels. Weir Mitchell's patient kept his feet wet in his boots to avoid jarring his body on walking. Even trivial external stimuli can elicit excruciating pain; a puff of air, banging of a door, a car starting up and emotional situations can be desperately painful. This is in marked contrast to the pain in plexus avulsion, where external stimuli have no effect. The part is cyanotic and cold, osteoporosis develops and the patient's whole life is taken up with his/her pain. Blocking the sympathetic by intravenous guanethidine or stellate ganglion block can dramatically relieve pain, but often only temporarily.

Success is usually taken as an indication to proceed to sympathectomy, but the sympathetic nervous system has an unrivalled penchant for regeneration and most pain specialists prefer repeated stellate or lumbar sympathetic blocks. It is essential to incorporate these techniques into a planned rehabilitation programme so that the patient uses the limb when pain-free and re-establishes normal patterns of neural activity.

What is the nature of causalgia? Clearly there must be a sympathetic disorder, for the symptoms and signs are those of sympathetic over-reaction, and there must also be the peripheral and central effects of deafferentation. The whole panoply of techniques for peripheral nerve pain relief may need to be deployed – sympathetic blocking, TNS, vibration, acupuncture and intensive rehabilitation. Recent research in this field, and results of treatment are discussed in Wynn Parry (1991).

Electrodiagnostic techniques

Electrodiagnostic techniques are of great value in the diagnosis and prognosis of peripheral nerve injuries. In clinical practice, the commonest situations where they are used are:

1 to assess if regeneration has begun at a time after suture when reinnervation could be expected, for electrical signs precede clinical signs of recovery by many weeks;

2 to decide if denervation is present when symp-

toms of nerve damage are present but there are no objective signs;

3 to assess the extent of damage in a partial lesion and, by serial studies, to determine if a lesion is remaining static, deteriorating or improving; this is of particular value in lesions suspected of being due to compression, e.g. entrapment neuropathies;

4 to establish if a brachial plexus lesion is pre-ganglionic or postganglionic;

5 to assess the presence of anomalous innervation;

6 to decide if neurological deficit is due to root or nerve involvement, e.g. distinguish in a patient with paraesthesiae in the thumb and index finger, between cervical spondylosis and median nerve compression at the wrist or, in a patient with paraesthesiae in the big toe, between L5 root pressure and a lateral popliteal palsy.

Electrodiagnosis uses two fundamental techniques: the activity of muscle at rest and on effort by recording with a needle electrode and displaying its electrical activity on the oscilloscope, and the response of motor and sensory nerves to electrical stimulation.

At rest a normal muscle is silent on EMG; on minimal contraction a few motor units fire, each unit comprising the axon and a variable number of terminal nerve fibres. Units are small in facial muscles (100 μV, 2–3 ms duration) and large in the proximal limb muscles (up to 5 mV and 10 ms in duration). As effort increases, so more units fire and their frequency increases until the whole baseline of the oscilloscope trace is obliterated to produce the so-called full interference pattern. If motor units have been damaged, then the interference pattern is incomplete.

Some 18–21 days after denervation, the muscle fibres no longer controlled by their nerve revert to their embryonic preinnervation behaviour and start to contract spontaneously. This activity is picked up on EMG as spontaneous fibrillation, potentials of amplitude 100 μV and duration 1 ms which, of course, cannot be detected by the naked eye. Thus the detection of these fibrillation potentials in a resting muscle is indicative of denervation. As the motor unit breaks up in active degeneration, the units are seen to be complex and polyphasic because the myelin is disintegrating, conduction in the distal terminals is slowed and temporal dispersion occurs. Exactly the same type of unit is seen

in early regeneration, for the nerve terminals in the newly formed unit also conduct slowly because the myelin is immature. The detection of a few polyphasic units of low amplitude and prolonged duration in a clinically paralysed muscle is a sure sign of recovery. In chronic partial denervation, denervated muscle fibres are incorporated into adjacent normal motor units by sprouts from normal nerve fibres, thus producing motor units of much greater amplitude than normal. These so-called giant units are another sign of denervation; units may be seen of amplitude 10 mV or even greater.

Motor nerves conduct at an average rate of 50 m/s and sensory nerves at a slightly faster rate. It is easy to measure conduction velocities by recording muscle activity with needle electrodes or from surface electrodes and stimulating the nerve at various accessible points. By using surface electrodes and stimulating beyond a point when no further current produces any increase in the size of response, one can gain an accurate idea of whether all the motor units are responding, as values are known for most muscles. In a suspected ulnar nerve lesion, for example, one can record over the abductor digit minimi and stimulate the ulnar nerve at the wrist, just below and just above the elbow and in the axilla. Latencies are thus obtained at each level and, by measuring the distances from the sites of stimulation, velocities are calculated for each segment of nerve. In this way, local slowing can be detected and the site of an entrapment neuropathy revealed.

Sensory conduction is measured in a similar manner. In the hand, sensory action potentials can be recorded by stimulating the digits with ring electrodes and recordings made over the appropriate nerves at the wrist. The radial sensory potential is obtained by stimulating the nerve antidromically in the mid-forearm over the radius and recording over the first dorsal interosseous space. The musculocutaneous nerve sensory potential is found by stimulating at the elbow and recording over the lateral border of the forearm. In the leg the sural potential is obtained by stimulating just lateral to the midline, 14 cm proximal to the Achilles tendon, and recording along the lateral malleolus. Two examples of the value of these techniques in assessing the site of entrapment may be given.

In a suspected compression lesion of the median nerve in the carpal tunnel, the sensory action potential may be smaller than normal and delayed in time (latency). The distal latency or time taken from stimulus at wrist to the abductor pollicis brevis (chosen for its virtually invariable median supply) may be prolonged, whilst the velocity in the forearm is normal. The normal latency from wrist to abductor pollicis brevis is 4 ms. A delay of more than 5 ms is significant of compression and more than 7 ms represents a severe lesion and needs surgical decompression. One of the earliest signs is reduction or loss of the median sensory action potential, which may occur well before there is any change in the motor response. These changes in conduction can occur before fibrillation appears or a substantial reduction in amplitude of the motor response.

In a suspected compression lesion of the ulnar nerve at the elbow, the sensory action potential from little finger to wrist may be reduced or absent and the mixed nerve action potential from wrist to above the elbow may also be abnormal, while the response from above the elbow to axilla is normal. With recording electrodes over the abductor digiti minimi, the response to supramaximal stimulation at the wrist might be 5 mV, just below the elbow 4.5 mV, just above the elbow and in the axilla 2.5 mV, thus indicating a pressure lesion at the elbow. The conduction velocities would be normal in the forearm but slowed across the elbow segment. If the lesion were more severe and involved a significant degree of Wallerian degeneration, the amplitude at the wrist would be markedly reduced and velocities slowed. Measurement of amplitudes is a helpful guide to the amount of denervation, and serial amplitude measurements will show recovery if they increase or deterioration if they diminish with time. We thus like to study conduction both by needles, which allow detection of denervation by showing fibrillation and giant units, and with surface electrodes, to allow quantification of the response.

The detection of local blocks to conduction due to local segmental demyelination can be demonstrated in all the accessible nerves. For example, in a suspected pressure lesion of the median nerve between the two heads of pronator teres, conduction velocities and amplitudes will be normal when stimulating at the wrist and recording over abductor pollicis brevis, while conduction will be prolonged

and amplitudes reduced when stimulating in the axilla.

Block of the lateral popliteal nerve will be shown at the knee by recording over extensor digitorum brevis and stimulating at the ankle, at the neck of the fibula and in the popliteal fossa.

Brachial plexus lesions

As discussed above, the key to prognosis is to distinguish the preganglionic lesion from the lesion distal to the posterior root ganglion, for in the preganglionic lesion the prognosis is hopeless, while in the latter there may be a prospect for recovery.

In preganglionic lesions, although there is total anaesthesia, the cell body of the sensory nerve is still intact and thus the peripheral sensory nerve will conduct an electrical impulse. Consequently sensory action potentials will still be present although sensation is absent. There is often some damage to the nerve in its postganglionic course and so the action potentials may be reduced in amplitude, but it remains true that any evoked action potential in sensory nerve in an anaesthetic area implies preganglionic involvement. Hence, recording sensory action potentials in the C5–T1 roots is an essential part of the investigation of plexus lesions.

It must, of course, be realized that if there is also a distal lesion, e.g. rupture or complete axonotmesis of nerves distal to the ganglion, the electrical findings will be those of a postganglionic lesion, i.e. absence of a sensory response.

Root lesions

Proximal nerve or root involvement by pressure, such as in cervical ribs and thoracic outlet syndromes or spondylosis or other causes of root pressure, result in local demyelination, but not changes in distal conduction. Thus in a cervical rib, denervation may be found in abductor pollicis brevis and also sometimes in an ulnar-supplied muscle, and yet sensory conduction, as judged by median and ulnar sensory action potentials, will be preserved and motor conduction will be normal. The same holds true in spondylosis; tinglings in the hand with preserved sensory and motor conduction with denervation in small hand muscles will suggest root involvement, as will preservation of sural and lateral popliteal nerve sensory potentials with tinglings in the foot and denervation in L5, S1-supplied muscles.

A lesion can be assigned to a particular root by demonstrating denervation (spontaneous fibrillation) in muscles supplied by that root but not in other muscles.

Facial nerve

There are certain situations when elaborate techniques, such as have been described, of measuring motor and sensory conduction are not necessary and when simple techniques provide the answer. This is particularly true of the neurapraxias. A good example is Bell's palsy. Here, there is complete paralysis of facial muscles on one side. EMG will be of no help 5–10 days after onset; denervation in the form of spontaneous fibrillation does not appear for 18 days and, because of the block, no units appear on effort on the oscilloscope.

However, if the facial nerve is stimulated at the stylomastoid foramen, contraction will be seen in all the facial muscles. The threshold can be compared with that on the normal side and should, in a non-degenerative case, be less than twice that of the affected side. Amplitudes to supramaximal stimulation can also be compared on the two sides by recording with surface electrodes over a facial muscle.

Wynn Parry & King (1977) showed that the vast majority of patients with complete palsies in whom nerve conduction was retained at 5 days recovered completely. However, a few cases showed late denervation – after 10 days – and the only way to pick these up is by serial conduction studies, so it is wise to study the response to nerve conduction, both qualitatively and quantitatively, up to 3 weeks after onset so as to detect these few patients who show late denervation. The same authors showed that if such patients had their facial nerves decompressed within 4 weeks there was a better chance of recovery than if treated conservatively. They also showed that electrical stimulation of the muscles when denervated in a degenerative lesion had no effect on the functional result, nor had splintage to lift the corner of the mouth any effect on the ultimate cosmetic or functional result.

Ideally, all patients in whom surgery for relief of pressure on peripheral nerves is planned should have EMG studies first to confirm the diagnosis. Many are the patients with pins and needles along the inner side of the forearm and in the ulnar two fingers whose ulnar nerves have been transposed at the elbow with no relief because their symptoms were due to a cervical rib or band, and many patients have had their carpal tunnels sectioned without relief of paraesthesiae in the median-supplied fingers because the cause was to be found in the neck. In many patients, too, the clinically obvious local pressure lesion was associated with a generalized neuropathy, the first signs being seen in sites vulnerable to pressure. In all these examples, careful EMG studies looking at motor and sensory conduction in both clinically affected and unaffected nerves would have given the answer.

However, there are vast numbers of such patients and few centres to provide EMG services, so selection is inevitable. In most patients, the diagnosis of compression of the median nerve in the carpal tunnel is obvious and EMG studies are not essential, but if there is any doubt operation should be delayed until EMG can be arranged. It is the author's view that no operation on the ulnar nerve should be undertaken without full EMG investigations; many patients have been made worse by unnecessary interference with the nerve.

The future

Clearly the most desirable advance will be in the field of prevention: reducing the frequency of motor-cycle accidents, preventing injuries in the home and banning glass from public doors. Far superior artificial limbs must be developed before it is justifiable to recommend amputation in a total preganglionic plexus lesion. More universal adoption of intensive rehabilitation programmes would certainly improve results.

References

Birch R. (1992) Advances in diagnosis and treatment on closed traction lesion of the supraclavicular brachial plexus. In Catterall A. (ed.) *Recent Advances in Orthopaedics*, No. 6, pp. 65–76. Churchill Livingstone, Edinburgh.

Bonnard C. & Narakas A. (1985) Syndromes douloureux et lésions post-traumatiques du plexus brachial. *Helvetica Chirurgica Acta* **52**, 621–632.

Cevero F., Iggo A. & Ogawa H. (1976) Nociceptor-driven dorsal horn neurones in the lumbar spinal cord of the cat. *Pain* **2**, 5–24.

Goldie B. & Coates C.J. (1992) A survey of closed supraclavicular injuries of the brachial plexus. *British Journal of Hand Surgery* **17B**, 84–86.

Goodman H.V. & Gilliatt R.W. (1961) The effect of treatment on median nerve conduction in patients with the carpal tunnel syndrome. *Annals of Physical Medicine, London* **6**, 137–155.

Loeser J.D., Ward A.A. Jr & White L.E. Jr (1968) Chronic deafferentation of spinal cord neurons. *Journal of Neurosurgery* **29**, 48–50.

Narakas A. (1977) Indications et résultats de traitement chirurical direct dans les lésions par élongation du plexus brachial. I – Les indications du traitement chirurical direct. *Revue de Chirurgie Orthopédique et Réparatrice de l'Appareil Moteur, Paris* **63**, 88–106.

Nashold B.S. & Ostdahl R.H. (1979) Dorsal root entry zone lesions for pain relief. *Journal of Neurosurgery* **57**, 59–69.

Ochoa J., Fowler T.J. & Gilliat R.W. (1977) Anatomic changes in peripheral nerve compressed by a pneumatic tourniquet. *Journal of Anatomy* **113**, 433–455.

Önne L. (1962) Recovery of sensibility and sudomotor activity in the hand after nerve suture. *Acta Chirurgica Scandinavica* Suppl. 300.

Ransford A.O. & Hughes S.P. (1977) Complete brachial plexus lesions: a ten-year follow-up of twenty cases.

Journal of Bone and Joint Surgery **59B**, 417–420.

Seddon H.J. (1972) *Surgical Disorders of the Peripheral Nerves.* Churchill Livingstone, Edinburgh.

Staal A. (1970) The entrapment neuropathies. In Vinken P.T. & Bruyn G.W. (eds) *Handbook of Clinical Neurology,* Vol. 7, pp. 285–325. North Holland Publishing Company, Amsterdam.

Sunderland S. (1991) *Nerve Injuries and Their Repair.* Churchill Livingstone, Edinburgh.

Thomas D.G.T. (1988) Dorsal root entry zone thermocoagulation. In Schmidek H.H. & Sweet W.H. (eds) *Operative Neurosurgical Techniques,* pp. 1169–1176. W.B. Saunders, Philadelphia.

Wall P.D. & Gutnick M. (1974) Properties of nerve impulses originating from a neuroma. *Nature, London* **248**, 740–743.

Wynn Parry C.B. (1974) The management of injuries to the brachial plexus. *Proceedings of the Royal Society of Medicine, London* **67**, 488–490.

Wynn Parry C.B. (1981) *Rehabilitation of the Hand,* 4th edn. Butterworths, London.

Wynn Parry C.B. & King P.F. (1977) Results of treatment in peripheral facial paralysis: a 25 year study. *Journal of Laryngology and Otology* **91**, 551–564.

Wynn Parry C.B. & Salter M. (1976) Sensory re-education after median nerve lesions: the hand. *Journal of the British Society for Surgery of the Hand* **8**, 250–257.

Wynn Parry C.B., Frampton V. & Monteith A. (1987) Rehabilitation of patients following traction lesions of the brachial plexus. In Terzis J.K. (ed.) *Microreconstruction of Nerve Injuries.* W.B. Saunders, Philadelphia.

20: Management of the AIDS Patient

H. OCHITILL AND D. McGUIRE

HIV infection in the CNS, 269
    Opportunistic infections of the nervous system, 271
    HIV-associated dementia, 273
    Clinical and pathological features, 273
    Evaluation, 273
    Epidemiology and natural history, 274
    Provision of services, 275
    General supportive approach, 275
    Environmental restructuring, 275
    Psychoactive medication, 276
Other HIV-associated mental and behavioural
    disorders, 277
    Anxiety states, 277
    Depressive disorder, 277
HIV-associated motor and sensory disorders, 278
    Myelopathy, 278
    Peripheral neuropathy, 278
    Myopathy, 279
Caring for the AIDS patient, 279

HIV infection in the CNS

The human immunodeficiency virus (HIV-1), the causative agent of the acquired immunodeficiency syndrome (AIDS), is a retrovirus which results in profound, and as yet, irreversible immunosuppression. Long-term survival with symptomatic HIV infection is rare. Death is usually due to overwhelming opportunistic infection with bacterial, fungal, viral or parasitic organisms, many of which are non-pathogenic in immunocompetent persons.

Infection with HIV-1 is emerging as a major cause of morbidity and mortality world-wide. The World Health Organization estimates that 500 000 Western Europeans are infected, and the infection rate among Western European males aged 15–49 is estimated at 1/200. There are approximately one million people infected in North America, and nearly six million in subSaharan Africa (Palca, 1991). The only 'cure' remains prevention.

The routes of HIV infection are well characterized. Transmission is via blood products or by intimate sexual contact. There is no risk of infection by non-intimate contact with HIV-infected persons. Needle-stick injuries are associated with a small but real risk, and direct skin contact with bodily fluids probably poses a risk in the presence of abraded skin. Gloves should be worn in the setting of exposure to blood and secretions, as well as masks and protective eyewear where there is a risk of contact with airborne secretions.

The groups at high risk for HIV infection vary to some extent among affected geographic regions. In North America and Western Europe, unprotected homosexual sex is a major risk factor, as is intravenous drug use with needle-sharing. In countries where clean needles are provided to intravenous drug users, infection rates in this group are low. In Africa, unprotected heterosexual sex is a major risk factor, as is infection via a contaminated blood supply and via unsterilized needles and other instruments reused in medical procedures. Vertical transmission *in utero* infects about one-third of children born to seropositive mothers.

Studies of the natural history and course of HIV infection have been conducted for the most part in North America and Western Europe. Whether the disease course varies significantly in developing countries remains to be determined. In West Africa, most reported cases of AIDS are not due to HIV-1, but to a related retrovirus HIV-2.

HIV is classified among the Lentiviridae — retroviruses which are cytopathic rather than oncogenic. The virus is cytopathic specifically for a subset of thymus-derived lymphocytes bearing the CD4 glycoprotein — that is, the T-helper–inducer phenotype. A viral coat protein designated gp120 binds to the CD4 receptor, and by this route virus is fused into the cell membrane and internalized. There is a microbiological latency of 5–10 years, on average, from infection to clinical disease, during which time an initially gradual but relentless destruction of T-helper cells occurs. B-cell mediated (humoral) immunity is also impaired, not by direct infection of B-cells but by dysregulation of B-cell function, the mechanisms of which are not yet well understood. A commonly used marker for the degree of immunosuppression is the CD4 count. The normal range is 400–1200/mm; when the CD4 count falls below 200, opportunistic infections are the rule. The fall in CD4 count may be associated with an increase in viral replication, measured by viral antigens such as P24 (MacDonell et al., 1990).

The most common opportunistic infections and neoplasms involve lung, gut, skin and central nervous system. The following reviews the neurological complications of HIV infection.

HIV-1 shares some genomic homologies with animal lentiviruses, such as Visna virus, known to target the nervous system of the host. The human brain is more heavily infected with HIV than is any other organ, possibly excepting the thymus, and neurological complications of HIV can manifest at all levels of the neuraxis, from brain and spinal cord to nerve and muscle (Levy et al., 1985).

HIV has been cultured from brain, cerebrospinal fluid (CSF) and nerve in patients at all stages of HIV disease; however, this is not in itself an indicator or predictor of neurological complications. Individuals who are neurologically asymptomatic and even those without detectable immune dysfunction have been culture-positive in CSF. Similarly, intrathecal synthesis of HIV-specific antibody, evidence of a CNS-specific immune response, is found early in infection, both in the presence and absence of neurological illness (Resnick et al., 1988).

Clearly, HIV enters the nervous system early, and usually without neurological morbidity. However, acute aseptic meningitis, acute encephalitis, and an acute inflammatory polyneuropathy indistinguishable from Guillain–Barré syndrome are all well described at the time of seroconversion.

HIV is cytopathic for CD4-expressing lymphocytes, but not for macrophages, which are the major infected cell group in the nervous system. The resistance to cell killing makes the macrophage a viral reservoir. Although the CD4 glycoprotein is present on neurons and astrocytes, direct, productive infection of the brain parenchyma appears to be rare. Rather, the intracytoplasmic vacuoles in macrophages contain the vast majority of virus in the CNS. Hence the macrophage is both a 'Trojan horse', purveying HIV from the periphery across the blood–brain barrier, and a reservoir for latent infection (Ho et al., 1987).

There is growing evidence that different strains of HIV with different cell tropisms exist within a single individual (Chiodi et al., 1989). In particular, strains which are highly efficient at replication in macrophages have been found in AIDS patients with severe cognitive impairment.

Having established latent infection within macrophages, it appears that HIV actually uses cytokines, secreted by activated immune cells to regulate the immune response, as the means by which it directs its own genetic expression and replication (Fauci, 1991).

The majority of AIDS patients have serious neurological signs and symptoms during their course, and 10–30% present with neurological dysfunction as the first manifestation of symptomatic HIV infection. The virus probably crosses the blood–brain barrier at the time of initial infection. Primary infection or seroconversion can be entirely asymptomatic, or associated with dysfunction at all levels of the neuraxis. Most common is an acute aseptic meningitis which is symptomatically self-limiting, but may result in a chronic CSF mononuclear pleocytosis (up to 450 WBCs) with mild to moderate protein elevation (up to 200 mg/dl). Neither CSF cellularity nor protein level distinguish seropositive patients with HIV-associated neurological disease from those without (Appleman et al., 1988).

Chronic infection, in the absence of opportunistic pathogens or neoplasia, can be associated with chronic symptomatic meningeal inflammation, with or without cranial neuropathies. Several distinct polyneuropathies and myopathies, both inflammatory and non-inflammatory, have been described, as has a myelopathy involving predominately posterior and lateral columns of the spinal cord. Less commonly, dorsal route ganglionitis or gracile tract degeneration has been reported, causing profound sensory ataxia. Autonomic neuropathy has been described, and may be underdiagnosed. Late in HIV disease, nearly always in the context of severe immunosuppression, a progressive cognitive decline, with or without disorder of motor function, is a cause of significant morbidity (Price *et al.*, 1988).

Therapy for primary HIV infection is in evolution as more of the viral genome is understood. Antiretroviral drugs are targeted at various points in the replication cycle. To date, most drugs developed are nucleoside inhibitors of viral reverse transcriptase, an RNA-dependent DNA polymerase which allows transcription of viral RNA into DNA which can then be integrated into the host genome. The most widely studied and used antiretroviral agent is the thymidine analogue, zidovudine. Zidovudine inhibits reverse transcriptase about one hundred times more efficiently than it inhibits cellular (host) DNA polymerase. However, it can cause a toxic mitochondrial myopathy due to inhibition of gamma DNA polymerase found only in the mitochondrial matrix. Zidovudine crosses the blood–brain barrier, and may slow initiation and progression of HIV-associated cognitive impairment. A dose of 500–600 mg/day is as effective as the higher dosages initially studied, and is associated with fewer toxic side-effects, especially the pancytopenia which can limit therapy. Current recommendation is that therapy should be initiated in seropositive persons with a CD4 count of 500 or less. Viral resistance develops in up to 90% of AIDS patients' isolates after one year of therapy; in asymptomatic patients, only 30% of viral isolates are zidovudine-resistant after one year. Preliminary studies suggest that these isolates remain sensitive to the other nucleoside analogues under major study, DDI and DDC. Combined chemotherapy with more than one antiretroviral agent is being investigated in order to control resistance and lessen toxicity associated with (higher dose) single agent use (Richman, 1991). Other investigative drugs include a non-nucleoside reverse transcriptase inhibitor, TIBO, immunomodulators such as alpha-interferon, and drugs which affect viral binding such as soluble CD4 and peptide-T.

Opportunistic infections of the nervous system

HIV-induced immunosuppression results in susceptibility to viral, bacterial, mycobacterial, fungal and parasitic opportunistic infections of the nervous system. Overall, the most common such infections encountered in AIDS patients in Western Europe and North America are those caused by *Toxoplasma gondii* and *Cryptococcus neoformans*. Meningitis and meningoencephalitis due to tuberculosis is a major opportunistic infection in developing countries and among immigrants with AIDS.

Toxoplasmosis

Toxoplasma gondii is an obligate intracellular protozoan found in raw meat and cat faeces, and causes a subclinical infection in man. In the immunosuppressed, however, dormant cysts in human brain can become activated. The replicating tachyzoites then invade brain parenchyma, causing cellular necrosis and vascular thrombosis. The symptoms may be those of a CNS mass lesion or of a meningoencephalitis. Common symptoms are headache, confusion and lethargy. Focal findings may include cranial nerve palsies. Up to 40% of patients present with seizures (Navia *et al.*, 1986).

Toxoplasma serologies are unreliable in establishing the diagnosis. CSF examination usually reveals elevated protein and a variable monocytic pleocytosis; glucose may be normal or low.

CT scan, even with contrast, may be normal. More commonly, single or multiple ring-enhancing lesions are seen. Uncommonly, the lesions show uniform enhancement or no enhancement at all. About one-half of patients have basal ganglia involvement. MRI is the study of choice, with a sensitivity of about 90%, compared with an 85% sensitivity with CT. Even if CT is positive, MRI can often demonstrate additional lesions, which may be important in establishing potential sites for biopsy.

Stereotaxic biopsy of accessible lesions is the gold standard for diagnosis, particularly to rule out polymicrobial infection or lymphoma. Alternatively, a ten-day to three-week trial of drugs effective against *T. gondii*, with ongoing clinical and radiological evaluation, is a possible approach.

Current treatments affect only the replicating tachyzoite; tissue cysts retain viable organisms. Initial therapy is with sulphadiazine 1–1.5 g orally every 6 hours, and pyrimethamine 75 mg orally as a loading dose, followed by 25 mg every day. Folinic acid, 10 mg/day, is added to decrease the marrow suppression caused by pyrimethamine. Duration of therapy is usually 6–8 weeks; however, recrudescence of infection occurs in 80% after therapy.

Current recommendations are for the continuation of therapy indefinitely. Clindamycin, 1200–2400 mg/day, is used either alone or in combination with pyrimethamine in patients with sulfa allergy.

Investigational drugs for *T. gondii* infection include trimetrexate, a dihydrofolate reductase inhibitor more potent than pyrimethamine, and roxithromycine, a macrolide antibiotic with a long half-life.

Patients on zidovudine may need to discontinue this antiviral therapy while on pyrimethamine, since bone marrow suppression can be exacerbated by the use of both drugs together.

Cryptococcal infection

The most common fungal CNS pathogen in AIDS patients is *Cryptococcus neoformans*, an unencapsulated yeast found in soil which infects via the respiratory route. Capsule formation takes place in the lung, and pulmonary infection can be followed by a basilar meningitis or meningoencephalitis, and, less commonly, by intraparenchymal or spinal cord granulomata (cryptococcoma).

Symptoms usually include fever and headache. Nausea and vomiting, photophobia, and mental status changes, including frank psychosis, occur in about 20–40% of patients. Papilloedema or optic neuritis occurs in up to a half of patients, while seizure and focal deficits (apart from cranial neuropathies) are seen in under 10%. Meningeal signs are absent in up to 80% of AIDS patients with cryptococcal meningitis.

Serology (cryptococcal antigen) is positive in about 95% of cases. CSF is entirely normal in 20% of patients, but may show a high opening pressure, low glucose, a mononuclear pleocytosis, and elevated protein. CSF cryptococcal antigen is positive in about 90% of cases, but immunocompetence appears to increase the frequency of false negative results. India ink is positive in only about 75% of cases, and should not be used as the only screening test.

Factors which suggest a poorer prognosis are high opening pressure, low glucose, very low CSF white blood cell count (<20 WBC/mm³), high titres of cryptococcal antigen (>1:32), a positive India ink stain, or cryptococcaemia.

CT scan may be normal, or show only atrophy and increased ventricles and basal cisterns. Focal lesions and areas of enhancement, as well as meningeal enhancement, are usually absent.

The yeast has a propensity to spread from the basal cisterns to the basal ganglia via the Virchow–Robin space; basal ganglia abnormalities may be detected on *T*2-weight MRI images. Cryptococcomas are seen in under 10%.

Treatment with amphotericin B, 0.3–0.6 mg/kg/day, with or without 5-flucytosine, 75–100 mg/kg/day, is the therapy of choice at this time. Combination therapy has been shown to be superior to monotherapy in non-AIDS patients. The neutropenia caused by flucytosine frequently necessitates its discontinuation. Optimal duration of therapy is unknown; 6–10 weeks therapy is usual, or until a cumulative total of 1.5 g of amphotericin has been administered. If flucytosine is used, serum levels of 50–100 g/ml are considered therapeutic. If the CSF opening pressure is extremely elevated (>350), or if CSF cultures remain positive, consideration can be given to placement of an Ommaya reservoir for intraventricular administration of amphotericin. After initial treatment of cryptococcal infection, maintenance therapy is recommended, either with amphotericin, 100 mg i.v. every week, or with ketoconazole, 800–100 mg/day (Chuck & Sande, 1989).

Itraconazole and fluconazole are now in clinical trials as investigational oral therapies for cryptococcal meningitis.

Other infections

Candida albicans, which commonly affects the oropharynx and oesophagus of AIDS patients, can cause a meningoencephalitis, as well as microabscesses in the cortex and brainstem. *Candida* may be part of polymicrobial CNS infection, or may infect intraventricular shunts, particularly in patients on broad-spectrum antibiotics and total parenteral nutrition. Fever, meningismus and elevated CSF pressure are seen in the majority of patients with CNS candidiasis. The CSF typically shows a pleocytosis (either polymorphonuclear or mononuclear), elevated protein and low CSF glucose. Diagnosis is made on culture of CSF, and treatment is that for systemic candidiasis: parenteral amphotericin B. Factors associated with poorer prognosis are delayed diagnosis (>2 weeks), intracranial hypertension, focal neurological deficits, and CSF glucose <35 mg/100 ml.

Among the opportunistic viral infections, the most important are the herpes viruses: herpes simplex 1 and 2, herpes zoster, and cytomegalovirus. Uncommon, but by no means rare, is symptomatic infection with papovavirus (JC), resulting in progressive multifocal leukoencephalopathy (PML). Reactivation of latent infection, rather than primary infection, is responsible for illness in these encephalitides. All can cause mental status changes and focal neurological findings; however, headache, fever and seizures should, in the absence of other clear aetiologies, create a high index of suspicion for a potentially treatable HSV infection. Intravenous acyclovir therapy should be initiated pending CSF culture and/or brain biopsy. Far from a fulminant illness, the course of HSV infection in the AIDS patient is often less dramatic and more chronic than in the immunocompetent host, making diagnosis highly dependent on suspicion. Infection with both HSV 1 and 2 has been reported, and in the majority of cases, skin or mucosal lesions are not present. MRI may reveal swelling in the characteristic locations: medial temporal lobes and inferior frontal lobes; however, diffuse lesions are also seen and definitive diagnosis may require brain biopsy (Glatt et al., 1988).

PML is not associated with signs of systemic illness; rather, confusion, pesonality change, aphasias, and focal neurological deficits are typical presenting features. CT and MRI show white-matter lesions without oedema or contrast enhancement (Krupp et al., 1985). There is no proven therapy; however, a few reported patients have stabilized or improved on zidovudine, and, most recently, cytosine arabinoside has been used intrathecally in a small number of patients with promising results.

HIV-associated dementia

Clinical and pathological features

As opportunistic infections become more manageable, and life expectancy lengthens, the severe cognitive impairment associated with HIV-1 is emerging as the major cause of neurological morbidity in AIDS in North America and Western Europe.

HIV-associated dementia, also called AIDS dementia complex or AIDS encephalopathy, is a clinical diagnosis and a diagnosis of exclusion. The criteria established by the Centers for Disease Control are the following: HIV seropositivity; cerebrospinal fluid examination which excludes other infection or neoplasm as the aetiology of cognitive impairment; a diagnostic image of the brain which is normal or demonstrated only atrophy or nonspecific white matter disease; and, clinically, disabling cognitive dysfunction, with or without motor dysfunction of a severity that interferes with work or activities of daily living. Neuropsychological testing may be required to distinguish early dementia from depression, since apathy, psychomotor retardation and dysphoria can be prominent early findings.

HIV-associated dementia has been called a 'subcortical' dementia: impairments in speed of information processing, retentive memory, and visuospatial skills are marked, while 'cortical' dysfunction, such as aphasia, dysnomia and agnosia, occurs late or not at all. Clumsiness of gait, slowed fine motor movements and tremor are common, and grasp reflexes or other release signs may be evident on examination. Corticospinal tract signs such as extensor plantar responses, hyperreflexia, and increased tone can be seen both in HIV-associated dementia alone or in association with the vacuolar myelopathy often found concomitantly.

Pathological changes in the brain can be remarkably bland relative to the degree of clinical dementia. Grossly, the brain can appear normal or profoundly atrophic. Microscopic changes range from a mild perivascular mononuclear infiltration to marked reactive astrocystosis and gliosis. Careful morphometric analysis suggests there is neuronal loss, at least in frontal cortex, but most studies have identified little change in cortical neurons overall. Although myelin loss can be prominent, oligodendroglial cells appear normal in number and morphology. Pathognomonic for HIV-encephalitis is the multinucleated giant cell, a synctitium of macrophages whose intracytoplasmic vacuoles contain most of the HIV virus found in the brain.

Evaluation

Careful evaluation and assessment are critical to the formulation of a management plan for the patient with HIV-associated dementia. Various facets of the patient's clinical status and function must be assessed. Evaluation is more than a single profile of the patient; rather it is an ongoing process of review informing management and influenced by patient response to interventions.

Cognitive capacity

Cognitive status and change in cognitive function are key clinical elements that require careful assessment. Cognitive dysfunction may herald, accompany, or complicate the course of AIDS. The special challenges for the clinician include sensitivity to early cognitive changes and their evolution as the course of the disorder unfolds.

Changes in patient mood, behaviour or personality should alert the clinician to the need for evaluation of cognitive capacity (Ostrow *et al.*, 1988). Early on, patients report forgetfulness, word confusion, or slowed mental activity. These complaints must be judged within the context of prior neuropsychiatric difficulties or substance abuse.

Systematic measures of cognitive performance are employed. All tests may be influenced by the patient's age, educational level, degree of anxiety and familiarity with the testing protocol. Most formal cognitive testing of AIDS patients has been done with white homosexual males living in Europe or North America – only a subset of AIDS patients.

The following tests have frequently been used:
1 attention – Trailmaking Test (TMT) A;
2 speed of information processing – TMT A and B, Wechsler Adult Intelligence Scale – Revised (WAIS-R) digit symbol subtest, Choice Reaction Time;
3 motor function – Finger Tapping Test, Grooved pegboard;
4 reasoning – Wisconsin Card Sort;
5 visuospatial skills – WAIS block design subtest;
6 memory/learning – Key Auditory Verbal Learning Test, Wechsler Memory Scale logical prose subtest;
7 speech/language – verbal fluency and Boston naming tests.

Functional level

All clinically significant neuropsychiatric disorders affect function. The extent of impaired work per-

formance and social function distinguishes among minor cognitive disorder and stages of dementia (Janssen *et al.*, 1989). Limitations of function determine rehabilitative needs.

Careful, systematic functional assessment helps to establish rehabilitative goals and measures of outcome. Any evaluation must account for the abilities of the individual and characteristics of the environment. Many assessment schemes are designed for institutional settings and some assess only basic daily activities such as eating, dressing, grooming and walking.

However, assessment schemes that review a broader range of impairments are available (Haffey & Johnston, 1990). Aside from self-care, mobility, and activities of daily living, evaluation of communication, memory, emotional, social-behavioural and occupational abilities is carried out as well. Such a comprehensive approach is vital for the care of the AIDS patient, in whom the latter capacities influence the overall level of disability.

Epidemiology and natural history

The prevalence and incidence of cognitive dysfunction and dementia in HIV-infected patients have not been precisely defined (Grant & Heaton, 1990). A number of cautions must be exercised in using the information available: many of the study samples have consisted solely of urban homosexual men from the United States or Western Europe; much information derives from anecdotal case reports and small samples in which varied evaluation procedures are used (Catalan, 1988).

The natural history of cognitive impairment in HIV infection remains to be clarified. Some individuals in early stages of HIV infection do demonstrate cognitive dysfunction (Grant & Heaton, 1990). While clinical studies suggest that a majority of HIV-infected patients will eventually develop a cognitive-behavioural disturbance (Fernandez *et al.*, 1989), frank dementia is felt to be infrequent among patients without general symptoms or immunocompromise (Janssen *et al.*, 1989). Based on clinical and pathological studies, dementia appears to be a relatively late complication in the course of HIV infection, with most cases occurring in the context of systemic AIDS (Price *et al.*, 1988). Price and co-workers (1988) reported that one-third of their sample demonstrated dementia at the point when AIDS was first diagnosed while two-thirds became demented at the preterminal stage of their illness.

The natural course of HIV-associated dementia is one of progressive worsening of mental status, though at varying rates. Individuals have progressed from the first signs of cognitive impairment to global severe dysfunction within months (Tross et al., 1988). One group (Navia & Price, 1987) reported a rapidly deteriorating course among dementia patients though 20% of the sample experienced a slower deterioration. Most of those in the sample died within one year.

Provision of services

The prevalence, severity and functional impact of HIV-associated dementia indicate that patients will require a range of neurological services, from outpatient services to in-patient, residential and terminal care. Health care providers, particularly in ambulatory care settings, need to be able to recognize the earliest stages of cognitive change in previously asymptomatic seropositive individuals. The clinician must be prepared to educate the family and 'significant others' of the patient about the nature, treatment options, and course of HIV-associated, neuropsychiatric disturbance; they should be assisted in realistically assessing the current and future burden of care.

With growing numbers of demented patients, the need for adequately staffed long-term residential care will become imperative. The staff of these institutions will need to manage a complex array of neurological, behavioural and medical difficulties. Community services are also needed to support care of the patient in a personal residence or an institutional setting.

General supportive approach

The neurological care provider should be familiar with approaches to several disabling aspects of dementia (Boccellari, 1990). Methods that promote clear-cut, explicit organization of information may buttress the patient's remaining memory capacity. Written aids that capture and organize significant information often prove helpful.

Though patients experience declining abilities, some form of continuing mental activity that does not frustrate the patient should be encouraged. Stressful tasks of any kind are likely to increase the patient's disorganization.

The schedule for the patient should include repetitive, relatively simple and familiar activities. Activities that require a critical time requirement should be avoided. There should be ample allowance for rest and sleep.

The provider should encourage the patient to maintain those activities that can be mastered and maintained while avoiding those that prove confusing or difficult. Circumstances that engender increased confusion and anxiety should be avoided. Significant others need to play a central role in constructing a schedule of activities and goals that are attainable and satisfying for the patient.

Increased anxiety and depression diminish cognitive capacity. Orientation, concentration and memory may all suffer from a developing mood disturbance. The health care provider should: (i) monitor ongoing mood levels; (ii) identify any mood decline with the patient and significant others; (iii) encourage all to identify and address apparent stressors; and (iv) consider mental health referral for any significant extended mood disorder.

Environmental restructuring

As the demented patient's mental abilities continue to decline, more emphasis should be placed on altering his/her environment to compensate for decreased ability and minimize frustration. Activities involving and surrounding the patient must be explicitly reviewed and altered in relation to the patient's residual functioning. Boccellari (1990) summarizes the management of several common problems including confusion, language difficulties, memory and safety issues.

There are a number of useful approaches for managing the patient's disorientation and confusion. Orientation cues include calendars, clocks, explicit written daily schedules and verbal reminders. Visual and hearing impairments may develop in the course of HIV disease and must be recognized and, when possible, treated. A night light may help to prevent nocturnal confusion. The level of stimulation must be modulated to avoid excessive or too little activity. Either extreme may heighten patient anxiety and confusion.

Surroundings, activities, and people should be familiar, predictable and clearly organized in relation to the patient. Change should be kept to a minimum with the patient assisted in coping with anticipated changes through forewarning, explanation and rehearsal.

Care providers should maintain calm behaviour in the face of the patient's confusion, and gently and firmly direct the patient away from inappropriate or unsafe behaviour. It is best to avoid questioning the patient regarding the motives for a particular action as the patient's insight is likely to be impaired.

While frank aphasia is not common in HIV-associated dementia, language difficulties may include receptive and expressive problems. In the case of the former, care providers should be encouraged to increase use of non-verbal cues, and to present information slowly and simply when the patient is fully attentive. The degree of comprehension should be checked by asking the patient to indicate what was understood.

Severely limited ability to retain and retrieve information may especially frustrate the patient's attempts to carry out daily activities safely and effectively. Again, a regular, consistent schedule of activities minimizes the need to adapt to the surprising and unknown; the patient's limited memory capacity is facilitated by simple repetition. Written and pictorial aids assist recollection of the daily routine and help the patient identify areas of the living environment.

A variety of behaviours represent special risks for the patient. The ambulatory patient with HIV-dementia may become disoriented or lost while moving about. Family members or other care-givers should ensure that the patient carries adequate identification, and should have on hand current photographs of the patient. It may be necessary to install less accessible outer door locks and an alerting system to indicate when the patient exits the house.

Various measures help to safeproof the patient's residence. Locks may be removed from inner doors to prevent accidental lock-ins. Sharp or dangerous household items should be inaccessible to the patient, including medication and other materials that may be misused. Valuable items and paperwork should be placed in a location removed from the patient. It may be necessary to render the stove and oven inoperable when a supervising individual is not around, thereby reducing the fire risk.

The patient's showers or baths should be supervised to prevent injuries. Physical alterations of the bathrooms may be necessary to assist the patient.

The HIV-demented individual is prone to difficulties with mood and judgement. Irritability and unpredictable changes in mood may be the rule. Decision-making, judgement of others, and recognition of one's own capacities and limitations are impaired. The neurologist should assist the home care-provider in understanding that these changes are part of the illness, and must be taken into account in planning the care of the patient. However, changes in mood or behaviour may also reflect worsening medical status or a reaction to medication.

Psychoactive medication

Patients with HIV-dementia may experience depressive symptoms including fatigue, apathy, sadness, reduced self-esteem, diminished appetite and disrupted sleep. The psychostimulants have proven effective and relatively well tolerated (Fernandez *et al.*, 1988). Medications such as methylphenidate or dextroamphetamine may improve mood, energy level and vegetative symptoms over a period of days or weeks. Treatment is begun with an equivalent of 5 mg of methylphenidate and the dosage is gradually increased to the point of significant clinical response or adverse effects. Conventional average dosage is 30–40 mg/day. Heterocyclic antidepressants may also be tried in the demented patient. However, these patients are especially susceptible to medication-induced confusion and seizures (see p. 277).

Paranoia, agitation, delusions or hallucinations may be features of HIV-associated dementia. Target symptoms may be managed with high potency antipsychotic agents. Gradual increase of low initial doses is the rule. The clinician should start with the equivalent of 1–2 mg of haloperidol in single or multiple doses. Dosage may be limited by worsening confusion or extrapyramidal symptoms. Also, neuroleptic malignant syndrome has been reported in the setting of HIV-associated dementia (Breithart et al., 1988).

Other HIV-associated mental and behavioural disorders

Anxiety states

Anxiety states are commonplace at various stages of HIV illness. Pre-existing factors such as personality and history as well as concurrent available social support influence patient response. Anxiety symptoms are evident with initial diagnosis, ongoing chronic disability and terminal illness.

The clinician discusses, reviews and reassures regarding the stressors specific to phases of the illness. Anxiety related to the diagnosis, neurological complications and functional impact is common and should be addressed by the neurological professional. Patients may have an overly fearful or grim understanding of possible neuropsychiatric difficulties.

Patients may profit from relaxation training, hypnosis or visualization techniques. Some find these activities are anxiety-reducing and enhance their sense of control of events.

Anxiolytics are especially helpful when used over relatively short time periods (days to weeks) to reduce significant levels of anxiety. They should be used in conjunction with other approaches to the anxious patient. Short- or intermediate-acting benzodiazepines are preferred to reduce the chance of toxic drug levels. The clinician remains vigilant for excessive sedation, coordination problems or confusion, all more problematic in a patient with cognitive impairment. Buspirone, a non-benzodiazepine anxiolytic, is relatively less sedating and prone to abuse. However, the response to this medication is slower than with the benzodiazepines.

There are no clear guidelines for chronic use of any anxiolytic drugs, therefore selective, episodic use is recommended. Possible complications of long-term use include compromised cognitive function and motor coordination.

Depressive disorder

Depressive symptoms of varying intensity, duration and functional impact are common among the mental disorders of HIV patients. Depressive responses are seen at various stages: seroconversion; onset of symptoms; symptom deterioration; and the terminal phase of the illness. The identification of depressive disorder is confounded by the developing panoply of medical symptoms in the symptomatic HIV patient; definition rests more heavily on the presence of cognitive and affective symptoms of depression.

Depressive symptoms related to illness transitions may respond to various approaches. Patient feelings of self-blame or guilt should be explored. The clinician encourages group involvement to reduce social estrangement and feelings of helplessness. The provider can assist the patient to accept the presence of his illness yet encourage continued meaningful activity; contact with other patients who have done so can be inspiring. When the patient experiences a decrement in functional ability, the clinician facilitates open expression of thoughts and feelings about the loss of ability. The provider should be available to consult with the patient and close relations regarding necessary adjustments in the patient's activities and living environment. Central concerns during the terminal phase of care include physical comfort and the continued presence of significant others. Therefore, the clinician can prevent unnecessary grief by encouraging the visitation of others and explicitly reviewing the measures to be taken to maximize patient comfort. The depressed HIV patient should be asked about suicidal ideas or intent. Such notions occur at any phase of the illness and should be carefully reviewed by the clinician. Those at serious risk may require a constant companion or hospitalization.

If a patient suffers sustained depressive symptoms with serious functional impact, the clinician should consider the use of an antidepressant. Personal or family history of positive response to antidepressant medication encourages a drug trial. Many symptomatic HIV patients are more sensitive to psychoactive medication and particularly to anticholinergic effects. Desipramine and trazadone are medications with low anticholinergic effects. The former medication is one of a group more useful with slowed withdrawn patients while the latter is one of several particularly useful with agitated, sleepless patients. The heterocyclic antidepressants, fluoxetine and bupropion, may prove helpful if other medications are poorly tolerated or clinically inadequate (Fernandez, 1990).

The starting dose is low (10–25 mg/day) with cautious, gradual increases. Measures of drug plasma levels assist in proper dosing. Once satisfactory improvement occurs, this therapeutic dose may be maintained for 3–6 months. Then, medication withdrawal can be carried out over a 1–2-month period.

Given difficulties with these agents, stimulant medication (methylphenidate, dextroamphetamine) is an option. This may be particularly appropriate in cognitively-impaired patients. Other medications include monoamine oxidase inhibitors and lithium carbonate. These agents should be considered for patients with a history of significant response to these drugs. Use of the former group requires special attention to diet while use of lithium calls for special attention to fluid and electrolyte status.

HIV-associated motor and sensory disorders

Myelopathy

Approximately 30% of patients with AIDS dementia will develop a vacuolar myelopathy resembling, clinically and pathologically, subacute combined degeneration of the spinal cord of vitamin B_{12} deficiency (Petito et al., 1985). The lateral and posterior columns, particularly of the thoracic cord, show white matter vacuolation, with relative sparing of axon cylinders. Patients develop a progressive, painless spastic paraparesis and ataxia, which may be associated with paraesthesias and incontinence. Dorsal column dysfunction, with impaired vibration and proprioception, may be evident on examination, but spasticity is generally the more prominent finding. While HIV has been cultured from affected spinal cords, there is no evidence that productive HIV infection is directly responsible; nor have secondary pathogens such as the herpes viruses been demonstrated. HIV-associated myelopathy can be seen in the absence of cognitive impairment, but, as in AIDS dementia, severe immunosuppression appears to be necessary before disease is clinically apparent. Apart from antiretroviral therapy, there is no specific treatment

as yet for this disorder; however, baclofen or dantrolene may provide some symptomatic relief of spasticity. Many patients remain ambulatory and stabilize clinically. Vitamin B_{12} deficiency and syphilis should be excluded in every patient.

Peripheral neuropathy

Peripheral neuropathies are common in association with HIV infection, and occur at all stages of disease. Subclinical neuropathic changes are found in 12–16% of asymptomatic seropositive patients (Hall et al., 1991) on electrophysiological testing. Early in the course of infection, an acute inflammatory demyelinating polyradiculoneuropathy can be seen. This syndrome is clinically indistinguishable from the Guillain–Barré syndrome (GBS); however, unlike GBS, a CSF mononuclear pleocytosis may be present, with as many as 50 cells per mm^3. A chronic inflammatory polyneuropathy (CIDP) is also not uncommon, and may involve significant axonal degeneration as well as demyelination. These neuropathies are probably immune-mediated; however, the inciting antigen has not been identified. Both tend to be self-limited, with good prognoses. Plasmapheresis is the current therapy of choice; however, gammaglobulin infusions are being investigated as an alternative treatment modality.

Mononeuritis multiplex (MM) is less common than the inflammatory demyelinating polyradiculoneuropathies, but also tends to occur early in HIV infection. Sensory or motor loss develops rapidly in the distribution of one or more nerves, nerve roots, or plexi. Electrophysiological studies reveal combined axonal loss and demyelination. MM can occur in the setting of a necrotizing vasculitis with systemic symptoms such as fever, weight loss, and anaemia, resembling polyarteritis nodosa, and with a similarly poor prognosis. More commonly, there are no systemic symptoms and the neuropathy is self-limited. However, progression to a confluent mononeuritis can occur, and may be difficult to distinguish from a distal symmetric polyneuropathy, or from CIDP (Parry, 1988).

The most common HIV-associated peripheral neuropathy usually occurs in the setting of severe immunosuppression and frank AIDS. This distal, predominantly sensory, polyneuropathy (DSPN) presents with numbness, burning or other painful dysaesthesias of the limbs, with feet more involved than hands. Sensory ataxia may be disabling. Features of both axonal loss and demyelination are present on electrophysiological testing, and nerve biopsy reveals large fibre drop out. Inflammation is absent or minimal, and there is no IgG or complement deposition. Mononuclear infiltration around blood vessels and within endoneurium has been described, with an increase in cytotoxic T-cells, leading to the hypothesis of a cell-mediated injury of nerve (Hogenhuis *et al.*, 1991). The most prominent alternative hypothesis is injury induced by cytomegalovirus, and CMV has been demonstrated by *in situ* hybridization in some endoneural macrophages. No HIV-1 viral genome has been found in injured nerve (Grafe & Wiley, 1989). Treatment is symptomatic, with tricyclic antidepressants as the mainstay of therapy. Mexiletine or lidocaine gel may also provide relief. Plasmapheresis is ineffective. An autonomic neuropathy may accompany DSPN, or be the dominant disorder and appear in early stages of infection, in which case use of tricyclics may be limited by orthostatic hypotension (Freeman *et al.*, 1990). Clinically similar syndromes have been reported in association with both sensory ganglionitis and gracile tract degeneration in AIDS patients.

The most serious, and potentially treatable, peripheral neuropathy in AIDS is a progressive polyradiculopathy resembling a *cauda equina* syndrome. Leg weakness, often asymmetric, is soon followed by urinary retention. Reflexes are hypoactive or absent. Weakness and sensory loss ascend over the course of days to weeks, and back pain or radicular pain may be severe. CSF is abnormal, with a pleocytosis that may show a predominance of polymorphonuclear cells. High CSF protein and hypoglychorrachia are usually present. Pathologically, inflammation and endoneural necrosis are seen. CMV has been cultured from CSF and nerve in some cases, and, while the prognosis is extremely poor, a few patients have responded to ganciclovir, an antiviral agent virostatic for CMV (Miller *et al.*, 1990).

Myopathy

Muscle involvement in HIV disease comprises a heterogeneous group of disorders clinically characterized by proximal greater than distal muscle weakness, increased fatigability, and myalgias, with mild to severe elevations in creatine kinase (CK). The most common myopathy, which occurs at any stage of HIV disease, is an immune-mediated inflammatory myopathy with muscle fibre necrosis and phagocytosis. This is a T-cell-mediated, MHC-1 restricted disease indistinguishable from polymyositis in seronegative individuals. Muscle is negative for HIV-1 by culture, and *in situ* hybridization has demonstrated no HIV-1 viral nucleic acids in affected muscle. While iatrogenic immunosuppression poses a risk for HIV-positive patients, treatment with prednisone can control the inflammatory process, and early treatment is advised since muscle fibrosis can limit the degree of recovery that can be achieved. Azathioprine or cyclophosphamide can also be used alone, or in combination with steroids.

Several other HIV-associated myopathies are less common. An acute necrotizing myopathy without inflammation, with no identifying myotoxic factor, has been described, as has a myopathy with rod bodies visualized on electron microscopy. The rods are thought to be comprised of actin and alpha-actinin, the Z-disk proteins which connect actin filaments. Denervation atrophy, disuse atrophy, and a type-II fibre atrophy similar to that seen in many chronic debilitating illnesses are more frequent findings at pathology (Wrzolek *et al.*, 1990).

An important, treatable cause of myopathy in HIV has been associated with zidovudine therapy. Zidovudine can cause a toxic mitochondropathy, probably due to inhibition of gamma-DNA polymerase, an enzyme found exclusively in the mitochondrial matrix. While clinically similar to polymyositis, the pathological picture is distinct: subsarcolemmal collections of abnormal mitochondria ('ragged red fibres') are seen in zidovudine-induced myopathy, which are absent from other HIV-associated myopathies. Weakness and myalgias are usually reversible with the discontinuation of zidovudine, and the mitochondria normalize on pathology. However, in some cases, weakness can persist (Chalmers *et al.*, 1991).

Caring for the AIDS patient

The care-provider should be aware of the special needs of the AIDS patient. Some patients are steeped in guilt and self-blame regarding their illness. The patient needs providers who are aware of their own stereotypic attitudes or feelings about homosexual orientation or drug-abusing behaviour. Through recognition of such biases, the provider will better be able to control, if not lessen, the introduction of anxiety, fear, or hostility into the relationship with the patient. Moreover, the provider may be able to ease the patient's burden of self-blame.

The patient's relative youth and contraction of an illness during prime productive years may be a special source of anguish. Younger care-providers may easily identify with the patient's distressing circumstances, heightening the provider's sense of vulnerability. This sense may be especially powerful if linked with a care-provider's fear of contagion. Care-givers may psychologically and literally distance themselves from the patient, thereby intensifying the patient's fear of isolation.

The patient's cognitive and behavioural problems may seriously hinder the patient–provider relationship. The care-provider may feel frustrated, alienated and exhausted in trying to manage these difficulties. As their efforts unfold, providers should attend to their own need for rest, relief, and support. Meeting regularly with other care-givers to share experiences and problem-solving strategies can be very helpful.

Finally, the provider caring for a patient with a highly complicated, ultimately terminal condition may often feel unhelpful to the patient and hopeless about the outcome. However, the continued presence of a familiar, committed care-provider is often central in easing the experience of the AIDS patient.

References

Appleman M., Marshall D., Brey *et al.* (1988) CSF abnormalities in patients without AIDS who are seropositive for human immunodeficiency virus. *Journal of Infectious Diseases* **158**, 193–199.

Boccellari A. (1990) Living and caring for the individual with AIDS dementia complex. In *AIDS Dementia Complex Training Manual*. Family Survival Project for Brain Injured Adults, pp. 99–123.

Breithart W., Marotla R.F. & Call P. (1988) AIDS and neuroleptic malignant syndrome. (letter) *Lancet* **2**, 1488–1489.

Catalan J. (1988) Psychosocial and neuropsychiatric aspects of HIV infection: review of their extent and implications for psychiatry. *Journal of Psychosomatic Research* **32**, 237–248.

Chalmers A., Greco C. & Miller R. (1991) Prognosis in AZT myopathies. *Neurology* **41**, 1181–1184.

Chiodi F., Valentin A., Keys B. *et al.* (1989) Biological characterization of paired human immunodeficiency virus type 1 isolates from blood and cerebrospinal fluid. *Virology* **173**, 178–187.

Chuck S. & Sande M. (1989) Infections with *Cryptococcus neoformans* in the acquired immunodeficiency syndrome. *New England Journal of Medicine* **321**, 794–799.

Fauci A. (1991) Immunopathogenic mechanisms in human immunodeficiency virus (HIV) infection. *Annals of Internal Medicine* **114**, 678–693.

Fernandez F. (1990) Psychopharmacological interventions in HIV infections. *New Directions for Mental Health Services* **48**, 43–53.

Fernandez F., Adams F., Levy J.K. *et al.* (1988) Cognitive impairment due to AIDS-related complex and its response to psychostimulants. *Psychosomatics* **29**, 38–46.

Fernandez F., Holmes V.F., Levy J.K. & Ruiz P. (1989) Consultation-liaison psychiatry and HIV-related disorders. *Hospital Community Psychiatry* **40**, 146–153.

Freeman R., Roberts M., Friedman L. (1990) Autonomic function and human immunodeficiency virus infection. *Neurology* **40**, 575–580.

Glatt M., Chirgwin K. & Landesman S. (1988) Treatment of infections associated with human immunodeficiency virus. *New England Journal of Medicine* **318**, 1439–1448.

Grafe M. & Wiley C. (1989) Spinal cord and peripheral nerve pathology in AIDS: the roles of cytomegalovirus and HIV. *Annals of Neurology* **25**, 561–566.

Grant I. & Heaton R.K. (1990) Human immunodeficiency virus-type 1 (HIV-1) and the brain. *Journal of Consulting and Clinical Psychology* **58**, 22–30.

Haffey W.J. & Johnston M.V. (1990) A functional assessment system for real-world rehabilitation outcomes. In Tupper D.E. & Cicerone K.D. (eds) *The Neuropsychology of Everyday Life: Assessment and Basic Competencies*, pp. 99–124. Kluwer Publishers, Boston.

Hall C., Snyder C.R., Messenheimer J.A. *et al.* (1991) Peripheral nerve function in HIV infected subjects. Abstract: *Neuroscience of HIV Infection Update*, p. 38. Padua, Italy.

Ho D., Pomerantz R. & Kaplan J. (1987) Pathogenesis of infection with human immunodeficiency virus. *New England Journal of Medicine* **317**, 278–286.

Hogenhuis J., Ratinahorana H., Henin D. *et al.* (1991) Cellular infiltrates in HIV-1 associated neuropathies. Abstract: *VII International Conference on AIDS*. Florence, Italy. MB 2015.

Janssen R.S., Cornblath D.R., Epstein L.G. *et al.* (1989) Human immunodeficiency virus (HIV) infection and the nervous system: Report from the American

Academy of Neurology AIDS Task Force, *Neurology* **39**, 119–122.

Krupp L., Lipton R., Swerdlow M. *et al.* (1985) Progressive multifocal leukoencephalopathy: clinical and radiographic features. *Annals of Neurology* **17**, 344–349.

Levy R., Bredesen D. & Rosenblum M. (1985) Neurological manifestations of the acquired immunodeficiency syndrome (AIDS): experience at UCSF and review of the literature. *Journal of Neurosurgery* **62**, 475–495.

MacDonell K.B., Chmiel J.S., Poggensee L. *et al.* (1990) Predicting progression to AIDS: combined usefulness of CD4 lymphocyte counts and p24 antigenemia. *American Journal of Medicine* **89**, 706–711.

Miller R., Storey J. & Greco C. (1990) Ganciclovir in the treatment of progressive AIDS-related polyradiculopathy. *Neurology* **40**, 569–574.

Navia B., Petit C., Gold J. *et al.* (1986) Cerebral toxoplasmosis complicating the acquired immunodeficiency syndrome: clinical and neuropathological findings in 27 patients. *Annals of Neurology* **19**, 224–238.

Navia B. & Price R.W. (1987) AIDS dementia complex as the presenting or sole manifestation of HIV infection. *Archives of Neurology* **44**, 65–69.

Ostrow D., Grant I. & Atkinson H. (1988) Assessment and management of the AIDS patient with neuropsychiatric disturbances. *Journal of Clinical Psychiatry* **49**, 14–22.

Palca J. (1991) The sobering geography of AIDS. *Science* **252**, 372–373.

Parry G. (1988) Peripheral neuropathies associated with human immunodeficiency virus infection. *Annals of Neurology* **23** (suppl.), S49–S53.

Petito C., Navia B., Cho E. *et al.* (1985) Vacuolar myelopathy pathologically resembling subacute combined degeneration in patients with acquired immunodeficiency syndrome. *New England Journal of Medicine* **312**, 874–879.

Price R.W., Brew B., Sidtis J. *et al.* (1988) The brain in AIDS: central nervous system HIV-1 infection and AIDS dementia complex. *Science* **239**, 586–592.

Resnick L., Berger J., Shapshak P. *et al.* (1988) Early penetration of the blood–brain-barrier by HIV. *Neurology* **38**, 9–14.

Richman D. (1991) Antiviral therapy of HIV infection. *Annual Review of Medicine* **42**, 69–90.

Tross S., Price R.W., Navia B. *et al.* (1988) Neurophysiological characterization of the AIDS dementia complex: a preliminary report. *AIDS* **2**, 81–88.

Wrzolek M., Sher J., Kozlowski P. *et al.* (1990) Skeletal muscle pathology in AIDS: an autopsy study. *Muscle & Nerve* **13**, 508–515.

21: Management of the Chronic Fatigue Syndrome

M. SHARPE AND T. CHALDER

Definitions, 282
  Fatigue, 282
  Neurasthenia and CFS, 283
  CFS and other syndromes, 283
Clinical description of CFS, 284
  Prevalence and prognosis, 284
  The clinical problem, 284
Aetiology of CFS, 284
  Viruses, 285
  Immune dysfunction, 285
  Muscle dysfunction, 285
  Psychiatric disorder, 285
  Effects of inactivity, 286
  Hyperventilation, 286
  Sleep disorder, 286
  Psychological factors, 286
  Social factors, 286
  Conclusions, 287
Treatment, 288
  Pharmacological therapies, 288
  Non-pharmacological therapy, 288
A rehabilitative programme, 289
  Assessment, 289
  Treatment, 290
  Cost of treatment, 292
  Evaluation of the rehabilitative approach, 292
Problems in treatment, 292
  Getting started, 292
  Failure to increase activity, 293
  Failure to accept the rehabilitative model, 293
  Invalidity benefit, 293
  Difficulty returning to work, 293
  Children, 293
Implications for medical services, 293
Future directions for research, 293

Patients complaining of chronic disabling fatigue frequently present to general practitioners and hospital physicians, especially neurologists. A small proportion of patients presenting in this way will be found to be suffering from well-recognized and treatable diseases. In the majority of cases, how-ever, no disease process is identified, and the disorder is then assumed either to be a consequence of previous infection or to be idiopathic. This syndrome has been given a number of names, including myalgic encephalomyelitis (ME), chronic Epstein–Barr virus (EBV) infection, postviral fatigue syndrome (PVFS), neurasthenia and, most recently, chronic fatigue syndrome (CFS).

Patients with unexplained fatigue are regarded as difficult to help. Whilst the patients are often severely disabled and may believe they have a physical disease called 'ME', the doctor can neither identify a disease process nor come to a firm conclusion about the status of 'ME' as an illness. Thus the patient wants a 'physical' diagnosis and 'medical' treatment and the doctor may feel that s/he can give neither. It is therefore not surprising that consultations often leave both parties dissatisfied.

In the following chapter we will first consider the definition of CFS, and briefly examine the evidence for each of the differing aetiological hypotheses. We go on to suggest a multifactorial model of causation that distinguishes between precipitating and perpetuating causes. After reviewing the treatment literature, we outline a rehabilitative approach based on our aetiological model. The problems likely to be encountered in the administration of this treatment are addressed. Finally, we consider some of the questions that future treatment research must seek to answer.

Definitions

Fatigue

Fatigue is a potentially confusing term. It is used here to refer to the subjective symptom of fatigue, rather than to objectively measured decrements in performance. Like other subjective states, the feeling of fatigue is difficult to define. Patients use a number of similar words to refer to it, including lack of energy, tiredness and weakness. The analysis of patients' complaints, however, suggests that at most two underlying concepts can be distinguished, namely physical fatigue and mental fatigue (Wessely & Powell, 1989).

Neurasthenia and CFS

In the early part of the twentieth century, unexplained fatigue was frequently ascribed to a disease called neurasthenia, the pathological basis of which was presumed to be due to weakness of the nervous system (Greenberg, 1990). However, the failure to identify a disease process and the increasing popularity of psychological explanations of fatigue led to the concept falling into disuse. In more recent years, a viral cause for unexplained fatigue has been postulated. Hence the terms PVFS, chronic EBV infection and ME have been coined. However, an infective aetiology has not been established and therefore the purely descriptive term CFS is preferable (Holmes *et al.*, 1988). The original clinical definition of CFS attempted to define a specific disease entity. It was consequently so complicated in application and restrictive in scope that it appeared to miss the point clinically. Most cases of unexplained fatigue were excluded, principally because they also met criteria for psychiatric disorders.

A simpler and wider definition was therefore proposed by a British consensus meeting in Oxford (see Table 21.1). This definition required that the patient's principal complaint was fatigue that had been present for at least 6 months' duration, was associated with impaired physical and mental functioning and was unexplained by physical disease (Sharpe *et al.*, 1991). This definition excluded patients suffering from physical diseases known to produce fatigue, but not patients with psychiatric diagnoses, except major mental illnesses (such as schizophrenia and manic depressive disorder). CFS defined in this way should be regarded as a *presenting syndrome* with multiple aetiologies. Hence individual cases should receive both a medical and a psychiatric assessment for a complete diagnosis to be made.

Table 21.1 Oxford consensus definitions (abbreviated). (From Sharpe *et al.*, 1991)

Chronic fatigue syndrome (CFS)
Inclusion
    Fatigue is the principal symptom
    Physical and mental functioning are impaired
    At least 6 months' duration
Exclusion
    Medical conditions known to produce chronic fatigue
    A current diagnosis of severe psychiatric illness (i.e. schizophrenia, manic depressive illness, substance abuse or proved organic brain disease)

Postinfectious fatigue syndrome (PIFS)
In addition to the above, there is definite evidence of infection at onset or presentation, corroborated by laboratory evidence

CFS and other syndromes

If the clinician is confident that there was an aetiologically relevant initiating infection, the term *postinfectious fatigue syndrome* or *PVFS* may be used (Behan *et al.*, 1985). However, in clinical practice it is difficult to establish the aetiological role of infection and the use of this term has, as yet, no clear implications for prognosis or treatment.

ME is a term introduced after an epidemic of unexplained symptoms and signs in medical and nursing staff of the Royal Free Hospital in London during an epidemic of polio in 1955. It therefore has little relevance to patients now presenting sporadically with fatigue, and furthermore is a misnomer as the inflammation of the central nervous system it implies has not been demonstrated. We refer to the term because it continues to be used by some doctors, patients, patient organizations and the media. 'ME' is often self-diagnosed and is therefore likely to represent an even more heterogeneous group of patients than those receiving a medical diagnosis of CFS. We would suggest, therefore, that CFS is the preferred term for those patients that meet the symptom criteria (above).

CFS overlaps with *fibromyalgia syndrome*, an idiopathic syndrome of generalized pain, fatigue, sleep disturbance and tender points on physical examination (Yunus, 1989). This similarity is worth noting because treatment research in fibromyalgia may offer helpful pointers to the management of CFS.

Clinical description of CFS

Patients with CFS complain that they feel exhausted and 'ill' and that they are unable to perform either physically or mentally. Many patients complain that the fatigue they experience is greatly exacerbated by activity, even minor exertion causing prolonged and overwhelming fatigue, resulting in days of severe disability. Patients with CFS commonly complain of a large number of additional symptoms; prominent amongst these are pain, depressed mood, sleep disturbance and subjective memory and concentration difficulties. Disability may be severe. Inability to work is common, and a significant proportion of patients have restricted mobility. Some become wheelchair-bound and a minority bed-bound.

Many patients adopt the view that a chronic virus infection or immunological disturbance underlies the symptoms and disability of CFS and that there is little that they can do about their condition. The research evidence is conflicting and such opinions remain essentially matters of belief. The patients' beliefs about their illness are a prominent aspect of the clinical picture, with considerable implications for management.

Prevalence and prognosis

The symptom of fatigue is extremely common in the general population. The number of people regarded as cases of CFS will depend on the threshold of duration and disability employed. Although approximately 20% of the population complain of troublesome fatigue (Chen, 1986), the prevalence of CFS is clearly very considerably lower. There are no UK epidemiological data. An Australian survey of general practice suggested a point prevalence of 40 cases per 100 000 (Lloyd et al., 1990). The prevalence of self-diagnosed 'ME' is also unknown, but it is probably more common than symptom-defined CFS. The largest patient organization, the ME Association, estimates that there are 150 000 sufferers in the UK.

The prognosis of CFS has received little systematic study. Clinical experience in tertiary referral centres has suggested a poor prognosis (Behan et al., 1985). Certainly the mean duration of illness in published case series suggests chronicity. A more optimistic prognosis is suggested by a follow-up study of patients seen in an infectious disease clinic. Only 30% had made a functional recovery by 2 years after assessment, but this rose to 66% by 4 years. However, many of these patients continued to complain of fatigue (Sharpe et al., 1992).

In summary, whilst we lack information concerning the prevalence and prognosis of CFS in the population, it is a significant clinical problem.

The clinical problem

The clinical problem is that of a patient presenting with chronic fatigue and disability, often with a strong belief in the presence of physical disease and antagonism to the suggestion of a psychological aetiology for his/her symptoms. Clinical assessment frequently reveals evidence of depression or anxiety, but rarely of neurological disease. Not surprisingly, the differing perceptions of the aetiology of the illness, the uncertainty about the facts, the differing opinions about treatment and the strong feelings on both sides result all too often in conflict between doctor and patient.

This regrettable situation arises, in part, because many doctors are bewildered by the controversy surrounding the aetiology and treatment of CFS. Some doctors believe that it is all depression and best treated by antidepressant drugs, others that it is a chronic virus infection and effective treatment must await the development of antiviral and/or immunological therapies, and yet others have been impressed by novel and 'alternative' treatments and advocate these. Few doctors, and consequently even fewer patients, take a multifactorial view of aetiology that takes all the clinical factors into account and leads to a positive management strategy. Before discussing treatment, the evidence for the various aetiological theories will be reviewed and a multifactorial model outlined.

Aetiology of CFS

The lack of agreed case definition, the disparate sources of patients and the lack of reliable and comparable measures have made much of the published research difficult to interpret (David et al., 1988). However, recent years have seen some improvement in the quality of research and there are now several coherent lines of evidence worthy of discussion. These include the role of virus infection, immune dysfunction, muscular dysfunction, depressive disorder and psychological causation. These factors will be reviewed in turn.

Viruses

Much of the earlier research in the USA sought evidence of chronic infection with EBV, the cause of glandular fever. Clinical experience suggested that glandular fever often resulted in a condition of chronic fatigue and disability. Hence it was hypothesized that chronic active infection was the cause of CFS. However, elevated antibody titres have been found to be non-specific and not to correlate with clinical state and therefore to be of doubtful significance (Schooley, 1988).

Viral research in the UK has focused on the role of Coxsackie viruses, which are known to produce myalgia. As with EBV, initial evidence of chronic infection has been found to lack specificity and relationship to clinical state and therefore to be of uncertain significance. More recently, advanced techniques of virus detection have been employed, and evidence of infection with other viruses has been sought. These studies suggest that persistent virus infection occurs in a proportion of cases, but the aetiological importance of these findings remains controversial (Wessely, 1991).

Immune dysfunction

Abnormalities in the immune system have been suggested to be of aetiological relevance because they may be the cause of failure to eradicate infection, may indicate persistent infection and may cause symptoms as a result of abnormal levels of immunological agents such as interferon or interleukins. Many publications have found evidence of relatively minor abnormalities in a proportion of patients. No consistent picture has been established. The possibility that the abnormalities observed are an epiphenomenon of other processes, such as depressive disorder and inactivity, has not been effectively excluded. Nor has an association of immune status and clinical state been established (Buchwald & Komaroff, 1991).

As with persistent virus infection, immune dys-

function may be shown by future research to be aetiologically important in a proportion of patients, but does not at present lead to effective and feasible treatment.

Muscle dysfunction

The symptoms of weakness and muscular pain have led investigators to examine muscle tissue and to test muscular function. Examination of muscle tissue has yielded evidence suggestive of persistent virus, but careful tests of muscle function have found this to be normal (Wessely, 1991). Both this finding and the complaint of subjectively impaired mental function have led investigators to turn from a peripheral (muscular) cause for fatigue to central (central nervous system) causes.

Psychiatric disorder

Very few of the above studies have carefully assessed the patients from a psychiatric standpoint. When this has been done, it has been found that most, but not all, patients meet criteria for a psychiatric diagnosis. The most common diagnosis is depressive disorder, with a prevalence much higher than that found in the general population. Other psychiatric diagnoses reported in case series include anxiety, panic disorder and somatization disorder (Lane et al., 1991).

It has been suggested that many cases of CFS are in fact suffering from primary depressive disorders (Greenberg, 1990). An alternative view is that depression is a secondary effect of the disability caused by CFS. On balance, the evidence suggests that depressive disorder accounts for the symptoms and disability attributed to CFS in many cases. First, both fatigue (physical and mental) and muscular pain are prominent symptoms of depressive disorder (Stoeckle & Davidson, 1962), so that the symptoms of patients with CFS cannot easily be distinguished from those of patients with depressive disorder (Wessely & Powell, 1989). Second, depressive disorder alone is sufficient to explain profound functional impairment (Wells et al., 1989). Third, the prevalence of depressive disorder in CFS is much higher than in similarly disabled controls (Wessely & Powell, 1989; Katon et al., 1991). Fourth, patients with CFS frequently have a previous history of depressive disorder (Katon *et al.*, 1991). Finally, the time of onset of the current episode of depression has been found to be coincident with or to precede that of CFS in many cases (Katon *et al.*, 1991).

The other symptoms of depressive disorder may not be obvious unless specifically enquired after. The importance of diagnosing a depressive (or anxiety disorder) lies in the implications for practical management.

Effects of inactivity

Clinical experience indicates that many, but not all, patients with CFS are profoundly inactive, some resorting to prolonged periods of complete bedrest. Research into the effects of inactivity in healthy young males indicates that complete bedrest produces muscle wasting, changes in the cardiovascular response to exertion and consequent intolerance of activity. Other changes include mental depression, altered autonomic regulation, with dizziness on standing, and impaired thermoregulation (Greenleaf & Kozlowski, 1982). Inactivity is, of course, treatable.

Hyperventilation

The increased subjective effort described by patients is a characteristic of the effort syndrome traditionally ascribed to the physiological and psychological effects of hyperventilation. Hyperventilation may play a role in symptom production in some cases of CFS, and is a treatable process.

Sleep disorder

Most patients with CFS complain of abnormal sleep, particularly feeling unrefreshed in the morning. Many have developed a pattern of sleeping during the day. Both overall sleep deprivation and excess sleep may lead to fatigue. Studies of sleep electro-encephalograms (EEG) have suggested the presence of an abnormal slow-wave sleep identified in patients with fibromyalgia (Whelton *et al.*, 1992). This abnormality requires further study. Insomnia, poor sleep and excess sleep all provide opportunities for therapeutic intervention.

Psychological factors

Psychological factors, which include a tendency to respond to illness with particular types of cognitions (attitudes, beliefs and thoughts) and behaviour, have been shown to perpetuate disability and to exacerbate symptoms in many chronic conditions (Sensky, 1990). These negative or unhelpful cognitions include the belief that activities that cause an increase in symptoms are damaging, that symptoms make activity impossible and that recovery from the illness is not under personal control. These beliefs also result in the patients focusing their attention on the symptoms, with a consequent increase in their awareness of them.

Thus, the patient's attempts to cope with symptoms may paradoxically perpetuate them. In the case of chronic pain, patients who cope with symptoms by avoiding the situations and activities that they associate with pain are reported to suffer more disability and more pain and to develop a feeling of loss of control (Philips, 1987). It has been suggested that such cognitions and behaviours interact with the physiological factors and the psychiatric disorders described above to perpetuate the symptoms and disability that comprise CFS (Wessely *et al.*, 1989; Sharpe, 1993).

The patients' and their families' beliefs about the cause of the illness determine their choice of treatment, and may make them hostile to treatments seen as 'psychiatric'. Thus psychiatric disorders often go untreated.

Social factors

Social factors have received less attention from researchers, but because of their likely importance they deserve discussion. One such factor is our cultural attitude to symptoms occurring in the absence of demonstrated physical disease. Such symptoms are frequently regarded as not resulting from 'real illness', as being 'all in the mind', as revealing personal weakness and as not being reason for exemption from daily demands (Greenberg, 1990). Physical disease, on the other hand, particularly if validated by a doctor, is rarely considered to be the responsibility of the afflicted, merits sympathy and excuses the sufferer from meeting the demands of others. Patients without a 'physical' label for their illness may consequently experience difficulty in explaining their disability to friends, family and employers and hence may request a 'physical' disease label from their doctors. In response to this lack of acceptance of the 'reality' of the symptoms and disability of CFS, patients have sought support for a physical disease called 'ME'. Whilst undoubtedly important in raising public awareness, the case for recognition of the reality of patients' suffering has become confounded with the less helpful view that psychological factors have no role in aetiology and that 'ME' is untreatable except by rest.

Other social factors may act as barriers to rehabilitation. An important factor is some employers' reluctance to facilitate a gradual return to work.

Conclusions

What are we to make of these contradictory aetiological hypotheses? We suggest that to determine which aetiological factors are relevant to rehabilitation the following principles should be applied:

1 *Focus on perpetuating causes* (see Table 21.2). The factors that perpetuate symptoms and disability in CFS should be separated from those that precipitated the illness. Thus, the condition may be precipitated by infection or by psychological stress. Chronicity is more likely to develop if perpetuating factors come into play and prevent recovery. A similar analysis has been made of the symptoms and disability consequent on head injury (Lishman, 1988).

2 *Focus on treatable causes.* Many of the potential perpetuating causes identified above are treatable. Others, such as possible occult viral infection and immune deficiency, have not so far proved to be so.

3 *Consider multiple factors.* As with other chronic conditions, the factors that perpetuate the condition are likely to be multiple. Hence, rather than search for a single cause, it is preferable to consider multiple perpetuating causes (see Table 21.2).

4 *Identify relevant factors by individual assessment.* CFS is a heterogeneous category. The principal perpetuating factors will differ between individuals, and hence should be identified in an individual assessment.

5 *Factors may interact.* It has been suggested that aetiological factors may interact in self-perpetuating vicious circles to perpetuate the condition (Wessely *et al.*, 1989). An example of how this interaction may occur is shown in Fig. 21.1. Thus fatigue may result initially from the physiological changes consequent on infection or as part of the emotional response to stress. The fatigue gives rise to negative thoughts of failure and inability to achieve tasks, which leads to further anxiety and depression. Thoughts of causing further harm lead to avoidance

Table 21.2 A model of causation

Precipitating	Perpetuating
Physiological	
Infection?	Infection?
Immune dysfunction?	Immune dysfunction?
	Inactivity
	Sleep disorders
	Depression
Psychological	
Stress	Focus on symptoms
	Belief in disease
	Depressed mood
	Avoidance behaviour
Social	
Conflict?	ME as a mystery illness
	Sick role
	Medical behaviour
	Social obstacles to recovery

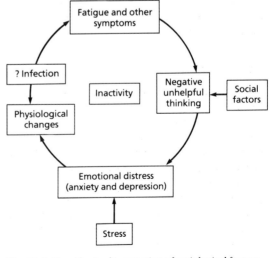

Fig. 21.1 Hypothesized interaction of aetiological factors in CFS.

of activity. Both inactivity and emotional arousal produce physiological changes that give rise to fatigue, poor concentration and muscular pain. Continuing stress and social influences also play a part. Thus the person becomes locked in a vicious circle of distress, disability and fatigue (see Fig. 21.1).

This aetiological model suggests a number of possible interventions. Before outlining a rehabilitative treatment, the existing evidence for the efficacy of specific treatment interventions will be reviewed.

Treatment

When evaluating treatments, adverse effects and feasibility of administration must be considered as well as efficacy. A wide variety of agents have been used in the management of CFS without adequate evaluation (Gantz & Holmes, 1989). Only those about which evidence of efficacy is available will be discussed.

Pharmacological therapies

Antiviral agents

The use of a specific antiviral drug, acyclovir, has been found to have no benefit over placebo and, at present, the cost, lack of efficacy and adverse effects of this and similar antiviral drugs prohibit their use (Gantz & Holmes, 1989).

Immunological agents

Other investigators have attempted to boost immune function by the administration of immunoglobulin. Two recent trials have come to opposite conclusions about efficacy (Straus, 1991). Even if shown to be beneficial, as with antiviral drugs such treatment is unlikely to be feasible on a wide scale because of cost and adverse effects.

Antidepressant drugs

Antidepressants may be used in either full dose (100–200 mg amitriptyline or equivalent) or low dose (less than 100 mg amitriptyline or equivalent). Although no controlled trials have yet been published, there are several lines of evidence supporting

their use in CFS. They are effective treatments (in full dose) for the depressive and anxiety disorders present in the majority of patients with CFS. Antidepressant drugs (used in low dose) are of established benefit in reducing sleep disturbance and pain in fibromyalgia. Finally, there are anecdotal reports of their efficacy in CFS itself, although there are as yet no controlled trials (Gantz & Holmes, 1989).

Against the use of antidepressants is the uncertainty about the degree of improvement they produce, and the frequent inability of patients with CFS to tolerate sedative and other side-effects. On balance, however, the evidence that these drugs can be helpful, considered together with their relative safety and ready availability, sanction their use. There are several types of antidepressant agent to choose from. Whilst tricyclic drugs are the most commonly used in the UK, there are arguments in favour of other types. The monoamine oxidase-inhibiting drugs (such as phenelzine) have been found to be superior to tricyclic antidepressants in patients with 'atypical depressive disorders', in which depressed mood is less sustained but lack of energy is prominent. The newer agents (such as fluoxetine) offer the advantage of causing less sedation and fewer side-effects.

Other agents

Several other agents have been assessed in controlled studies. These include magnesium injections and high-dose essential fatty acids. Although both agents produced symptomatic improvement over placebo, it remains to be established whether the benefits persist at longer follow-up and whether the studies can be replicated (Gantz & Holmes, 1989; Shafran, 1991). At present, we would not recommend these treatments.

Non-pharmacological therapy

Planned activity and rest

A graded increase in activity is an established means of improving functioning in many disabling illnesses, including chronic neurological disorders (Vignos, 1983). Activity does not necessarily mean vigorous exercise. None the less, the role of increasing activity in the treatment of CFS is controversial because it has been regarded by some as harmful to patients with this condition (Dowsett *et al.*, 1990). Whilst increasing activity may cause a temporary increase in symptoms, we are not aware of any evidence to support the suggestion that *gradual* increases in activity, interspersed with proper rest, cause harm to patients with CFS. On the contrary, graded increases in physical activity are used successfully by many clinicians in their management of CFS.

There may also be a place for more vigorous exercise in the rehabilitation of patients with CFS. Many patients with CFS are unfit and might therefore be expected to benefit from exercise. Furthermore, fitness training has been shown to reduce fatigue and pain and improve sleep in fibromyalgia (Yunus, 1989). In the authors' view, however, graded increases in activity alone are unlikely to be either effective or acceptable to the majority of patients if psychological factors are neglected.

Psychological treatments

In addition to showing the positive support that is part of every good doctor–patient relationship, psychological treatments include highly developed techniques of individual, group, couple and family therapy. Individual cognitive behaviour therapy (CBT) has been applied specifically to CFS and will therefore be discussed further. Other therapies are likely to have a role in helping some patients with CFS but their place remains to be established.

CBT is a form of psychotherapy first developed for use in phobic and depressed patients (Hawton *et al.*, 1989). This form of treatment has been shown to be effective in treating both depressive and anxiety disorders, and has also been adapted for use in patients with predominantly physical complaints. The efficacy of CBT in the treatment of CFS has been evaluated at the National Hospital for Nervous Diseases in London (Butler *et al.*, 1991). Patients with depressive disorders were also given antidepressants. Fifty severely disabled patients were offered treatment. Eighteen refused, but of the 32 patients treated there was a significant improvement in symptoms and functioning for 22/32 (69%), which was maintained at 3 months follow-

up. The improvements in many cases were dramatic and included effective 'cure' with a return to work and normal lifestyle. However, five patients dropped out before treatment was completed and four were unchanged. One patient who completed treatment was clearly worse at the end, a deterioration that the authors ascribe to a worsening depressive disorder. This study did not include a control group or independent assessment of outcome, and the high refusal rate and high drop-out rates were unsatisfactory. However, the study was carefully conducted and the results encouraging for those patients who accepted treatment. Furthermore, effective psychological treatments exist for depression and for anxiety, and are an alternative to antidepressant drugs (Hawton *et al.*, 1989). Thus there would appear to be a role for psychological treatments in patients with CFS. Skilled therapists are, however, not widely available.

A rehabilitative programme

In our opinion the existing evidence suggests that an effective approach to treatment of CFS must consider the role of a number of factors, including depression and anxiety, the physiological effects of inactivity and the patients' thinking about their symptoms. The following description is based on our own treatment programmes. They rely heavily on the techniques of CBT. A full account of the principles of this form of treatment can be found in Hawton *et al.* (1989) and a practical guide to its use in patients with unexplained physical symptoms in Sharpe *et al.* (1992). In our experience effective treatment is possible in the majority of cases. Treatment in some cases may be difficult, however, and can be time-consuming.

Assessment

The assessing doctor's first priority is to ensure that the patient with CFS is not suffering from a treatable medical disease. This can be achieved by means of a careful history and examination. Investigations should include full blood count, erythrocyte sedimentation rate (ESR), biochemistry and thyroid function as a minimum. Other investigations should be performed as indicated, although viral serology is unlikely to be helpful in established cases. The use of extensive laboratory investigation has been found to be unrewarding (Lane *et al.*, 1990). Unnecessary investigation is not only expensive but may be psychologically harmful to the patient.

The second task is to identify psychiatric disorder. A psychiatric assessment is therefore necessary and, as patients with CFS may minimize psychological symptoms, these should be specifically sought. The use of a simple self-rating scale may be useful in detecting symptoms of anxiety and depression, although for psychiatric diagnosis a full psychiatric interview is preferred. Both these techniques have proved acceptable in research studies.

The third task is to assess both the degree and pattern of functional impairment. It is useful to go through a typical day hour by hour. Measurement of both function and symptoms is important to determine progress. Simple rating scales are appropriate (see Butler *et al.*, 1991). The results of such measurements can be used to provide accurate feedback to patients on progress and can also highlight specific areas of difficulty.

Finally, the assessment of a patient with CFS should aim to identify the most important illness-perpetuating factors for that individual. Those to be considered are listed in Table 21.2.

Treatment

Getting started

The initial assessment is also an opportunity to build a therapeutic relationship with the patient. This is an essential part of treatment. Previous encounters with doctors may have left them feeling that the doctor considered their symptoms to be 'all in the mind'. Indeed, this view is sometimes expressed by doctors. It is therefore easy for the therapist to become embroiled in an argument with patients about whether their condition is 'physical' or 'psychological'. This debate is sterile and should be avoided. Rather, the doctor should emphasize his/her acceptance of the reality of their symptoms, listen to their views about the nature of the illness, and then focus on a pragmatic approach to rehabilitation.

Without a clear understanding of why this type of treatment is being tried, it is doubtful that the patient will engage in it. It is the authors' experience, however, that it is not necessary for patients to wholly agree with what is being said, as long as they are willing to try this approach. It can be useful to ask patients to list the pros and cons of trying out the rehabilitative approach, and to compare this with their experience of previous treatments. Many patients will have spent a considerable amount of time looking for a specific physical cause for their fatigue in the hope that this will lead to a 'cure'. The therapist may ask how productive this has been so far and then suggest that the patient tries rehabilitation for a set period of time (say 3 months), after which the benefits of this approach can be assessed.

The treatment 'contract'

The aims of treatment should be explicitly negotiated and agreed with the patient. These aims are best defined in terms of specific and realistic achievements (such as going back to work, or swimming a certain number of lengths of a pool).

It is also important to discuss the role of continuing medical investigation and parallel treatments. The continuation of these is likely to be a distraction from the rehabilitation and may increase preoccupation with illness. Therefore, before negotiating treatment, all physical investigations should have been completed and a positive diagnosis of CFS made. If patients are engaged in some other form of treatment, this should be terminated.

Who should treat?

Although this chapter is aimed at the neurological specialist, in many cases general practitioners can offer effective management. Out-patient treatment may be administered by the neurologist, or alternatively by a psychologist, nurse-therapist, physiotherapist or a combination of these. Whatever the therapist's discipline, it is necessary that they possess basic skills in psychological treatment. The involvement of a psychiatrist may be appropriate for those patients with severe psychiatric problems or where the psychiatrist has a special interest in CFS.

In-patient or out-patient?

Most patients can be treated as out-patients. However, if the patient lives too far away or is bed-bound, in-patient treatment may be required. There are difficulties in using medical wards for this purpose, unless nurses are trained in rehabilitative techniques. The principles of treatment of in-patients are the same as those used in the treatment of out-patients. Goals for activity may have to be initially very modest, e.g. getting out of bed for meals. If the patient has been severely dependent on family members, they may need to be helped to allow increasing independence.

The role of the family

The therapist spends a relatively small amount of time with the patient. Out-patient appointments usually occur once weekly or fortnightly and it is therefore helpful to have a close relative or friend involved in the treatment, acting as a co-therapist. The rationale for treatment should be explained to him/her and, with the agreement of the patient, he/she should be encouraged to attend some treatment sessions. The consequence of not involving significant others may be disastrous, as their mis-understandings about therapy may influence the patient.

Specific techniques

The rehabilitative approach advocated employs specific techniques to reduce emotional disorder, and to change patterns of thinking and behaviour that perpetuate illness. For clarity these will be described separately although they are usually employed in combination.

Treatment of emotional disorders

Depressive and anxiety disorders, including panic, may be a major cause of the patient's symptoms and may impede rehabilitation. Depressive disorder merits treatment, regardless of whether it is considered to be a primary cause or secondary consequence of the illness. Antidepressant drugs can be used in full dose to treat depression anxiety and panic. Alternatively, specific psychological therapy for these emotional disorders may be included in treatment. Milder depression and anxiety will tend to improve with increasing activity and may not require specific treatment.

Increasing activity

Assessment will indicate not only the patient's total level of activity but also specific patterns of impairment. One common pattern is an overall reduction in activity, and avoidance of specific activities associated with an increase in symptoms. Episodic bouts of increased activity are also common. This 'boom and bust' pattern prevents cumulative improvements, tends to confirm illness beliefs and is demoralizing. Treatment aims to show the patient that increased activity can be achieved without harm. The emphasis is on practising activities at regular intervals regardless of the occurrence of symptoms. The activities should be consistent with the patient's goals and consist initially of everyday physical activities such as walking, domestic tasks and socializing. Tasks are graded in terms of how difficult they are, and introduced in stages. They may gradually progress to more vigorous exercise.

During the early stages of treatment, the patient is likely to experience an increase in symptoms. It is imperative that the therapist predicts this and offers an explanation in terms of the effects of previous inactivity. The increase in symptoms is transient, but may take days and sometimes weeks to subside. However, as long as planned increases are set at a low enough level, this increase should be tolerable.

In addition to carrying out planned activity, planned rest is also prescribed, and should be recommended even if the patient feels that on a particular day it is not required. Activity should only be increased when the current level can be achieved without severe symptoms. Although symptom intensity usually reduces, symptoms do not always disappear altogether. This should be discussed with the patient.

Modifying negative and unhelpful thinking

The main aim of this component is to prevent negative and unhelpful thinking from causing distress and from blocking progressive increases in activity. The first step is to provide education about the nature of the condition. CFS patients have often read a great deal about their condition (CFS and 'ME'), not all of which is either accurate or helpful. It is important to explain that, whilst infection may cause acute symptoms, chronic symptoms are likely to have multiple contributory causes. This explanation provides alternative explanations for the patient's symptoms which are amenable to treatment. These explanations will include the physiological effects of depression anxiety and in-activity. The patient is assured of the safety of gradual increases in activity. Hand-out information sheets are useful.

The second step is to elicit and to try and change inaccurate or unhelpful thoughts. It is important to address each thought specifically. An example is: 'If I go for a walk today, I'll cause lasting damage to my muscles so I won't go.' In order to identify these thoughts, patients are asked to keep a record of 'what goes through their mind' when attempting activity. This is not as easy as it may seem. Patients may find keeping a record of such thoughts dis-tressing. It should therefore be explained that re-cording thoughts is a first step to controlling them.

Once the patient is able to record thoughts and can see the negative effects they have on mood and activity, they can be shown how to question and alter them as they arise. There are several ways of doing this. First, alternative explanations, such as 'My muscles are bound to hurt simply because I have become unused to exercise; I needn't worry and I should persevere', can be introduced. Second, the evidence both for and against the alternative and the original thought should be listed. If evidence is lacking, experiments can be performed to decide between alternative explanations for symptoms — for example, recording pain in the legs and distance walked whilst gradually increasing activity to deter-mine whether an increased level of activity pro-duces a persistently increased level of pain or whether it subsides with time.

Helping with psychosocial problems

Psychological and social problems will often emerge as important issues during treatment. If it is necess-ary that they be dealt with before further progress can be made, conventional problem-solving tech-niques can be employed (Hawton *et al.*, 1989). However, it is important to avoid unnecessary dis-tractions from the agreed treatment programme, and some issues may be best deferred. The im-provement in self-confidence which results from overcoming symptoms and disability may enable

the patient to make substantial life changes without the therapist's direct intervention.

Sleep and hyperventilation

Both sleep problems and hyperventilation are treat-able causes of fatigue and other symptoms. Treating them may not only reduce symptoms but also show the patient that symptoms have readily under-standable manageable causes. Difficulty getting to sleep or waking in the night may be improved by increasing daytime activity. Antidepressant drugs may also help. Excess sleep should be gradually reduced.

The effect of hyperventilation can be demon-strated to the patients by voluntary overbreathing, and, if it is contributing to symptoms, it can be managed with breathing exercises.

Cost of treatment

In our treatment programme, treatment is given in individual sessions, and usually takes between five and 20 1-hour sessions spread over several months. Treatment could in theory be given in groups, however, with some saving in therapist time.

Evaluation of the rehabilitative approach

The initial evaluation of combined CBT and anti-depressant treatment discussed above (Butler *et al.*, 1991) is encouraging, and the problem of getting patients to participate in this form of treatment is potentially soluble by paying greater attention to the beliefs of patients and their families. Controlled trials are in progress (see Sharpe, 1993).

Problems in treatment

There are many pitfalls in treatment, some of which are discussed below.

Getting started

The first problem is therapeutic nihilism. Treatment may not even be attempted if the doctor shares the patient's feeling of helplessness and mystery re-garding the illness. Alternatively, expecting too much too soon from the patient is likely to result in disillusionment. Even if treatment is offered, some patients will refuse. Sometimes the best one can do is to follow patients up. A similar strategy may be adopted for patients who drop out of treatment in the early stages. Clinical experience suggests that involving the patient's partner in treatment minimizes this problem.

Failure to increase activity

The most likely reasons for the patient failing to increase their activity level are: (i) too large an increase in activity was planned; (ii) the patient has doubts about the safety or value of the treatment; or (iii) there is some other block to increasing activity, such as severe depression. This problem is best managed by reviewing the level of activity planned and also the patient's beliefs and thoughts about the effect of activity. Fear of possible harmful effects of treatment is a common problem.

Failure to accept the rehabilitative model

There is some evidence that patients who believe very strongly that psychological factors are not relevant to their illness respond less well to the treatment described (Butler *et al.*, 1991). If the patient is resistant to accepting the multifactorial model, repeated arguments about the scientific evidence are unlikely to be helpful, and indeed may serve to strengthen the patient's beliefs. Rather, the therapist should re-emphasize his/her open-mindedness about the cause of symptoms whilst advocating a pragmatic approach to rehabilitation.

Invalidity benefit

Problems may arise if the patient requests a diagnosis the doctor feels is inappropriate, or wants certification of permanent invalidity. If the doctor feels unable to agree to the diagnosis of 'ME', then CFS or PVFS are usually mutually acceptable alternatives. Whilst many patients are severely disabled, this should not be regarded as a permanent state until an adequate trial of appropriate treatment has been undertaken.

Difficulty returning to work

The patient may have difficulty in achieving a level of function that feels adequate to permit a return to work. Work pressure may have been an important aetiological factor for the illness. If a gradual return is negotiable, this is likely to be of benefit. Alternatively, voluntary work may be used to build confidence. Some patients choose to change their premorbid employment or studies.

Children

CFS is being diagnosed in children by both parents and doctors. It is an important clinical problem, often associated with considerable amounts of time off school. The principles of management are similar but with particular attention being paid to the beliefs and behaviour of the parents (Lask & Dillon, 1990).

Implications for medical services

The full implications for medical services are difficult to calculate because of inadequate epidemiological data. Many cases may be manageable in general practice, using the principles described above. Hospital services would be best organized as joint medical and psychiatric clinics. At present, the main obstacles to providing an effective service is the relative unavailability of specialized psychological treatment. The bed-bound patient may be particularly badly served, with neither medical nor psychiatric units being suitable. Combined medical–psychiatry units are, unfortunately, rare in the UK, and rehabilitation and pain treatment units may offer the best alternative service for such patients.

Future directions for research

Clearly, further studies are needed to inform clinical treatment. Such studies will be of most use if they use agreed case definitions, specify how patients were selected and report details of both medical and psychiatric assessments. Substantial spontaneous remission and placebo response rates highlight the need for untreated controls and adequate periods of follow-up.

References

Behan P.O., Behan W.M.H. & Bell E.J. (1985) The postviral fatigue syndrome — an analysis of the findings in 50 cases. *Journal of Infection* **10**, 211–222.

Buchwald D. & Komaroff A.L. (1991) Review of laboratory findings for patients with chronic fatigue syndrome. *Reviews of Infectious Diseases* **13** (Suppl. 1), S12–S18.

Butler S., Chalder T., Ron M. & Wessely S. (1991) Cognitive behaviour therapy in chronic fatigue syndrome. *Journal of Neurology, Neurosurgery and Psychiatry* **54**, 153–158.

Chen M.K. (1986) The epidemiology of self-perceived fatigue among adults. *Preventative Medicine* **15**, 74–81.

David A.S., Wessely S. & Pelosi A.J. (1988) Postviral fatigue syndrome: time for a new approach. *British Medical Journal* **296**, 696–698.

Dowsett E.G., Ramsay A.M., McCartney R.A. & Bell E.J. (1990) Myalgic encephalomyelitis — a persistent enteroviral infection? *Postgraduate Medical Journal* **66**, 526–530.

Gantz N.M. & Holmes G.P. (1989) Treatment of patients with chronic fatigue syndrome. *Drugs* **38**, 855–862.

Greenberg D. (1990) Neurasthenia in the 1980s: chronic mononucleosis, chronic fatigue syndrome, and anxiety and depressive disorders. *Psychosomatics* **31**, 129–137.

Greenleaf J.E. & Kozlowski S. (1982) Physiological consequences of reduced physical activity during bed rest. *Exercise and Sport Sciences Reviews* **10**, 84–119.

Hawton K., Salkovskis P., Kirk J. & Clark D. (eds) (1989) *Cognitive Behaviour Therapy for Psychiatric Problems: a Practical Guide*. Oxford Medical Publications, Oxford.

Holmes G.P., Kaplan J.E., Gantz N.M. *et al.* (1988) Chronic fatigue syndrome: a working case definition. *Annals of Internal Medicine* **108**, 387–389.

Katon W.J., Buchwald D., Simon G.E., Russo J. & Mease P. (1991) Psychiatric illness in patients with chronic fatigue and rheumatoid arthritis. *Journal of General Internal Medicine* **6**, 277–285.

Lane T.J., Matthews D.A. & Manu P. (1990) The low yield of physical examinations and laboratory investigations of patients with chronic fatigue. *American Journal of the Medical Sciences* **299**, 313–318.

Lane T.J., Manu P. & Matthews D.A. (1991) Depression and somatization in the chronic fatigue syndrome. *American Journal of Medicine* **91**, 335–344.

Lask B. & Dillon M.J. (1990) Postviral fatigue syndrome. *Archives of Diseases in Childhood* **65**, 1198.

Lishman W.A. (1988) Physiogenesis and psychogenesis in the postconcussional syndrome. *British Journal of Psychiatry* **153**, 460–469.

Lloyd A.R., Hickie I., Boughton C.R., Spencer O. & Wakefield D. (1990) Prevalence of chronic fatigue syndrome in an Australian population. *Medical Journal of Australia* **153**, 522–528.

Philips H.C. (1987) Avoidance behaviour and its role in sustaining chronic pain. *Behaviour Research and Therapy* **25**, 273–279.

Schooley R.T. (1988) Chronic fatigue syndrome: a manifestation of Epstein–Barr virus infection? *Current Clinical Topics in Infectious Diseases* **9**, 126–146.

Sensky T. (1990) Patients' reactions to illness. *British Medical Journal* **300**, 622–623.

Shafran S.D. (1991) The chronic fatigue syndrome. *American Journal of Medicine* **90**, 730–739.

Sharpe M.C. (1993) Non-pharmacological approaches to treatment. In *Chronic Fatigue Syndrome*. CIBA Symposium, **173**, pp. 298–317. Wiley, Chichester.

Sharpe M.C., Archard L.C., Banatvala J.E. *et al.* (1991) A report — chronic fatigue syndrome: guidelines for research. *Journal of the Royal Society of Medicine* **84**, 118–121.

Sharpe M.C., Hawton K.E., Seagroatt V. & Pasvol G. (1992) Patients who present with fatigue: a follow-up of referrals to an infectious diseases clinic. *British Medical Journal* **305**, 147–152.

Sharpe M.C., Peveler R. & Mayou R. (1992) Psychological treatment of functional somatic symptoms: a practical guide. *Journal of Psychosomatic Research* **36**, 515–529.

Stoeckle J.D. & Davidson G.E. (1962) Bodily complaints and other symptoms of depressive reaction. *Journal of the American Medical Association* **180**, 134–139.

Straus S.E. (1991) Intravenous immunoglobulin treatment for the chronic fatigue syndrome. *American Journal of Medicine* **89**, 551–552.

Vignos P.J. (1983) Physical models of rehabilitation in neuromuscular disease. *Muscle and Nerve* **5**, 323–338.

Wells K.B., Stewart A., Hays R.D. *et al.* (1989) The functioning and well-being of depressed patients. *Journal of the American Medical Association* **262**, 914–919.

Wessely S. (1991) Chronic fatigue syndrome. *Journal of Neurology, Neurosurgery and Psychiatry* **54**, 669–671.

Wessely S. & Powell R. (1989) Fatigue syndromes: a comparison of chronic 'postviral' fatigue with neuromuscular and affective disorder. *Journal of Neurology, Neurosurgery and Psychiatry* **52**, 940–948.

Wessely S., David A.S., Butler S. & Chalder T. (1989) Management of chronic (post-viral) fatigue syndrome. *Journal of the Royal College of General Practitioners* **39**, 26–29.

Whelton C., Saskin P., Salit H. & Moldofsky H. (1988) Post-viral fatigue syndrome and sleep. *Sleep Research* **17**, 307.

Whetton C., Salit L. & Moldofsky H. (1992) Sleep, Epstein–Barr virus infection, musculoskeletal pain, and depressive symptoms in chronic fatigue syndrome. *Journal of Rheumatology* **19**, 939–943.

Yunus M.B. (1989) Fibromyalgia syndrome: new research on an old malady. *British Medical Journal* **298**, 474–475.

22: Management of Children with Neuromuscular Disorders

L. MERLINI AND C. GRANATA

Intermediate spinal muscular atrophy, 295
    Management, 298
Duchenne muscular dystrophy, 302
    Natural history, 302
    Management, 305
Acknowledgements, 310

Patients with neuromuscular disorders, their parents and the doctors who attend them are going through a phase of great expectations but also of confusion. The cure for muscular dystrophy is round the corner and the cure for other muscular disorders is on the way, so why bother about management? With the same line of reasoning, the bulk of research resources is being channelled into basic science, especially genetics, and only crumbs find their way into rehabilitation research. Is it sensible? Every week in the muscle clinic we see neuromuscular patients without a rehabilitation programme or already past the right moment for surgical treatment for scoliosis or with symptoms of hypoventilation who have never been told of the possibility of mechanical ventilation. Is it right? Taking care of children with neuromuscular disease means bearing in mind two levels of intervention that are complementary to one another: what can be achieved today, maybe partial but practical, and what we may be able to offer tomorrow, the real final cure. We can already offer the neuromuscular patient effective treatments that significantly lengthen life, keep the patient walking and halt the progression of scoliosis. The patients or carers should be made aware of this, should take part, if they can, in the decisions and should take advantage of the therapeutic possibilities. They and their parents will have more confidence in the attending physician, we doctors will feel more help-

ful and, last but not least, the child will be in the fittest condition to reach the winning-post that we all hope is near.

Management can be properly planned only when the natural history of the disease is known precisely; this rule, true for all diseases, is particularly so for neuromuscular disorders. There are two neuromuscular disorders that, both because of their frequency and because they present with varying degrees of muscle weakness, deserve to be discussed separately: the intermediate form of spinal muscular atrophy (SMA) and Duchenne muscular dystrophy (DMD). They represent a frame of reference for rehabilitation in neuromuscular disorders; in one, intermediate SMA, the muscle weakness is so great from the start that the patient never stands, but the course thereafter is relatively static, whereas in DMD strength is near-normal to start with and then the course is rapidly downhill, with loss of walking and respiratory and cardiac failure. They therefore constitute a point of reference for the treatment of other muscular disorders.

After outlining the natural history of intermediate SMA and DMD, we shall then turn to the rehabilitation measures that we normally offer and the results we have obtained in our patients.

Intermediate spinal muscular atrophy

SMA is an autosomal recessive disorder in which there is a degeneration of the anterior horn cells of the spinal cord, with associated muscle weakness and atrophy. This is symmetrical and affects the legs more than the arms and the proximal more than the distal muscles. The gene of SMA has recently been mapped to 5q11.2–q13.3 (Brzustowicz et al., 1990; Melki et al., 1990). Further,

Table 22.1 International SMA Collaboration classification of spinal muscular atrophy (Munsat, 1991)

Designation	Symptom onset (months)	Course	Death (years)
I (severe)	0–6	Never sits	<2
II (intermediate)	<18	Never stands	>2
III (mild)	>18	Stands alone	Adult

consensus (Munsat, 1991) has been reached regarding the classification of the disease in three principal forms according to age at onset, maximum functional capacity and life expectancy, as in Table 22.1.

Intermediate SMA is characterized by weakness, predominantly of the legs, with ability to sit unsupported but not to stand, onset before the age of 18 months, and a long-term prognosis depending on respiratory function (Dubowitz, 1989a). The intermediate and mild form of SMA have a prevalence among children as high as 40×10^{-6} and around 12×10^{-6} in the general population (Emery, 1991). We have found (Marri et al., 1991) an incidence of intermediate SMA as high (48.1×10^{-6}) as the one reported for the severe form of SMA. A possible explanation of the higher incidence of intermediate SMA in our area could be a better recognition of this form, which is still poorly diagnosed (Dubowitz, 1991).

Muscle weakness is apparent at birth or in the first months of life in 15% of cases and between 4 and 18 months in 85% (Merlini et al., 1989), sometimes after a free interval of some months during which the baby is thought to be completely normal, both by parents and by the doctor. Not infrequently the weakness is acute in onset, following vaccination or a febrile episode. At 12 months the weakness

of the leg muscles is so great that the child cannot stand (Fig. 22.1). The weakness of the trunk muscles is not so severe at this age and the child, when placed in the sitting position, can maintain it pretty well. The arms are less affected; some range of abduction of the shoulders is possible and hand movements are well preserved. Facial muscles are spared, but there may be atrophy or fasciculation of the tongue and tremors of the hands. Of the respiratory muscles, the intercostal and abdominal muscles are more markedly affected, while the diaphragm is spared. On inspiration, the rib cage has restricted expansion, because of the weakness of the intercostal muscles, while the effect of aspiration of the diaphragm is conserved, with resulting paradoxical breathing. Children affected with SMA have normal intelligence.

The course of the disease is marked by a progressive spine collapse, initially in kyphosis and later in kyphoscoliosis. We have reviewed the incidence and severity of scoliosis in 49 patients with intermediate SMA (Fig. 22.2). Scoliosis had an early onset and rapid progression before puberty; pelvic obliquity and vertebral rotation were proportional to the severity of the curvature (Granata et al., 1989b), which went on worsening after puberty until complete collapse of the spine with the ribs resting on the pelvis. All patients were fitted with a

Fig. 22.1 (*opposite*) Pedigree (a) of a family with intermediate spinal muscular atrophy, in which the parents are first cousins. The disease appeared in the index case (subject III-2, marked by arrow) at age 7 months, when the patient ceased to take weight on her legs. At 16 months, in 1956, she (b) was admitted to Istituto Ortopedico Rizzoli because she could not stand. Later she could sit unsupported. At age 5 she was found to have scoliosis. At age 27 (c) she could no longer sit unsupported because of the unbalance of the trunk due to severe scoliosis (more than 150° from supine) and marked pelvic obliquity. She had never had bronchopulmonary infections. Her brother (d) (subject III-3) ceased to take weight on his legs at 9 months and at 19 months was admitted to Istituto Ortopedico Rizzoli because he could sit but could not stand. He later had numerous bronchopulmonary episodes and died at the age of 7. *Comment*. These two familial cases illustrate well the natural history of intermediate SMA, which may be quite different in the same sibship: onset before the age of 1 year and course complicated by bronchopulmonary episodes with death in infancy in one case; in the other case no respiratory complications with survival into adulthood and development of progressive scoliosis not controlled by orthopaedic treatment.

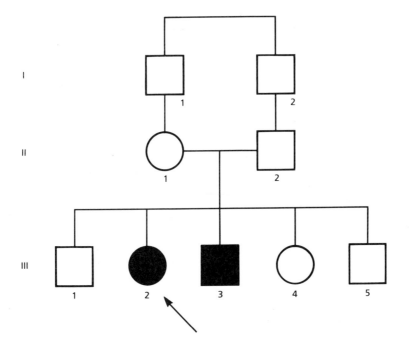

(a)

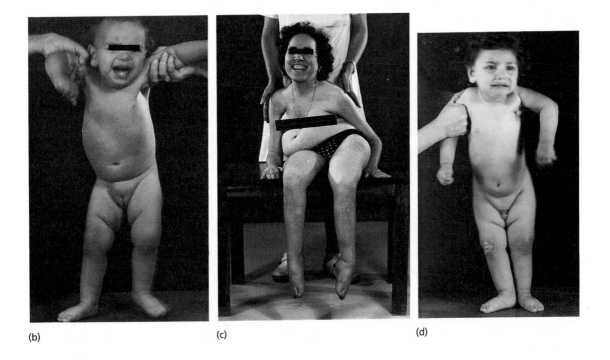

(b)　　　　　　　(c)　　　　　　　(d)

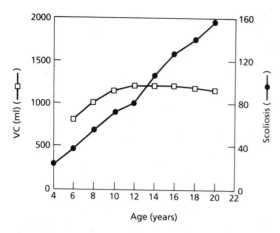

Fig. 22.2 Spinal muscular atrophy. The graph shows the changes in average vital capacity (VC) and scoliosis with age in 49 patients with intermediate SMA. Note the peculiar trend of VC with age: between 6 and 12 years VC is low and increases little but it tends to remain static throughout the second decade of life. Scoliosis is early in onset, is already severe before onset of puberty and continues to worsen during puberty, later to end in spinal collapse. In this group of patients the VC trend is clearly not affected by the scoliosis: VC continues to be static after age 12 despite the progressive worsening of the scoliosis. Note the difference of VC and scoliosis patterns between SMA and DMD (Fig. 22.6). Data from Istituto Ortopedico Rizzoli.

spinal brace from the onset of scoliosis but, even so, the curvature continued to worsen. Admittedly, the brace was not worn continuously, because it was poorly tolerated. In 18 of our patients who had worn the brace continuously for a period ranging from 4 months to 4 years, the mean worsening of scoliosis was 12° per year despite the treatment. Further, the brace, especially in patients with very weak costal musculature, compresses the rib cage and restricts vital capacity (Noble-Jamieson et al., 1986).

Vital capacity runs a characteristic course in intermediate SMA (Merlini & Granata, 1990). It increases (Fig. 22.2) very little with growth and attains its peak (1200 ml ± 400) at 12 years, remaining on a plateau for several years. Normal alveolar multiplication, which occurs in the first years of life and is facilitated by expansion of the rib cage, is inhibited in SMA by the paralysis of the thoracic muscles (Duval-Beaupère et al., 1985).

Episodes of respiratory obstruction are common in children with intermediate SMA; these, combined with the restrictive syndrome and the reduced capacity to cough, can be life-threatening.

Hip dislocation is a common feature in SMA, its frequency and severity tending to increase with age and severity of scoliosis (Granata et al., 1990). More than 90% of patients with some degree of scoliosis have hip dislocation, the severity of the dislocation correlating with the severity of the scoliosis. In a review at the Hammersmith Hospital, it was found that the side of the hip dislocation corresponded to the concavity of the curve in 77% of the cases (Rodillo et al., 1989). Although the dislocation is associated with a severe scoliosis, it seems to be a secondary phenomenon, as the side of dislocation usually corresponded to the concave side of the curve. So the dislocation seems more likely to be the result than the cause of the pelvic tilt.

Some children with intermediate SMA are overweight. Obesity is not desirable in this condition because it adversely affects functional ability, respiratory function and scoliosis. Estimation of body composition by anthropometry has shown that children who appeared excessively slender and underweight with respect to their ideal weight were really normal in terms of desirable bodyweight, because the underweight condition was due to loss of lean mass (Ballestrazzi et al., 1989).

The course is reported static in many cases (Dubowitz, 1974) or progressive in most (Russman et al., 1983). These patients have scant residual functional capacity and their strength is barely measurable. Our impression is that the course is static in many cases. We have, however, noted in older patients very reduced capacity for movement, practically confined to the hand muscles; this suggests a further loss of strength over the years. Patients may expect to reach adulthood in the intermediate form of SMA. Death before the age of 20 is infrequent and is, as a rule, related to the severity of the respiratory involvement (Merlini et al., 1989).

Management

Patients are followed up every 4–6 months after first examination. Assessment includes evaluation of functional capacity and of joint mobility, monitoring of respiratory function as from age 5, and sitting X-rays of the spine at the first sign of scoliosis and every year thereafter. Estimation of body composition is done by plicometry or bioelectrical impedance analysis.

Walking with calipers can be promoted in children with intermediate SMA. In five patients with mild SMA who had ceased walking, the provision of lightweight, long leg braces and crutches prolonged walking for up to 5 years in one patient (Evans *et al.*, 1981). The reciprocal hinge brace allows mobility and in some children seems to delay rapidly developing scoliosis (Eng *et al.*, 1984). We have shown that walking can be promoted in intermediate SMA (Granata *et al.*, 1987) and that there are important advantages in the early fitting of orthoses for SMA children (Fig. 22.3). Twelve children were fitted with calipers at mean age 2.2 years (range 1.1–4.3); at a mean follow-up age of 9.5 (range 6.9–13.6), orthoses had improved functional performance in all patients. All achieved unsupported standing, eight of the 12 assisted ambulation and four of these were eventually able to ambulate independently. These results are remark-

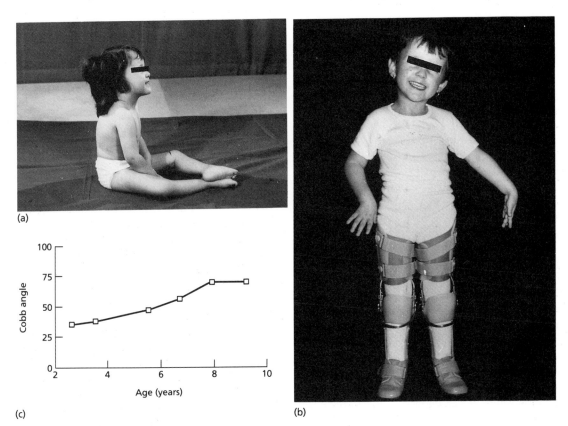

(a)

(c)

(b)

Fig. 22.3 Girl with intermediate SMA, sporadic case. Parents unrelated. The disease was noted at 9 months when the patient no longer tried to stand. Her mother reported that during gestation the child moved less than her healthy firstborn son. At the age of 12 months she was able to sit unsupported but not to stand. At age 2.5 years (a) she was still making no progress and so she was fitted with polyethylene calipers. With the calipers she managed to stand unsupported and rapidly began to move around independently. Since she already had an incipient scoliosis (graph (c)), she was supplied at the same time with a brace to wear in the sitting position. At the age of 7 (b) she continued to use calipers from 2 to 4 h a day, partly at school and partly at home. From age 2.5 to age 8 her scoliosis (c) worsened despite the use of the brace. At last follow-up at age 9 the scoliosis was stationary and the child was still walking with calipers and support. The graph (c) shows the trend of scoliosis during the period of observation during which she wore calipers and spinal brace.

able, since it has been assumed up to now that children with intermediate SMA cannot even stand unaided. Functional regression was observed at later follow-up: one child could no longer sit because of severe scoliosis, four could sit unaided, four could stand unsupported, three could walk with assistance and one at the age of 8.4 was still able to walk with calipers. During the follow-up period, hip dislocation remained steady in seven and deteriorated in five. At the follow-up, scoliosis was in the same range as in the children treated with spinal brace only. Children with intermediate SMA can be fitted with calipers once over the age of 1, with functional advantages, for some manage to move a few steps unaided and all can stand unsupported (Granata *et al.*, 1987).

We do not offer any treatment for hip dislocation, which is usually well tolerated without pain and does not involve functional deterioration (Granata *et al.*, 1990). The findings of Rodillo *et al.* (1989) contradict those of Shapiro & Bresnan (1982), who suggested that hip dislocation causes pelvic tilt, which will adversely affect an existing or developing scoliosis. Thus, surgical correction of hip dislocation is unlikely to have any effect on the scoliosis. Moreover, in SMA patients who had undergone surgical correction, the dislocation recurred (Thompson & Larsen, 1990).

Scoliosis or kyphosis in these patients invariably progresses and therefore requires treatment (Bradford, 1987). In the age range 4–10 years, for curvatures of over 20° and under 70° there are two options: no treatment and continued observation or bracing in order to delay the inevitable progression. There are arguments for both and the choice depends on the patient's age and his/her parents' readiness to co-operate. The first option is usually proposed for very young children or when the curve is minor, in the knowledge that bracing will not stop progression of the deformity and is poorly tolerated and from fear that bracing may lead to chest restriction and deformity in its own right. The second option, bracing in the attempt to slow curve progressing, allowing more spinal growth and delaying the inevitable surgical procedure, is offered to older children or to those with more marked curvature. When, between 6 and 8–9 years, the curvature is greater than 70–80° and rapidly progressive, provisional surgery with a Harrington rod

without fusion to allow further spinal growth is offered. After the age of 10 in children with curves exceeding 50–60°, there is nothing to be gained from waiting and surgery with fusion is indicated. Surgery remains the definitive treatment of choice in these patients. This calls for preoperative assessment of respiratory function, including vital capacity (VC) and blood-gas analysis. In the majority of cases a posterior approach alone is sufficient, and Luque's segmental instrumentation (Fig. 22.4) is preferred by the surgeons at the Rizzoli Institute (Cervellati *et al.*, 1989). Spinal fusion from the upper thoracic spine to the pelvis is required and banked bone is used. Anterior surgery (Dwyer's technique (see Table 22.2)) in combination with Luque's posterior instrumentation may be needed in patients with severe lumbar scoliosis and pelvic obliquity. Postoperative immobilization in a brace is necessary for a few months.

In our series (see Table 22.2) the mean age at surgery was 13 years and the mean Cobb angle 110°. The mean percentage correction was 50.5 (range, 27–59%). Patients had a preoperative VC of 1178 ml (range 700–1920 ml) but none had severe postoperative respiratory complications. Immediately after the operation, there was some loss of VC but during follow-up the values tended to regain the preoperative VC and stabilize. Good results like ours were obtained with the Luque instrumentation plus fusion in two SMA patients by Daher *et al.* (1985), in six by Brown *et al.* (1989) and in five by Phillip *et al.* (1990). In addition, two younger patients of ours, both aged 7 years, with very severe and progressive scoliosis, received provisional treatment with a subcutaneous Harrington rod without fusion. This, combined with bracing, allowed good correction and control of the curvature until the permanent fusion operation.

Table 22.2 Spinal surgery in intermediate spinal muscular atrophy ($n = 11$, 4 Harrington–Luque, 2 Luque + Dwyer, 5 Luque)

Age at surgery	13.7	(10.5–21.3)
Scoliosis preop.	110°	(55–180°)
Scoliosis postop.	48°	(32–90°)
Scoliosis F/U	53°	(42–100°)
F/U (years)	3.3	(1–7)

F/U = follow-up.

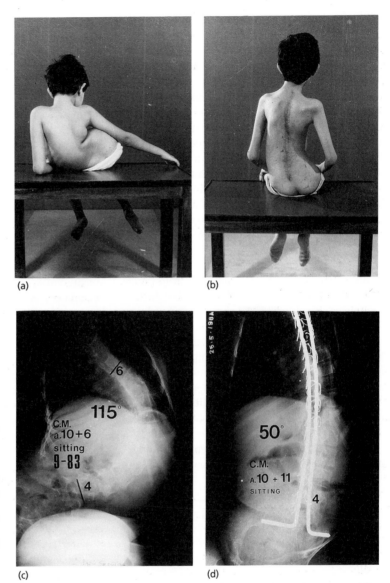

Fig. 22.4 Intermediate SMA. This 10-year-old boy sat at 12 months but was never able to stand or walk. Apart from a progressive scoliosis, his condition remained static. At the age of 10 (a) he had a very severe kyphoscoliosis and could not sit unsupported any more. After the Luque instrumentation and fusion (b) from upper thoracic spine to the pelvis, he was again able to sit unsupported. X-rays before (c) and after surgery (d).

On the respiratory front, the aim is: (i) to allow pulmonary growth, mainly through preventive ventilation (Delmas & Berard, 1990), and (ii) to prevent life-threatening respiratory failure. Duval-Beaupère *et al.* (1985) recommend assisted respiration with a Bird respirator early on, even before the age of 4, in order to favour normal multiplication of the alveoli, which requires correct chest expansion. Poor results are reported in children in whom treatment is started after the age of 4 years, while results are encouraging, though still preli-

minary, in those in whom assisted respiration is started earlier (Duval-Beaupère *et al.*, 1985). Episodes of bronchial obstruction must be dealt with quickly and actively by postural drainage, aspiration of the secretions, antibiotics and mucolytics. Gilgoff *et al.* (1989) suggested that, before ethical issues regarding prolonging life in patients with degenerative disease can be considered, the quality of life with medical intervention must be delineated. They have followed 15 patients with SMA treated with mechanical ventilation and found that ventilatory support was useful in prolonging life without significantly interfering with these patient's plans and expectations.

Some recreational activities have been proposed for children with severe muscle weakness. Eng *et al.* (1984) have found adaptative horseback riding and swimming acceptable.

Duchenne muscular dystrophy

The gene that, when defective, results in DMD was recently mapped to Xp21 and isolated. Then came the discovery of the protein product of the gene, most appropriately called dystrophin (for references, see Dubowitz, 1989b). Rowland (1988) quickly pointed out that any myopathy due to mutation at Xp21 is a variant of DMD, with an expected continuous clinical spectrum from severe to mild and minimal expression of the disease. Dubowitz (1989b) called for some degree of international consensus on the definition of the different grades of severity of Xp21 disease, for at least two good reasons: to be able to compare data from different centres and laboratories and to be able to give some sort of prognosis and appropriate supportive therapy to the patient and his/her family. He proposed separating the two main phenotypes by age at loss of walking: loss of independent walking by age 12 years for the Duchenne and maintenance of independent walking beyond the 16th

birthday as a definition for the Becker. This leaves an 'intermediate' group of patients who lose walking between 13 and 16 years and also allows for considerable variability within the two main groups. This simple definition of what DMD means enables us to trace the natural history of the disease, which underlies the treatment proposed and its evaluation.

Natural history

DMD is present at birth, the muscle weakness presenting later but anyway by the 5th year of life, leading to loss of independent walking between 6 and 13 years and death in the second–third decade. The heart muscle is affected but clinically significant cardiomyopathy is infrequent. Contractures of the limbs, scoliosis and above all the restrictive respiratory syndrome, which is the most frequent cause of death, invariably complicate the progressive and tumultuous course of the disease (Fig. 22.5).

The signal moments of the disease are: age at clinical onset, age at loss of walking and age at death.

Although present from birth, the disease does not manifest itself until the 2nd–3rd year of life and in a few cases as late as 4–6 years. The parents become aware of the first abnormalities when the child begins to stand and walk, the first mile-

Fig. 22.5 (*opposite*) Familial DMD (natural history), index case (subject III-1, marked by arrow in a). This boy learned to walk at a normal age but was never able to run. His parents noted that at age 3 years he had difficulty in getting up from the floor, fell often and had difficulty in climbing stairs. He was first seen at Istituto Ortopedico Rizzoli when he was 5.5 years old. Creatine kinase was 9050 (normal values up to 70) and EMG myopathic. The muscle biopsy showed typical dystrophic features. At the age of 8 (b, c) he showed increasing muscle weakness, lumbar lordosis (b) and broadening of the support base (c). The boy ceased to walk at 8.5 years. After he became chair-bound, a 10° T12–L5 scoliosis appeared at age 10 and at age 12 the scoliosis was 75°. At 13.7 years he could no longer sit unsupported (d, e) and the scoliosis in the supine position measured 64°. At 14.5 (f) the scoliosis was 91° (supine) worsening to 116° (supine), with 90° kyphosis at age 16. From the age of 10 he had worn several types of brace, which he tolerated poorly and which anyway did not hinder the relentless progression of kyphoscoliosis. VC reached its peak at 13 years and declined rapidly thereafter (g). At age 17 he was hospitalized elsewhere as an emergency case in respiratory failure and was tracheostomized. He was then treated with positive-pressure ventilation via the tracheostomy at home. He died at the age of 19 of complications related to the tracheostomy. The proband's uncle (II-3 in a) walked at 15 months. At age 4 he had frequent falls and his walking was unsteady. He ceased to walk at 8 years. In 1957 at age 8.5 he was admitted to Istituto Ortopedico Rizzoli, where he received medical (glycine, vitamin E) and physical treatment. He died at 16. *Comment*: The proband (III-1) with familial DMD with X-linked heredity had a typical 'natural' history unaffected by the physiotherapy given (gymnastic, swimming, passive mobilization, night splints, spinal braces and so on): loss of walking at 8.5 years, progressive scoliosis, evolving restrictive ventilatory syndrome. Only emergency tracheostomy proved effective in that it prolonged the patient's life for 2 years.

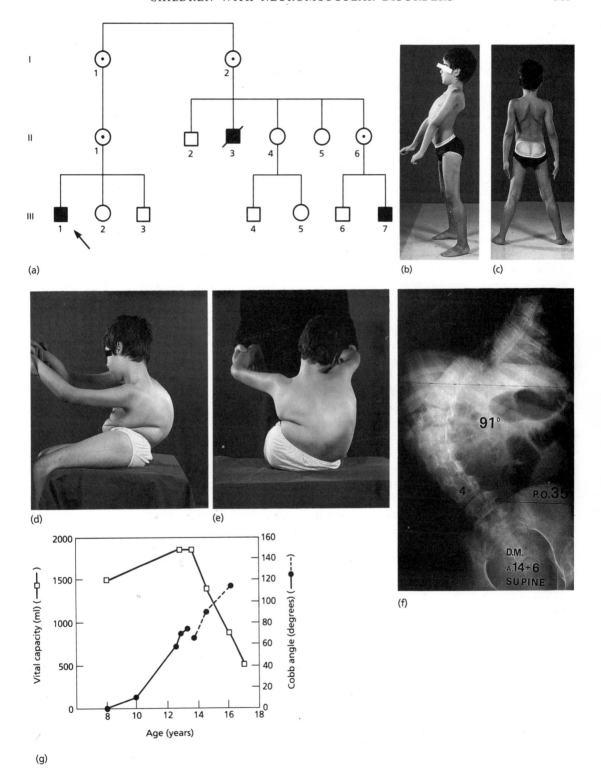

(a)

(b)

(c)

(d)

(e)

(f)

(g)

Table 22.3 Natural history of 43 patients with 'familial' Duchenne muscular dystrophy seen at the Istituto Ortopedico Rizzoli

	Mean	Range
First steps	16 m	11 m–30 m
First symptoms	3 y	1 y–5 y
Diagnosis	3 y + 6 m	0 m–7 y
Stops climbing stairs	8 y + 6 m	6 y–11 y
Stops independent walking	9 y + 6 m	7 y–13 y

y = years, m = months.

stone being attained normally according to Brooke (1986). In our experience of 43 cases of 'familial'* DMD, the first steps were taken at the age of 16 months on average (mean 11–30 months), a fair number of these patients never even managing to crawl (Table 22.3). When the child is 2–3 years old, the parents note that he falls easily, rises from the ground with difficulty and tends to have a clumsy walk. They often say that they have thought the child to be simply 'quieter' or 'lazier' than his peers or siblings. At 3–4 years the effect of muscle weakness is clear: the child cannot run, has difficulty in climbing stairs (usually one at a time) and falls a lot. At the age of 5 years the disease is overt. The stance is broad with equinus of the feet and lumbar lordosis. The muscles of the calves and buttocks and sometimes also the deltoids may be hypertrophic. The child has a waddling gait and cannot run. In getting up from the supine position he first gets on all fours and then pushes his hand against his knee (Gowers' sign). By this manoeuvre he takes 2–3 seconds to get up while a normal child of 4–5 gets on his feet in less than a second and with no need to push. Very early on, at the age of 4–5 years, it is possible to demonstrate a weakness of the gluteal and quadriceps muscles and of the extensors of the foot and to detect incipient contractures, resulting in equinus of the foot, flexion of the knee and flexion–abduction of the hip. Progression of the disease is later marked by inability to rise from the ground and climb stairs. Walking is lost at some

* Familial Duchenne with X-linked heredity ('familial' for short) denotes a patient with an affected maternal male cousin or uncle or two or more affected brothers or one affected brother and mother or sister with high CK values.

point between the ages of 7 and 13 years. In the last period of walking, falls are frequent and the asymmetry of the lower limb contractures becomes more pronounced.

In all cases DMD involves pathological changes in the statics and dynamics of the spine, responsible for major aesthetic damage and, what is worse, increasing discomfort in the sitting position and probably adverse repercussions on respiratory function. Three patterns of spinal deformity emerged in our series: kyphoscoliosis with collapse of the spine, lordoscoliosis and hyperlordosis with rigid spine (Granata *et al.*, 1982). Initially, while the patient is still ambulant, the spine remains straight and fully movable in flexion and extension. When the child ceases to walk because of the progressive loss of strength in the lower limbs, the spine is still on its axis in the frontal plane, though in the sitting position an incipient kyphotic collapse of the lumbar spine is often already evident. Gradually, partly because of the presence of asymmetrical contractures of the pelvis and lower limbs and partly because of increasing paralysis of the axial muscles, kyphoscoliosis develops. Occurring in the phase of fast pubertal growth of the spine, this deformity evolves rapidly. The kyphoscoliosis presents the typical characteristics of the neuromuscular curves, namely, a single long thoracolumbar curve with pelvic obliquity as associated component, marked correction with traction and collapse of the spine. In a small number of cases, there is no deformity on the frontal plane but a sagittal curve marked by accentuation of the lumbar lordosis and flattening or reversal of the thoracic kyphosis. This hyperlordosis is accompanied by marked limitation of spinal flexibility (rigid spine). An intermediate situation is the lordoscoliosis deformity, which combines the frontal and sagittal deformities in scoliosis and lordosis respectively. This pattern may be primary or may represent the evolution of both of the former. Indeed, in kyphoscoliosis the progressive rotation of the vertebral bodies may result in a lordoscoliosis while hyperlordosis may in the advanced stages be accompanied by a scoliotic deviation.

In this disease the respiratory pump mechanism is steadily undermined by the primary change in the muscles. The outcome is a restrictive ventilatory syndrome with dwindling VC, alveolar hypo-

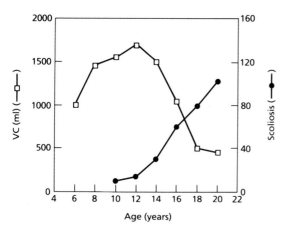

Fig. 22.6 Duchenne muscular dystrophy. The graph shows the changes in mean vital capacity (VC) and scoliosis with age in 39 patients with DMD (familial cases only). Note the characteristic bell-shaped trend of the VC with age: an ascending phase up to the age of 12 years and rapidly progressive descending phase thereafter. Absent during the ambulatory phase of the disease, scoliosis developed at around the age of 12 years, when most of the children were already chair-bound and, despite the use of a spinal brace, it rapidly worsened with age, especially during puberty. Our policy at Istituto Ortopedico Rizzoli is to recommend spine surgery as soon as the curve is apparent, if possible before it progresses beyond 40°, when VC is just beginning to decline. Compare the trends of mean VC and scoliosis in DMD with those of SMA (Fig. 22.2). Data from Istituto Ortopedico Rizzoli.

ventilation, hypoxia and hypercapnia. There is a peculiar trend of VC with advancing age (Fig. 22.6): ascending phase up to 12 years, descending phase with a very rapid loss after the age of 13–14 years. The progressive restrictive syndrome is such a constant feature of the advancing disease that, in our view, a patient who does not develop it at the appropriate stage of the disease cannot be classed as a case of DMD. Awareness of this fact is far from universal, even among specialists.* Respiratory failure develops in two stages: the first 'asymptomatic',

lasting for years, in which the loss of VC is gradual and hypoxaemia occurs during sleep, known as the phase of asymptomatic nocturnal hypoventilation, and a 'symptomatic' end stage featuring alteration of the blood gases, even during the day, and severe symptoms of suffocation and of cardiorespiratory failure. Alexander et al. (1979) found that respiratory failure becomes symptomatic after patients lose the capacity to cough effectively, which happens shortly after the age of 15 on average (range 10–20 years). When the VC falls below 700 ml, the signs of nocturnal hypoventilation are always present and the risk of death is imminent.

Mean age at death varies according to series from 15 to 18 years (Emery, 1987); the cause of death in 90% of cases is respiratory failure.

Management

Patients are followed up every 4–6 months after first examination. Assessment includes evaluation of functional capacity and of joint mobility, manual muscle test, isokinetic muscle testing, monitoring of respiratory function as from age 5, sitting X-rays of the spine at the first sign of scoliosis and every year thereafter, and cardiological evaluation as appropriate. Estimation of body composition is done by bioelectrical impedance analysis.

The manual muscle test (MMT) is the most widely used method for evaluating muscle strength in the neuromuscular patient. It requires no equipment but it is time-consuming and the test values (Medical Research Council, 1976), being descriptors of strength and not absolute measures, do not lend themselves to parametric statistical evaluation. Quantitative myometry, hand-held myometry and isokinetics do not have these limitations. Hand-held myometry measures an isometric muscular force and so depends on the point of force application and on the joint position, conditions that are difficult to reproduce in successive tests in the same patient (Delitto, 1990). Isokinetic muscle testing (IMT) does not have these drawbacks and permits the precise and repeatable description of the force produced by the skeletal muscle during exercise at constant velocity and accommodating resistance. Merlini et al. (1991) investigated the repeatability of IMT of the knee in eight neuromuscular patients with a marked reduction of force in the quadriceps

*In a recent study designed to test the power of therapeutic trials in DMD, based on the natural history of the disease, as many as 15 of the 114 patients included in the study had VC values of between 3500 and 5000 ml at ages of between 12 and 17 years (Brooke et al., 1983). These patients clearly did not have the typical form of DMD.

(less than antigravity at the MMT). Test—retest over a 4-day period yielded a coefficient of correlation of 0.99 for the extensors and 0.95 for the flexors. In this study, IMT was performed by a special method (continuous passive motion plus gravity compensation, at the angular velocity of 30°/s), which allowed the measurement of very weak forces: range 1–18 N.m for extensors and 8–28 N.m for flexors. The improper use of MMT in research has been clearly pointed out in the review of Cook & Glass (1987) and again recently by Delitto (1990); and yet it keeps on being proposed for the assessment of trials in neuromuscular disease (Bertorini *et al.*, 1991). The isokinetic test does not have these drawbacks and the particular method we have devised ('active' gravity compensation plus continuous passive motion produced by the robot) ensures the reliable measurement of even very weak forces in children from the age of 6 years (Merlini *et al.*, 1991). The disadvantages of the isokinetic method are that only the movements of the principal joints (hip, knee, ankle, shoulder and trunk) can be tested easily and the high cost of the machine. There is no doubt, however, that especially in the research setting in the field of neuromuscular disorders, when even the tiniest variations in strength up or down can be extremely important, an investment of this kind is justified.

Proposed treatments for DMD have been and continue to be numerous, as numerous as ineffective when not actually counterproductive (Emery, 1987). Both physical treatment (heat, massage, active and passive exercise, night splints, spinal brace) and pharmacological treatments (glycine, amino acids, anabolic steroids, vitamins E and B6, growth hormone inhibitor, calcium channel blockers, steroids, vasodilators and so on) have all proved powerless to affect the natural history of the disease (loss of walking before 13 years, progressive scoliosis, respiratory failure, death in the second decade). Recently, thanks to the thrilling succession of discoveries in genetics, there is a growing expectation, indeed conviction, among patients, relatives and medical staff that the discovery of a cure of DMD is at hand. In the hope that this expectation will soon be fulfilled, it is up to us in the meantime to do all we can to help the DMD sufferers now, at whatever stage of the disease they may find themselves. If there is not yet a cure for DMD, effective treatments are available to help all patients at every stage of the disease. The time has come to spread the news and promote the use of these treatments, whose efficacy has been amply proved. These treatments appreciably modify the progressive course, that is, the natural history, of DMD.

In recent years Rideau *et al.* (1983) have developed a surgical procedure designed to improve and preserve the Duchenne boy's walking and hence his independence for as long as possible. From the age of 4 onwards, the range of motion in leg joints undergoes increasing limitation, which physiotherapy cannot counter. Rideau's procedure consists in releasing hip, knee and ankle contractures in the early stages of the disease, optimally between the ages of 4 and 6. He claims that this resulted in an improvement in the boys' ability to rise from the ground with improvement or stabilization of the time taken to do so. They are also able to walk more normally and a few of them to run. The contractures have not recurred and no passive stretching was necessary. Several centres, including our own, have followed this protocol in uncontrolled trials, and Dubowitz (1989b) has set up a prospective randomized controlled trial. Of the eight patients operated on at our centre according to Rideau's protocol, four ceased to walk between the ages of 9 and 11 years and another two ceased to get up from the ground at 8 and 9 years (Fig. 22.7). In our experience, correction of the contractures has been very good and persistent, with recurrence only just before loss of walking. As to functional performance, none of our patients managed to run after the operation but their walking was more normal and confident, the time taken to rise from the ground was shorter in the year after the operation only to lengthen later, as in the boys who did not undergo operation. On our evidence the operation proved safe and effective in correcting contractures, but we think it best to await the conclusion of the controlled trials before evaluating the functional advantages.

Independent walking, which is lost between the ages of 7 and 13, can be restored for 2–3 years on average (Heckmatt *et al.*, 1985; Granata *et al.*, 1988) by fitting lightweight calipers for the lower limbs after subcutaneous tenotomy of the Achilles tendon only (Heckmatt *et al.*, 1985) or of the Achilles tendon, the superficial flexors of the hip and the

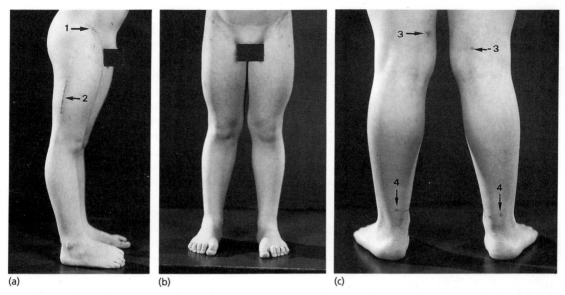

(a)   (b)   (c)

Fig. 22.7 This boy, never able to crawl, walked at 13 months. He was considered 'slow' by his parents. At 2 years he was found incidentally to have a very high CK. After the diagnosis of dystrophy he underwent multiple tenotomies according to Rideau's technique at age 5. The procedure includes (a) tenotomy of the hip flexors (scar marked by arrow 1), removal of the tensor of the fascia lata (long scar marked by arrow 2), subcutaneous release (c) of the medial flexor tendons of knee (arrow 3) and of the Achilles tendon (arrow 4). Note the expansion of the muscles (b) on the lateral side of the thigh 6 months after the operation. We have been following this child for 4 years: he has maintained good correction of the orthopaedic deformities, ceased to rise from the floor at 7.5 years; now at 9.5 he no longer climbs stairs on his own, falls only three or four times a week, still walks, slowly but fairly safely, and has only mild flexor contractures of the hips, knees and ankles. Deletion in exons between 3 and 17 was found.

medial hamstrings (Granata *et al.*, 1988) or by open surgery (Williams *et al.*, 1984). In our experience the outcome of this treatment, which should be given on loss of walking or within 3–6 months at most, is very successful. We have fitted 40 Duchenne patients aged from 8 to 13 years with calipers (lightweight knee–ankle–foot orthoses) on loss of independent walking: 35 after surgical correction of lower limb contractures (Fig. 22.8) and five without. Surgery consisted in subcutaneous release of hip flexors, medial hamstrings and Achilles tendon bilaterally. All 40 children succeeded in walking unaided with calipers. In the 13 boys who ended up in a wheelchair, independent walking was prolonged for 2.8 years on average (range 1 to 4 years). The other 27 are still walking, nine of them for more than 2 years. We feel that all Duchenne children should be offered this treatment, which has definitive functional and psychological advantages, as soon as they cease to walk.

The progression of scoliosis in DMD can be avoided only by early stabilization of the spine at the very first sign of deviation (Rideau *et al.*, 1984). It is significant that authors (Gibson & Wilkins, 1975; Drennan *et al.*, 1979) who once argued for orthopaedic treatment are now convinced that the prevention of deterioration of the spinal deformity should be entrusted to the surgeon (Gibson *et al.*, 1978; Cambridge & Drennan, 1987). Until the early 1970s, the surgical procedure was based on the Harrington instrumentation and spinal fusion (Swank *et al.*, 1982). The mechanical complications were numerous and postoperative immobilization in a cast for 12 months was required. The advent of segmental fixation (Luque, 1981) replaced every other technique for treating neuromuscular scoliosis: segmental spinal instrumentation and fusion yield good correction and provide rigid internal stabilization, eliminating the need for postoperative external immobilization. Rideau and associates

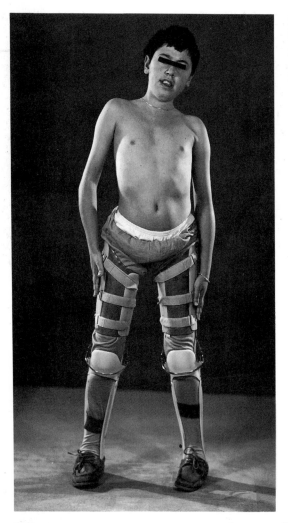

Fig. 22.8 This 13-year-old Duchenne boy continued to walk in calipers for 3.5 years after loss of walking. A maternal uncle and brother were affected. Following the loss of walking at age 9.5 he underwent percutaneous tenotomy of the Achilles tendon bilaterally and was fitted with lightweight polyethylene orthoses. His younger brother ceased to walk at 10 but remained ambulant in calipers for 2 years.

(1984) reported good results with segmental spinal instrumentation without fusion in five Duchenne patients. Moseley & Mosca in 1986 reported on 17 patients who had undergone the Luque procedure: there were no mechanical complications and the correction achieved was 52%. At the Istituto Ortopedico Rizzoli between 1985 and 1990 Luque instrumentation and fusion were performed on 15 boys with DMD (Fig. 22.9). The mean age of the nine with more than 1 year's follow-up was 13 years; the preoperative scoliosis was 42° (range 10–80°) and mean VC 1842 ml (range 1250–2100). Postoperatively, the average scoliosis was 14° (range 0–43°) and mean VC 1693 ml (range 1250–2100). Our policy now is to advise surgery in all non-ambulant Duchenne patients between 10 and 13 years when the VC is not less than 40% of the predicted value and the curve is less than 40°. In these conditions the operation is easier and quicker and carries less risk. The Luque procedure with arthrodesis is still the method of choice, because it affords good correction and restores balance to the trunk and pelvis, allowing a more comfortable seated position and releasing the hands, which no longer have to hold up the trunk, for other activities. Our results likewise show that it is possible to operate on these patients early and that the correction is sufficiently stable through time; in cases in which loss of correction occurred, it was found to be slight and after long follow-up VC is not significantly affected by the operation and the fall observed in the postoperative period and in follow-up (Fig. 22.9) lies within the descending limb of the curve that characterizes the disease (Miller *et al.*, 1991). Very mild deformities in patients up to the age of 12 can be corrected without arthrodesis, which shortens the operating time and allows some further growth of the spine (Rideau *et al.*, 1984).

The respiratory failure of DMD can be treated effectively, both in the end stage, with severe symptoms and altered blood gases at rest, and in the asymptomatic phase, marked by sleep hypoxia and decreasing VC with no daytime symptoms of hypoventilation. The rationale of mechanical ventilation is the demonstration supplied by Rochester *et al.* (1977) that it rests the respiratory muscles and diaphragm of patients with chronic restrictive syndrome, as shown by the absence of electrical activity on electromyography (EMG). It was shown that mechanical ventilation at night significantly improved the gas exchange, not only during the period of nocturnal ventilation but also during the day. This prolonging of the effect of ventilation was attributed by Curran (1981) to the resting of the respiratory muscles during the night and to their better oxygenation.

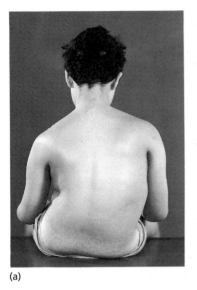 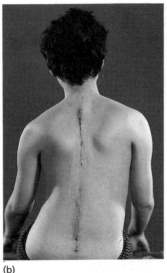 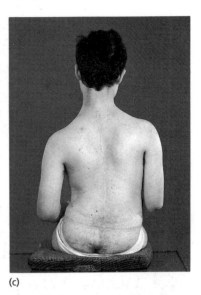

(a) (b) (c)

Fig. 22.9 This Duchenne boy ceased walking at age 10, and at age 12 showed (a) thoracolumbar scoliosis of 35° and a kyphosis of 40° with pelvic obliquity; his VC was 1500 ml (62%). He underwent Luque segmental spinal instrumentation plus fusion. Four months after surgery (b) at 13 years of age he could sit with a good balance and a straight spine. Postoperative scoliosis measured 20° and kyphosis 10°; VC was 1500 ml (56%). At 19 years of age (c), 6 years after surgery, the spine remained stable and VC was 1200 ml (29%). Early stabilization of the spine allows a long-lasting control of the curve but does not modify the progressive deterioration of VC.

Alexander *et al.* (1979) reported on 10 Duchenne patients with caring families who had a meaningful average survival of 3.4 years, using a combination of positive and negative ventilatory aids at home, after allegedly reaching the end stage of ventilatory insufficiency. Curran (1981) in nine late-stage Duchenne boys found that night ventilation by body respirators provided a constant significant improvement in daytime gas exchange for periods averaging up to 2 years following the occurrence of respiratory failure. On this evidence he recommends aggressive early conservative measures, including body respirators, postural drainage, chest physiotherapy with abdominal-assisted coughing, intratracheal suctioning and bronchoscopy to combat respiratory infection and decrease the need of tracheostomy and volume ventilators, which can be so disabling to the chronic restrictive disease patient. By means of positive-pressure ventilators, Bach *et al.* (1981) were able to prolong the lives of 29 patients with muscular dystrophy, 10 of whom had permanent tracheostomies, by an average of 7 years. The reporting of these results did not change

the prevalent attitude of the international medical community of no action to prolong the lives of Duchenne patients. Rideau and associates (1983) criticized this position, which perhaps stemmed from the conviction that prolonging Duchenne life 'simply prolongs an unacceptable condition of living'. They argued that, given technological improvements and better social and educational opportunities, premature death from respiratory failure was no longer to be considered an inevitable event but was 'simply a therapeutic failure'. In a survey conducted in the USA (Colbert & Schock, 1985) on the use of respirators for progressive neuromuscular diseases, it was found that only 495 patients in 132 Muscular Dystrophy Association clinics received some form of assisted ventilation (43% of whom had permanent tracheostomies), but neither patient selection nor protocol for respirator use was standardized.

The recently introduced intermittent positive-pressure ventilation via nasal mask has revolutionized the management of 'symptomatic' hypoventilation in neuromuscular, including

Duchenne, patients (Bach *et al.*, 1987; Ellis *et al.*, 1987; Kerby *et al.*, 1987; Granata *et al.*, 1989a; Heckmatt *et al.*, 1990). This technique is non-invasive, well tolerated and suitable for use at home. Symptoms of chronic hypoventilation, such as headache, insomnia and/or somnolence and impaired intellectual capacity, rapidly disappear with overnight ventilation. Good oxygen saturations are achieved during night-time ventilation, and daytime arterial Po_2 and Pco_2 improve with treatment.

Rideau & Delaubier (1987) have suggested that nasal ventilation should be given as a form of 'prophylaxis' to Duchenne patients to prevent symptoms of suffocation, preserve lung function and allow the patient to live a more enjoyable life to his full capacity. Using this method in 30 patients Rideau & Delaubier (1987) managed to keep the annual loss of VC down to 39 ml/year compared with 206 ml/year before treatment. Our own approach is to start nasal ventilation at night as soon as the Duchenne boy begins to lose VC, which happens after the age of 13–15 years, when he is already chair-bound. Since 1986 we have treated 21 Duchenne patients in this way (Granata *et al.*, 1989a). Of these, 12 have a follow-up of more than a year. The mean age of the latter patients when first seen was 14.3 years (range 11.7–19) and their mean VC 1659 (range 696–2160). At the start of treatment, the mean age was 15.9 years (range 13–20) and their mean VC was 1219 ml (range 480–1680). In the meantime they had lost VC at the rate of 333 ml/year. All but one had normal blood-gas values when awake. At a mean follow-up of 2.4 years, their mean VC was 1073 ml (range 300–1740), with a mean loss of VC of 46 ml/year only (range −222 to +187). In view of these encouraging results, we now start night-time nasal ventilation as soon as sleep hypoxia is apparent, without waiting to demonstrate a tendency to loss of VC.

All neuromuscular patients followed by the authors at the Istituto Ortopedico Rizzoli receive the treatments mentioned in this review. With thorough knowledge of the natural history of the disease, expected complications such as progressive scoliosis in DMD can be prevented by means of early surgery on the spine. Independent ambulation can be prolonged significantly by fitting long leg orthoses in young children with intermediate SMA or in boys with DMD on loss of walking. Surgical correction of scoliosis in intermediate SMA appreciably enhances the quality of life by making the sitting position comfortable and the child's appearance more pleasing. Mechanical ventilation can prolong life indefinitely. While we hope that advances in the basic sciences, especially genetics, will lead to the final defeat of these diseases one day, the rehabilitative measures now available have immense value for patients suffering here and now.

Acknowledgements

The work of the Muscle Clinic Laboratory is supported by the Istituto Ortopedico Rizzoli and by grants from the Italian Telethon (project no. 340) and the NATO Scientific Affairs Division.

References

Alexander M.A., Johnson E.W., Petty J. & Stauch D. (1979) Mechanical ventilation of patients with late stage Duchenne muscular dystrophy: management in the home. *Archives of Physical and Medical Rehabilitation* **60**, 289–292.

Bach J., Alba A., Pilkington L.A. & Lee M. (1981) Long-term rehabilitation in advanced stage of childhood onset, rapidly progressive muscular dystrophy. *Archives of Physical and Medical Rehabilitation* **62**, 328–331.

Bach J.R., Alba A., Mosher R. & Delaubier A. (1987) Intermittent positive pressure ventilation via nasal access in the management of respiratory insufficiency. *Chest* **92**, 169–170.

Ballestrazzi A., Ballardini D., Battistini N. & Merlini L. (1989) Growth pattern and body composition in spinal muscular atrophy. In Merlini L., Granata C. & Dubowitz V. (eds) *Current Concepts in Childhood Spinal Muscular Atrophy*, pp. 221–226. Springer-Verlag, Vienna.

Bertorini T.E., Palmieri G.M., Griffin J., Igarashi M., Hinton A. & Karas J.G. (1991) Effect of dantrolene in Duchenne muscular dystrophy. *Muscle and Nerve* **14** (6), 503–507.

Bradford D.S. (1987) In Bradford D.S., Lonstein J.E., Moe J.H., Olgivie J.W. & Winter R.B. (eds) *Moe's Textbook of Scoliosis and Other Spinal Deformities*. W.B. Saunders, Philadelphia.

Brooke M.H. (1986) *A Clinician's View of Neuromuscular Diseases*. Williams and Wilkins, Baltimore.

Brooke M.H., Fenichel G.M., Gripp R.C. *et al.* (1983) Clinical investigation in Duchenne dystrophy: 2. Determination of the power of therapeutic trials based on the natural history. *Muscle and Nerve* **6**, 91–103.

Brown J.C., Zeller J.L., Swank S.M., Furumasu J. & Warath S.L. (1989) Surgical and functional results of spine fusion in spinal muscular atrophy. *Spine* **14** (7), 763–770.

Brzustowicz L.M., Lehner T., Castilla L.H. *et al.* (1990) Genetic mapping of chronic childhood-onset spinal muscular atrophy to chromosome 5q11.2–13.3. *Nature* **344** (6266), 540–541.

Cambridge W. & Drennan J.C. (1987) Scoliosis associated with Duchenne muscular dystrophy. *Journal of Pediatric Orthopedists* **7**, 436–440.

Cervellati S., Palmisani M., Bonfiglioli S. & Savini R. (1989) Surgical treatment of scoliosis in spinal muscular atrophy. In Merlini L., Granata C. & Dubowitz V. (eds) *Current Concepts in Childhood Spinal Muscular Atrophy*, pp. 175–192. Springer-Verlag, Vienna.

Colbert A.P. & Schock N.C. (1985) Respirator use in progressive neuromuscular diseases. *Archives of Physical and Medical Rehabilitation* **66**, 760–762.

Cook J.D. & Glass D.S. (1987) Strength evaluation in neuromuscular disease. *Neurological Clinics* **5**, 101–123.

Curran F.J. (1981) Night ventilation by body respirators for patients in chronic respiratory failure due to late stage Duchenne muscular dystrophy. *Archives of Physical and Medical Rehabilitation* **62**, 270–274.

Daher Y.H., Lonstein J.E., Winter R.B. & Bradford D.S. (1985) Spinal surgery in spinal muscular atrophy. *Journal of Pediatric Orthopedists* **5**, 391–395.

Delitto A. (1990) Isokinetic dynamometry. *Muscle and Nerve* Suppl., 53–57.

Delmas M.C. & Berard C. (1990) Prise en charge globale de l'amyotrophie spinale infantile. Guide pratique pour les équipes médicales. *Pédiatrie* **45** (7–8), 457–464.

Drennan J.C., Renshaw T.S. & Curtis H.H. (1979) The thoracic suspension orthosis. *Clinics in Orthopedics* **139**, 39–41.

Dubowitz V. (1974) Benign infantile muscular atrophy. *Developmental and Medical Child Neurology* **16**, 672–675.

Dubowtiz V. (1989a) *A Colour Atlas of Muscle Disorders in Childhood*. Wolfe Medical Publications, London.

Dubowitz V. (1989b) The Duchenne dystrophy story: from phenotype to gene and potential treatment. *Journal of Child Neurology* **4**, 240–250.

Dubowitz V. (1991) Chaos in classification of the spinal muscular atrophies of childhood. *Neuromuscular Disorders* **1** (2), 77–80.

Duval-Beaupère G., Barois A., Quinet I. & Estournet B. (1985) Les problèmes thoracique rachidiens et respiratoires de l'enfant attent d'amyotrophie spinale infantile à évolution prolongée. *Archives Françaises Pédiatriques* **42**, 625–634.

Ellis E.R., Bye P.T., Bruderer J.W. *et al.* (1987) Treatment of respiratory failure during sleep in patients with neuromuscular disease: positive-pressure ventilation through a nose mask. *American Reviews of Respiratory Disease* **135**, 148–152.

Emery A.E.H. (1987) *Duchenne Muscular Dystrophy*. Oxford University Press, Oxford.

Emery A.E.H. (1991) Population frequencies of inherited neuromuscular diseases – a world survey. *Neuromuscular Disorders* **1** (1), 19–30.

Eng G.D., Binder H. & Koch B. (1984) Spinal muscular atrophy: experience in diagnosis and rehabilitation management of 60 patients. *Archives of Physical and Medical Rehabilitation* **65**, 549–553.

Evans G.A., Drennan J.C. & Russman B.S. (1981) Functional classification and orthopaedic management of spinal muscular atrophy. *Journal of Bone and Joint Surgery* **63B**, 516–522.

Gibson D.A. & Wilkins K.E. (1975) The management of spinal deformities in Duchenne muscular dystrophy. *Clinics in Orthopedics* **108**, 41–51.

Gibson D.A., Koreska J., Eng P., Robertson D., Kahn A. & Albisser A.M. (1978) The management of spinal deformity in Duchenne's muscular dystrophy. *Orthopedic Clinics of North America* **9** (2), 437–450.

Gilgoff I.S., Kahlstrom E., MacLaughlin E. & Keens T.G. (1989) Long-term ventilatory support in spinal muscular atrophy. *Journal of Pediatrics* **115** (6), 904–909.

Granata C., Merlini L., Parisini P. & Savini R. (1982) Spinal deformity in Duchenne muscular dystrophy. *Cardiomyology* **1**, 117–126.

Granata C., Cornelio F., Bonfiglioli S., Mattutini P. & Merlini L. (1987) Promotion of ambulation of patients with spinal muscular atrophy by early fitting of knee–ankle–foot orthoses. *Developmental and Medical Child Neurology* **29**, 221–224.

Granata C., Giannini S., Rubbini L., Corbascio M., Bonfiglioli S., Sabattini L. & Merlini L. (1988) La chirurgia ortopedica per prolungare il cammino nella distrofia muscolare di Duchenne. *Chirurgia degli Organi di Movimento* **73**, 237–248.

Granata C., Capelli T., Schiavina M., Fabiani A. *et al.* (1989a) Ventilation mécanique dans la dystrophie musculaire de Duchenne. *Semaine des Hôpitaux* **65**, 1037–1041.

Granata C., Merlini L., Magni E., Marini M.L. & Stagni S.B. (1989b) Spinal muscular atrophy: natural history and orthopaedic treatment of scoliosis. *Spine* **14** (7), 760–762.

Granata C., Magni E., Merlini L. & Cervellati S. (1990) Hip dislocation in spinal muscular atrophy. *Chirurgia degli Organi di Movimento* **75**, 177–184.

Heckmatt J.Z., Hyde S.A., Florence J., Gabain A.C. & Thompson N. (1985) Prolongation of walking in Duchenne muscular dystrophy with lightweight orthoses: review of 57 cases. *Development and Medical Child Neurology* **27**, 149–154.

Heckmatt J.Z., Loh L. & Dubowitz V. (1990) Night-time nasal ventilation in neuromuscular disease. *Lancet* **335**, 579–582.

Kerby G.R., Mayer L.S. & Pingleton S.K. (1987) Nocturnal

positive pressure ventilation via nasal mask. *American Reviews of Respiratory Disease* **135**, 738–740.

Luque E.R. (1981) Segmental spinal instrumentation in the treatment of paralytic scoliosis. *Orthopedic Transactions* **5**, 409–410.

Marri E., Calabria M.A., Granata C., Bonfiglioli Stagni S. & Merlini L. (1991) Le malattie neuromuscolari a Bologna e provincia. Aspetti epidemiologici. *Epidemiologia per la Salute* **4**, 36–40.

Medical Research Council (1976) *Aids to the Investigation of Peripheral Nerve Injuries.* Her Majesty's Stationery Office, London.

Melki J., Abdelhak S., Sheth P. *et al.* (1990) Gene for chronic proximal spinal muscular atrophies maps to chromosome 5q. *Nature* **344** (6268), 767–768.

Merlini L. & Granata C. (1990) Rehabilitation of children with muscle disease. *Current Opinion in Neurology and Neurosurgery* **3**, 738–741.

Merlini L., Granata C., Capelli T., Mattutini P. & Colombo C. (1989) Natural history of infantile and childhood spinal muscular atrophy. In Merlini L., Granata C. & Dubowitz V. (eds) *Current Concepts in Childhood Spinal Muscular Atrophy*, pp. 95–100. Springer-Verlag, Vienna.

Merlini L., Dell'Accio D., Bonoldi S. & Monti D. (1991) Isokinetic evaluation in neuromuscular patient. *International Society of Electrophysiological Kinesiology* Abs. 20.

Miller R.G., Chalmers A.G., Dao H., Filler-Katz A., Holman D. & Bost F. (1991) The effect of spine fusion on respiratory function in Duchenne muscular dystrophy. *Neurology* **41**, 38–40.

Moseley C.F. & Mosca V. (1986) The Duchenne muscular dystrophy child: recent development in spinal fusion. *Muscle and Nerve* Suppl. 9, 86–87.

Munsat T.L. (1991) Workshop report: International SMA Collaboration. *Neuromuscular Disorders* **1** (2), 81.

Noble-Jamieson C.M., Heckmatt J.Z., Dubowitz V. & Silverman M. (1986) The effect of posture and spinal bracing on respiratory function in neuromuscular disease. *Archives of Disease in Childhood* **61**, 168–171.

Phillip D.P., Roye D.P. Jr, Farcy J.P., Leet A. & Shelton Y.A. (1990) Surgical treatment of scoliosis in a spinal muscular atrophy population. *Spine* **15** (9), 942–945.

Rideau Y. & Delaubier A. (1987) Neuromuscular respiratory deficit: setting back mortality. *Seminars in Orthopaedics* **2**, 203–210.

Rideau Y., Glorion B. & Duport G. (1983) Prolongation of ambulation in the muscular dystrophies. *Acta Neurologica* **5**, 390–397.

Rideau Y., Glorion B., Delaubier A., Tarlé O. & Bach J. (1984) The treatment of scoliosis in Duchenne muscular dystrophy. *Muscle and Nerve* **7**, 281–286.

Rochester D., Braun N. & Laine S. (1977) Diaphragm energy expenditure in chronic respiratory failure: effect of assisted ventilation with body respirators. *American Journal of Medicine* **63**, 223–232.

Rodillo E., Marini M.L., Heckmatt J.Z. & Dubowitz V. (1989) Scoliosis in spinal muscular atrophy: review of 63 cases. *Journal of Child Neurology* **4** (2), 118–123.

Rowland L.P. (1988) Clinical concepts of Duchenne muscular dystrophy. *Brain* **111**, 479–495.

Russman B.S., Melchreit R. & Drennan J.C. (1983) Spinal muscular atrophy: the natural course of the disease. *Muscle and Nerve* **6**, 179–181.

Shapiro F. & Bresnan J.M. (1982) Orthopaedic management of childhood neuromuscular disease. *Journal of Bone and Joint Surgery* **64A**, 785–789.

Swank S.M., Brown J.C. & Perry E.R. (1982) Spinal fusion in Duchenne's muscular dystrophy. *Spine* **7** (5), 484–491.

Thompson C.E. & Larsen L.J. (1990) Recurrent hip dislocation in intermediate spinal atrophy. *Journal of Pediatric Orthopedics* **10** (5), 638–641.

Williams E.A., Read L., Ellis A., Galasko C.S.B. & Morris P. (1984) The management of equinus deformity in Duchenne muscular dystrophy. *Journal of Bone and Joint Surgery* **66**, 546–550.

23: Neurological Rehabilitation in the Elderly

R.C. TALLIS

The need for a rehabilitative approach throughout the medicine of old age, 313
  The burden of chronic disabling disease, 313
  Global impact of focal disease in the biologically aged, 315
  Multiple pathology, 315
  The vicious spiral of immobility, 315
  Adverse social circumstances, 316
  The situation of the disabled elderly person, 316
Rehabilitation in old age: some general principles, 316
  Definition of rehabilitation, 316
  Principles of rehabilitation in old age, 317
  The multidisciplinary team, 318
  Multidimensional assessment, 320
Medication as a cause of chronic disability in old age, 322
Aids, 323
  Principles of provision, 323
  What is available, 324
  Problems, 324
The organization of rehabilitation services for the elderly, 324
  Progressive patient care, 325
  The problems and perils of hospital admission for an elderly person, 325
  Geriatric day hospitals, 326
  Domiciliary care, 327
The needs of carers, 327
Rehabilitation in long-term care, 329
Geriatric rehabilitation: an infant science, 329

Many of the general principles and the particular techniques used in neurological rehabilitation apply equally to young and old patients. Moreover, the conditions that account for the greatest burden of neurological disability in old age (stroke, parkinsonism and dementia) have been dealt with in earlier chapters. In order, therefore, to avoid duplication of coverage, the scope of the present chapter will be limited, with an emphasis on the issues that are particularly relevant to the elderly. Nevertheless, some general points will be reiterated.

The need for a rehabilitative approach throughout the medicine of old age

There are many reasons why rehabilitation should be at the centre of the medicine of old age and why, increasingly, the elderly are, or should be, of central importance to rehabilitationists.

The burden of chronic disabling disease

The elderly bear the heaviest burden of chronic disabling disease. According to a recent major survey in the United Kingdom (OPCS, 1988a), there is a more than 20-fold increase in the prevalence of disability between the twenties and the eighties. The strong relationship between age and disability is dramatically illustrated in Fig. 23.1. The prevalence of major and minor disabilities rises to over 700 per 1000 in people over the age of 80; and the vast majority of individuals with the most severe (grade 9–10) disabilities are over the age of 65. Even though one might quarrel with the threshold for defining disability in the OPCS survey, the steep age trend in both prevalence and severity of disability is beyond question. Other surveys have shown that chronic disability is common in old age and is commoner in the old elderly compared with the young elderly. For example, while 5% of those between 65 and 69 are unable to go out and walk unaided, this figure rises to 48% for those over 85. The corresponding figures for those unable to climb stairs are 3% and 31% (General Household Survey, 1980). The steep relationship between increasing age and dependency within the elderly population is demonstrated vividly in the data from Vetter *et al.*

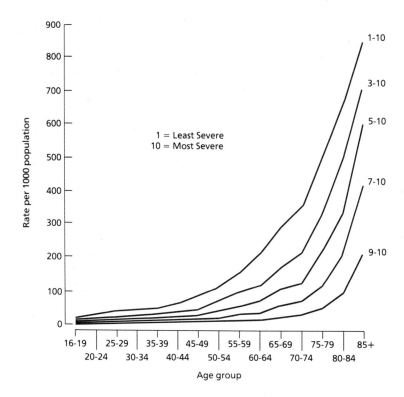

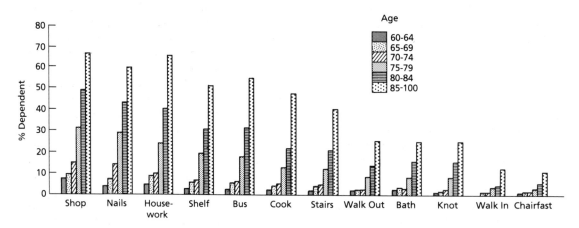

Fig. 23.1 Estimates of the prevalence of disability among adults in Great Britain by age and severity category. Source: OPCS, 1988a.

(1990), reproduced in Fig. 23.2. A recent survey of people aged over 75 living in their own homes in South Wales found that 15% were severely disabled (Salvage *et al.*, 1988).

These findings are hardly surprising as many chronic disabling conditions are strongly age-related. This particularly applies to neurological problems, such as stroke (Bamford *et al.*, 1988), Parkinson's disease (Mutch *et al.*, 1986), dementia (Kay, 1991) and epilepsy (Tallis *et al.*, 1991). For example, the Oxford Community Stroke Project (Bamford *et al.*, 1988) found that the steep age-

Fig. 23.2 Dependency profile of elderly people by age. Source: Vetter *et al.*, 1990.

associated rise in incidence is maintained into extreme old age, with rates as high as 20 per 1000 being reached in the over-85s, compared with an overall population incidence of 2 per 1000. The same study showed that the likelihood of permanent disability following stroke was also strongly age-related. Whereas only about 30% of those who survive a first stroke under the age of 65 are dependent after 6 months, the dependency rates in those aged 75–84 are 50% and in those over 85 70–80%. The projected ageing of the elderly population, with a disproportionate increase in the very old (US Bureau of the Census), implies a further increase in the absolute numbers of disabled elderly people, though this may not be as great as expected (Malmgren et al., 1989; see also the discussion at the end of this chapter).

Global impact of focal disease in the biologically aged

Another important reason why rehabilitation is central to old age medicine is connected with the atypical way in which acute illnesses present in the biologically aged (Horan, 1992). Even focal, reversible conditions may have a global impact and present with certain non-specific symptoms that are common to many conditions. For example, a chest infection may cause an elderly person to become confused, to lose continence, to be prone to falls or to become immobile, with the consequent risk of the complex negative effects of immobility (see below). This global impact reflects in part the impaired adaptative response to adverse events that is seen in the ageing body and in part the fact that aged patients frequently have concurrent diseases in other organs.

Multiple pathology (Wilson et al., 1962)

In old age, 'When sorrows come, they come not single spies, But in battalions' (Shakespeare, Hamlet). Patients with neurological problems will often have other disabling conditions. Of these, the most important are bone and joint disease. Osteoarthritis is strongly age-related (Lawrence et al., 1969) and about 80% of people over 60 have some evidence of osteoarthritis (Favour et al., 1956). A painful knee will provide a major barrier to the restoration of mobility in a stroke patient, and painful arthritic hands, as well as being demoralizing in their own right, may predispose to upper limb spasticity. Osteoporosis, also strongly age-associated (Francis, 1992), will mean that falls associated with neurological disease will be more likely to be associated with fracture. The age-dependency of both osteoporosis and neurological causes of instability explains some of the spectacular rise in fractured neck of femur with age (Sainsbury, 1991). Andrews (1985) reported that 35% of successive patients admitted to his rehabilitation unit had four or more chronic conditions.

The recognition and treatment of concurrent diseases (for example, the cardiac failure that is presenting atypically as fatigue and lethargy) are crucial to successful geriatric rehabilitation. It is equally important to ensure that this treatment does not itself interfere with rehabilitation of the primary neurological problem (for example, postural hypotension making it impossible for the stroke patient to tolerate standing).

The vicious spiral of immobility

The common occurrence of combinations of illnesses can readily lead to a vicious spiral of muscular weakness, immobility, dependency and loss of confidence. Consider the situation of an elderly stroke patient who, as frequently happens, develops a chest infection. Let us suppose also that he/she has co-existent osteoarthritis. As a result of the chest infection, he/she may go off his/her legs. This will rapidly lead to disuse atrophy of the muscles (Rennie, 1985). Wasting of the quadriceps, in particular, will cause destabilization of the knee joint, an increase in arthritis-associated pain and a disinclination to walk or even stand. This further immobilization will cause further weakness and wasting and add to the mobility problems arising from the stroke. All of these adverse changes will take place against the background of a pre-existing age-related impairment in muscle function (Young et al., 1985; Bruce et al., 1989). A positive feedback mechanism, whereby even minor locomotor disability sets in train a cascade of adverse events inexorably leading to progressive loss of ambulatory function and eventual total immobility, is thus readily envisaged. This process would be greatly accelerated in the case of a neurologically disabled individual who had a fall – a common occurrence in stroke, epilepsy and Parkinson's disease – and, due to osteoporosis (itself perhaps the result of reduced mobility), sustained a fractured neck of femur. The adverse effect of age on adaptative responses to trauma (Horan *et al.*, 1988) will further predispose to the vicious spiral whereby decreased mobility leads to increasing weakness and further immobility and loss of confidence.

Adverse social circumstances

The impact of acute and chronic physical impairments may be exacerbated by adverse social circumstances. In old age, isolation (General Household Survey, 1980) and material deprivation (OPCS, 1988b) are not uncommon. Isolation is not just a simple matter of living alone. Poor mobility, associated with non-neurological as well as neurological problems and with fear of injury and assault, may lead to an individual becoming housebound. This will severely limit socialization and the development and maintenance of social support networks. To this may be added the isolating effects of visual and hearing impairment, both of which are steeply age-dependent (Herbst & Humphrey, 1981; Jones *et al.*, 1984; Warren, 1985). Physical impairments may also take place against the background of chronic cognitive deficits, which also rise sharply with age (Kay, 1991). The impact of sensory impairment on cognitive function has been carefully investigated: deafness or a cataract may bring an individual with mild cognitive impairment closer to cognitive breakdown, failure of function and dependency.

The situation of the disabled elderly person

The situation of many disabled elderly patients, depicted in Fig. 23.3, is thus very complex and indicates the need for a response that is as complex.

Rehabilitation in old age: some general principles

The medicine of old age is thus concerned not only with the diagnosis and treatment of disease but also

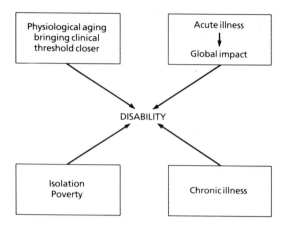

Fig. 23.3 The complex situation of the biologically aged ill person.

with assessing and reversing their functional and social consequences, using a variety of professional help and support services. This, in essence, is the rehabilitation approach. Although the principles are similar in younger and older patients, it is worth reiterating these before focusing on more specific issues relevant to the elderly.

Definition of rehabilitation

Rehabilitation is difficult to define succinctly. It means different things to different people, or, rather, different aspects of it are emphasized in different definitions. It may be characterized in terms of its context, its procedures and its goal.

As regards *context*, rehabilitation as an approach to management predominates when the pathological processes underlying a disease prove unresponsive, or only partially responsive, to would-be cure. This is unhelpfully non-specific but it does draw attention to the fact that, although rehabilitation is a part of all medicine, it comes to the fore in our dealings with chronic or incurable disease and so in the management of many elderly patients.

Rehabilitation may be defined in terms of its *procedures* and strategies. According to Hirschberg (1983), 'the basic concept of medical rehabilitation is to have the healthy part of the body take over functions that the diseased part cannot handle'. This may involve retraining in daily living skills and may be helped by the judicious deployment of aids and appliances. Rehabilitation will also include manipulating the extracorporeal world to make it more user-friendly for the disabled person; such manoeuvres range from provision of adapted clothing to making shops more accessible, for example by the provision of special transport or a mobility allowance. Rehabilitation also includes the gradual withdrawal of support to minimize disability. More narrowly, 'rehabilitation' refers to certain procedures carried out mainly by remedial therapists, such as ploys to reduce spasticity, retraining of gait and teaching activities of daily living (ADL) with or without the help of aids and appliances.

Finally, rehabilitation may be defined in terms of its *goal*, which has been characterized as 'restoring a disabled person to a condition in which he or she is able, as early as possible, to resume a normal life'. From this rather vague description we may salvage the idea of rehabilitation as all the things that are done to minimize the adverse impact of what is irreversible in pathological processes upon the patient's life.

Clarifying the distinction between impairment, disability and handicap has sharpened our conception of rehabilitation. We may think of the impairment as essentially a deficiency in the body; the disability as a limitation in ADL; and the handicap as the social disadvantage and dependency that result. The handicap is the 'cash value' of the impairment or the disease. The fundamental insight behind rehabilitation is *that the amount of handicap need not be proportional to the amount of impairment.* An individual may have only a small impairment and yet be enormously handicapped, or, on the other hand, may be severely impaired and yet be relatively free of handicap. Most rehabilitation at present is about intervening between impairments and disabilities and between disabilities and handicaps. With advancing knowledge of, for example, neurophysiology and plasticity in the nervous system, the neurological rehabilitation of the future may increasingly include reversing impairments (Fig. 23.4).

Principles of rehabilitation in old age

The approach to the rehabilitation of the elderly (which, as I have indicated, differs only in emphasis from the principles of rehabilitation applicable to any age) is symbolized in Fig. 23.5. This figure could be summarized in the statement that successful rehabilitation will require that we take notice not only of what has happened to the 'organism' (or the organ) but also of the environment of the person. It is necessary, therefore, to treat not only the damaged system, if such treatment is available (for example the injury to the brain as in a stroke, or the infected lungs as in pneumonia), but also the rest of the body. The latter will be at risk in the elderly for several reasons: the global impact of focal diseases (discussed above); the increased likelihood of concurrent pathology; and the secondary effects of non-specific manifestation of disease in old age, such as immobility and incontinence. It will be necessary to counter adverse psychological attitudes in patients and in both informal and professional carers; pessimism has a tendency to be self-fulfilling. As discussed below, many institutions are themselves potentially disabling for elderly people and a

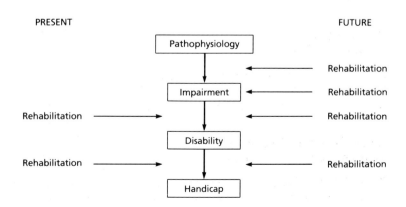

Fig. 23.4 Rehabilitation – present and future.

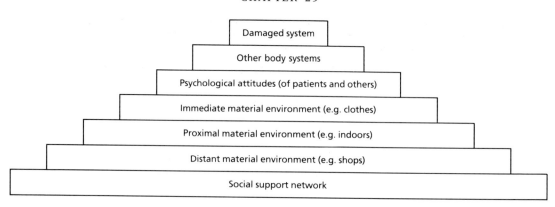

Fig. 23.5 Rehabilitation targets.

conscious policy which actively encourages independence by a gradual withdrawal of support when it is not required is essential. The material environment may be considered in layers, extending outside from the patient's clothes: the bed, toilet and chairs; access to work surfaces; mobility within, into and out of, and outside the house; and finally access to facilities such as shops. The material environment should be modified in the patient's favour with retraining in ADL, modification of commodities, the provision of aids to living, the adaptation of living spaces and the provision of allowances. Finally, existing social networks should be mobilized to provide most effective and least intrusive support and supplemented where necessary by various services and statutory agencies (see Table 23.1).

The multidisciplinary team

This complex response to the complex needs of elderly people clearly cannot be the responsibility of one group of professionals alone. The multidisciplinary team is consequently a ubiquitous feature of geriatric services. The core members of the team are patients and carers, nurses, therapists, social workers and doctors. In the case of a particular patient, the team may be augmented by, for example, a clinical psychologist, psychiatrist or orthopaedic surgeon. Successful teamwork depends upon respect for each other's expertise and good communication between team members.

Mutual respect is less of a problem than it was. Interprofessional rivalry between, for example, occupational therapists and physiotherapists has been replaced by recognition that the work of the latter in retraining ADL is dependent upon the success of the former in restoring upper limb mobility and ambulation. The rival claims of the medical and the social models of disability have been laid to rest in the recognition that disability (or, at any rate, handicap) is the social consequence of medical illness and that the two approaches are not mutually exclusive but complementary.

If there is less debate about the 'socialization' and the 'medicalization' of disability (Kane, 1982), it may be because the role of the doctor in geriatric rehabilitation is perhaps less problematic than in other areas of rehabilitation. Multiple pathology is a feature of old age and there are usually enough ongoing medical problems to prevent the physician from feeling sidelined by the central work of the therapists into becoming a 'medically qualified amateur social worker' or, worse still, trying to reassume control of the case by gratuitous interference with the duration and nature of remedial therapy. The physician should be responsible for ensuring that the management is guided by an accurate diagnosis of the initial problems, that appropriate medical treatment is instituted, that medication is constantly reviewed, that new medical problems are diagnosed and treated, that a full assessment has been carried out, that explicit goals are set and progress towards them is monitored and

Table 23.1 Examples of services which should be available to support elderly people in the community

Domiciliary services

Home help	People requiring help with personal care, housework and shopping
Meals on wheels	People unable to prepare a meal for themselves, usually living alone, usually housebound
Bath attendant	People unable to bath themselves
Laundry service	Incontinent people
Home-nursing aids	People being nursed at home
Aids to daily living, adaptations to home	People requiring aids or adaptations to achieve maximum independence
Sheltered housing	People requiring alarm system, oversight system, oversight by a warden (N.B. not a personal care service)
District nurse	People requiring nursing at home or in residential care
Community psychiatric nurse	Mentally ill people needing nursing support, carers needing advice regarding management
Health visitor	People at home needing advice about diet, general health care
Chiropody	People in any setting needing foot care
Social worker	People requiring practical help and support, and counselling
Occupational therapist (OT)	People needing rehabilitation advice or treatment

Day care services

Day centre	Those requiring social stimulation or personal care
Geriatric day hospital	Mentally ill or frail people requiring rehabilitation or medical treatment
Psychogeriatric day hospital	Mentally ill or infirm people requiring rehabilitation or maintenance
Luncheon club	People able to make their own way to a centre, benefiting from company and having a meal provided

that plans for discharge or discontinuation of therapy are made when appropriate. This should be sufficient to keep even the most role-sensitive doctor from feeling marginalized.

The problem of satisfactory communication – crucial to the multidisciplinary, multiagency management of elderly people – is less easily solved. Within hospital-based teams, this is relatively straightforward: the team should meet on a weekly basis at a case conference. At such a meeting, progress should be reported in the following areas: the treatment of medical problems; recovery of mobility skills; restoration of independence in ADL; and the outcome of discussions with patients (and possibly carers) regarding the setting and attainment of the goals of rehabilitation. Observations about the patient's moods, wishes, hopes and fears can also be reported. The case conference is also the forum where more detailed social enquiries and home assessment visits can be planned and their findings fed back and where discharge from hospital can be planned. A successful discharge will require a clear appreciation of the patient's capabilities, knowledge of the support that is available and of the particular strengths and weaknesses of the material and social home environment, and the timely provision of aids, appliances and social support and of appropriate adaptations. Discharge may fail because of a walking aid that arrives 24 hours too late, a promised home help that does not materialize or inadequate warning of informal carers. Ensuring this does not happen requires good communication, not only within the immediate rehabilitation team but also between members of the team and their counterparts elsewhere. District nurses, general practitioners, community therapists and district social workers will all need to be informed of 'the story so far' if they are going to be involved in future management. This may raise problems of communication, as it is often difficult, and not very cost-effective, for community-based professionals to attend case conferences whose time and place are determined for the convenience of their hospital-based colleagues.

Different methods of circumventing this problem have been tried. The use of hospital–community liaison personnel (such as district nurse liaison officers) who attend case conferences is one solution. Another is the identification of an individual (such as the community nurse for the elderly) whose responsibility is to monitor fragile discharges that involve complex packages of care and to report to both community and hospital personnel. The most ambitious and potentially the most successful approach is the identification of hospital-based and community-based key workers or case managers who will requisition the relevant resources for individual patients and will liaise with one another at times of admission or discharge. There still remains the question of who the key worker should be, especially when different professionals are central to the patient's care at different times. Close multidisciplinary working with free exchange of information also raises issues of confidentiality.

Multidimensional assessment
(see also Wade, Chapter 10)

Successful multidisciplinary management will be based on multidimensional assessment of the patient (see Table 23.2). It is essential not only to make a precise diagnosis of the underlying medical problem (or more usually problems) but also to determine its functional impact – on mobility, postural control and the ability to perform ADL.

Mobility may be graded very simply, in such a way as to give some idea of the social implication of limitations. For example, Andrews (1989) has suggested the following:
1 Fully mobile.
2 Activities limited but can get away from neighbourhood.
3 Activities limited to the immediate neighbourhood.
4 Activities limited to the home or one floor of the home.
5 Activities limited to one room.
6 Chair-fast.
7 Bed-bound.
It is important not to deceive oneself into believing that scales such as these are 'scientific' or that they

Table 23.2 Multidimensional assessment of the elderly patient

Precise medical diagnosis(es)
Functional impact of disease
  on mobility
  on postural control
  on the ability to perform activities of daily living
    in institution
    in 'realistic' setting
    at home
Exercise tolerance
Cognitive function
'Motivation' (see text)
Home circumstances
Social support network

are necessarily an improvement on a precise account of the patient's limitations. In any case, they will not supersede an observation of the patient actually walking, which, in addition to its diagnostic value, will also give some idea of postural stability. The latter is particularly important as falls may not only lead to injury (even fractures in an osteoporotic elderly patient) but also to fear of further falls, loss of confidence and severe self-limitation.

The ability to perform ADL can also be recorded, using a variety of standardized protocols, the most commonly used being the Barthel index (Table 23.3). Such an index is a useful prompt but its status as a scientific instrument is controversial (Wade *et al.*, 1985; Tallis, 1991). All ADL assessments should encompass the ability to transfer from bed to chair, feeding, grooming, walking, continence, and managing the toilet and the stairs and, where appropriate, aids such as wheelchairs. Extended ADL assessments (for example, the Nottingham scale (Nouri & Lincoln, 1987)) look beyond mere survival to recreational and other activities.

Before discharge, patients should be assessed outside of institutions: their own homes may not be as easy to negotiate as a ward and there may be less on-line help available there. It is often observed that patients who are quite competent at 'playing' ADL in hospital do not actually perform them once they get home (Andrews & Stewart, 1979). This may be due to more difficult material circumstances but also to different interpersonal relations. Wives who have never seen their husbands make a cup of tea are gape-mouthed with amazement to see them perform this action for the first time in an occupational therapy kitchen after they have had a stroke. With the return home, however, the customary helplessness is soon resumed.

It is important to assess exercise tolerance. In an elderly stroke patient, for example, walking may be limited by cardiorespiratory disease, exercise-associated or postural hypotension, and arthritis. Severe limitations in maximum energy expenditure may be particularly significant since even single disabilities markedly increase energy requirements; for example, hemiplegia increases the energy consumption on walking by 50–100% (Corcoran *et al.*, 1970).

Only a proportion of patients will require expert assessment of cognitive function by a clinical psy-

Table 23.3 The Barthel index of activities of daily living

Activity	Score	Criteria
Feeding	2	Independent
	1	Needs help
	0	Dependent
Grooming	1	Independent
	0	Dependent
Bowels	2	Fully continent
	1	Occasional accident
	0	Incontinent
Bladder	2	Fully continent
	1	Occasional accident
	0	Incontinent
Dressing	2	Independent
	1	Needs help
	0	Dependent
Chair/bed transfer	3	Independent
	2	Minimal help
	1	Able to sit
	0	Dependent
Toilet	2	Independent
	1	Needs help
	0	Dependent
Mobility	3	Independent walking
	2	Minimal help
	1	Independent in wheelchair
	0	Immobile
Stairs	2	Independent
	1	Needs help
	0	Unable
Bathing	1	Independent
	0	Dependent
Total = (maximum) 20	. . . .	

chologist; all patients, however, should have some simple test of mental functions such as the 10-item abbreviated mental test score (Hodkinson, 1972), or the short orientation, memory and concentration test (see Wade, Chapter 10). This will give at least some idea whether or not there is likely to be difficulty in co-operating with therapy, in understanding instructions and learning new techniques and understanding and agreeing to shared goals.

One parameter that tends to be assessed rather casually and unhelpfully is so-called 'motivation'. The 'motivation' of the patient usually tends to become an issue when it is thought to be missing or inadequate. This is usually when progress falls short of expectation and the team is itself becoming a little undermotivated. Motivation *per se* is actually difficult to assess (soul biopsy is the only method) and the claim of 'poor motivation' should not be accepted uncritically. Some of the reasons why a patient may underachieve and so appear – or be accused of being – 'poorly motivated' include: subtle neurological problems (such as perceptual deficits in a patient with reasonably preserved power); undiagnosed depression; metabolic, endocrine, infectious or other overlooked diseases; the adverse effects of medication (sedatives, diuretics, etc.); a dislike (not always entirely without justification) of the attitudes, manner or manners of the staff; the intrusive presence of other patients or of the regime or material environment of the institution; and a difference of perception between patient and team members as to what are sensible and/or worthwhile goals and what is required to achieve them.

Whether or not it is realistic to consider discharging a patient home will depend not only on the level of independence he or she has achieved but also on the level of support that is, and is likely to remain, available. Assessment of the social support network is, therefore, a crucial part of the assessment process. In determining how much help is likely to be forthcoming from potential carers, it is necessary to know how committed they are to helping, how good the premorbid relationship has been, what other commitments they have, what the state of their own health is, and how much they understand of the burden of caring that they are going to be required to carry out.

Medication as a cause of chronic disability in old age

Rehabilitation should include a critical examination of current medication and a high index of suspicion regarding its role in the production of or exacerbation of disability. Adverse drug reactions (ADRs) are very common in the elderly population: a recent survey of community-dwelling elderly people found that about 10% felt they were suffering from the adverse effects of medication (Cartwright & Smith, 1988). The proportion is even higher in hospital populations, where the elderly were long ago shown to be up to seven times as likely to suffer from ADRs as young patients (Hurwitz, 1969) and 15% of patients on prescribed medication admitted to geriatric units were suffering from ADRs (Williamson & Chopin, 1980). In this latter study, ADRs had been a contributory factor to admission in 10% of cases. These observations are not altogether surprising in the light of the fact that elderly people are often prescribed inappropriate medication: contraindicated and·interacting drugs (Gosney & Tallis, 1984; Adams *et al.*, 1987; Gosney *et al.*, 1989) or unnecessary medications (Lindley *et al.*, 1992). That this iatrogenic toll is not an inevitable consequence of age- and illness-related changes in drug-handling and drug sensitivity, of multiple pathology or of poor compliance (the reasons usually given) was shown by Lindley *et al.* (1992), who found that nearly half of ADRs and of drug-related admissions were due to unnecessary or contraindicated drugs.

There are two major reasons why drug-related iatrogenic disease is of particular importance in the neurological rehabilitation of the elderly.

The first and most obvious is that chronic neurological disease is not uncommonly caused by prescribed medication. This has been reviewed by Swift (1989). Drugs may produce disturbances of higher mental function. Some of these are predictable; for example, anticholinergic agents may cause severe memory impairment, hallucinations and global cognitive failure indistinguishable from dementia; sedatives may cause confusion and progressive loss of independence. Others are less predictable; for example, H2 receptor antagonists have been incriminated in producing drowsiness, impaired orientation and loss of cognitive function. Drugs are a major cause of disturbances of locomotion, including postural instability and falls (Prudham & Evans, 1981), cerebellar ataxia and parkinsonism. The latter is especially worrying: Stephen & Williamson (1984) found that over half of the elderly patients referred to a Parkinson's clinic had drug-induced parkinsonism. In the vast majority of cases, the drug incriminated was prochlorperazine given for the non-indication of non-specific dizziness.

(Prochlorperazine also causes postural hypotension, further undermining the tenability of the vertical position.) Drug-induced myopathy and neuropathy may also occasionally occur – especially in elderly patients whose impaired drug-handling may lead to high blood levels. Finally, drug-induced seizures (Chadwick, 1983) are important causes of neurological morbidity in a population at increased risk from seizures (Tallis *et al.*, 1991).

The second reason why drugs are important is that they may interfere drastically with rehabilitation. First, they may exacerbate existing neurological problems: the damaged nervous system is particularly vulnerable to neurological ADRs. Secondly, they may interfere with co-operation. A patient who has drug-induced postural hypotension will not be very keen to stand. Likewise an elderly man with prostatism who has a severe diuresis from frusemide will not relish a trip to the physiotherapy department as it may be associated with the humiliation of incontinence. Drug-induced depression will not improve a patient's interest in the advice of an occupational therapist. And so on. The adverse effects of medication are often very complex (such as when a diuretic causes hyponatraemia and hypovolaemia – and so may lead to postural hypotension, falls and possible fracture – uraemia, constipation, other electrolyte disturbances, incontinence and confusion). Equally, ADRs may often present in a rather non-specific way, so that their causative role is not suspected.

In the light of the above, it will come as no surprise that frequently the most effective intervention in an elderly person who has gone off her/his feet, has become confused or cannot cope is the careful and considered withdrawal of medication. Although the elderly are potentially the greatest beneficiaries of drug therapy, one could be forgiven for sometimes believing that allowing oneself to be disabled by a doctor is part of the job description of a septuagenarian.

Aids

This topic is central to rehabilitation; but it is a huge one and it would be inappropriate to attempt to cover it in any detail here. The reader is referred to two recent definitive reviews by Mulley (1989, 1991) and I shall confine myself only to some general observations and a brief overview of what is – or should be – available. (I shall use 'aids' in the extended sense of 'tools to assist living', encompassing accessories, adaptations and appliances.)

Principles of provision

Aids should not be provided without a diagnosis of the underlying cause of the disability; for example, pads and pants should not be issued without the cause (or more usually causes) of incontinence being determined. The prescription of aids should be as precise as the prescription of drugs; it is not enough to prescribe a walking-stick – it has to be of the right length (equal to the vertical distance from the ground to the wrist crease with the elbow slightly flexed and the patient wearing everyday shoes). The prescriber should ensure not only that the aid is appropriate (in other words, there is no better solution) but also that it is acceptable (cosmetically) and easy to use. The patient (and/or carer) should be trained in its use and a check made as to whether or not it is being used. If it is not, the reason for this should be sought; it may be uncomfortable, an embarrassment, too much trouble, too complicated, or useless because inappropriate or incorrectly used. Sometimes the environment where an aid is tried out is not the same as that in which it is to be used. A wheelchair that gives a patient ward mobility may be unmanoeuvrable at home; a wheeled zimmer that functions on a smooth hospital floor gets bogged down in a carpet at home and is consequently used as an auxiliary towel rail. A patient's need for aids should be reviewed regularly; disability rarely remains stable and recovery or progression may mean that some aids become redundant or inadequate. There should also be some kind of overview of the aids with which a patient has been provided. As Mulley (1992a) has pointed out:

> different health and social service professionals may focus on certain disabilities and not recognise others. The doctor may examine the spectacles and hearing aid; the physiotherapist the walking stick or frame; the occupational therapist the chair, bed, toilet and bathing aids and items to help in the kitchen or feeding; the nurse may consider the need for incontinence

aids; the social worker the suitability of a telephone or alarm system.

This may be a healthy reflection of the differentiation of expertise but the right hand should know what the left hand is doing. It is important, finally, not to think of aids in a narrowly medical sense; tools for living include not merely tools for survival and self-care but also tools for enjoying life, such as those which will help the pursuit of pleasurable pastimes, such as fishing, golf or gardening. Contrary to popular belief, these are as important in the elderly as in younger people.

What is available

Patients present with complex disabilities which may limit them in many aspects of life. The range of aids is correspondingly enormous and almost as daunting and baffling to providers as to users. Some kind of classification of aids and the needs they meet is therefore useful. Table 23.4, which is based on Mulley (1992a), provides a shell in which different needs can be considered. The shell approach, or a check-list matched against observed skills in daily living, may be useful. A 24-hour period of observation of need and dependency in the ward or a hospital assessment flat will also help; so, too,

Table 23.4 Aids and appliances for the elderly

To compensate for sensory impairment
  Vision
  Hearing

To permit performance of everyday living activities
  Activities outside the home
    Getting outside the house (e.g. ramps)
    Movement outside the house (e.g. footwear, transport)
    Recreation (e.g. gardening aids, holidays)
  Activities inside the home
    Aids to home-making (e.g. tap turners, labour-saving equipment)
    Aids to mobility (e.g. stair rails, seating the patient can get out of without help, walking sticks and frames, wheelchairs)
    Aids to recreation (e.g. reading aids)
  Personal care activities
    Bath aids (e.g. mats, boards, seats)
    Toilet aids (e.g. raised seats, frames)
    Dressing aids (e.g. stocking aids, velcro fasteners)

will observations made on a home visit, when difficulties and barriers not apparent in hospital may be identified and solved.

Problems

Despite the existence of large numbers of aids that could greatly alleviate dependency and distress, they do not always reach those who need them. Mulley (1992a) has identified some of the reasons for this. Perhaps the most important is the fact that, even amongst geriatricians, knowledge of what is available and how it should be used is not regarded as a proper part of medicine. History-taking often fails to include reference to aids such as glasses. Moreover, doctors are often unimpressed by the value of some aids. In addition to the lack of leadership from doctors, who are often in the strongest position to requisition aids for their patients, there is the problem of the complexity of the system through which they are provided, and the question of who funds them. At the very least, this may lead to unacceptable delays in their provision; this is particularly unsatisfactory in patients with progressive conditions (so that the aid is inadequate by the time it arrives), in elderly patients in whom non-provision creates the risk of injury, and in patients whose hospital stays are prolonged while the aid is awaited. Finally, there are problems arising from the fact that the patient may, for reasons discussed earlier, find the aid unacceptable or unusable. We may, with Mulley, look forward to a future in which better (easier to use, more aesthetically appealing, more effective) aids (which have been fully evaluated) are made more widely available through a less cumbersome system operated by better-educated professionals. There is much to be done before this future is realized.

The organization of rehabilitation services for the elderly

The services that should be provided for elderly patients within a district have been described by Horrocks (1986). While there is no dissent over the belief that rehabilitation services should have a central place, there are several areas of discussion.

Progressive patient care

In most geriatric units in the UK, acute, rehabilitation and long-stay facilities tend to be separated – an arrangement called 'progressive patient care' (Exton-Smith, 1962).

The separation of rehabilitation from acute wards may seem inappropriate in the light of the earlier assertion that the vast majority of geriatric patients – including those who present with an acute illness – require rehabilitation as well as medical and nursing treatment in the narrower sense. (Indeed, one could define a geriatric patient as one who would benefit from the multidisciplinary approach.)

Some authors (e.g. Whitehead, 1981; Horrocks, 1986) have argued for a single facility in which acute, rehabilitation and continuing-care patients are all together. In this way, all patients benefit from a wider range of expertise, time is not wasted waiting for a bed in another part of the service, patients do not get confused by being shuffled around the system and long-stay patients are not separated from adequate medical care.

Despite these arguments, most geriatric units practise progressive patient care. Though the distinction between acute and rehabilitation wards is not absolute – rehabilitation is available on acute wards and acute care if necessary on rehabilitation wards – there is a crucial difference of emphasis. On the acute ward, acute management – diagnosis and medical treatment – of largely acute illness has central place. In a rehabilitation ward, the emphasis is on restoration of function, using the multidisciplinary team approach already described. The reason for separating the two facilities may be summarized in an aphorism: the urgent drives out the important. On an acute geriatric ward, urgent problems – the management of the patient with an overwhelming chest infection, cardiac failure or gastrointestinal haemorrhage, etc. – tend to take precedence over merely important ones – such as restoring the function of a patient with a stroke. The virtue of a designated rehabilitation ward is that the latter is central and not merely an optional extra to be undertaken when more pressing problems have been dealt with.

The problems and perils of hospital admission for an elderly person

'Lasciate ogni speranza, voi ch'entrate' (Abandon all hope, you who enter) – the motto inscribed over the gates of hell – might justifiably be placed over the entrance to some hospital wards where elderly people receive medical treatment. Although there have been enormous improvements over the last few decades in attitudes towards elderly patients, there is still a long way to go. The effect of better staff training has been counteracted by 'cost improvement programmes', which, combined with more intensive medical care, have increased the pressure on all professionals, especially nurses and doctors. Overburdened staff may be less inclined to struggle against the tactlessness and insensitivity with which we are all congenitally afflicted and which is inevitably exacerbated by the institutional mores that emerge when professionals become accustomed to contact with other people's suffering. Admission to hospital cuts across the routines of a lifetime and other things will conspire to make the patient if not helpless, at least lacking in initiative. For example, he/she will often have been separated from his/her spectacles, hearing-aid and walking-stick and this will make it difficult to negotiate the new environment. There are other ways in which hospital life will undermine rather than restore independence: drug treatment may cause confusion, incontinence and instability; sleep deprivation due to noise and anxiety will sap morale; an unfamiliar environment will predispose to accidents (there is no furniture to hang on to in the wide open spaces of the ward); and nosocomial infection will take its toll. Rosin & Boyd (1966) found that 70% of elderly patients admitted to hospital experienced some complication and half of these were occasioned by the hospital stay itself, with respiratory infections, falls, ADRs and pressure sores heading the list. Things have certainly improved since then, but hospital admission remains hazardous.

Even if a patient does not fall victim to any of the hazards mentioned above, hospital admission may cause such a catastrophic loss of confidence that a patient who was initially reluctant to be admitted is reluctant to be discharged. Two things may combine to make discharge difficult: the patient may have lost some of the skills necessary for independent living; and the ecological niche to which he/she was previously adapted may have disintegrated. The social support network may have frayed, with perhaps a hardening of attitudes by relatives and neighbours, who may be unwilling to resume the burden of support; accommodation may decay, or be burgled or vandalized; and so on.

A successful rehabilitation service, therefore, must begin with the premise that hospital care is potentially disabling. This should be combated by a positive attitude from the day of admission, by clearly setting out the goals of the admission as negotiated with the patient, by identifying what has to be achieved in order to make discharge possible, and by monitoring progress towards these goals. There should be an explicit policy of the gradual withdrawal of support as the patient recovers independence. Although it may be more time-consuming to supervise a patient making his/her own way to the toilet than pushing him/her there in a wheelchair, the former will contribute to rehabilitation, while the latter will confirm disability.

The ward environment should be user-friendly, with grab rails in corridors, clearly signposted, accessible toilets and a reasonable amount of personal – and personalized – space. There should be day-room facilities and opportunities to participate in recreational and diversional activities. A television that is switched off only when it breaks down and unremitting pop music that appeals only to the nursing staff – not uncommon features of hospital wards – are not therapeutic. Patients who wish to read or to engage in hobbies should not find this impossible. They should not be prevented from doing so by being deprived of their spectacles, hearing-aids or walking aids.

Return to the community should not be sprung on the patient (or carers) but signalled well in advance. In most cases, a home visit of a few hours accompanied by a therapist and involving important carers will be essential. This will permit assessment of function in the environment in which the patient is actually going to live, and enable unrecognized daily living problems to be picked up, the need for aids and support services to be determined and the anxieties of patients and carers to be addressed. Successful discharge requires that the care package

is in place, that aids are available and that adaptations are implemented before discharge. Ideally, a designated individual – a health visitor, community nurse for the elderly or social worker – should be responsible for checking that all the elements of the package are ready and should report back to the team if things are not going according to plan.

Geriatric day hospitals
(Brocklehurst & Tucker, 1980)

The problems associated with hospital admission are a good reason for looking for alternatives to hospital care for those patients who are sufficiently independent or have sufficiently good support to be able to remain in the community. Day hospitals are an important adjunct to in-patient care in most geriatric units in the UK. Ideally, they should provide all the facilities of in-patient rehabilitation without the perils and financial costs associated with hospital stay. They separate the investigational and therapeutic aspects of treatment from the hotel aspect, which often requires patients to remain in hospital in the evening, at night and at the weekend when nothing of therapeutic benefit is taking place. They are multipurpose, catering for a wide range of patients, from those who require out-patient diagnosis and management of medical problems to those who attend to give their carers relief. However, their central role is to provide multidisciplinary rehabilitation for patients with chronic disability. Accordingly, they are staffed with therapists and social workers as well as doctors and nurses.

Patients may be referred directly from the community or following discharge from hospital. They attend for one or more days a week, for several weeks, and typically arrive in the morning by ambulance, stay for the day, during which they receive whatever treatment or advice they need, and return home in the late afternoon. Day hospitals are usually – and ideally should be – near to the in-patient rehabilitation facilities, allowing shared resources. The latter should include staff, thus ensuring continuity of care and consistent management.

On the whole, day hospitals have been found useful. There are problems, however. First, some patients find attending several times a week as disruptive and intrusive as being an in-patient. Often attendance requires both patient and/or carer to rise early to be ready in time for an ambulance whose arrival may be somewhat unpredictable; involves a journey that in 20% of cases (Stokoe & Zuccollo, 1985) is associated with some degree of travel sickness (to which neurological patients are particularly susceptible), and other discomforts (including worsening of spasticity); includes a long period of waiting for therapy in a setting and amongst company that may be uncongenial; and means a return after a further ambulance journey to a home that may be increasingly neglected due to the time taken up by therapy. Assuming that there are adequate staff to give more than token therapy, the key to a successful day hospital is a flexible and reliable transport system that can bring patients on time for the treatment they require and return them when they have been treated.

Secondly, it has been difficult to prove that day hospitals do save costs. Brocklehurst (1985) summarizes the evidence that day hospitals do seem to diminish the number of in-patient days and allow earlier discharge from hospital. However, a patient supported in the community is also consuming resources, and Opit (1977) showed that even without day hospital attendance there was little financial advantage; as so often, an apparent saving is merely the shift of cost from one budget to another. The most important function of a day hospital may, however, be to spare patients who do not wish it the experience of in-patient care.

Domiciliary care (Andrews, 1987)

Another approach that has much to commend it is the use of domiciliary services. Rehabilitation comes to the patient and not the other way round. As well as being less disruptive for the patient, who may be frail as well as disabled, it also has the advantage that the patient recovers mobility and relearns daily living skills in the setting where they are to be used. Relatives can be trained in the appropriate levels of assistance and realistic goal-setting is easier where the goal is actually visible. On the other hand, it is less convenient for staff, who have to travel and who can see fewer patients in a given time. There is also a limit to the amount of specialized equipment that can be transported

to the patient. Domiciliary treatment provides no social outlet for the patient and no relief for the carer.

The question of home or hospital remains unresolved. As Andrews (1989) points out, most of the published research is descriptive and there have been very few controlled trials. Frazer (1980) found that home treatment was cheaper than day hospital treatment but others have not found this and there are many hidden costs that have to be taken into account. There will never be an unambiguous, comprehensive answer regarding comparative costs, let alone effectiveness. Different patients in different social circumstances and different geographical areas will have different needs. This is illustrated by two recent studies (Young & Foster, 1992; Gladman et al., 1994) which have shown conflicting results in patients receiving post-discharge rehabilitation at home compared to rehabilitation in day hospitals. Any study done at the present time will inevitably be forced to compare unsatisfactory hospital with inadequate domiciliary services. In an ideal world, we should have sufficiently well-developed services in both hospital and community for patients to have a genuine choice and for those electing for initial hospital management to return early to the community if they wish to do so.

The needs of carers

It is easy for those working within a rehabilitation service to become intoxicated by their own rhetoric of optimism and to have an exaggerated idea of the effectiveness of the service. This is in part because patients who do badly tend to move on – either into long-term care or to the care of their families. In many cases, professional intervention is only a small episode in a long story that continues for many years after discharge. There has over the last decade been an increased awareness of the 'unremitting burden' carried by many of those looking after disabled elderly people. Kruse (1991) has described the physical and psychological strains of having sole responsibility for another adult, who may make enormous physical and psychological demands. The price of being a carer may be loss of one's own freedom and independence. The costs may be reflected in poor health (Kinsella & Duffy,

1979; Gallagher *et al.*, 1989): carers tend to neglect their own health needs and problems, focusing on those of the person they are caring for. There are often adverse impacts on their relationships with others – in particular, other family members. Spouses may resent the time the carer spends in caring for an aged dependent, thus deflecting attention from themselves. Children may feel neglected. Marriages of couples who no longer have time to consider each other's needs may end in divorce. Being a carer may damage career prospects or even make it impossible to hold down a job. The adverse financial consequences of this will create further problems. The dependent may be, or come to be viewed as, impossibly demanding. This in turn may lead to a progressively deteriorating relationship between carer and cared for: anger, exasperation and fatigue may lead to verbal, physical or psychological abuse, followed perhaps by guilt and even depression. (Kinsella & Duffy (1979) found that 42% of spouses of disabled stroke patients were depressed.) In a relatively short period of time the burden of caring may have impaired the carer's physical and mental health, damaged family and social relationships, ruined career and financial prospects and irreversibly wounded his or her self-esteem.

A rehabilitation service for the elderly should therefore concern itself with the needs of carers. From the beginning, carers have the right to be informed about the nature of the condition from which the patient suffers. Symptoms may require explanation – especially in complex conditions such as stroke. This in itself may provide some relief, as Mulley (1992b) has pointed out. As far as possible they should be given an idea of the patient's prognosis – for survival, for deterioration and for improvement. They should be taught basic skills – such as transferring and dressing the patient, the use of aids, etc. – and should be given adequate opportunity to ask questions. (To this end, they should participate actively in the rehabilitation process.) Anxieties – 'What should I do if . . . ?' – should be identified and answered. Carers should be involved, along with the patient, in planning the package of care. They should be given advice about the relevant benefits without having to ask for it themselves. Finally, they should be put in touch with relevant patient and support groups, such as the Alzheimer's Disease Society or the local carers' group.

In many cases, relief will be required to enable the carer to get on with household and organizational tasks unhindered, to enjoy a bit of time to him/herself and to recharge batteries. This may be provided on a daily basis through the patient's attendance at a local authority day centre or (in the case of severely disabled patient) at a geriatric day hospital, though the unpredictability of transport and the reluctance of the patient to attend may make this not altogether satisfactory for the carer. The use of a day hospital for social relief may seem to be a waste of a scarce resource whose primary function is medical treatment and active rehabilitation. At my own hospital we have established an Elderwell Unit, where patients who are too disabled to be accommodated at a day centre attend for primarily social purposes. With earmarked transport and meaningful social activities, it is very popular with both patients and their carers. Day relief may be insufficient and provision of regular relief admissions in a residential home, hospital or nursing home may provide a much needed break, especially for carers whose sleep is disturbed. Such relief is also provided in hospital and this may be more acceptable to patients and offers the opportunity to review medication and the need for further rehabilitation. The recent Royal College of Physicians (1990) study should allay fears raised by earlier studies that relief admission to hospital is associated with increased morbidity and mortality due to nosocomial infection and other mishaps.

Eventually, intermittent relief admission may be insufficient and nursing home or long-term hospital care may be required. It is an important part of the team's work to help carers to come to terms with the guilt they often feel when this happens. (Ironically, it is usually those who have done the most who are most likely to reproach themselves with 'abandoning' their dependant.) Anticipating and discussing these feelings is an essential part of the rehabilitation of a family whose life may have revolved round the care of one individual over many years. It is important to recognize – and to support – their need to play a continuing role in looking after the individual, even after the latter has been admitted to a long-term care facility. They will also need to talk over, and to come to terms with, the events that have taken place in the years of unremitting responsibility. Carers should be entitled to counselling support at every stage in the process. It is not usually possible for this to be provided by full-time professional counsellors. This may not be appropriate anyway: those of us who look after patients and their families are not especially enthusiastic about 'handing over' patients to experts for dealing with the emotional consequences of illness. A better arrangement is that those who are already working with the patient and family should be aware of the feelings experienced by carers – shock, unrealistic hope, anger, guilt, despair – and deal with these opportunistically as they manifest themselves. The counsellor at any time should be the professional who is most involved – the primary nurse, the therapist, the doctor, the social worker – and this will change at different times in the illness. All members of the team should be sufficiently experienced to detect serious problems – abuse by or depression in the carer – and to seek advice accordingly.

Rehabilitation in long-term care

Many disabled elderly people will not regain sufficient independence to return to living in the community. Admission to a nursing home or a continuing-care ward in hospital does not mean that rehabilitation has been a waste of time or even that it has failed. A rehabilitation service that uses place of discharge as a measure of its effectiveness has an excessively narrow and economistic interpretation of its role. Small improvements – regaining the ability to feed oneself, greater ease of transfer from bed to chair – may mean a lot in terms of quality of life. Moreover, the rehabilitation team will have the opportunity to educate the staff in the nursing home or other long-term care facility to which the patient is being discharged.

It is important, also, to appreciate that a patient in a long-term care facility is not beyond benefiting from further rehabilitation. Many conditions are progressive and require reassessment and a 'brush-up' course of treatment – for example, a patient with Parkinson's disease who may benefit from further speech therapy, an individual with cerebrovascular disease whose apraxic gait requires retraining, or a hemiplegic sufferer who requires

treatment to reduce spasticity. However, this should not be taken to imply that all disabled people should be given active therapy indefinitely. This is a waste of resources, may reinforce a patient's sense of failure and may interfere with the process of adaptation to disability by prolonging expectation of a miracle cure. Unfortunately, at present, disabled patients in institutions tend to be denied therapy because their needs seem less pressing than those of patients in the community and scarce resources have to be allocated where they are seemingly most needed.

Geriatric rehabilitation: an infant science

I have outlined some of the principles of geriatric rehabilitation and, in particular, of the way in which services are organized. Many of the elements in the rehabilitation package have not been evaluated (Tallis, 1989) and the way they are put together is often uncoordinated, equally confusing for patients, for their families and for professionals. That geriatric rehabilitation is an infant science is self-evident; however, it has adult spending habits. The need for a major research offensive in this area is paramount, especially in view of the implications of the population trends discussed at the beginning of this chapter. Progress will depend on making evaluation a routine part of everyday practice, avoiding misleading or unilluminating outcome measures (Tallis, 1991), increasingly rooting rehabilitation techniques in neuroscience and weeding out techniques that have no rational or empirical basis. Every rehabilitation centre should be a rehabilitation research centre, just as every oncology centre is an oncology research centre.

From this point of view, politico-economic trends could not be more unfavourable. The fear of uncontrolled expenditure on health care and of an increasingly ungrateful electorate has triggered recent legislation, whose overt purpose is to improve the way money is spent but whose actual purpose is to distance central government from responsibility for shortfalls in health and social services provision. *Working for Patients* (1989) will encourage the prudent manager or budget-holder to have as little to do with expensive disabled elderly patients as possible. *Caring for People* (1990) will ensure that provision of care for disabled elderly people will be a battleground between budget-holders wishing to shift the cost of care from health to social services and vice versa. The emphasis on competition will deal a death blow to the inter-agency co-operation so essential to the successful management of elderly patients and to the honest evaluation of alternative approaches. The distance between the literature dealing with the evaluation of NHS nursing homes and the rhetoric of private-sector brochures gives a clear idea of the impact the market ethos will have on science in this area. A throughput-besotted service conducted in a blizzard of invoices will have little spare capacity to look critically at what it is doing or to advance the science of geriatric rehabilitation to the point where it becomes as grown-up as its spending habits.

Nevertheless, it is important not to be pessimistic. There is considerable controversy as to whether the future holds an increase or a decrease in the level of disability in old age (Fries, 1980; Grundy, 1987; Bury, 1992). It has been suggested that increased survival into extreme old age will be associated with an increased prolongation of the period of disability before death – that extra years will be bought at the cost of extra years of disability. There is little in recent trends to support this gloomy suggestion: if anything, disability-free life expect-ancy as a proportion of overall life expectancy or of life expectancy after retirement is slightly increasing in most advanced countries (Robine & Ritchie, 1991). A conservative estimate of likely progress in the prevention and treatment of those conditions that contribute most to neurological disability in old age (stroke, dementia, Parkinson's disease) would encourage the belief that the elderly in fu-ture will be less, not more, disabled than their predecessors. While the dream of 'a health co-terminous with the lifespan' is rather too optimistic, that of a progressive compression the period of morbidity before death (Fries, 1980) does not seem out of the question. It remains the 'regulative idea' (in the Kantian sense) of geriatric medicine – indeed, of medicine as a whole.

References

Adams K., Al-Hamouz S., Edmond E., Tallis R.C., Vellodi C. & Lye M.D.W. (1987) Inappropriate prescribing in the elderly. *Journal of the Royal College of Physicians* **21** (1), 39–41.

Andrews K. (1985) Rehabilitation. In Brocklehurst J.C. (ed.) *Textbook of Geriatric Medicine and Gerontology*, 3rd edn. Churchill Livingstone, Edinburgh.

Andrews K. (1987) Organisation of rehabilitation services. In Andrews K. (ed.) *The Rehabilitation of the Older Adult*. Edward Arnold, London.

Andrews K. (1989) Rehabilitation. In Tallis R.C. (ed.) *The Clinical Neurology of Old Age*. John Wiley, Chichester.

Andrews K. & Stewart J. (1979) Stroke recovery: He can but does he? *Rheumatology Rehabilitation* **18**, 43–48.

Bamford J., Sandercock P., Dennis M. *et al.* (1988) A prospective study of acute cerebrovascular disease in the community: the Oxfordshire Community Stroke Project 1981–1986. 1. Methodology, demography and incident cases of first-ever stroke. *Journal of Neurology, Neurosurgery and Psychiatry* **51**, 1373–1380.

Brocklehurst J.C. (1985) The geriatric service and the day hospital. In Brocklehurst J.C. (ed.) *Textbook of Geriatric Medicine and Gerontology*, 3rd edn. Churchill Livingstone, Edinburgh.

Brocklehurst J.C. & Tucker J.S. (1980) *Progress in Geriatric Day Care*. King Edward's Hospital Fund for London, London.

Bruce S.A., Newton D. & Woledge R.C. (1989) Effect of age on voluntary force and cross-sectional area of human adductor pollicis muscle. *Quarterly Journal of Experimental Physiology* **74**, 359–362.

Bury M. (1992) The future of ageing. In Brocklehurst J.C., Tallis R.C. & Fillet H. (eds) *Textbook of Geriatric Medi-cine and Gerontology*, 4th edn. Churchill Livingstone, Edinburgh.

Caring for People (1989) Community care: the next decade and beyond. HMSO, London.

Cartwright A. & Smith C. (1988) *Elderly People, their Medicines and their Doctors*. Routledge, London.

Chadwick D.W. (1983) Convulsions associated with drug therapy. *Adverse Drug Reaction Bulletin* **87**, 316–319.

Corcoran P.J. & Brengelemann G.L. (1970) Oxygen uptake in normal and handicapped subjects in relation to speed of walking beside velocity controlled cart. *Archives of Physical and Medical Rehabilitation* **51**, 78–87.

Exton-Smith A.N. (1962) Progressive patient care in geriatrics. *Lancet* i, 260–263.

Favour C.B., Ritts R.E.J. & Bayles T.B. (1956) Arthritis research. *New England Journal of Medicine* **254**, 1078–1080.

Francis R.M. (1992) Osteoporosis. In Brocklehurst J.C., Tallis R.C. & Fillet H. (eds) *Textbook of Geriatric Medicine and Gerontology*, 4th edn. Churchill Livingstone, Edinburgh.

Frazer F.W. (1980) Domiciliary physiotherapy: cost and benefit. *Physiotherapy* **66**, 2–7.

Fries J.F. (1980) Ageing, natural death and the compres-sion of morbidity. *New England Journal of Medicine* **303**, 130–135.

Gallagher D., Ros J., Rivera P. *et al.* (1989) Prevalence of depression in family caregivers. *Gerontologist* **29**, 449–456.

General Household Survey (1980) HMSO, London.

Gladman J.R.F., Lincoln N.S. & Barer D.H. (1994) A randomised controlled trial of domiciliary and hospital based rehabilitation for stroke patients after discharge from hospital. *Journal of Neurology, Neurosurgery and Psychiatry* (in press).

Gosney M. & Tallis R.C. (1984) Prescription of contra-indicated and interacting drugs in elderly patients admitted to hospital. *Lancet* **i**, 564–567.

Gosney M., Vellodi C., Tallis R., Edmond E. & Al-Hamouz S. (1989) Inappropriate prescribing in Part 3 residential homes for the elderly. *Health Trends* **21** (4), 129–131.

Grundy E. (1987) Future patterns of morbidity in old age. In Caird F.I. & Grimley Evans J. (eds) *Advanced Geriatric Medicine*, Vol. 6. Wright, Bristol.

Herbst K.G. & Humphrey C. (1981) Prevalence of hearing impairments in the elderly living alone. *Journal of the Royal College of General Practitioners* **31**, 155–160.

Hirschberg G. (1983) Foreword. In Sine R.D., Holcomb J.D., Roush R.E. *et al.* (eds) *Basic Rehabilitation Techniques*, 2nd edn. Aspen, Maryland.

Hodkinson H.M. (1972) Evaluation of a mental test score for assessment of mental impairment in the elderly. *Age and Ageing* **1**, 233–238.

Horan M.A. (1992) The atypical presentation of disease. In Brocklehurst J.C., Tallis R.C. & Fillet H. (eds) *Textbook of Geriatric Medicine and Gerontology*, 4th edn. Churchill Livingstone, Edinburgh.

Horan M.A., Barton R.N. & Little R.A. (1988) Ageing and the response to injury. In Grimley Evans J. & Caird F.I. (eds) *Advanced Geriatric Medicine*. Wright, London.

Horrocks P. (1986) The components of a comprehensive district health service for elderly people – a personal view. *Age and Ageing* **15**, 321–342.

Hurwitz N. (1969) Predisposing factors in adverse reactions to drugs. *British Medical Journal* **i**, 536–539.

Jones D.A., Victor C.R. & Vetter N.J. (1984) Hearing difficulty and its psychological implications for the elderly. *Journal of Epidemiology and Community Health* **38**, 75–78.

Kane R.A. (1982) Lessons for social work from the medical model: a viewpoint for practice. *Social Work*, 315–321.

Kay D.W.K. (1991) The epidemiology of dementia: a review of recent work. *Reviews in Clinical Gerontology* **1**, 55–66.

Kinsella G.J. & Duffy F.D. (1979) Psychosocial readjustment in the spouses of aphasic patients. *Scandinavian Journal of Rehabilitation Medicine* **11**, 129–132.

Kruse A. (1991) Caregivers coping with chronic disease, dying and death of an aged family member. *Reviews in Clinical Gerontology* **1**, 411–415.

Lawrence J.S. (1969) Generalised osteoarthrosis in a population sample. *American Journal of Epidemiology* **90**, 381–384.

Lindley C.M., Tully M.P., Paramsothy V. & Tallis R.C. (1992) Adverse drug reactions in the elderly: the contribution of inappropriate prescribing. *Age and Ageing* **21**, 294–300.

Malmgren R., Warlow C., Bamford J. *et al.* (1989) Projecting the number of first-ever strokes and patients newly handicapped by strokes in England and Wales. *British Medical Journal* **20**, 333–339.

Mulley G.P. (1989) *Everyday Aids and Appliances*. BMJ, London.

Mulley G.P. (1991) *More Everyday Aids and Appliances*. BMJ, London.

Mulley G.P. (1992a) Aids for old people living at home. *Reviews in Clinical Gerontology* **II** (2), 157–169.

Mulley G.P. (1992b) Stroke. In Brocklehurst J.C., Tallis R.C. & Fillet H. (eds) *Textbook of Geriatric Medicine and Gerontology*, 4th edn. Churchill Livingstone, Edinburgh.

Mutch W.J., Dingwall-Fordyce I., Downie A.W. *et al.* (1986) Parkinson's disease in a Scottish city. *British Medical Journal* **292**, 534–536.

Nouri F.M. & Lincoln N.B. (1987) An extended activities of daily living scale for stroke patients. *Clinical Rehabilitation* **1**, 301–305.

OPCS (1988a) *Surveys of Disability in Great Britain, Report 1. The Prevalence of Disability Among Adults*. HMSO, London.

OPCS (1988b) *Surveys of Disability in Great Britain, Report 2.* HMSO, London.

Opit L.J. (1977) Domiciliary care of the elderly sick: economy or neglect? *British Medical Journal* **i**, 30–33.

Prudham D. & Evans J.G. (1981) Factors associated with falls in the elderly: a community study. *Age and Ageing* **10**, 141–146.

Rennie M. (1985) Muscle protein turnover and wasting due to injury and disease. *British Medical Bulletin* **41**, 257–264.

Robine J.M. & Ritchie K. (1991) Healthy life expectancy: an evaluation of global indicators of change in population health. *British Medical Journal* **302**, 457–460.

Rosin A.J. & Boyd R.V. (1966) Complications of illness in geriatric hospital patients. *Journal of Chronic Diseases* **19**, 307–313.

Royal College of Physicians (1990) *Study of relief admissions.*

Sainsbury R. (1991) Hip fracture. *Reviews in Clinical Gerontology* **1**, 67–80.

Salvage A.V., Jones D.A. & Vetter N.J. (1988) Awareness of and satisfaction with community services in a random sample of over 75s. *Health Trends* **20**, 88–92.

Stephen P.J. & Williamson J. (1984) Drug-induced parkinsonism in the elderly. *Lancet* **ii**, 1082–1083.

Stokoe D. & Zuccollo G. (1985) Travel sickness in patients attending a geriatric day hospital. *Age and Ageing* **14**, 308–311.

Swift C. (1989) Drug-induced neurological disease. In Tallis R.C. (ed.) *The Clinical Neurology of Old Age*. John Wiley, Chichester.

Tallis R.C. (1989) Measurement and the future of rehabilitation. *Geriatric Medicine* **19**, 31–40.

Tallis R.C. (1991) Assessing outcome in rehabilitation. In Seymour C.A. & Summerfield J.A. (eds) *Horizons in Medicine No. 3*. Transmedica, London.

Tallis R., Hall G., Craig I. & Dean A. (1991) How common are epileptic seizures in old age? *Age and Ageing* **20**, 442–448.

US Bureau of the Census (1987) *An Ageing World*. Torrey B.B., Kinsella K. & Taeuber C.M., eds. International Population Reports **78**, 95. US Government Printing Office, Washington.

Vetter N.J., Lewis P.A. & Ford D. (1990) The relationship between symptoms of chronic disease and dependence. *International Disability Studies* **12**, 22–27.

Wade D.T., Langton Hewer R., Skilbeck C.E. & David R.M. (1985) *Stroke: a Critical Approach to Diagnosis, Treatment and Management*. Chapman and Hall, London.

Warren M.D. (1985) The Canterbury study of disablement in the community: prevalence, needs and attitudes. *International Journal of Rehabilitation Research* **8**, 3–18.

Whitehead J.A. (1981) A single ward approach to the elderly mentally ill. *Health Trends* **13**, 99–100.

Williamson J. & Chopin J.M. (1980) Adverse reactions to prescribed drugs in the elderly: a multicentre investi-gation. *Age and Ageing* **9**, 73–80.

Wilson L.A., Lawson I.R. & Brass W. (1962) Multiple disorders in the elderly – clinical and statistical study. *Lancet* **ii**, 841–843.

Working for Patients (1989) HMSO, London.

Young A., Stokes M. & Crowe M. (1985) The size and strength of the quadriceps muscles of old and young men. *Clinical Physiology* **5**, 145–154.

Young J.B. & Foster A. (1992) The Bradford Community Stroke Trial. Results at six months. *British Medical Journal* **304**, 1085–1089.

Further reading

Andrews K. (1989) *The Rehabilitation of the Older Adult*. Edward Arnold, London.

Mulley P.G. (1989) *Everyday Aids and Appliances*. BMJ Publications, London.

Mulley P.G. (1991) *More Everyday Aids and Appliances*. BMJ Publications, London.

Reviews in Clinical Gerontology. This journal has a section devoted to geriatric rehabilitation, covering the main topics on a cyclical basis.

Part 5
Specific Problems

24: Management of Spasticity

L.S. ILLIS

The role of muscle tone in movement: anatomical
    considerations, 335
Clinical features, 336
    Evolution of spasticity in a transverse lesion of the
        spinal cord, 336
    Evolution of spasticity in lesions of the primary motor
        area and internal capsule, 337
    Does spasticity interfere with movement?, 338
Treatment of spasticity, 338
    General management, 339
    Physical therapy, 339
    Drug treatment, 339
    Intrathecal drug treatment, 341
    Chemical interruption of the reflex arc, 342
    Surgical treatment, 342
    Peripheral functional stimulation, 343
    Central functional stimulation, 343
Summary, 345

To the clinician spasticity indicates abnormally increased muscle tone, usually with other manifestations of abnormal motor function, including loss of voluntary power and co-ordination, increased tendon reflexes, altered cutaneous reflexes, spread of reflexes, clonus and spontaneous spasms. Fluctuations in spasticity may be spontaneous or in response to some stimulus. The stimuli which may alter spasticity include a change in emotional state or a change in internal stimuli such as from a distended bladder.

To the physiologist, spasticity is a motor disorder with a velocity-dependent increase in muscle tone (tonic stretch reflexes) with exaggerated monosynaptic tendon reflexes. The physiologist's attention is focused on the stretch reflex. However, to the experimental anatomist, spasticity is simply one result of the reorganization of the intact central nervous system (CNS) after a lesion.

The patient is not concerned with the clinical or physiological or anatomical niceties of spasticity. To the patient the disabilities that categorize spasticity include negative symptoms of weakness, fatiguability and lack of dexterity; and positive symptoms of flexor spasms and dystonic rigidity. The positive symptoms are presumed to be due to the release of segmental reflexes from higher control.

Spasticity is further complicated by the fact that, in patients with chronic spinal lesions, the clinical features differ from spasticity resulting from cerebral lesions. Although the two groups, brain stem and spinal, share the similarity of exaggerated tendon jerks and phasic spasticity, Dimitrijevic & Nathan (1967) and Dimitrijevic et al. (1980) have shown waxing and waning of excitability of phasic and tonic stretch reflexes, habituation, and sensitization of segmental reflexes by stimulus-induced activation of latent propriospinal inhibitory and excitatory mechanisms. In those cases where there is brain stem impairment and there is preservation of ascending and descending pathways, this does not occur. These differences indicate that spasticity is not a single phenomenon but the complex result of alteration of an integrated control system.

The role of muscle tone in movement: anatomical considerations

Muscle possesses some elasticity but most of the resting condition of muscle tone or tension is of a reflex nature and is maintained by afferent impulses which arise in the muscle spindles. The spindles form part of a servo-mechanism signalling to the CNS information about the length of the muscle. More information which is available to central processors includes information about the speed with which lengthening occurs, and the CNS (spinal cord) is also able to adjust the sensitivity of the muscle spindles.

The normal resting tone is maintained by the tonic stretch reflex. On moving the limb, as in testing tone clinically, the muscle is suddenly stretched and this elicits the phasic stretch reflex. The difference between the tonic stretch reflex and the phasic stretch reflex is due chiefly to the rapidity of stretching, and the differences between muscle tension tested by palpation and by passive stretching are probably best explained, again, by the tonic stretch versus the phasic stretch reflex. For example, in capsular hemiplegia the tone tested by palpation may be reduced, whereas tone tested by passive stretch is increased.

Gamma-loop and alpha motor neurons collaborate in the execution of movement and are subject to supraspinal control. For example, clinical neurological signs of the state of tone and myotatic reflexes may show subtle differences at the beginning and at the end of the clinical examination and are a reflection of the patient's mood and state of relaxation; unusually brisk jerks at the beginning of clinical examination are not necessarily pathological.

The organization of the spinal cord adds further understanding and further complexity to the CNS control and the interaction between the gamma and alpha neuron systems. Not only are nerve cells organized in columnar and somatotopical arrangements, but dendrites are arranged in specific patterns. For example, some dendrites are arranged longitudinally within the cell column to which the cell belongs (Scheibel & Scheibel, 1966). A single dorsal root supplying monosynaptic afferents may spread collaterals over several segments rostrally and caudally and also to contralateral dendrites (Illis, 1967b, 1973a, b). In this way the effects of spindles in a single muscle may activate motor neurons in several spinal cord segments, including contralateral segments. The endings of dorsal root collaterals are different in different sites. For example, up to 50% of terminals on the ipsilateral cell surface are from monosynaptic afferents, whereas less than 30% of terminals on ipsilateral dendrites are from dorsal root monosynaptic afferents. On the contralateral side of the spinal cord, less than 10% of terminals on cells are from crossed monosynaptic afferents and not more than 15% of terminals on dendrites are from crossed monosynaptic afferent fibres. At least four times as many

monosynaptic afferent fibres end on the ipsilateral side compared with the contralateral side (Illis, 1967b – in the cat spinal cord). A similar differential arrangement is valid for descending supraspinal afferents (corticospinal). The total effect is that of a network of a number of motor units distributed over several segments of the spinal cord supplying many different muscles, giving an anatomical substrate for the functional organization of muscle tone and movement. Alteration of the substrate by a lesion alters both impulse traffic and anatomical organization (see Illis, 1988), producing a change in muscle tone, power and movement. Since an anatomical substrate exists, the pattern of disturbance will reflect the pattern of connection. For example, corticospinal and rubrospinal tracts activate flexor neurons and inhibit extensor neurons, whilst vestibulospinal activity has the opposite effect. Fibre systems end in different parts of the spinal cord: those concerned with facilitation of flexor neurons end in V–VI and dorsal VII, and those concerned with extensor facilitation end in ventral VII and VIII, ending therefore on different sets of interneurons (see Brodal, 1969). This simplified view is complicated further by the fact that there are several supraspinal descending pathways within each group and there are interactions between descending afferents in the intact spinal cord and anatomical disturbances in the partially damaged cord.

Clinical features

Evolution of spasticity in a transverse lesion of the spinal cord

In a complete lesion of the spinal cord (nearly always traumatic), there is complete paralysis and anaesthesia below the level of the lesion. Immediately after the lesion, tone is flaccid and all reflexes absent. This is the initial stage of spinal shock, and it is followed by the stage of reorganization, during which autonomous activity of the severed cord appears, with the reappearance of sweating and of automatic reflex activity of the bladder and rectum. Later, muscles regain tone and reflexes simultaneously appear. This reorganization, which may include paraplegia in flexion with severe spasticity, usually requires several months to evolve. Animals lower in the phylogenetic scale regain automatic and reflex behaviour more rapidly, as though the spinal reflex apparatus is more independent of descending control in lower evolutionary species. At the spinal level there is a disorganization of the 'synaptic zone', which may account for the cessation and then reduction of spinal neuron excitability, with an ensuing reorganization, which may explain the return of reflex activity in an altered form (Illis, 1963; see also Chapter 5). This clinical picture is different at different levels of cord transection and is altered by infection or by the development of pressure sores.

In a gradually progressive partial lesion, as opposed to the acute lesion described above, the evolution is different although the final result may be the same.

Spasticity is one of the inevitable consequences of a spinal cord lesion. In man spasticity usually begins about 3 weeks after the lesion, in both complete and incomplete disturbances (i.e. spinal shock lasts something like 3 weeks). However, there are many exceptions to this. Spasticity tends to occur later in high cervical lesions, much earlier in some incomplete lesions, and may not occur at all where a transverse lesion is combined with a longitudinal lesion or where there are two lesions present and the lower lesion is in the cauda equina. The spasticity, which is entirely secondary to the lesion itself, is sometimes called 'basic spasticity' as opposed to 'excess spasticity', thought to be due to imposed afferent stimuli, which can be prevented by appropriate management (Michaelis, 1976). Michaelis suggests that the basic type of spasticity has some advantages in that the patient may use spasticity in order to initiate emptying of automatic bladder or flexion of the leg at hip and knee. This degree of spasticity rarely needs medical treatment, as opposed to excess spasticity, which has considerable disadvantages and complications. The major complication is the development of contractures, which appears to impose more severe spasticity, which in turn increases the contracture defect. All abnormalities below the level of the spinal cord lesion are likely to increase spasticity. Such processes include constipation, infection, pressure sores or any other kind of damage, fractures and dislocations.

Particularly in high lesions, sudden change of temperature will alter the degree of spasticity, as will physical or emotional stress.

Evolution of spasticity in lesions of the primary motor area and internal capsule

Although spasticity is usually described as being due to pyramidal lesions, and the term 'pyramidal hypertonia' is sometimes used to distinguish the increase in tone from rigidity which is of extrapyramidal origin, this is not strictly true clinically. Although the two types of increase of tone are distinct clinical entities with different clinical features, it is impossible to designate a definite pathophysiology to each type, and many of the underlying mechanisms are common to both. Moreover, the term 'pyramidal hypertonia' is confusing since lesions of the pyramidal tract do not cause hypertonia; it is parapyramidal lesions, such as lesions of the suppressor strip area 4S which produces hypertonia or lesions of area 6, the para- or juxtapyramidal area, which may be responsible.

Further levels involved in the control of muscle tone include the basal ganglia, the midbrain, the vestibular apparatus, the spinal cord and the neuromuscular system. The brain stem reticular formation contains both inhibitory and facilitatory areas. The cerebral cortex (suppressor strips), the basal ganglia and the anterior lobe of the cerebellum connect with bulbar inhibitory areas. Facilitatory pathways include reticulospinal and vestibulospinal.

In acute lesions, flaccid paralysis with absent reflexes is present, as in the initial stage of spinal shock. Much earlier (usually a matter of hours) in spinal lesions, plantar responses appear, but tendon reflexes usually take a number of days to return. Simultaneously, muscle tone increases, with the development of spasticity, which is usually more evident in the leg than in the arm. Muscle tone is greater in extensor muscles of the leg, but tends to be more marked, in the upper limb, in shoulder abductors, elbow flexors and hand pronators. This gives the characteristic pattern seen in patients with a chronic hemiplegia and is presumably a reflection of the pattern of endings of supraspinal pathways on interneurons.

Although some fine voluntary as well as crude flexor synergy and extensor synergy may appear (Foerster, 1936), this is frequently masked by the pronounced spasticity. Improvement in spasticity may result in improved movement, as described below.

Does spasticity interfere with movement?

The relationship between spasticity and motor control has been the subject of unresolved debate since the last century. Landau argues that motor control and function cannot be altered by procedures which reduce spasticity. Landau & Hunt (1990) believe that negative and positive phenomena are dissociated, and cite variations in spasticity and motor disability in relation to acute and chronic lesions and during recovery and the abolition of stretch reflex without loss of strength. They also state that pharmacological depression of spasticity has never been shown to improve functional motor performance (see below).

Peacock & Standt (1991) contest this view and point out that spasticity has been implicated as an interfering factor in gait as well as other functional tasks, and it is a common clinical experience that improvement in spasticity frequently results in improvement in gait, posture and transfer. This does not contest the probably correct view that the major functional defect is inappropriate or absent motor function, but leaves open the possibility of modulating motor performance by altering spasticity.

In spastic patients the stretch reflex is altered and is hyperexcitable. Does this produce or trigger inappropriate activity? Dimitrijevic & Nathan (1967) demonstrated that antagonists may be activated and thus produce movements opposite to those intended. McLellan (1977) showed that reflex activity may be altered by the degree of spasticity and the vigour of activity. Deterioration of performance may be produced by inappropriate activity (Pierrot-Deseilligny, 1983; Corcos et al., 1986). Conversely, spastic activity may keep paralysed or partially paralysed muscles in a satisfactory condition, so that, for example, FES-induced activities such as standing and reciprocal walking need no introductory training (see Chapters 34 and 35).

After intrathecal baclofen, suppression of spasticity may be accompanied by more selective voluntary muscle activation and tonic co-activation of antagonists and distant muscle groups is decreased (Latash et al., 1990). A similar effect may be seen with spinal cord stimulation.

In a much earlier paper, Foerster (1936) demonstrated how spasticity may affect movement. He described in detail the problems facing a hemiplegic patient. In the legs spasticity is most developed in extensors and in the plantar flexors. Isolated dorsiflexion is opposed by the spasticity. The spasticity is of a reflex nature and can be diminished by section of some of the dorsal roots subserving plantar flexors, with the result that dorsiflexion is no longer opposed.

The argument will continue as long as procedures are carried out without controlled studies; however, as indicated below excess spasticity needs treatment and may result in improved motor control.

Treatment of spasticity

This section is not intended as a bench guide to specific treatments, and practical details of techniques and precise drug regimens and dosages are not given. This information is readily available and, for example, the doses of any particular drug will vary from patient to patient and from time to time.

One of the problems with treatment of spasticity is the difficulty in assessment and the unpredictability of pharmacological manipulation. Clinical assessment is accurate for gross changes but is hardly susceptible to quantification. Neurophysiological assessment relies on some form of quantitative electromyography (EMG) or force measurements and the techniques are not universally accepted or applied. The neuropharmacological problem is best summed up by the fact that there are many neurotransmitters identified but only one disease in which the responsible neurotransmitter has been established (dopamine depletion).

The primary aim of treatment is to prevent spasticity occurring or to keep it within tolerable limits. Michaelis's (1976) concepts of basic and excess spasticity are useful in this context, as mentioned above. Basic spasticity shows little or no wasting of muscles, helps to prevent secondary complications such as osteoporosis and is useful in triggering emptying of bladder or flexion of knee and ankle joints. In contrast, excess spasticity is excessive and is due to superimposed stimuli, such as those produced by contractures. Spasticity may act as a stabilizing factor on otherwise uncontrolled joints, but excessive spasticity is associated with excessive co-activation of muscles, fatigue and severe walking difficulties. Improvement in spasticity and spasms is, therefore, likely to result in improved motor control.

General management

Poor position of the limbs or failure of treatment with passive movements from the onset of paralysis will result in semifixed flexion or, less commonly, extension contractures, which will increase spasticity, and this will, in turn, increase the contracture deformities. Relatively simple physiotherapeutic manoeuvres will prevent this complication. The development of contractures is the most important contributory factor to excess spasticity, but any pathological process resulting, in effect, in an increase in afferent stimulation below the level of the lesion is likely to alter basic spasticity to excess spasticity. These factors include constipation, pressure sores, burns, any skin disease, urinary tract infection, unrecognized fractures or dislocations, sudden alteration of temperature or humidity and mental or physical stress. Removal or prevention of the causes of excess spasticity must precede any specific treatment.

Spasms are a serious obstacle to rehabilitation, particularly because they are often so uncontrollable. Severe spasm occurs in about one-third of patients with spinal injury and is not unusual in the late stages of multiple sclerosis.

Preventing the progression of spasticity to a degree which would produce secondary handicaps in terms of immobility of joints with severe postural changes is as important, if not more important, than any other therapeutic technique.

Physical therapy

Physiotherapy

The aim of physiotherapy is to reduce spasticity and to improve voluntary motor control as a result. Increased afferent stimulation and active movement almost certainly bring inhibitory systems into action, and hopefully this will result in the better understanding of physiotherapy as a preventive and as a therapeutic measure. Several programmes for physiotherapy have been elaborated which include the elicitation of stretch reflexes and the inhibition and reciprocal inhibition of antagonist reflexes, often with marked improvement. However, in severe cases physiotherapy by itself is unlikely to succeed.

Cryotherapy

Cryotherapy, ice therapy or cooling therapy is a technique in which icepacks are used, and this probably produces depression of stretch reflexes. This may be beneficial when applied before physiotherapy.

Drug treatment

There are innumerable drugs which are not only useless but may be addictive (opiates) or have unacceptable side-effects (e.g. chlorpromazine) or are potentially harmful.

The first drug to be of real value was diazepam.

Diazepam

This is a member of the benzodiazepine group, widely used as tranquillizers and sedatives and, to a lesser extent, as anticonvulsants. Neurophysiological effects include inhibition of brain stem-activating systems (Przybyla & Wang, 1968), increase in presynaptic inhibition (Stratten & Barnes, 1971), suppression of polysynaptic spinal reflexes and inhibition of fusimotor firing (Brausch et al., 1973).

Clinically, diazepam alleviates both spasticity and flexor spasms, probably by reducing abnormal excitation in antagonists (Pinelli, 1973), and since benefit is seen in complete lesions (Cook & Nathan, 1967) the therapeutic action must be at the spinal level. If the beneficial effect is produced by reducing abnormal excitation, then this gives further weight to the concept of excess versus basic spasticity.

Benzodiazepines act at benzodiazepine receptors, which are associated with gamma-aminobutyric acid (GABA) receptors. Dependency may occur and benzodiazepine withdrawal syndrome (insomnia, anxiety, loss of appetite, tremor, perspiration and perceptual disturbances) is a potential danger. Diazepam must, therefore, be used with caution. It is contraindicated in respiratory depression.

Baclofen

This drug is a derivative of GABA, a neurotransmitter acting predominantly at inhibitory synapses. GABA itself is not effective since it cannot cross the blood−brain barrier. Baclofen is readily absorbed, reaches a peak blood level in 2−3 hours and is mainly excreted via the kidneys. It has been shown to decrease experimental spasticity and to be effective in man (e.g. Sachais *et al.*, 1977). It may act by inhibiting alpha motor neurons and fusimotor neurons or by facilitating Renshaw feedback inhibition. Baclofen acts as an agonist at the presynaptic GABA receptor, causing hyperpolarization and decreasing the release of neurotransmitters, such as glutamate, catecholamines and substance P. There appears to be a selective reduction in excitability of the monosynaptic reflex arc (McLellan, 1973) and a decrease in substance P release or a blocking of take-up by postsynaptic receptors (Kato *et al.*, 1978). An interesting effect is the report of improvement of bladder function (Jones, 1971).

Side-effects include hallucinations, mood change and mental symptoms (excitation, depression, confusion, anxiety). Liu *et al.* (1991) reported an interesting case of a frontal lobe syndrome apparently induced by baclofen. Baclofen and diazepam are said not to be effective in spasticity of cerebral origin (but see below).

Progabide

Enhancement of GABA neurotransmission is often very effective in the treatment of spasticity, but not all patients respond. Progabide (a GABA agonist) appears to have no interaction with other neurotransmitters (Bowery *et al.*, 1982) and no effect on GABA synthesis or degradation (Bartholini *et al.*, 1979; Kaplan *et al.*, 1980). The drug probably binds to GABA receptors.

Mondrup & Pedersen (1984) reported a reduction in spasticity and flexor spasms in patients with spasticity, and Rudick *et al.* (1987) investigated the effect of progabide in a double-blind placebo-controlled crossover trial in patients with multiple sclerosis. There was improvement in spasticity as measured by the Ashworth scale, no change as regards spasms and no loss of motor power. Adverse effects were common and included relatively minor gastrointestinal symptoms, motor weakness and urinary tract symptoms, but also some serious effects: fever, rash and elevation of aminotransferase levels. All reactions resolved when treatment was stopped. However, 28% of patients showed some evidence of hepatotoxicity.

Dantrolene

This appears to act distally to the neuromuscular junction, probably by interfering with calcium ion release from the sarcoplasmic reticulum. In addition, it suppresses the excitation of primary muscle spindle afferents. The effect of dantrolene as a relaxant of muscle is seen in both fast and slow muscle fibres. Dantrolene appears to have an effect irrespective of the site of abnormality and may be effective in spasticity of cerebral origin, where baclofen is unlikely to produce a worthwhile result.

It should be used with caution in patients with cardiac, pulmonary or liver disease. It is advisable to test liver function before and during treatment. Full therapeutic effect may take some weeks to develop.

Tizanidine

Tizanidine is an $alpha_2$-adrenergic agonist. Mathias *et al.* (1989) reported reduction of spasticity in patients with paraplegia. Medici *et al.* (1989) compared tizanidine with baclofen in patients suffering from spasticity secondary to cerebrovascular disease and showed a rather better improvement in the patients treated with tizanidine. This is interesting because baclofen is usually described as not being effective in spasticity in cerebral origin. Clearly more information is needed about this drug, but it appears to improve the symptoms of spasticity in about 75% or more of patients. Adverse effects seem to be infrequent.

Botulinum toxin

Botulinum toxin may control spasm and spasticity without producing untoward systemic effects or weakness. Botulinum toxin type A, a protein, is one of the serologically distinct neurotoxins produced by *Clostridium botulinum*. The toxin binds to the motor nerve endplate, causing presynaptic neuromuscular blockade, and produces a dose-related weakness of skeletal muscle by impairing acetylcholine release at the neuromuscular junction. Weakness occurs within 2–20 days, but new terminal axons sprout and recovery takes 2–4 months as neuromuscular transmission is restored. In the UK the product licence is currently restricted to treatment of hemifacial spasm and blepharospasm.

The technique has shown benefit in blepharospasm (Scott *et al.*, 1985), strabismus (Scott, 1981), hemifacial spasm (Mauriello, 1985), spasmodic torticollis (Tsui *et al.*, 1986) and spasmodic dysphonia (Ludlow *et al.*, 1988).

Adductor spasm and spasticity may be particularly resistant to treatment. Snow *et al.* (1990) report a double-blind study on nine patients who were either chair-bound or bed-bound with chronic multiple sclerosis. Botulinum toxin produced a significant improvement in the ease of nursing care and a significant reduction in spasticity. There were no adverse effects.

Intrathecal drug treatment

The technique of intrathecal administration of drugs via a catheter connected to a reservoir and pump has been in use since it was first employed to relieve intractable pain (see Penn & Kroin, 1987). It is clear that spinal cord processes may be pharmacologically manipulated by this method. Drugs such as morphine, clonidine and baclofen have been used and have been shown to have an effect on pain, spasticity and bladder function. Presumably this is via an action on specific receptors in the dorsal horn of the spinal cord, leading to alteration in spinal modulatory systems and central sensory transmission and processing. Examples of such pharmacological manipulation include enhancement of flexor reflexes by intrathecal noradrenaline (Dhawan & Sharma, 1970), enhancement of Renshaw recurrent inhibition (Roby *et al.*, 1981), alteration in polysynaptic flexor reflex activity (Willer & Bussel, 1980) and suppression of spasticity (Struppler *et al.*, 1983; Erickson *et al.*, 1985). Bolus

doses of morphine cause naloxone-reversible alterations in bladder function and spasticity (Wainberg *et al.*, 1987; Herman *et al.*, 1988).

Direct infusion of drugs into the cerebrospinal fluid (CSF) of the subarachnoid space prevents problems encountered by systemic administration. For example, severe side-effects, peripheral drug deactivation, impaired drug absorption, protein binding, inadequate penetration of the blood–brain barrier and poor patient compliance are all reduced by intrathecal drug delivery systems.

The extent of penetration of the drug into the nervous system depends on a number of factors, including the agent to be used and the method of administration. Bolus injections into the subarachnoid initially result in high CSF drug concentration and relatively limited parenchymal penetration. Serial bolus injections of low concentration of an agent are more effective and less toxic than a single large dose, but, for longer-duration action and deeper diffusion into the parenchyma (for example, the ventral horn), continuous infusion is necessary and the pharmacological agent is then concentrated at the site which is presumed to be the anatomical location of the sensory processes that subserve enhanced somatic reflexes (spasticity) and autonomic reflexes (detrusor hyperactivity).

When neurotransmitters or their agonists or precursors are applied in this way, the neurological action is limited to that particular region. That is, there is little direct distribution to higher levels of the CNS. The duration of action and the clinical effectiveness of any particular drug is due, in part, to the efficiency of the drug–receptor interaction. As metabolism makes a relatively minor contribution, the rate at which drugs are redistributed into the peripheral circulation would be a limiting factor, and this is largely dependent on the lipid solubility coefficient of the agent and the binding capacity once it is within the tissue. Drugs with a low lipid solubility, for example neuropeptides, will produce a behavioural effect at concentrations which are virtually inactive systemically. They are also much better candidates for deeper parenchymal penetration than pharmacological agents which readily cross the blood–brain barrier. Lazorthes *et al.* (1990), in a careful study of 18 patients with severe spasticity, found marked improvement, particularly in traumatic cases.

It is likely that intrathecal drug delivery systems will be the most effective way of treating spasticity and they may well have other beneficial effects, such as suppression of pain and improvement of bladder function.

Chemical interruption of the reflex arc

If the reflex arc is interrupted, then spasticity can no longer be a clinical manifestation. Direct interruption by the local injection of toxic substances may be carried out at the motor point, at the nerve, at the nerve root at or near the root exit, by subarachnoid or intrathecal injection affecting several nerve roots or in the spinal cord.

Procaine

Procaine is used for short-acting effects such as localizing the site of subsequent injections.

Phenol and alcohol

These are used for long-acting or possibly permanent interruption of the reflex arc. Nathan (1959) introduced phenol injections in the belief that injection produces destruction of small nerve fibres and thus a selective reduction in fusimotor activity. In a later paper (Nathan, 1965), he suggested that in fact phenol destroys nerve fibres in a non-selective manner. Phenol probably produces its effect by decreasing afferent bombardment to the spinal segmental neurons and thereby reducing excessive motor neuron activity and allowing latent patterns of co-ordination to emerge.

These substances, introduced, as for lumbar puncture, with the patient adjusted to ensure that the solution collects in the area of the appropriate nerve root, may reduce spasticity for many years. The technique should only be used where other methods of treatment have failed and where no spontaneous improvement is likely to occur. Contractures are unlikely to benefit and there is a risk of producing incontinence in patients who previously had intact sphincters. The increased sensory deficit raises the risk of dangers of pressure sores and constipation. Bladder automatism and potency may be abolished and it is clear that these blocks are only indicated as an ultimate treatment.

Surgical treatment

Effective early medical treatment has resulted in a considerable decrease in surgery for spasticity, and probably only about 1–2% of patients need surgical procedures. On the whole, surgical procedures are not without risk and spasticity may recur.

Rhizotomy

This technique can be carried out by surgical means or by radio frequency or chemical methods. In the early part of this century, Foerster (1911) described section of the posterior roots and for many years this was the only partially effective procedure for the treatment of spasticity. Spasticity usually recurred eventually. A refinement of this technique is to use intraoperative stimulation to define those roots which are responsible for the spasticity. The aim of this was to try to avoid the complete loss of muscle tone and, therefore, to spare some of the useful spasticity. Another variation is by producing a dorsal root entry zone (DREZ) lesion. The original observation of the use of DREZ lesions in the treatment of spasticity was made by Sindou when treating intractable pain. Sindou (1992) has reported 75% and 88% improvement in spasticity and spasms respectively. There is still considerable argument about the efficacy of rhizotomy, not so much as regards the effect on spasticity, but whether or not it has any effect on functional motor disability.

Chemical rhizotomy depends on the use of either alcohol or phenol and has been discussed above.

Myelotomy

The rationale here is the interruption of spinal reflex pathways by separating the anterior horn from the posterior horn of the spinal cord. The operation is now rarely performed. It can only be carried out for paraplegic patients with no voluntary movement and no bladder function. A variety is longitudinal myelotomy as opposed to transverse myelotomy.

Orthopaedic treatment

These procedures are not so much involved in the treatment of spasticity as in the treatment or prevention of complications and bony deformation

caused by spasticity. Results are likely to be unfavourable unless the imbalance of muscular tone
has been treated since if severe spasticity persists
then the results of surgery will be destroyed. The
aims of surgery are to prevent or correct deformity,
or to stabilize or to remove any specific handicap
to rehabilitation. Procedures include tenotomy,
Achilles tendon lengthening, myotomy, muscle
slides and capsulotomy. In addition, bony protu-
berances or abnormal ossification may be removed.

Peripheral functional stimulation

Neuromuscular stimulation

Neuromuscular stimulation may be used in spastic
conditions. This is a technique using surface stimulation with electrodes placed over the belly of the
muscle (cathode distally placed). The strength of
the stimulus used must be below that which would
elicit hypertonia or spasms. Spasticity may respond
to stimulation of affected muscles or of cutaneous
nerves, usually at 20–50 Hz for up to 20 minutes
twice a day until skin tolerance has developed.
If spasticity is severe, then stimulation may be
gradually increased up to 3 hours two or three
times per day (Bajd et al., 1985; Dimitrijevic et al.,
1987).

Franek et al. (1988) carried out a trial in a group
of patients with spinal injury and spasticity. They
compared two groups, treated with transcutaneous
nerve stimulation (TNS) (44 patients) and antispastic drugs (35 patients) respectively. Measurements were made using a clinical scale, muscle
strength, response of muscle to mechanical stimulus, vital capacity, blood pressure, range of
movement, stretch reflexes, pendulum test for
spasticity and bladder function (cystomanometry
and sphincterometry). The results of both groups
seemed remarkably good (Table 24.1).

Other effects of the TNS group included increased

Table 24.1 Results of treatment in patients with spinal
injury and spasticity

	TNS	Non-electrical treatment
Spasticity abolished	50%	25%
Spasticity decreased	22%	75%

strength, reappearance of some stretch reflexes and
improvement in vital capacity. The beneficial effect
of electrical stimulation continues after stopping
stimulation, for hours or days, or even months.
Stimulation was via three pairs of symmetrical
points over upper hip adductors, anterior thighs
and central areas of the buttocks, using triangular
pulses at a frequency of 5–7 Hz and an amplitude
of 10–15 V.

Central functional stimulation
(see also Chapter 36)

One of the earliest demonstrations of the effect of
spinal cord stimulation was Frolich & Sherrington's
(1902) demonstration of inhibition of muscular
rigidity. Table 24.2 indicates some of the experimental work, which has demonstrated alteration
in spinal segmental mechanisms, and also the work
on spinal cord stimulation in man, which has
shown alteration of presynaptic inhibition, alteration of stretch reflexes and suppression of spasms.
Illis et al. (1976) and Thoden et al. (1977) demonstrated changes in the H reflex after spinal cord
stimulation in man. This was confirmed by Feeney
& Gold (1980) and Dimitrijevic & Sherwood (1980),
who demonstrated alteration in stretch reflexes.
Shimoji et al. (1982) reported presynaptic inhibition in spinal cord stimulation in man, and Laitinen
& Fugl-Meyer (1981) measured improvement in
spasticity, using isokinetic dynamometry, and
demonstrated reduction in spasticity and inhibition
of spasms, with concomitant EMG changes. H-reflex
alteration was reported by Siegfried et al. (1981),
Rossi et al. (1984), Nakamura & Tsubokawa (1985),
Barolat-Romana et al. (1985) and Gottlieb et al.
(1985), and alteration of segmental reflexes was
demonstrated by Dimitrijevic et al. (1986a,b). In
Dimitrijevic's studies (Dimitrijevic et al., 1986a, b),
improvement was noted in spasticity in two-thirds
of patients with spinal cord injury. The effects were
more marked in those patients with incomplete
injuries and better results were found with stimulation below the lesion rather than above. In some
cases the effect on spasticity was immediate, in
others it took several days or weeks before benefit
was seen. As spasms improved, motor control may
also benefit. After a period of spinal cord stimulation, voluntary activity tends to be more controlled with less inadvertent co-activation of

Table 24.2 Some reported physiological changes with spinal cord stimulation (for Specific Vascular Changes see Chapter 36)

Author	Animal	Effect
Frolich & Sherrington, 1902	Cat Dog Monkey	Inhibition of muscular rigidity
Larson *et al.*, 1974	Man	Changes in evoked responses
Bantli *et al.*, 1975	Monkey	Evoked responses in thalamic nuclei
Foreman *et al.*, 1976	Primate	Changes in spinothalamic tract neurons; post-synaptic inhibition
Siegfried *et al.*, 1981	Cat Man	Inhibition of monosynaptic reflex activity Decrease in tonic stretch reflex; changes in H-reflex
Saade *et al.*, 1984	Cat	Modulation of spinal segmental mechanisms: primary afferent depolarization; depression of polysynaptic reflexes; facilitation of monosynaptic reflexes
Weisendanger *et al.*, 1985	Cat Monkey	Depression of stretch reflexes (or facilitation, depending on electrode position)
Maiman *et al.*, 1987	Cat	Suppression of spasms: EMG
Illis *et al.*, 1976	Man	Changes in H-reflex
Thoden *et al.*, 1977	Man	Changes in H-reflex
Abbate *et al.*, 1977	Man	Improvement in urodynamic studies
Sedgwick *et al.*, 1980	Man	Changes in cervical and brainstem evoked responses
Feeney & Gold, 1980	Man	Changes in H-reflex
Illis *et al.*, 1980	Man	Improvement in urodynamic studies
Read *et al.*, 1980	Man	Improvement in urodynamic studies
Hawkes *et al.*, 1980	Man	Improvement in urodynamic studies
Meglio *et al.*, 1980	Man	Improvement in urodynamic studies
Dimitrijevic & Sherwood, 1980	Man	Alteration of stretch reflexes
Berg *et al.*, 1982	Man	Improvement in urodynamic studies
Shimoji *et al.*, 1982	Man	Pre-synaptic inhibition; facilitation of primary afferent depolarization
Laitinen & Fugl-Meyer, 1981	Man	Improvement in spasticity (isokinetic dynamometry measurement)
Scerrati *et al.*, 1982	Man	Changes in H-reflex
Tallis *et al.*, 1983a,b	Man	Increase in skin and muscle blood flow
Read *et al.*, 1985	Man	Improvement in urodynamic studies
Nakamura & Tsubokawa, 1985	Man	Changes in H-reflex; reduction in spasticity
Barolat-Romano *et al.*, 1985	Man	Inhibition of spasms: EMG changes
Gottleib *et al.*, 1985	Man	Alteration of stretch reflexes; changes in joint compliance
Dimitrijevic *et al.*, 1986	Man	Alteration of segmental reflexes (polyEMG)

inappropriate muscle groups. Possibly repetitive stimulation via spinal cord stimulation activates dorsal columns and related brain stem structures, which in turn modify descending motor volleys and thus influence segmental reflexes (see Sherwood, 1985).

In animal experiments (cat), Krainick et al. (1977) demonstrated inhibition of monosynaptic reflexes of lumbar extensor and flexor muscles by 20% of control value; an alteration in H-reflex recovery time; alteration in inhibition; and increase in threshold for the extensor reflex. Inhibition of H reflex occurs during spinal cord stimulation. Maiman et al. (1987) undertook an experimental study of spinal cord stimulation in cats. Dorsal spinal impact injuries at T8 produced paraplegia and spasticity, and spinal cord stimulation was carried out above and below the lesion. Stimulation above the lesion aggravated spasticity, which was relieved with stimulation below the lesion. Suppression was maximal with the cathode applied to the cord (monopolar stimulation), and less marked stimulation was seen with bipolar currents.

Read et al. (1980), after a very careful and comprehensive study of 15 patients with multiple sclerosis, concluded: 'Voluntary reduction of spasticity in MS must be regarded as almost impossible. We were impressed by the remarkable decrease in leg spasticity . . . and the frequent reports of the abolition of nocturnal flexor spasms.'

Barolat et al. (1988) studied 16 patients with spasticity and spasms refractory to medical and physical therapy. All had been on large doses of diazepam and baclofen for at least 6 months with no significant benefit or with intolerable side-effects. Fifteen of the patients were traumatic (C4 to T1) and one had cervical myelopathy. Assessment was on the basis of neurological examination, EMG polygraphic recordings, H reflex and H-reflex recovery curves, recording of voluntary movements and spasms with the Cybex isokinetic dynamometer, videotape recording and urodynamic measurements. In 14 of the 16 patients there was significant therapeutic benefit. In eight cases there was an immediate (few seconds) response on starting and stopping stimulation. In some cases, response took several days, and in one patient benefit was not seen until 4–5 weeks of stimulation. The reason for the variation in this time course

is not clear. The almost immediate response suggests the removal of inhibition. Other effects were noted: in one patient there was rapid improvement in bladder function with urodynamic changes, in two cases there was symptomatic bladder improvement, and in most cases there was concomitant improvement in voluntary motor function as spasms were controlled. There were no adverse effects and complications were minor (displacement of electrodes, and one case of infection in the receiver pocket).

Twenty patients with movement disorders and spasticity were studied by Koulousakis et al. (1987). Twelve of the patients had multiple sclerosis. This group reported quantitative changes in spasticity and bladder function, with improvement maintained for up to 4 years. Where technical breakdown of stimulation occurred, there was an increase in spasticity and deterioration of gait.

Krainick et al. (1988) assessed patients by measuring walking speed, H reflex, polygraphic EMG, electrogoniometer and joint compliance. Although the patient's motivation cannot be ignored, the use of objective measures of assessment are obligatory and, as in this study, demonstrates objective evidence of improvement.

Mode of action

In the large group of patients studied by Dimitrijevic et al. (1986a) there was a very much greater chance of improvement in patients with incomplete lesions, and the best effects were in a patient who reported paraesthesiae in the area where he had spasticity. This suggests that partial preservation of long tracts is essential and that long-loop spinal–brain–spinal mechanisms are involved. It was suggested that stimulation modulates brain stem activity, which in turn suppresses segmental excitability. Saade et al. (1984) showed, in decerebrate adult cats, modulation of segmental mechanisms by activating the dorsal column–brain stem–spinal loop.

Summary

There is abundant evidence for the effect of spinal cord stimulation on spinal cord reflex activity in experimental animals and in man. Spinal cord stimulation is a method of treating spasticity and spasms secondary to myelopathy. It is a safe and effective form of treatment in those patients where medical treatment and physiotherapy are ineffective or drug dosage produces unacceptable side-effects. Abnormal hyperactivity to cutaneous stimuli are reduced, pathological spread of activity to other muscle groups is reduced, clonus is reduced, spastic bladder disturbance may be reduced and voluntary motor activity may be enhanced as spasms and spasticity are controlled. Other invasive techniques such as myelotomy or rhizotomy produce neurological deficit. However, intrathecal drug delivery (see p. 341) may be even more effective.

References

Abbate A.D., Cook A.W. & Attalah N. (1977) The effect of electrical stimulation of the thoracic spinal cord on function of the bladder in multiple sclerosis. *Journal of Urology* **117**, 285–288.

Bajd T., Gregoric M., Vodovnick L. & Benko H. (1985) Electrical stimulation in treating spasticity due to spinal cord injury. *Archives of Physical Medicine* **66**, 515–517.

Bantli H., Bloedel J.R. & Thienprasit P. (1975) Supraspinal interactions resulting from experimental dorsal column stimulation. *Journal of Neurosurgery* **42**, 296–300.

Barolat-Romano G., Myklebust J.B., Hemmy D.C., Myklebust R. & Wenninger W. (1985) Immediate effects of spinal cord stimulation in spinal spasticity. *Journal of Neurosurgery* **62**, 558–562.

Barolat G., Myklebust J.B. & Wenninger W. (1988) Effects of spinal cord stimulation on spasticity and spasms secondary to myelopathy. *Applied Neurophysiology* **51**, 29–44.

Bartholini G., Scatton B., Zivkovic B. *et al.* (1979) On the mode of action of SL76002, a new GABA receptor agonist. In Krogsgaard-Larsen P., Scheel-Kruger J. & Kofold H. (eds) *GABA-Neurotransmitters*, pp. 363–340. Munksgaard, Copenhagen.

Bowery N., Hill D. & Hudson A. (1982) Evidence that SL75102 is an agonist at GABA-B as well as GABA-A receptors. *Neuropharmacology* **21**, 391–395.

Brausch U., Henatsch H.D., Student D. & Takano K. (1973) The effect of diazepam on development of stretch reflex tension. In Garattini S., Mussini E. & Randall L.O. (eds) *The Benzodiazepines*, pp. 530–543. Raven Press, New York.

Brodal A. (1969) *Neurological Anatomy*, pp. 151–255. Oxford University Press, London.

Cook J.B. & Nathan P.W. (1967) On the site of action of diazepam in spasticity in man. *Journal of Neurological Science* **5**, 33–37.

Corcos D.M., Gottlieb G.L., Penn R.D., Myklebust B. &
Agarwal G.C. (1986) Movement deficits caused by hyperexcitable stretch reflexes in spastic humans. *Brain* **109**, 1043–1058.

Dhawan B.N. & Sharma J.N. (1970) Facilitation of the flexor reflex in the cat by the intrathecal injection of catecholamines. *British Journal of Pharmacology* **40**, 237–248.

Dimitrijevic M.R. & Nathan P.W. (1967) Studies of spasticity in man. *Brain* **90**, 1–30.

Dimitrijevic M.R. & Sherwood A.M. (1980) Spasticity: medical and surgical treatment. *Neurology* **30**, 19–27.

Dimitrijevic M.R., Nathan P.W. & Sherwood A.M. (1980) Clonus: the role of central mechanisms. *Journal of Neurology, Neurosurgery and Psychiatry* **43**, 321–331.

Dimitrijevic M.M., Dimitrijevic M.R., Illis L.S., Nakajima K., Sharkey P.C. & Sherwood A.M. (1986a) Spinal cord stimulation for the control of spasticity in patients with chronic spinal cord injury. I. Clinical observations. *Central Nervous System Trauma* **3**, 129–144.

Dimitrijevic M.R., Illis L.S., Nakajima K., Sharkey P.C. & Sherwood A.M. (1986b) Spinal cord stimulation for the control of spasticity in patients with chronic spinal cord injury. II: Neurophysiological observations. *Central Nervous System Trauma* **3**, 145–152.

Dimitrijevic M.R., Halter J.A., Sharkey P.C. & Sherwood A.M. (1987) Epidural spinal cord stimulation and carryover effect in chronic spinal cord injury patients. *Applied Neurophysiology* **50**, 449–450.

Erickson D.L., Blacklock J.B., Michaelson M., Sperling K.B. & Lo J.N. (1985) Control of spasticity by implantable continuous flow morphine pump. *Neurosurgery* **16**, 215–217.

Feeney D.M. & Gold G.N. (1980) Chronic dorsal column stimulation: effect of H reflex and symptoms in a patient with multiple sclerosis. *Neurosurgery* **6**, 564–566.

Foerster O. (1911) Restriction of the posterior nerve roots of the spinal cord. *Lancet* **ii**, 76–79.

Foerster O. (1936) Motorische Felder und Bahnen. In Bumke O. & Foerster O. (eds) *Handbuch der Neurologie*, Vol. 6, pp. 1–357. Springer-Verlag, Berlin.

Foreman R.D., Beall J.E., Applebaum A.E., Coulter J.D. & Willis W.D. (1976) Effects of dorsal column stimulation on primate spinothalamic tract neurons. *Journal of Neurophysiology* **39**, 534–546.

Franek A., Turczynski B. & Opara J. (1988) Treatment of spinal spasticity by electrical stimulation. *Journal of Biomedical Engineering* **10**, 266–270.

Frolich A. & Sherrington C.S. (1902) Path of impulses for inhibition under decerebrate rigidity. *Journal of Physiology* **28**, 14–19.

Gottlieb G.L., Myklebust B.M., Stefoksi D., Groth K., Kroin J. & Penn R.D. (1985) Evaluation of cervical stimulation for chronic treatment of spasticity. *Neurology* **35**, 699–704.

Hawkes C.H., Wyke M., Desmond A., Bultitude M.I. & Kanegaonkar G.S. (1980) Stimulation of dorsal column in multiple sclerosis. *British Medical Journal* **1**, 889–891.

Herman R.M., Wainberg M.D., Delguidice P.F. & Willscher M.K. (1988) The effect of low dose intrathecal morphine on impaired micturition reflexes in human subjects with spinal cord lesions. *Anesthesiology* **69**, 313–318.

Illis L.S. (1963) Changes in spinal cord synapses and a possible explanation for spinal shock. *Experimental Neurology* **8**, 328–335.

Illis L.S. (1967a) The motoneurone surface and spinal shock. In Williams D. (ed.) *Modern Trends in Neurology*, Chapter 3. Butterworths, London.

Illis L.S. (1967b) The relative densities of monosynaptic pathways to cells and dendrites in the ventral horn. *Journal of Neurological Sciences* **4**, 259–270.

Illis L.S. (1973a) An experimental model of regeneration in the CNS. I: Synaptic changes. *Brain* **96**, 47–60.

Illis L.S. (1973b) An experimental model of regeneration in the CNS. II: Glial changes. *Brain* **96**, 61–68.

Illis L.S. (1988) Clinical evaluation and pathophysiology of the spinal cord in the chronic stage. In Illis L.S. (ed.) *Spinal Cord Dysfunction: Assessment*, pp. 107–128. Oxford University Press, Oxford.

Illis L.S., Sedgwick E.M., Oygar A.E. & Awadalla M.A.S. (1976) Dorsal column stimulation in the rehabilitation of patients with multiple sclerosis. *Lancet* **i**, 1383–1386.

Illis L.S., Sedgwick E.M. & Tallis R. (1980) Spinal cord stimulation in multiple sclerosis: clinical results. *Journal of Neurology Neurosurgery and Psychiatry* **43**, 1–14.

Jones R.F. (1971) Lioresal in the control of spasticity. In Birkmeyer W. (ed.) *Spasticity – a Topical Survey*, pp. 110–112. Hans Huber, Vienna.

Kaplan J.P., Raizon B.M. & Desarmenien M. *et al.* (1980) New anticonvulsants. Schiff bases of gamma-aminobutyric acid and gamma-aminobutyramide. *Medical Chemistry* **23**, 702–704.

Kato M., Waldmann U. & Murakami S. (1978) Effects of baclofen on spinal neurones of cats. *Neuropharmacology* **17**, 827–833.

Koulousakis A., Buckhaas U. & Nittner K. (1987) Application of spinal cord stimulation for movement disorders and spasticity. *Acta Neurochirurgica (Suppl.)* **39**, 112–116.

Krainick J.-U., Thoden U., Strassburg H.M. & Wenzel D. (1977) The effects of electrical spinal cord stimulation on spastic movement disorders. *Advances in Neurosurgery 4*, pp. 257–260. Springer, Berlin, Heidelberg, New York.

Krainick J.-U., Waisbrod H. & Gerbershagen H.U. (1988) The value of spinal cord stimulation (SCS) in treatment of disorders of the motor system. In Müller H., Zierski J. & Penn R.D. (eds) *Local Spinal Therapy of Spasticity*, pp. 245–252. Springer-Verlag, Berlin.

Laitinen L.V. & Fugl-Meyer A.R. (1981) Assessment of function effect of epidural electrostimulation and selective posterior rhizotomy in spasticity. *Applied Neurophysiology* **45**, 331–334.

Landau W.M. & Hunt C.C. (1990) Dorsal rhizotomy, a treatment of unproven efficacy. *Journal of Child Neurology* **5**, 174–178.

Larson S.J., Sances A., Riegel D.H., Meyer G.A., Dallman D.E. & Swiontek T.J. (1974) Neurophysiological effects of dorsal column stimulation in Man and monkey. *Journal of Neurosurgery* **41**, 217–223.

Latash M.L., Penn R.D., Corcos D.M. & Gottlieb G.L. (1990) Effects of intrathecal baclofen on voluntary motor control in spastic paresis. *Journal of Neurosurgery* **72**, 388–392.

Lazorthes Y., Sallerin-Caute B., Verdie J.-C., Bastide R. & Carillo J.-P. (1990) Chronic intrathecal baclofen administration for control of severe spasticity. *Journal of Neurosurgery* **72**, 393–402.

Liu H.-C., Tsai S.-C., Liu T.-Y. & Chi C.-W. (1991) Baclofen induced frontal lobe syndrome: case report. *Paraplegia* **29**, 554–556.

Ludlow C.L., Naunton R.F., Sedory S.E. *et al.* (1988) Effects of botulinum toxin on speech in adductor spasmodic dystonia. *Neurology* **38**, 1220–1225.

McLellan D.L. (1973) Effect of baclofen upon monosynaptic and tonic vibration reflexes in patients with spasticity. *Journal of Neurology, Neurosurgery and Psychiatry* **36**, 555–560.

McLellan D.L. (1977) Co-contraction and stretch reflexes in spasticity during treatment with baclofen. *Journal of Neurology, Neurosurgery and Psychiatry* **40**, 30–38.

Maiman D.J., Myklebust J.B. & Barolat-Romana G. (1987) Spinal cord stimulation for amelioration of spasticity: experimental results. *Neurosurgery* **21**, 331–333.

Mathias C.J., Luckitt J., Desa P., Baker H., El-Masri W. & Frankel H.L. (1989) Pharmacodynamics and pharmacokinetics of the oral antispastic agent tizanidine in patients with spinal cord injury. *Journal of Rehabilitation, Research and Development* **26**, 9–16.

Mauriello J.A. Jr (1985) Blepharospasm, Meige syndrome, and hemifacial spasm: treatment with botulinum toxin. *Neurology* **35**, 1499–1500.

Medici M., Pebet M. & Siblis D. (1989) A double-blind long-term study of tizanidine (Sirdalud) in spasticity due to cerebrovascular lesions. *Current Medical Research Opinion* **11**, 398–407.

Meglio M., Cioni B., d'Amico E., Ronzoni G. & Rossi G.F. (1980) Epidural spinal cord stimulation for the treatment of neurogenic bladder. *Acta Neurochirurgica* **54**, 191–199.

Michaelis L.S. (1976) Spasticity in spinal cord injuries. In Vinken P.J. & Bruyn G.W. (eds) *Handbook of Clinical Neurology*, pp. 447–487 (Chapter 26). North-Holland, Amsterdam.

Mondrup K. & Pedersen E. (1984) The clinical effect of the GABA-agonist, progabide, on spasticity. *Acta Neurologica Scandinavica* **69**, 200–206.

Nakamura S. & Tsubokawa T. (1985) Evaluation of spinal cord stimulation for post-apopletic spastic hemiplegia. *Neurosurgery* **17**, 253–259.

Nathan P.W. (1959) Intrathecal phenol to relieve spasticity in paraplegia. *Lancet* **ii**, 1099–1102.

Nathan P.W. (1965) Relief of spasticity. *British Medical Journal* i, 1096–1100.

Peacock W.J. & Standt L.A. (1991) Selective posterior rhizotomy: further comments. *Journal of Child Neurology* 6, 173C–174C.

Penn R.D. & Kroin J.S. (1987) Long-term intrathecal baclofen infusion for treatment of spasticity. *Journal of Neurosurgery* 66, 181–185.

Pierrot-Deseilligny E. (1983) Pathophysiology of spasticity. *Triangle* 22, 165–174.

Pinelli P. (1973) Electromyographic evaluation of drug-induced muscle relaxation. In Garattini S., Mussini E. & Randall L.O. (eds) *The Benzodiazepine*, pp. 559–564. Raven Press, New York.

Przybyla A.C. & Wang S.C. (1968) Locus of central depressant action of diazepam. *Journal of Pharmacological and Experimental Therapy* 163, 439–447.

Read D.J., James E.D. & Shaldon C. (1985) The effect of spinal cord stimulation on idiopathic destrusor instability and incontinence: a case report. *Journal of Neurology, Neurosurgery and Psychiatry* 48, 832–834.

Read D.J., Matthews W.D. & Higson R.H. (1980) The effect of spinal cord stimulation on patients with multiple sclerosis. *Brain* 103, 803–833.

Roby A., Bussel B. & Willer J.C. (1981) Morphine reinforces post-discharge inhibition of alpha motoneurons in man. *Brain Research* 222, 209–212.

Rossi L., Rasella M. & Ubiali E. (1984) Method of measuring spasticity: studies of 12 cases of spastic patients treated with chronic epidural implanted electrodes. *Rivista Di Neurologia (Roma)* 54, 87–93.

Rudick R.A., Breton D. & Krail R.L. (1987) The GABA-agonist progabide for spasticity in multiple sclerosis. *Archives of Neurology* 44, 1033–1036.

Saade N.E., Tabet M.S., Atweh S.F. & Jabbur S.J. (1984) Modulation of segmental mechanisms by activation of a dorsal column brainstem spinal loop. *Brain Research* 310, 180–184.

Sachais B.A., Logue J.N. & Carey M.S. (1977) Baclofen: a new antispastic drug. *Archives of Neurology (Chicago)* 34, 422–428.

Scerrati M., Onofrj M. & Pola P. (1982) Effects of spinal cord stimulation on spasticity: H-reflex study. *Applied Neurophysiology* 45, 62–67.

Scheibel M.E. & Scheibel A.B. (1966) Spinal motorneurons, interneurons and Renshaw cells. *Archives of Italian Biology* 104, 328–353.

Scott A.B. (1981) Botulinum toxin injection of eye muscles to correct strabismus. *Transactions of the American Ophthalmological Society* 79, 7334–7770.

Scott A.B., Kennedy R.A. & Stubbs H.A. (1985) Botulinum toxin injection as a treatment for blepharospasm. *Archives of Ophthalmology* 103, 347–350.

Sedgwick E.M., Illis L.S., Tallis R.C., Thornton A.R.D., Abraham P., El-Negamy E., Doherty T.B., Soar J.S., Spencer S.C. & Taylor F.M. (1980) Evoked potentials and contingent negative variation during treatment of multiple sclerosis with spinal cord stimulation. *Journal of Neurology, Neurosurgery and Psychiatry* 43, 14–24.

Sherwood A. (1985) Electrical stimulation of the spinal cord in movement disorders. In Myklebust J.B., Cusick J.F., Sances A. & Larson S.J. (eds) *Neural Stimulation*, pp. 111–146. CRC Press, Boca Raton, Florida.

Shimoji K., Shimizu H., Maruyama Y., Matsuki M., Kurirayashi H. & Rjioka H. (1982) Dorsal column stimulation in man: facilitation of primary afferent depolarization. *Anaesthesia and Analgesia* 61, 410–413.

Siegfried J., Lazorthes Y. & Broggi G. (1981) Electrical spinal cord stimulation for spastic movement disorders. *Applied Neurophysiology* 44, 77–92.

Sindou M. (1992) Microsurgical DREZ-tomy for the treatment of pain and spasticity. In Young R.R. & Delwaide P.J. (eds) *Principles and Practice of Restorative Neurology*, pp. 144–151. Butterworth Heinemann, Oxford.

Snow B.J., Tsui J.K.C., Bhatt M.H., Varelas M., Hashimoto S.A. & Calne D.B. (1990) Treatment of spasticity with botulinum toxin: a double-blind study. *Annals of Neurology* 28, 512–515.

Stratten W. & Barnes C.D. (1971) Diazepam and presynaptic inhibition. *Neuropharmacology* 10, 685–696.

Struppler A., Burgmayer G., Ochs G.B. & Pfeiffere H.G. (1983) The effect of epidural application of opioids on spasticity of spinal origin. *Life Sciences* 33 (Suppl. 1), 607–610.

Tallis R.C., Illis L.S., Sedgwick E.M., Hardwidge C. & Garfield J.S. (1983a) Spinal cord stimulation in peripheral vascular disease. *Journal of Neurology, Neurosurgery and Psychiatry* 46, 476–484.

Tallis R.C., Illis L.S., Sedgwick E.M., Hardwidge C. & Kennedy K. (1983b) The effect of spinal cord stimulation upon periphral blood flow in patients with chronic neurological disease. *International Rehabilitation Medicine* 5, 4–9.

Thoden U., Krainick J.-U., Strassburg H.M. & Zimmerman H. (1977) Influence of dorsal column stimulation on spastic movement disorders. *Acta Neurochirurgica* 39, 233–240.

Tsui J.K., Eisen A., Stoessel J. *et al.* (1986) Double-blind study of botulinum toxin in spasmodic torticollis. *Lancet* ii, 245–257.

Wainberg M.C., Herman R.M., Willscher M.K. & Delguidice P.F. (1987) The effect of low-dose intrathecal morphine on bladder capacity in human subjects with spinal cord lesions. *Society for Neuroscience Abstracts* 13, 1302.

Weisendanger M., Chapman C.E., Marini G. & Schorderet D. (1985) Experimental studies of dorsal cord stimulation in animal models of spasticity. In Delwaide P.J. & Young R.R. (eds) *Clinical Neurophysiology in Spasticity* pp. 205–219. Elsevier, Amsterdam.

Willer J.C. & Bussel B. (1980) Evidence for a direct spinal mechanism in a morphine-induced inhibition of nociceptive reflexes in humans. *Brain Research* 187, 212–215.

25: Rehabilitation and Management of the Neuropathic Bladder

K.F. PARSONS, R.C.L. FENELEY AND M.J. TORRENS

Theoretic considerations, 349
  Vesico-urethral structure and innervation, 350
  Central nervous influences, 352
Functional considerations, 354
Clinical assessment, 355
  Urological history, 355
  Clinical examination, 356
Investigation, 357
  Urinary infection, 357
  Direct assessment of vesico-urethral function, 358
  Urodynamic techniques, 358
Classification of the neuropathic bladder, 363
  Classification of the neurological condition, 363
  Classification by symptoms, 364
  Functional classification, 364
Management of the neuropathic bladder, 364
  Management of long-term vesico-urethral neuropathy, 366
  Improvement of bladder function, 367
  Hyperactive urethra (high outflow resistance), 370
  Catheterization, 372
  Urethral incompetence, 374
  Cutaneous urinary diversion, 375
Complications of the neuropathic bladder, 376
Palliation of incontinence, 377
  Incontinence appliances, 377

Classification and terminology of the neuropathic bladder can be inordinately complex and confusing. It is bedevilled by inexact assessment methods, empirical attitudes and an illogical overemphasis on the neurological lesion. Indeed management has often been described solely in relation to a particular disease or on the site of the clinically demonstrable neurological level. This approach is fortunately changing, largely for two reasons. First, as a more functional view of the urinary tract has developed, it has become evident that it is difficult to predict from the neurological signs how the bladder will behave. Second, close observation has shown that function changes considerably at different stages of the same disease, and also in response to environmental factors, notably infection. Optimal management in neuropathic cases thus requires proper functional investigation, and treatment directed appropriately.

In this chapter the principles of treatment will be described in relation to what is pathophysiologically *observed* rather than expected. The first section therefore concentrates on the structure and innervation of the bladder and urethra and on the principles of functional investigation. The second section of the chapter discusses practical management in relation to physiological principles. Such management is governed by an overriding prerequisite that everything appropriate must be done to preserve renal and ureteric function. If that is so, then a second consideration can be entertained that continence may be restored or incontinence palliated provided that renal function is not compromised.

Theoretic considerations

An understanding of how the system works is always a necessary prerequisite for putting it right. Because of continuing research into the area of vesico-urethral function, much of it stimulated by the activities of the International Continence Society, understanding of the mechanisms of normal micturition is improving, and the abnormalities in neuropathic vesicourethral dysfunction are much better understood. The pivotal investigation which has produced these advances is the *urodynamic* assessment of bladder function during which the pressure flow relationships of the bladder during both filling and emptying are measured, usually combined with radiographic screening or other imaging technique designed synchronously to observe the bladder neck. The following accounts must be regarded not as definitive statements of fact, but as a physiological stimulus to more rational treatment. Indeed perhaps the greatest single contribution which urodynamics has made has been to provoke thought about therapeutic dogma.

Vesico-urethral structure and innervation

The structure and innervation of the bladder and urethra in humans has been studied extensively by Gosling and his co-workers (Gosling *et al.*, 1977; Gosling, 1979), and the following account is based largely on their work.

Detrusor

The bladder can be considered to be a simple sphere of muscle in continuity with the tubular outflow conduit, the urethra. The main bulk of the detrusor, including the condensation around the bladder neck, is a meshwork of smooth muscle. This is not layered as in the intestine. It is relatively rich in acetylcholine esterase, evidence for a dominant cholinergic innervation. There are few noradrenergic neurons.

Excitatory motor nerves to the detrusor arise from the parasympathetic (cholinergic) ganglion cells in the pelvic plexus. The preganglionic fibres run in the sacral roots 2, 3 and 4. Nerve-mediated detrusor inhibition has been described, occurring after stimulation of the perianal area, and it is suggested that such relaxation may be induced by β-sympathetic action (Sundin & Dahlstrom, 1973). Bladder relaxation evoked by bladder wall stretch (accommodation) may be similarly mediated. As little significant sympathetic innervation reaches the bladder dome in humans it is suggested by Gosling that such inhibition may occur at the neurons in the pelvic ganglia where noradrenergic axosomatic terminals have been observed. These sympathetic nerves leave the cord at the T10–L2 level and run in the pre-sacral nerves and hypogastric plexus. There is some evidence that the cell bodies of these neurons lie in the sacral cord and that the fibres ascend to leave at the thoracolumbar outflow (Laruelle, 1948).

Around the bladder neck the detrusor muscle is arranged in various loops and slings. No doubt these are involved in the mechanisms of closure and opening of the bladder neck and several mechanical theories of function have been elaborated. All are presumptive and none gained general acceptance such that the precise mechanism of bladder neck opening remains enigmatic.

Urethral smooth muscle

At and below the vesicourethral junction the smooth muscle of the proximal or preprostatic urethra is histochemically distinct from that of the detrusor. In the male (Fig. 25.1) this muscle also forms the prostatic capsule and is richly provided with noradrenergic terminals, but relatively little acetylcholine esterase is found. In the female (Fig. 25.2) the fibres are longitudinally arranged along the urethra, and in contrast to the male the dominant innervation is cholinergic. In both sexes experimental studies using α-adrenoreceptor blocking agents (Donker *et al.*, 1972) suggest that up to 80% of the resting urethral pressure depends on α-adrenergic activity. As with the detrusor it is likely that the sympathetic influence on the urethra occurs in part at the pelvic ganglia, especially in the female. In the male the role of the sympathetic system coordinates seminal emission and the closure of the preprostatic urethra so that the 'genital sphincter' prevents seminal reflux into the bladder. Stimulation of sacral nerves, perhaps involving preganglionic parasympathetic fibres, has been shown to cause urethral relaxation (Torrens, 1978). These and other studies suggest that the autonomic innervation regulates reciprocal activity between the bladder and urethra.

Urethral striated muscle

There are two groups of striated muscle in relation to the urethra, called by Gosling intramural and periurethral. Intramural fibre bundles are found close to the urethral lumen, sometimes interdigitating with smooth muscle and known as the intrinsic urethral sphincter mechanism. In the male (Fig. 25.1) these fibres are orientated circularly around the postprostatic 'membranous' urethra. The muscle cells are smaller than general striated muscle and almost all are of the 'slow twitch' type, rich in myosin ATPase. No muscle spindles have been seen. Evidently these fibres are adapted to

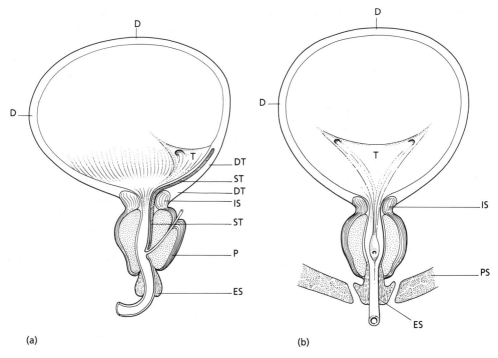

Fig. 25.1 (a) The male lower urinary tract in midline sagittal section. The detrusor (D) is condensed behind the bladder neck as the deep trigone (DT). This is distinct from the superficial trigone (ST). The smooth muscle at the bladder neck (IS) forms the proximal part of the urethral sphincter mechanism and is continuous with the prostatic capsule (P). The intramural striated muscle (ES) is condensed around the postprostatic urethra and forms the striated part of the distal urethral sphincter mechanism, or 'external sphincter'. (b) Viewed from the front the intramural (ES) and periurethral (PS) striated muscles are separated by a connective tissue septum. (From Gosling, 1979, with permission.)

maintain tone over a relatively long period of time. In the female (Fig. 25.2) the fibres are similar in type but form no such sphincter. Their density is greatest anteriorly and laterally in the middle third of the urethra. The intramural striated muscle is supplied by myelinated nerve fibres from S2–4 passing through the pelvic plexus *not* running in the pudendal nerve. This explains why pudendal neurectomy does not abolish sphincter spasm.

The periurethral striated muscle of the pelvic floor is relatively remote from the urethra, separated from the intramural muscle by a connective tissue septum. The muscle is a mixture of slow and fast twitch fibres and is supplied by the pudendal nerves (S2–4). This muscle is part of the levator ani complex or pelvic diaphragm. It can contract quickly, as on coughing or voluntary interruption of the urinary stream, but cannot maintain a long

sustained contraction and thus has little contribution to general continence.

The urethra should not be regarded as a collection of sphincters, but as an integrated closure system relying not only upon the active neuromuscular components described above but also on passive factors such as urethral elasticity, mural tension and abdominal compression not dissimilar to the intra-abdominal oesophagus.

Receptor sites

Much recent effort has been directed towards the analysis of sympathetic receptors in the urinary tract. The distinction between experimentally demonstrable α and β adrenergic receptor sites and innervation is not always made clear. α-Adrenoreceptors, causing smooth muscle contraction when

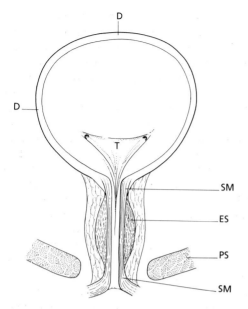

Fig. 25.2 The female lower urinary tract in coronal section. A thin layer of smooth muscle (SM) extends the full length of the urethra. The intramural striated muscle (ES) is thickest in the middle one-third of the urethra, and is anatomically separate from the periurethral striated muscle (PS). (From Gosling, 1979, with permission.)

stimulated, are located mainly in the region of the bladder neck and proximal 4 cm of urethra in both sexes. β-Receptors are very few in this area, being present mainly over the bladder dome. β Stimulation encourages bladder relaxation. Appreciation of these functions aids the understanding of the action of drugs on the urinary tract.

The complex interrelation of nerves, transmitter substances and receptor sites are, after years of controversy, revealing the relative roles of the sympathetic and parasympathetic systems (Caine, 1984). Radioligand studies have confirmed the presence of cholinergic receptors throughout the detrusor, and pharmacological testing shows the postganglionic nerve endings to be muscarinic. Stimulation to the muscarinic receptors results in an increase in tone or as contraction of the muscle fibre. Adrenoreceptor sites, however, are not fixed and immutable entities and changes can occur from one type to another (i.e. α to β) under certain circumstances, for example in response to temperature changes (Kunos & Nickerson, 1976) or in

the detrusor adrenoreceptors, to chronic stretching (Rohner et al., 1978). Adrenoreceptors can be divided into subtypes α_1, the effector cell receptor, and α_2, a presynaptic receptor site on the nerve terminal itself. This second receptor seems to have an autoregulatory function whereby stimulation of it acts as a type of negative feedback mechanism (Bertelsen & Pettinger, 1977). Nergardh (1975) has shown that while acetylcholine always leads to contraction of the detrusor fibres, resistance at the bladder neck may either decrease or increase. By selective blocking of receptor sites he demonstrated that the actions of acetylcholine may be mediated by adrenergic receptors. It appears that a single transmitter substance can act on two adrenergic receptors producing opposite muscular responses. Despite these complex interactions understanding of the autonomic control of the smooth muscle of the lower urinary tract does allow rational pharmacotherapy to be planned (Diokno & Sonda, 1984), particularly in neuropathic conditions where receptor function may be exaggerated by decentralization supersensitivity, and the response to pharmacological agents more impressive.

Central nervous influences

The seminal work of Nathan (1976) and Fletcher and Bradley (1978) from the foundation of the understanding of the central nervous control of micturition. Recent developments in neurological investigation using electrical (Thiry & Deltenre, 1989) or magnetic stimulation (Barker et al., 1985; Hess et al., 1986) of the motor cortex holds great promise in further understanding of the relationship between the vesicourethral apparatus and the somatically innervated pelvic floor.

Sensation

In general there are no specialized sensory endings peripherally. Endings from the muscle (presumed mechanoreceptors) enter through the sacral roots (S2–4). Afferents in the hypogastric nerve and thoraco-lumbar roots (T12–L2) are most likely to originate in the submucosal layer. Clinical studies confirm that discriminatory sensation, both proprioceptive and enteroceptive, is mediated by sacral roots. Afferents with the sympathetic component of the thoraco-lumbar nerves produce a poorly localized feeling of distension or pain, but this underlines the importance of blocking nerve roots as high as T12 when local anaesthetic techniques are used in endoscopic lower urinary tract surgery.

There is some dispute as to the pathways of sensation centripetally in the spinal cord. Most observations have been made on patients who have undergone anterolateral cordotomy. Nathan (1976) believes that all intrinsic sensations from the bladder and urethra ascend in the spinothalamic tracts. If these are sectioned the patient may retain both the feeling that micturition is imminent and other sensations from the pelvic floor mediated by the posterior columns. Others (Hitchcock et al., 1974) have shown preservation of bladder sensation after spinothalamic tractotomy producing bilateral sacral anaesthesia. Certainly experiments in animals suggest that some bladder afferents pass in the medial part of the posterior columns (Kuru, 1965), but the spinothalamic tract is the more significant conduit.

Techniques using cortical evoked potentials from direct stimulation within the lower urinary tract have demonstrated that, for example, the proximal and distal urethra are innervated by different peripheral afferents (Sarica & Karacan, 1988). However, these data showed that somatosensory evoked potentials mediated by pelvic afferents demonstrated much inter-individual variation in normal subjects. Furthermore, this technique may excite several (extero- and proprio-ceptive) types of sensory receptors or fibres (Bradley & Sundin, 1982) which project centrally in both the dorsal columns and the spinothalamic tracts. Afferent vesical pathways thus might be better studied by measuring cortical evoked potentials in response to mechanical bladder distension rather than electrical stimulation (Deltenre & Thiry, 1989) and the development of this technique is awaited.

Brain centres

Stimulation studies in animals and analysis of the effects of ablation and tumours in man have revealed a number of areas in the brain with an influence on micturition.

Since micturition is subject to social constraint the cortical control of lower autonomic centres is highly developed in social animals. The areas involved in man are the superior frontal gyrus and the adjacent anterior cingulate gyrus. Lesions here diminish the awareness of vesical events, allowing the lower centres to act autonomously. This is the territory supplied by the anterior cerebral/pericallosal artery, spasm or occlusion of which promotes incontinence. Otherwise local tumours may have the same effect, and similar manifestations occur in more generalized cerebral disorders such as cerebral atrophy and hydrocephalus. Lesions more posteriorly in the frontal region (paracentral lobule) may result in spasticity of the striated sphincters and levatores ani producing urinary retention.

In the subcortical brain are various areas that between them produce the balanced facilitation and inhibition necessary for coordinated bladder function. The organization is summarized diagrammatically in Fig. 25.3. The principal areas involved are the septal region and anterior hypothalamus, the pontine reticular formation and the cerebellum. This descending system is controlled not only by the frontal cortex but also by the limbic system, the reason why bladder function is so influenced by emotion.

Efferent tracts

Efferent fibres from the reticular formation of the brain stem, concerned with bladder control, pass caudally in relation to the lateral corticospinal tract. Several authors place them laterally, and Kuru (1965) suggests that the vesico-constrictor and vesico-relax or fibres are separate in the lateral and ventral reticulospinal tracts, respectively. In man the position may be laterally close to the insertion of the dentate ligaments (Hitchcock et al., 1974) or medially between the lateral corticospinal tract and the intermediolateral grey matter of the cord (Nathan, 1976). The fact that tract localization in the cord is difficult may suggest individual variability, or perhaps that the tracts are not localized to the expected extent.

Sacral micturition centre

The so-called 'sacral micturition centre' (Lapides et al., 1976) in the conus medullaris can also act autonomously. Unlike the centres in the brain,

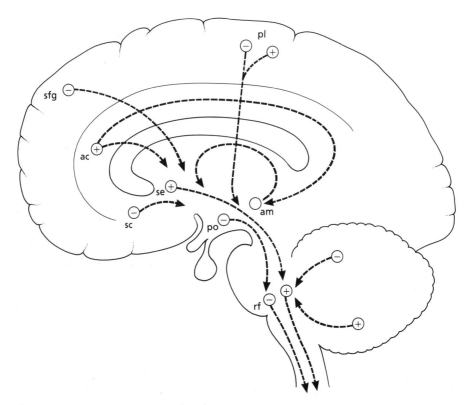

Fig. 25.3 Higher nervous influences on bladder function. ⊕ = facilitation, ⊖ = inhibition. ac – anterior cingulate gyrus, am – amygdala, pl – paracentral lobule, po – preoptic nucleus, rf – reticular formation, sc – subcallosal cingulate gyrus, se – septal area, sfg – superior frontal gyrus.

however, it cannot fully coordinate parasympathetic, sympathetic and somatic activity. This discoordination, or 'dyssynergia', is the basis of many of the complications to be described in more detail below. Under normal circumstances the reciprocal and integrated action of the autonomic and somatic systems, suggested by the observed peripheral innervation described above, is mediated in the conus. This activity is summarized in Fig. 25.4 which must be regarded as an oversimplification.

Functional considerations

Normal urinary continence and voiding may be regarded as the balanced reciprocal interaction of the forces of expulsion and the forces of retention. These have been discussed by many authors (Bates, 1971; Yeates, 1972) and for simplicity they are listed in Table 25.1.

Table 25.1 Forces involved in urinary function

Forces of expulsion	Forces of retention
Detrusor contraction Abdominal muscle contraction Diaphragmatic contraction	Detrusor relaxation
Bladder neck funnelling	Bladder neck closure Intra-abdominal urethra Urethral tension and elasticity
Urethral relaxation	Distal urethral closure: involuntary voluntary

These various forces do not depend solely upon normal nervous control. Physical and hormonal factors are of great importance, influencing how the muscle and supporting tissue can respond. For

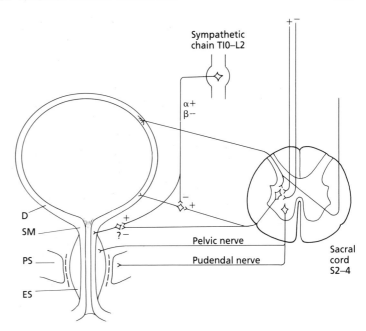

Fig. 25.4 The peripheral innervation of the bladder and urethra. Abbreviations as in Fig. 25.1.

example, detrusor relaxation (accommodation) depends upon distensibility (compliance). Contractility depends upon undamaged muscle. Sensation, and urethral contraction vary with the hormonal state, especially in females. Muscle hypertrophy can influence physically the way that muscle behaves.

Bearing in mind the complexity of the situation, it is facile to classify the neuropathic bladder based only on the type or level of neurological lesion. It is obligatory to measure the various factors and build up a picture of bladder dysfunction, as each case is different. This then enables a much more rational functional classification to be established. In order for this to be done, appropriate urodynamic investigation has to be performed and interpreted in conjunction with the neurological diagnosis.

Clinical assessment

Urological history

This may help in the assessment of the patient with neurological disease but rarely will add to the neurological diagnosis. The pre-morbid history of bladder function may influence greatly the response to disease, and the subsequent management of the neuropathic bladder, thus special note should be made of previous urological surgery or other relevant treatment. The onset and progress of the current complaints are recorded, bearing in mind the most significant problem for the patient.

Sensation of bladder filling is quite separate from that of imminent micturition, the latter occurring after the bladder neck has opened. Deficient bladder sensation often contributes to incontinence and thus enquiry of it should always be made.

Voiding may take place on volition, spontaneously with or without sensation, reflexly to stimulation, or on voluntary straining only. A series of questions pertinent to vesico-urethral function may be asked. Can the urinary stream be interrupted briskly by voluntary sphincter contraction? Is the stream interrupted involuntarily? On all occasions what force of stream is possible? Under which circumstances does incontinence occur? What steps are being taken to manage it? What degree of social or other disruption does it cause? Not only are the answers important in themselves but they will provide help in interpretation of subsequent urodynamic investigation to be sure that this test does reflect accurately what happens under more normal circumstances for the patient.

Complications such as infection, pain, autonomic dysreflexia, and developing obstruction must be excluded. Infection must be taken very seriously, especially if accompanied by stones, debris or blood. As the patient may be unable to sense uralgia a subjective history of freedom from infection cannot be accepted.

Bowel dysfunction may parallel bladder dysfunction, and a similar sort of history should be obtained. Special emphasis may be paid to sensory discrimination, questioning whether the patient is able to tell the difference between solid, liquid or gaseous material in the anal canal.

The *sexual history* can be of diagnostic value. It should be determined whether erection is absent, reflex or psychogenic. If ejaculation is preserved, is it forceful and clonic or weak, which might reflect only the presence of seminal emission. Is there evidence of retrograde ejaculation? What is the character and acuity of orgasm if present?

Reflex erection is mediated by sacral roots and pelvic nerves whereas psychogenic erection may occur through the cholinergic fibres in the hypogastric nerves. Seminal emission into the posterior urethra depends upon an intact sympathetic efferent and ejaculation requires coordinated action of the somatic musculature of the pelvic floor and therefore the pudendal nerves. Closure of the bladder neck is necessary to prevent retrograde ejaculation, and orgasmic sensation is a combined afferent bombardment through the hypogastric (sympathetic) and pudendal nerves. Careful inquisition of sexual function thus has the potential to differentiate subtle differences in pelvic neuropathy.

The significance of all these and other urological symptoms is summarised in Table 25.2.

Clinical examination

The clinical assessment of the neurological patient in whom vesico-urethropathy is anticipated must include a full physical examination with careful suprapubic palpation to determine whether the bladder is full or overdistended. In acute spinal transection the onset of spinal shock guarantees that the detrusor becomes acontractile, and urgent decompression of the bladder by catheterization in this circumstance is mandatory. The period of recovery of contractility is dependent upon the length of time that the detrusor is overstretched and acontractility may persist for up to 12 months even with the return of other reflex activity if the overdistension is prolonged. Where there is any doubt as to whether the bladder is overdistended, which may occur particularly in those cases where the distension may be chronic and the bladder 'floppy', an ultrasound examination should be per-

Table 25.2 The significance of urological symptoms

Lesion	Storage	Voiding	Sexual history
Complete UMN* lesion	Reflex incontinence, autonomic dysreflexia	Reflex voiding, intermittent spurting stream	Reflex erection (80%), no ejaculation, no orgasm
Incomplete UMN* lesion	Urgency, urge incontinence, storage decreased	Precipitate voiding	Variable
Complete LMN* lesion	Retention, overflow/stress incontinence, may feel abdominal sensation of fullness	Voiding by strain, unable to stop stream except by relaxing	Psychogenic erection (30%), no ejaculation, weak emission, no orgasm
Incomplete LMN* lesion	Storage increased, often continent	Infrequent slow stream, may feel bladder never empties	Variable, often impotent
Peripheral autonomic lesion (e.g. abdomino-perineal resection)	Stress incontinence, storage increased	Infrequent slow stream, may strain, feel urine passing	No erection, ejaculation possible, diminished orgasm

* UMN – upper motoneuron; LMN – lower motoneuron.

formed. This examination can also easily determine the integrity of the upper urinary tracts, which is of critical importance when the bladder is neuropathic.

A full and detailed neurological examination should be performed and perhaps the most pertinent aspect of that examination is the neurological level of the lesion as judged by sensory testing. This will allow some assessment to be made of the relationship between the level of the lesion to the sacral micturition and in this respect it is crucial to recognize the normal sensory distribution of the sacral nerves. Indeed accurate knowledge of sensory distribution can avoid the common clinical error which assumes in those cases where sensation is preserved over the clavicles and upper thorax, that there is neurological preservation of T1 and above; whereas the lesion is indeed much higher for the area involved is supplied by the second and third cervical nerves.

There are specific clinical signs pertinent to vesico-urethral neuropathy which are of critical importance and which will help to determine the neurological level that relates to bladder function.

The bulbocavernosus reflex

The presence of this reflex can be used to infer that the conus micturition centre is intact for it relies upon integrity of the lower sacral segments. The reflex is elicited by a brisk pinching of the glans penis which provokes a contraction of the perianal muscles. In females it can be observed by gently pinching the clitoris or rather more easily by a single tug on a balloon catheter. The afferent and efferent limbs are in the pudendal nerves and for it to be present the S2−4 sacral segments must be intact.

The bulbocavernosus reflex is absent in conus and cauda equina lesions. In higher lesions the reflex returns within the first 12 hours or so following acute spinal injury following the general principle that the more peripheral the reflex the sooner it is likely to return as spinal shock abates. It is therefore important to test this reflex within the first day after spinal injury for it may help to predict the type of bladder dysfunction anticipated. The limitation of the reflex is that it is absent in perhaps 30% of neurologically intact individuals.

The anocutaneous reflex

This reflex can be seen by pricking the perianal skin with a needle and observing a contraction of the perianal muscles similar to that seen in the bulbocavernosus reflex. It also demonstrates presence of the S2−4 reflex arcs. The advantage of looking carefully for this reflex is that it can be used to detect laterality of a lesion in the lower spinal segments depending upon which side of the anal skin evokes the response.

The anal reflex

The third of the three anal responses can be demonstrated by brief finger dilatation of the anus at rectal examination. If the conus reflexes are intact this manoeuvre will produce an immediate contraction of the anal ring.

A clear demonstration of the sensory level and testing of the conus reflexes will indicate the level of the neurological defect and allows some anticipation of the type of bladder dysfunction to be anticipated. Indeed in patients with congenital vesico-urethral neuropathy the conus reflexes have been the most accurate predicator of both bladder dysfunction, and of upper urinary tract dilatation.

Investigation

Urological investigation of the patient with neurological disease concentrates on three main fields: urinary infection; a direct assessment of vesico-urethral function; and upper urinary tract morphology and function.

Urinary infection

It is always necessary to rely on regular urinary culture for the absolute diagnosis of urinary infection because disorders of sensation may prevent the appreciation of uralgia which would signify infection. Routine urine culture specimens frequently become contaminated and interpretation may be difficult. For this reason, a dip inoculum in midstream is suggested. However, the significance of bacterial counts in neuropathic cases may be different to that which is significant in the neurologically intact patient, and the case may be made to withhold therapy unless the infection produces systemic signs. This is certainly so in those patients in whom a permanent indwelling catheter is *in situ*.

Suprapubic needle aspiration of the bladder is probably the most reliable method of obtaining accurate bacteriological data relating to urinary infection, particularly in patients who carry a residual urine.

Direct assessment of vesico-urethral function

Post-micturitional residual urine

The simplest method of assessing the adequacy and efficiency of bladder emptying is to measure the post-micturitional residual urine. This can be performed either directly by catheterization, by ultrasonography or deduced from the post-micturition film of an intravenous urogram. Voiding efficiency can be expressed as a percentage of the ratio of residual urine to bladder capacity (Bors & Comarr, 1971). This principle was developed to define a 'balanced' bladder and to differentiate from that which was unbalanced. An arbitrary percentage residual urine was used to make the differentiation. Unfortunately this does not separate several significantly different voiding patterns. An elevated residual urine in a suprasacral lesion may imply an acontractile bladder, insufficient reflex bladder contractility, or detrusor sphincter dyssynergia, where despite adequate detrusor contraction, voiding is obstructed by uncoordinated distal sphincteric activity. In an infrasacral lesion, the inability to produce significant abdominal straining or the inability to overcome outlet resistance may also produce a residual urine. Of rather more fundamental importance is the inability of the measurement of post-micturitional residual urine to reflect intravesical pressure during voiding or during urinary storage between voiding episodes.

Assessment of detrusor function during filling and emptying is therefore mandatory in the management of neuropathic vesico-urethral dysfunction.

Urodynamic techniques

Perhaps the most basic urodynamic assessment that can be made is a simple test for the presence or absence of detrusor contraction. This can be per-

formed merely by using the catheter tubing as an elementary manometer and observing fluctuations which may, especially in the paralysed patient, be assumed to be due to detrusor contraction. This may provide the barest minimum of information. Most clinicians would, however, find this inadequate and a full urodynamic assessment of the patient is normally required before treatment can be planned.

A full synchronous videocystographic pressure flow study (Thomas, 1979) should be used as this obtains as much information as possible about bladder function albeit that it is, for the patient, an invasive investigation. The components of the investigative technique will be described in detail.

The crux of the investigation determines detrusor function with great accuracy; records it during bladder filling and emptying; relates it to the urinary flow rate during micturition; whilst the bladder and outflow are synchronously imaged by radiographic screening. Where this facility is not available, the bladder neck and proximal urethra can be visualized by transrectal ultrasound scanning and this provides a reasonably satisfactory alternative imaging (Fellows *et al.*, 1987; Shabsigh *et al.*, 1988).

Detrusor function

The contribution to total bladder pressure made by the detrusor can be recorded relatively easily. The pressure within the bladder is a summation of the intrinsic pressure of the muscle within its wall, generated largely by the contractility of the detrusor muscle and, because the organ is intraperitoneal, an extrinsic element of intraperitoneal pressure. Detrusor function may thus be obtained by recording total intravesical pressure and subtracting abdominal pressure from it. This is done in practice by recording total bladder pressure by a fine pressure line inserted either by suprapubic stab, or transurethrally, into the bladder. Intra-abdominal pressure is measured by a similar rectal pressure line passed *per anum*. Intrinsic rectal activity potentially might produce recording artefacts, but in practice this is not a problem. The abdominal (intra-rectal) pressure is subtracted electronically from the total bladder pressure to record intrinsic or detrusor pressure continuously. The bladder is filled with radiographic contrast via a filling catheter under X-

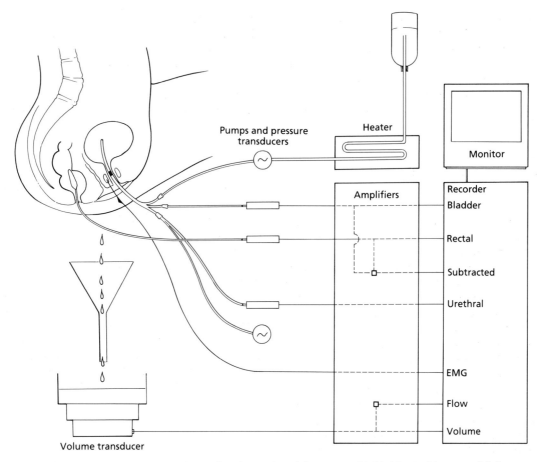

Fig. 25.5 The arrangement of apparatus for urodynamic testing of the neuropathic bladder. In this case a triple lumen Portex 'Rossier' catheter is in place recording both bladder and urethral pressure. X-ray equipment is not included in this diagram.

ray screening and the filling limb of the micturitional cycle is recorded, during which the detrusor pressure can be measured. Once capacity is reached, micturition can take place and the pressures similarly monitored, and the cystogram viewed. Indeed it was in an effort to reduce the screening time at cystography, and to try to identify pertinent episodes during the micturition filling and voiding phases, that the technique of pressure flow video urodynamics was developed (Fig. 25.5).

Uroflow measurement

It is crucial to know the *rate* at which the bladder empties once the pressure responsible is determined and characteristic flow patterns can be recognized (Fig. 25.6). There are a variety of methods by which this can be done but all depend upon measurement of mass per unit time of urine passed from the bladder.

The transducers used to measure this rely on different principles, and each is ingenious, reliable and holds no particular advantage over another. Any of the uroflowmeters can be incorporated into the schema of urodynamic investigation so that the relationship between detrusor pressure and the flow rate that the pressure produces can be analysed. This is the essence of urodynamic investigation and allows the differentiation between the obstructed and the non-obstructed bladder, whilst

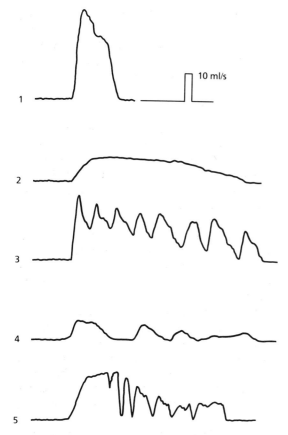

Fig. 25.6 Urinary flow rate tracings to demonstrate both quantitative and qualitative variations. **1** Normal. **2** Obstructed, prostatic hyperplasia. **3** Abdominal straining. **4** Intermittent weak detrusor contractions. **5** Obstructed detrusor–sphincter dyssynergia.

the radiographic screening identifies the site of obstruction. Furthermore detrusor function can be recognized as normal or abnormal and the cause of incontinence, if present, accurately identified.

Urodynamic results

The results of urodynamic studies allow objective measurement of a variety of parameters. Bladder sensation, capacity, compliance (the ability to accommodate increasing volume), contractility and uroflow may be increased, normal or reduced (Torrens & Abrams, 1979). Bladder sensation is twofold: (i) the sensation when filling is first ap-

preciated; and (ii) the point during filling at which a normal sensation to void is experienced. Each is marked as an absolute value on the filling cystometrogram but there is no 'normal' value for either. However, the patient who has deficient sensation will be easily recognized, as will one with a hypersensitive bladder. The maximum cystometric capacity is the point at which the patient feels a normal strong desire to micturate. The bladder should not be overfilled during cystometry because this will influence contractility. Compliance is the volume increment for a given change in pressure. This is a defined parameter which describes the slope of the filling cystometrogram. Previously this may have been referred to as bladder 'tone', but this confusing concept is best abandoned. Indeed the slope of the filling cystometrogram of the normal bladder should be virtually flat at a low filling rate over the normal range. The normal bladder should not contract under provocation until the patient wishes to void and the increase in intrinsic detrusor pressure should not exceed 10–15 cmH$_2$O. Fluctuations in intra-abdominal pressure may be wide and of course will alter total bladder pressure, underlining the importance of recording subtracted or detrusor pressure.

Spontaneous bladder contractions during the filling phase have been given many names of which *detrusor instability* is reserved for those cases in which no identifiable aetiology is recognized and *uninhibited* or *hyper-reflexic* applied to cases with a neuropathic cause. These contractions may lead to involuntary incontinence; whether or not the patient is aware of this will depend upon the sensation.

When compliance is low as recorded by standard cystometric techniques, continuous ambulatory urodynamic monitoring has shown the pressure rise within the bladder generally to be less. Phasic contractions over and above the inexorable bladder pressure increase are recorded and it is these which seem positively to correlate with a threat to the upper urinary tracts (Webb *et al.*, 1989) (Fig. 25.7).

Detrusor contractility is assessed upon the result of an effort to initiate micturition. The pressure required to generate a normal urinary flow rate (see below) should not exceed 50 cmH$_2$O and thus outflow obstruction can be diagnosed if the detrusor pressure peaks beyond this point. An acontractile

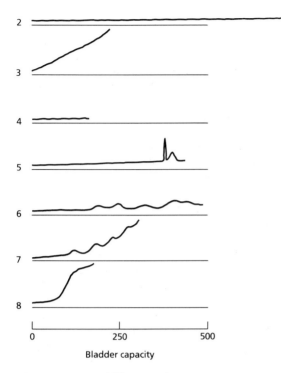

Fig. 25.7 Pattern of filling cystometrograms. Types 5 and 8 show various stages in the development of hypercontractility. (After Torrens & Abrams, 1979.)
1 The normal situation, compliant and with no contractions until the patient voids voluntarily.
2 Capacity large, highly compliant, with no contraction on voluntary effort and reduced sensation: the denervated or overstretched bladder. **3** Capacity small, low but constant compliance: the physically indistensible bladder. **4** Capacity small because of increased sensitivity, compliant, no involuntary contraction: the inflamed or idiopathically hypersensitive bladder. **5** Capacity normal or a little reduced, compliance normal, abnormal contractions provoked by coughing and physical activity. **6** Capacity normal or a little reduced, compliance normal, contractions appear spontaneously. **7** Capacity reduced, compliance reduced progressively as capacity increases, contractions appear spontaneously but relaxation occurs. This usually indicates a hypertrophic bladder. **8** Capacity very reduced, compliance difficult to assess as the bladder contracts spontaneously at low volume and only relaxes slightly, maintaining a high pressure.

bladder can be recognized easily though it is one of the failings of urodynamic analysis that the patient who is profoundly inhibited by the circumstance of the test may find it impossible to initiate a detrusor

contraction though the bladder may be absolutely normal. Deficient contraction is rather more subjective and depends upon the uroflow analysis and decompensation of the detrusor is judged by measurement of post-micturitional residual urine.

Pharmacological tests

An extension of cystometric urodynamic techniques is to differentiate acontractility due to detrusor failure from that due to denervation or decentralization. Lapides reported a test for peripheral denervation of the bladder based upon Cannon's law that a denervated structure becomes supersensitive to its neurohumoral transmitter (Lapides *et al.*, 1962). This test is thus useful to determine in those cases where the bladder is acontractile, whether this is due to nerve injury. The Glahn modification of the test (Glahn, 1970) is the simplest to perform. The bladder is filled after cystometry to a volume of 100 ml and the pressure within it monitored continuously. A subcutaneous injection of bethanechol 2.5 mg is given and if a pressure rise is recorded in the bladder over the subsequent 20 min of more than 15 cmH$_2$O, the test is positive. Others have used prostaglandin as an alternative provocation for this response in neuropathic cases (Kondo *et al.*, 1980).

False positive results have been attributed to cystitis, emotional stress and rapid diuresis during the monitoring period, and false negative results to myogenic failure, poor absorption of bethanechol, and a delay in conversion of the denervated bladder until some 6 months after the neurological insult. Accepting these limitations, the test is most useful in differentiating neuropathic from non-neuropathic causes of the non-contractile detrusor.

Urethral pressure profilometry – urostatics

This technique depends upon the principle that if a side-holed catheter is perfused at a constant yet slow rate, the pressure required to maintain the fluid flow will vary depending upon the wall pressure of the urethra upon the side holes. Thus if the catheter is withdrawn slowly from bladder to external meatus, a profile of pressure can be drawn on an X–Y plotter (Fig. 25.8).

Urethral pressure profiles in isolation can give only the broadest indication of abnormal ureth-

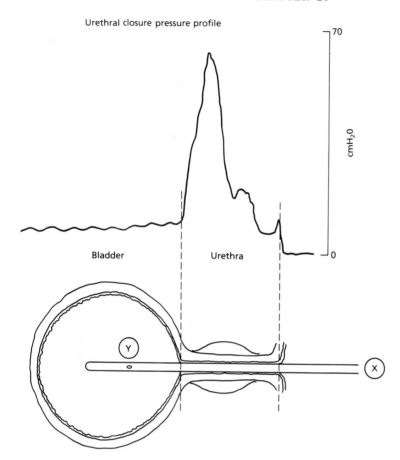

Urethral closure pressure profile

Bladder   Urethra

cmH₂0

Fig. 25.8 Urethral closure pressure profile and a diagram of the recording catheter. At ⊗ is situated the pressure transducer and the constant perfusion pump. Perfusion may be with water (2 ml/min) or carbon dioxide (130 ml/min). The perfusate escapes through small holes at Ⓨ, which is the point from which the pressure is recorded as the catheter is slowly withdrawn down the urethra.

ral function and as such are relatively uninformative. The test can be useful in three circumstances. Firstly, sequential profiles can be drawn over time to identify changes in urethral pressure resistance. This is crucial in cases of vesico-urethral neuropathy where midline neuropathic urethral obstruction may have a devastating effect upon the urinary tract. Secondly, by using pharmacological blocking agents, it is possible to determine which element of the urethral sphincteric mechanism behaves abnormally. Specifically, use of an α-adrenoreceptor blocker can demonstrate the phenomenon of isolated distal sphincter obstruction. In this condition, there is abnormal activity of the intrinsic urethral muscle innervated by the sympathetic nervous system. This phenomenon is found in conus and cauda equina neuropathy. In cases of higher lesions, the contribution of the α-adrenergically innervated

intrinsic urethral muscle within a dyssynergic sphincter can be identified. Finally, using a modified technique of *voiding urethral pressure profilometry* (Desmond & Ramayya, 1988), a baseline profile is drawn to allow accurate localization of the bladder neck and the urethral sphincter. These are marked by cursor on an oscilloscope. A second profile is then drawn whilst the patient is micturating and this is compared to the pressure constantly recorded in the bladder. Where the two pressure curves separate indicates the site of obstruction within the lower urinary tract. This test can thus distinguish whether obstruction in a neuropathic case is at the bladder neck or at the level of the distal urethral mechanism. This distinction can otherwise prove to be difficult when only video-cystography is used.

Urethral pressure has been measured directly

by micro-transducers mounted on a catheter and placed at the pressure active area of the urethra (Bary *et al.*, 1982). Urethral activity is thus monitored during voiding and a dynamic assessment of urethral function made.

Electromyography

Direct recording of the EMG activity within the urethral mechanism is difficult (Blaivas *et al.*, 1977) but has been reported to be useful. A bipolar needle is inserted directly into the periurethral area and specific patterns of EMG potentials are recognized.

It has been rather more common for electromyograms to be recorded either by anal plug electrodes, skin electrodes, or needle electrodes inserted into the levator ani muscle. Patterns of abnormal activity can be seen in those cases with a dyssynergic pelvic floor which produces urethral obstruction. In practical terms EMG recordings have rarely added significantly to urodynamic data but are a useful adjunct to pressure flow tests.

Sacral evoked potentials

A useful application of electromyographic technique is direct recording of the conus reflexes (Rockswold & Bradley, 1977; Galloway *et al.*, 1985). The nerve transmission time between the urethral sphincter, the anal sphincter and the dorsal nerve of the penis (or clitoris) is measured. Multiple stimuli are given to ascertain the sensory threshold, and multiple recordings are analysed by an electronic averager. A single evoked potential for each of the reflexes can then be drawn and the reflex latency measured. Normal values are available for comparison with those recorded in neuropathic cases.

The technique is little more than an electrophysiological analysis of the bulbocavernosus (Siroky *et al.*, 1979) and anal reflexes but its strength is that it allows a degree of objectivity in the assessment of neurological injury. In overt neuropathic cases it adds little to essential data relating to the urinary tract (Lucas & Thomas, 1989) but in cases of subtle or even perhaps disputed neuropathy recording of sacral evoked potentials can be of critical importance (Fidas *et al.*, 1989). This would certainly apply to cases of vesico-urethral neuropathy, but it also can be of crucial importance in those cases of mild to moderate spinal trauma with little overt evidence of neuropathy who, for example, subsequently complain of impotence, or of an otherwise inexplicable alteration in bladder function.

Classification of the neuropathic bladder

The classification of the neuropathic bladder has been bedevilled by complexity and confusion between the neurological condition and classification of bladder function when the two may not be the same. It is thus important to use terms capable of definition, and to distinguish clearly between the neurological lesion and its level and the functional urodynamic diagnosis.

Classification of the neurological condition

The options are outlined in Table 25.3. In all cases it is necessary to quote the neurological level and anatomical position of the lesion remembering the relationship between the vertebral bodies and the corresponding neurological segments and nerve roots. This may influence the effects of interaction of sympathetic, parasympathetic and somatic systems.

A clear demonstration of the sensory level and testing of the conus reflexes will indicate the level of the neurological deficit, and allow some anticipation of the type of bladder dysfunction which is to be expected. Bors & Comarr (1971) classified neurological lesions as either upper or lower motor

Table 25.3 Classification of the neurological condition

	Complete	Incomplete
Lower motoneuron lesion		
Sensory		
Motor		
Upper motoneuron lesion		
Sensory		
Motor		
Mixed lesions		
Sensory		
Motor		

neuron lesions in respect of the anatomical relationship of the injury to the sacral cord reflex centres. An upper motor neuron lesion involved disruption of the descending pathways to the bladder and somatic pathways to the lower extremities. Suprasacral spinal cord lesions would thus be expected to result in reflex spasticity of the bladder and the lower extremities. This has been described as a 'reflex' or 'automatic' bladder, but these terms are better abandoned because of the confusion which results from their use, particularly with the 'autonomous' bladder, a term also to be abandoned, used to describe a lower motor neuron lesion involving pre- and post-ganglionic fibres to the bladder. In these cases the somatic nerves to the lower extremities are involved and this would be expected to produce vesical and lower extremities flaccidity. A 'mixed lesion' group accounts for the exceptions: lower extremity spasticity with an acontractile bladder, and normal or flaccid lower extremities with a hypercontractile bladder. The neurological classification can thus be summarized into broadly three groups: *suprasacral; sacral* and *mixed* lesions.

Unfortunately, neurological examination alone is insufficient to classify bladder behaviour, particularly if the lesion is in the T10 to L2 area. The urological presentation may vary depending upon the involvement of the micturition centre or segments immediately above this level. This may lead to a mixed neurological presentation secondary to direct injury to the sacral cord or by descending cord infarction. It is indeed possible to see absence of conus reflexes and acontractility of the bladder with a cord lesion as high as T6 which would normally be associated with a suprasacral type of bladder dysfunction. This is due to vascular injury to the cord below the level of the lesion.

Classification by symptoms

This is the least accurate way of representing function, but is very important if the patient's problem is to be viewed in perspective.

Functional classification

The aim of diagnosis is to bring together the clinical features and the results of investigations to provide a rational basis for management. The urodynamic patterns in vesico-urethral neuropathy which determine treatment can pragmatically be categorized into relatively simple groups, and they occur whether the neurological lesion is complete or partial and whether it is congenital or acquired.

The phenomena are: whether the detrusor exhibits contractility; whether that contractility satisfactorily opens the bladder neck; and whether urethral resistance to flow, be that by intermittent discoordinated pelvic floor contractions or by a similar unwanted intrinsic urethral muscular contraction, exceeds the contractile force of the detrusor; and finally whether the outflow resistance is incompetent.

In lower motor neuron lesions with a 'sacral' bladder, the expulsive force is provided by abdominal straining and inappropriate urethral resistance results from contraction of intrinsic urethral muscle, whereas in higher lesions, the detrusor will usually, if not always, regain uninhibited contractility whilst urethral resistance is a combination of striated and intrinsic muscular contraction which is out of synchrony with the detrusor contraction.

Therefore the *neuropathic urethra* is the critical element which merits specific consideration. If the expulsive force is sufficient, the resistance in the urethra is the crucial and fundamental factor (Gibbon *et al.*, 1980; Mundy *et al.*, 1985) in vesico-urethral neuropathy.

Management of the neuropathic bladder

The objectives and aims of management must be to minimize the social and medical consequences of disordered bladder function. With these aims in mind the urological management may best be conducted in a unit coordinating this aspect of care with that of the patient as a whole. A suggested scheme of management is outlined in Fig. 25.9.

General and social factors

The mental state, mobility and dexterity of the patient have a profound influence on management. Are they well motivated? Can the patient manage an appliance? Would they be continent if more mobile and able to reach the toilet? Will they cooperate with follow-up or take medication reliably?

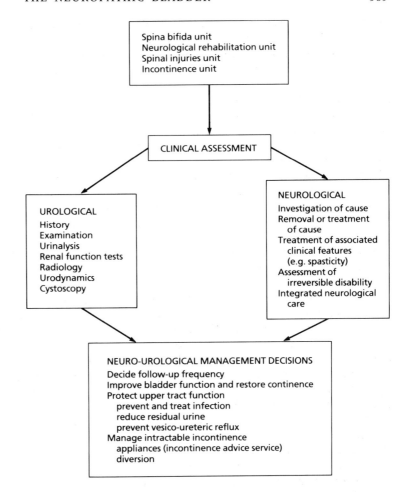

Fig. 25.9 Management of
neuropathic bladder dysfunction.

Such factors modify the approach to the patient to such a great extent that it is appropriate that they should be considered first.

Much of the management of vesico-urethral neuropathy has evolved from the treatment of spinal cord injury patients and these cases do pose rather specific problems for which a system of care has been worked out, even though the mechanisms of abnormal bladder function now seem more complex than had previously been supposed.

In these cases, satisfactory micturition differs from that in neurologically intact individuals because the emphasis shifts from a function which has to be socially acceptable, to that which is mandatory for preservation of the upper urinary tracts and avoidance of urinary infection.

There is no doubt that the attention paid to the urinary tract has improved that survival of spinal cord injured patients, by the prevention of urosepsis. This gratifying change in the mortality has been carefully recorded over the last 30 years. In 1961 it was found to be around 50% (Breithaupt *et al.*, 1961); by 1968 it had dropped to 36% (Jousse *et al.*, 1968) and yet a further drop was found in 1973 (Geisler *et al.*, 1977). The marked decrease in renal deaths continued when in 1983 it stood at 15.3% (Geisler *et al.*, 1983).

The concurrent advent of renal replacement therapy, which is available to spinal cord injured patients, will have had a significant effect on mortality figures, but none the less careful urological management has had a substantial impact to the

Table 25.4 Incidence of neuropathic bladder disorders

Abdomino-perineal resection	10 (44%)
Radical hysterectomy	7 (80%)
Polio (almost always recovers)	4 (42%)
Diabetic neuropathy	2 (83%)
Lumbar disc disease	6 (18%)
Multiple sclerosis	
Presenting symptom	2 (12%)
Overall incidence	33 (78%)
Parkinsonism	37 (70%)
Stroke	34 (53%)
Meningomyelocele	(97%)

point where in the nineties, renal compromise is a rarity, possibly no more prevalent than 1% of cases and certainly not the common cause of death that it once was.

Recent developments have allowed a further dimension to be added to the management of the neuropathic bladder. Whereas previously continence might have been sacrificed for the preservation of renal function and urinary sterility, the current aim of treatment should always include consideration of techniques which preserve or restore continence, providing that they neither

provoke infection nor put the upper urinary tracts in jeopardy.

The incidence of neuropathic bladder disorders in neurological disease is high. The exact incidence, however, seems very variably reported and is summarized in Table 25.4.

Management of long-term vesico-urethral neuropathy

There are in simple terms four particular areas of abnormality of vesico-urethral function produced by chronic neuropathy which may or may not co-exist and to which treatment must be addressed (Fig. 25.10). The functional classification of the neuropathic bladder is based upon them, and this can be correlated to the level of neurological lesion. The *bladder* may be: (i) hyperactive – producing high pressures, or (ii) hypoactive – at low pressure and acontractile; and the *urethra* or *outlet* may be: (iii) hyperactive – increasing outlet resistance, or (iv) hypoactive – reducing the resistance.

Clearly, the diagnosis of these abnormalities can only be made by a careful urodynamic assessment and, bearing in mind the delicate balance that

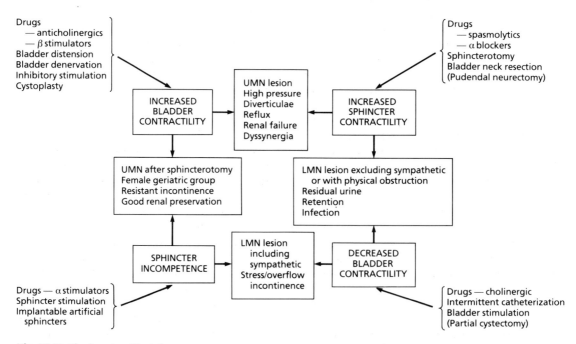

Fig. 25.10 The functional basis for treatment.

pertains between the detrusor and the outflow in neuropathic states and indeed the potential for any subtle change in the neurological condition profoundly to upset this balance, urodynamic assessments should be repeated regularly.

Management should be in relation to three areas: that designed to improve bladder and urethral function; that designed to prevent complications and especially to protect renal function; and that to palliate incontinence if it is inevitable.

Substantial disturbance in function can occur before the bladder fails in its purpose of storage and voiding. Investigation must indicate therefore whether the bladder still functions acceptably in this respect. The parameters that must be subserved are that the urine should remain uninfected and the upper tracts undilated. Whether a residual urine is 'acceptable' is a moot point and is determined by the previous two absolute prerequisites.

Improvement of bladder function

Bladder hyperactivity

The failure of the normal storage function of the bladder usually occurs because of increased phasic or tonic contractility. This reduces bladder capacity and produces either a high intra-vesical pressure or urinary leakage, or both depending on the function of the outflow tract. When bladder hypercontractility is associated with a hyperactive obstructive sphincter which contracts dyssynergically with the detrusor, the bladder wall will hypertrophy and become trabeculated. This hypertrophy affects particularly the bladder neck, sometimes to the extent of producing a secondary obstructive element. As the bladder pressure increases and the detrusor fails, diverticula and ureteric reflux develop and the residual urine increases. Muscle hypertrophy makes the bladder wall physically less distensible, a phenomenon exacerbated by fibrosis produced by chronic infection.

Overactivity of the bladder can be controlled or modified either pharmacologically or by surgical intervention.

The concept of using drugs to control neuropathic vesico-urethral dysfunction is not new but new pharmacological agents that are now available broaden the treatment options. These agents have specific target sites and a combination of therapeutic modalities may be necessary in order to achieve the desired effect.

Drugs which inhibit detrusor activity

These agents can be used to reduce unwanted detrusor pressure, increase capacity, or inhibit uninhibited reflex activity. Pure anticholinergic agents can be subdivided into: (i) belladonna alkaloids (tincture of belladonna); (ii) quaternary ammonium derivatives of the belladonna alkaloids (methscopolamine bromide); and (iii) synthetic substitutes (propantheline, methantheline and emepronium bromide). They all block the effect of acetylcholine at postganglionic cholinergic nerve endings yet have to be given in relatively high doses for a significant effect to be recorded and at a level at which side-effects are often noticed.

Anticholinergic/antispasmodic agents are perhaps better suited to control uninhibited detrusor contractions (Vinson & Diokno, 1976), of which oxybutynin hydrochloride, now available on prescription in the United Kingdom, and dicyclomine chloride are both antimuscarinic and have an additional direct effect on the detrusor smooth muscle membrane.

All the anticholinergic agents have similar side-effects, of which a dry mouth and blurred vision are the commonest. Not all the 'bladder relaxants' work equally well but in practice oxybutynin seems to have the greatest beneficial effect.

Surgical inhibition of detrusor contractility

In those cases where the detrusor is shown urodynamically to be uninhibited and hyperreflexic, a procedure to inhibit the contractility might be considered. Ablation of the vesical pelvic nerves is an attractive option and pudendal neurectomy, sacral rhizotomy, intrathecal phenol injection or conectomy have all been advocated and should be considered particularly when the exaggerated bladder activity is associated with peripheral mass somatic spasms. In the male, impotence is invariably produced by these operations. A more peripheral denervation, or more correctly decentralization procedure, has been tried and transvaginal neurotomy seems excellent in controlling idiopathic detrusor instability in women, but strangely proves to be ineffective in neuropathic cases. Similarly, transtrigonal injection of phenol should produce a satisfactory neurotomy in neuropathic cases but fails to do so, except in demyelinating disease (Ewing *et al.*, 1983). Bladder transection (Gibbon, 1973), which is a procedure designed to reduce detrusor contractility in neurologically intact patients, also seems ineffective in neuropathic cases.

A less destructive and physiologically much more attractive option is the use of inhibitory perineal stimulation. Inhibition of bladder contraction has been noted following anal distension and electrical stimulation of the anal canal (Kock & Pompeius, 1963) and the vagina (Fall, 1977). Fall has worked out the optimal parameters for electrical stimulation and reports (Fall, 1979, personal communication) that the majority of his patients were cured or greatly improved by this technique, though benefit sometimes appeared only after several weeks. Others have confirmed this work (Godec *et al.*, 1976). A recent report (Ohlsson *et al.*, 1989) reiterated the technique and found it to be beneficial in patients with idiopathic detrusor overactivity, yet the method has not gained popularity and is rarely, if ever, used in clinical practice.

Interpositional cystoplasty is perhaps the most effective operation to increase bladder capacity and to reduce contractility. A segment of ileum, isolated upon its mesentery, is laid into the bladder opened coronally, in the 'Clam' operation (Bramble, 1982, 1990) or sagittally. The very presence of the bowel segment increases bladder capacity, but has the added benefit of preventing transmission of a contractile wave from bladder base to fundus, whilst presenting also a barrier to potential reinnervation.

This procedure is particularly effective in increasing compliance in the congenital neuropathic bladder seen in patients with meningomyelocele (Parry *et al.*, 1990). It is important to ensure that in any neuropathic vesico-urethral dysfunction, the intrinsic bladder pressure is not elevated for prolonged periods for this will adversely affect the upper urinary tracts. Long-term follow-up in neuropathic cases showed that continence was maintained in 93% of cases (Fenn *et al.*, 1992). Interpositional cystoplasty can be used in combination with a procedure to increase outflow resistance (see later) in those cases who are able thereafter to catheterize intermittently (Rickwood *et al.*, 1982; McRae *et al.*, 1987). Interestingly, however, it is unusual if not exceptional for this type of combined procedure ever to be needed in spinal injured patients, which is perhaps a reflection that the growing, decentralized bladder exhibits different visco-elastic properties than does the normal bladder deprived acutely of its innervation.

Bladder hypoactivity

Decreased contractility may be consequent upon denervation or over-distension, or more often both. Because the parasympathetic motoneurons are located peripherally near the bladder, true denervation almost never occurs. The interruption of preganglionic parasympathetic fibres could more properly be termed a decentralization. This explains why the bladder retains intrinsic contractility after lesions of the cauda equina or pelvic nerves though the tone and feeble uncoordinated contractions seldom are able to empty the bladder largely due to sustained urethral resistance as a result of urethral 'denervation' or decentralization supersensitivity (Gibbon, 1980). This phenomenon also applies to the detrusor devoid of its central nervous connections and the supersensitivity (Lapides *et al.*, 1962; Glahn, 1970) does mean that drugs have a better chance of working.

It is possible that efficient bladder emptying may be achieved even in the acute stage by Crede expression of the bladder. This will only apply to those male patients who have previously had a prostatectomy and in whom the urethral outflow resistance is solely constituted by muscle activity in the region of the external urethral sphincter. This resistance inevitably is reduced in acute spinal injury allowing, when appropriate, Crede expression of the bladder to be used. In all other cases the bladder neck closure mechanism precludes Crede expression as a treatment option.

Drugs that enhance detrusor activity

Cholinergic agents may improve bladder emptying by increasing the efficiency of detrusor contractility;

indeed parasympatheticomimetics are only likely to increase contractility of *neuropathic* muscle because unless smooth muscle is deprived of its innervation it will not respond to pharmacological stimulation and this is the basis of the pharmacological tests for denervation or decentralization. It is an interesting speculation that the effect of this group of drugs in neurologically intact patients is mediated only through the parasympathetic sensory system. If cholinergic stimulants are to be used where detrusor dyssynergia is present then some method of reducing sphincteric activity must also be employed for potentially they might increase urethral resistance in addition to increasing detrusor contraction.

Bethanechol hydrochloride is a choline ester that acts directly on the effector cells and probably is the most potent cholinergic agent available.

Distigmine bromide is an anticholinesterase that relies upon enhancement of endogenous acetylcholine to exert its effect.

Recent reports of the use of prostaglandin F2α in patients with neuropathic bladder dysfunction have shown that the drug given intravesically produces contractions that can induce voiding in patients with suprasacral lesions but not in patients with complete denervation, detrusor-sphincter dyssynergia or spinal shock (Vaidyanathan *et al.*, 1981).

Detrusor stimulation/urethral relaxation

A logical method of provoking micturition in patients with vesico-urethral neuropathy would be artificially to stimulate the bladder. Direct stimulation by electrodes implanted into the bladder wall was first reported in 1964 (Boyce *et al.*, 1964) and several others tried the technique, which failed, however, to gain clinical acceptance. Movement often led to fractured cables; infection was common; electrodes tended to erode into the bladder; and current spread led to pain and stimulation of the outlet resistance during voiding.

As an alternative, nerve stimulation techniques have been developed, designed to provoke detrusor contraction. Conus medullaris electrodes positioned in the intermedio-lateral grey columns of the cord at S1 or lower have produced successful long-term results in three of five paraplegics (Nashold *et al.*, 1972).

The sacral anterior root stimulator

The most efficient electrostimulation of micturition in patients with complete spinal cord section and neuropathic bladder dysfunction has been by the sacral anterior root stimulator popularized by Brindley (Brindley, 1973, 1977).

Stimulation of the S2, S3 or S4 anterior root causes contraction of the pelvic floor producing unwanted outflow resistance. To overcome this, intermittent bursts of stimulation are used whereby the detrusor and pelvic floor initially contract in unison. When stimulation ceases, pelvic floor relaxation is instantaneous whereas the detrusor pressure decays much more slowly such that during this period of pressure differential, post-stimulation voiding occurs. Thus good bladder emptying is achieved whilst continence is often maintained.

Surgical technique. An intradural approach via laminectomy is required. The anterior roots of S2, S3 and S4 are identified on each side in the cauda equina and the function of each is ratified by electrical stimulation monitoring bladder, rectal and pelvic floor activity. The anterior is separated from the posterior root and each is laid within the stimulator booklet. From it, cables are led subcutaneously to a radio receiver buried in the subcutaneous tissues of the antero-lateral chest wall. Within the buried receiver there are three radio receivers of differing frequency tunings, one for each pair of nerve roots.

Following operation when voiding is required, a small triradiate transmitter is placed over the receiver so that its three coils correspond to those that stimulate the nerve roots. The transmitter can then be tuned to stimulate whichever nerve root has been shown predominantly to effect micturition. It can also be used to stimulate erection, largely a function of the S2 root, or assist bowel emptying by S4 root stimulation.

In order to abolish uninhibited detrusor contraction, the posterior roots of S3 and S4 are divided. This has the advantage of increasing functional bladder capacity and enhancing continence, and will also abolish pain associated with electromicturition (MacDonagh *et al.*, 1990).

The advantage of this type of implanted device is

that satisfactory micturition can be achieved with reasonable continence and no need for an external collecting device. The incidence of urinary infection is reduced because residual urine is reduced to virtually nil, and the self image and dignity of the patient is greatly enhanced.

Other options

Partial resection of the bladder should be mentioned if only to be dismissed. For some time large atonic bladders have been electively reduced in size by excision or infolding of part of the bladder wall. The object, in theory, was to make the remaining muscle more efficient in its action. Though the muscle may work more effectively for a short while, sooner or later further bladder distension occurs and the situation reverts to its previous state.

Despite all that has been written above, many patients with inadequate detrusor contraction require no intervention. Voiding may be facilitated by raising intra-abdominal pressure, with or without manual compression. In any case the presence of an uninfected residual urine does not make treatment obligatory, though close observation must be maintained.

Hyperactive urethra (high outflow resistance)

The neuropathic urethra produces a dynamic obstruction implying phasic or tonic hypercontractility of the sphincteric apparatus which can be treated either pharmacologically or by surgery.

Drugs that reduce outlet resistance

Outlet resistance in vesico-urethral neuropathy is composed of a striated and an intrinsic muscular element.

Skeletal muscle relaxants can therefore be utilized and are grouped according to the site of action. Centrally acting *benzodiazepines*, either diazepam or baclofen, have both been shown to enhance bladder emptying by reducing outlet resistance (Leyson *et al.*, 1980) whereas *dantrolene* can produce a similar effect by a direct action on skeletal muscle (Pedersen *et al.*, 1978).

Intrinsic urethral muscle can be relaxed by α-adrenolytic agents and of all the pharmacological manipulations this is probably the most reliably effective. *Phenoxybenzamine* was the first used and was shown to be effective alone in reducing residual urine (Krane & Olsson, 1973), or in combination with cholinergic agents (Khanna, 1976). Unfortunately, subsequent studies have shown a tiny carcinogenic potential of this agent in mice and thus its use has been curtailed, but other α-blocking agents *prazosin* and *indoramin* have more specific α-receptor blocking effect and do not block presynaptic receptors so they are more specific to urethral responses (Anderson *et al.*, 1981) and produce less cardiovascular side-effects.

Surgical relief of midline outflow obstruction

Suprasacral lesions

Detrusor contractility in these cases is usually regained in an uninhibited and hyperreflexic fashion. Urine is thus only retained within the bladder if the midline outflow resistance exceeds the intravesical pressure. This midline resistance is exerted at the level of the bladder neck, at the level of the membranous urethra, or both. Bladder neck closure may be maintained despite a powerful detrusor contraction and thus it is important always to determine whether this is the case. The forces that produce the pressure resistance at the level of the membranous urethra comprise intrinsic urethral muscle contractility; dyssynergic pelvic floor striated muscle activity or a combination of the two.

The level of obstruction therefore has to be determined and the contribution of each potential obstructing element assessed so that appropriate surgical correction can be undertaken.

In female patients it is unusual to be able satisfactorily to reduce outflow resistance without provoking incontinence and thus high lesions are probably best treated by long-term catheterization. Similarly, bladder neck resection in the female with an acontractile bladder should rarely be countenanced because of the risk of incontinence (Delaere *et al.*, 1983), but fortunately the option of intermittent catheterization (see later) makes this operation obsolete in these cases.

In males, the treatment options are greater but a fundamental decision must first be taken whether to leave the midline vesico-urethral apparatus untouched and artificially to provoke micturition using a sacral anterior root stimulator (Brindley et al., 1986) or whether to reduce or ablate the midline resistance and produce unobstructed, uninhibited voiding *per urethram* into a condom collecting device.

When the latter is chosen, there are three surgical options: incision or resection of the bladder neck; incision of the distal urethral mechanism (external sphincterotomy); or both.

Bladder neck resection. The correction of bladder outflow obstruction should only be undertaken by surgeons well practised in endoscopic surgical techniques and all the usual prerequisites for this type of surgery are mandatory. Antibacterial prophylaxis should always be used whether or not preoperative urine cultures are positive because patients with vesico-urethral neuropathy who have had any type of instrumentation whatever, at any stage, seem always to have a significantly higher tendency to bacteraemia, endotoxaemia or septicaemia following endoscopic surgery. The patient should be placed in the relaxed lithotomy position which usually means that paralysis under anaesthesia with positive pressure ventilation will be needed. In some circumstances, controlled hypotension can be useful.

Ablation of bladder neck resistance can be either by incision or resection. Bladder neck incision, however, does not seem totally to relieve obstruction in neuropathic cases and a formal resection is preferable. Furthermore, though uncommonly seen in patients with chronic neuropathy, prostatic hyperplasia may also be present and any obstructing adenoma needs also to be resected.

A circumferential resection of the bladder neck is unnecessary and will increase the incidence of postoperative bladder neck sclerosis. An anterior mucosal bridge should thus be retained to prevent this tedious complication. The resection should be deep leaving only a thin rim of circumferentially orientated bladder neck fibres without a prominent ridge on which a catheter may catch.

Postoperative catheterization with irrigation, either by a three-way catheter or augmented diuresis, should be used because it is vital that blockage by clots should never occur for this may induce autonomic dysreflexia.

On removal of the catheter, the output from the bladder must be monitored carefully and the residual urine checked, preferably by ultrasound examination. If a satisfactory voiding pattern is not quickly established the catheter should be replaced for a day or two.

Incision of the distal urethral mechanism — external sphincterotomy. This operation is designed to abolish any obstructing element at the level of the distal urethral mechanism whether it is due to overactivity of the intrinsic urethral muscle, or due to a hyperreflexic striated pelvic floor, or both. Antibacterial prophylaxis is mandatory, and the patient should be crossmatched for a blood transfusion because the site at which the operation is done is exceptionally vascular and replacement of blood may be necessary. As with bladder neck surgery this operation is not for the occasional operator.

The 'external urethral sphincter' presents itself to the endoscopic operator as a circular ring below the level of the prostatic verumontanum. Incision of it, therefore, can be single or multiple, and in various anatomical orientations. If a single incision is to be used it is preferable not to orientate it posteriorly or posterolaterally for this seems to encourage restoration of sphincteric activity perhaps by encouraging early healing of the disrupted muscular ring. Incision at the midline, 12 o'clock position avoids this complication (Madersbacher & Scott, 1976; Whitmore et al., 1978).

Posterobilateral incisions are effective in totally abolishing sphincteric activity and relieving obstruction (Gibbon, 1973), but carry the disadvantage that the incisions are precisely at the point where the nerves to the corpora cavernosa traverse the membranous region (Walsh & Donker, 1982) and thus erectile failure is a potential complication. Median sphincterotomy is therefore preferable in the younger male patient.

The surgery is relatively simple but requires accurate and confident identification of endoscopic landmarks. All the muscle layers of the urethra must be divided from a point just above the verumontanum to some 2–3 cm below it. The incision is made with a 'Collins' diathermy electrode in a resectoscope using the cutting current. Care has to be taken not to cut too deeply at the distal end of the incision for at this point the corpus spongiosum of the urethra is close by, and if opened will bleed alarmingly and persistently despite all endoscopic attempts to stop it. The haemorrhage can be arrested relatively easily utilizing tamponade by a large diameter (24Ch) urethral catheter, augmented if needed by compression through the perineum.

The indwelling catheter should be retained for 6–7 days and upon removal strict attention paid to the adequacy of voiding.

Sacral lesions

The first cases of external sphincterotomy were performed on patients with sacral neuropathy and an acontractile detrusor in whom micturition by straining was obstructed within the urethra (Ross *et al.*, 1957). The cause of the obstruction was not realized but subsequently it has been recognized that in these cases the urethral obstruction is due to activity in the intrinsic urethral muscle. Bladder emptying was satisfactory once this obstruction had been dealt with by sphincterotomy.

In adult female patients, and in children, both male and female, with sacral neuropathy, unwanted excess pressure generated by the intrinsic urethral mechanism can be modified by simple urethral overdilatation or urethrotomy (Rickwood, 1982). The physical overdistension disrupts the integrity of the intrinsic urethral spiral muscle fibres and thus reduces the resistance which they impart. If the bladder neck is competent, this will not provoke incontinence, but paradoxically may cure stress-induced leakage from a chronically overdistended bladder in which the bladder neck is constantly pulled open by the excessive volume by allowing complete emptying by abdominal straining.

Other options

Endoscopic resection of the bladder neck or incision of the distal urethral mechanism is designed to reduce the outflow resistance pressure. This can theoretically at least be achieved by stenting the urethra open. Early work has shown that this is a realistic treatment option and a recently introduced 'Wallstent' (AMS Medical, UK Ltd), designed for the treatment of urethral strictures, has been successfully used to maintain an open urethra in vesico-

urethral neuropathy (McInerney *et al.*, 1990; Shaw *et al.*, 1990).

Catheterization

Indwelling urethral catheterization

Whilst acute vesico-urethral neuropathy demands immediate bladder decompression by catheterization this technique of bladder management may also be used in long-term neuropathy. Indeed in high female tetraplegic patients often it is the only treatment option available as it may also be in some wheelchair-bound female invalids.

Fine-diameter catheters should always be used, with a high ratio of internal to external diameter. Thought must be given to the time that the catheter is likely to be in place and if this is to be prolonged, a silicone catheter should be used and can remain *in situ* for up to 2 months. Unfortunately these catheters do not have a particularly large internal diameter, but the diminished reaction which they provoke within the urethra, when compared to latex catheters, provides a great advantage. It is as well to remember that *silicone-coated latex* catheters, produced in an attempt to match the properties of a pure silicone catheter, lose the coating within 24 hours within the urethra negating any advantage which the silicone coating may have (Blacklock, 1986).

The weight of the tubing and the drainage bag must always be supported, especially in females. If attention is not paid to this simple detail, damage by pressure necrosis at the bladder neck in females, progressing ultimately to complete destruction of the whole urethra, will occur. In males, if the catheter and tubing are not supported, a 'bow-string' of the urethra will produce a urethral stricture at the site of maximum pressure against the urethral wall.

It must be accepted that the intravesical foreign body of an indwelling catheter will provoke lower urinary tract infection if present for more than three days or so (O'Flynn, 1974), but antibacterial therapy should be withheld unless systemic effects of the infection become manifest. It is likely, however, that in the acute phase, antibacterials will be administered for other indications.

Long-term catheterization has an important place

in the management of the chronic invalid with urinary incontinence, and there is no doubt that with better catheter materials, better use of appropriate antibacterial therapy where indicated, and better catheter care the incidence of complications can be considerably reduced.

The management of the patient on long-term catheter drainage is not a procedure that can be described on the basis of a standardized regimen. It must be undertaken as a trial on an individual basis, and the frequency of catheter change adapted to suit the individual patient.

Leakage around a catheter is a major problem with patients who have a small capacity or hyperactive bladder. This may be aggravated by constipation and can be helped by the judicious use of enemata to evacuate the distal colon and rectum. A familiar mistake in such cases is the use of a progressively larger catheter, so that the urethra becomes grossly dilated and patulous, and this should be avoided. Furthermore, the quantity of fluid used to fill the retaining balloon should initially be kept low, to avoid the bladder trying to expel by contraction the foreign body within it. Bladder contraction in this circumstance can be controlled by oxybutynin therapy or, if severe, the contraction can be abolished by subtrigonal phenol injections. This technique is particularly effective in patients with multiple sclerosis.

Intermittent catheterization

It is relatively easy to implement intermittent catheterization in patients with lesions at, or below, T12 even in acute spinal injury. The benefit of this method of drainage was realized when it was appreciated that urinary infection was rendered less likely when the bladder was drained regularly and completely (Guttman & Frankel, 1966), in the absence of an indwelling foreign body. Furthermore, it was realized that when these prerequisites were met, it was unnecessary always to use a sterile catheter passed under aseptic conditions but that a *clean intermittent self-catheterizing* (*CISC*) technique could be adopted (Lapides et al., 1972). In patients with higher lesions the technique may still be used but will involve organizational problems as these patients are unable to catheterize themselves. As the spinal cord injury evolves, these patients de-

velop peculiar urinary output patterns which make it more difficult to adhere to a rigid timed schedule of catheterization.

The technique, though simple in concept, has to be carefully taught and practised with great diligence. Once adopted there can be no respite, for the bladder must be emptied regularly with adjustment of the schedule to prevent volumes in excess of 600 ml. In tetraplegics typically the urinary output is small during the day when the patient is upright in a chair, and the interval between catheterization can be increased, but on assumption of the supine position a diuresis occurs which may require hourly catheterization.

It is perfectly practical to continue intermittent catheterization indefinitely in many patients (Herr, 1975; McGuire & Brady, 1979). However, with recovery of reflex activity as spinal shock recedes, both sphincteric and bladder pressure increase in virtually all patients with spinal cord or spinal root lesions. Urodynamic assessment should therefore be undertaken to answer the simple question whether urine is stored to those volumes recorded at catheterization at low pressure. Absolute pressure values are relatively arbitrary but should be less than 20 cmH$_2$O. If so, intermittent catheterization can be continued. If not, some means of decreasing intravesical pressure is needed. In those cases with detrusor areflexia an important observation is the pressure at which leakage occurs. This leak point pressure is governed by the urethral resistance, which will need to be reduced if the leak point pressure is high. In practice, in patients with sacral spinal cord, or root lesions, the intravesical pressure only rises as high as the urethral resistance will allow.

The same principles of pressure relationships govern the adequacy of intermittent catheterization in patients with suprasacral lesions. In these cases reflex vesical activity returns and this is frequently associated with discoordinate urethral activity producing 'detrusor–sphincter dyssynergia'. In this circumstance it is necessary to reduce detrusor activity by medication, then to judge the safety of intermittent catheterization by assessing the peaks of intravesical pressure urodynamically to ensure that they remain within the safety limits. Ingenious devices have been designed to assist intermittent catheterization in female wheelchair-bound patients who otherwise would find the practice difficult (Hunt & Whitaker, 1990).

Suprapubic catheterization

Suprapubic catheterization might appear a logical solution to the acutely paralysed bladder because it will leave the urethra uninstrumented and theoretically uncontaminated. However, it requires skill to perform and carries with it a certain morbidity. The colon and peritoneum are both vulnerable to perforation, yet serious damage fortunately is rare.

Frustratingly, a suprapubic tube may not always keeps the bladder entirely empty and as a result some small quantity of urethral leakage may occur. Finally, theoretically at least, the tract may re-open if, once voiding is re-established, the bladder develops outflow obstruction as it may potentially do in a spinal injured patient.

Urethral incompetence

A totally inadequate urethra is relatively less common in neurological disease though sadly is all too common as a result of treatment by catheterization in female patients.

Drugs that increase urethral resistance

Urethral intrinsic muscular tone can be increased by α-adrenergic stimulants of which two are commonly prescribed for this purpose, but both are contraindicated in patients with hypertension and thus should be avoided in cases where autonomic dysreflexia is a possibility.

Ephedrine has both α- and β-adrenoreceptor stimulating properties. In addition to a direct effect on receptors it has the ability to release noradrenaline from storage sites in the sympathetic nerves. The primary use is to control sphincter weakness incontinence, and in mild to moderately severe cases this can be achieved in perhaps 73% (Diokno & Taub, 1975).

Phenylpropanolamine hydrochloride has similar pharmacological effects to ephedrine yet causes less central stimulant effect (Awad *et al.*, 1978). These two agents are often found in proprietary cold cures and are worth using particularly in patients

with a neuropathic bladder secondary to spina bifida where the outlet is paralysed yet some reasonable expulsive force can be generated.

Theoretically at least, β-adrenoreceptor blockers should increase urethral intrinsic muscle tone and thus increase urethral outflow resistance. In practice, however, this proves not to be the case, and in any event the cardiovascular side-effect militates against their use (Khanna, 1976).

Surgical restoration of urethral resistance

Loss of support of the pelvic floor which will allow transmitted abdominal pressure to be deflected away from the urethra may in time render the closure mechanism in the urethra incompetent and stress-induced leakage of urine will occur. This is particularly prevalent in congenital neuropathy, and in this circumstance may be associated with persistence of detrusor contractility. In these cases it is necessary to reduce detrusor pressure prior to restoring urethral resistance.

In females, surgical repositioning of the bladder neck and proximal urethra to ensure that the compressive influence of abdominal pressure is maintained, can be achieved by an open suprapubic colposuspension operation. A simple 'Stamey' endoscopic needle suspension is an attractive alternative which achieves a similar elevation of the bladder neck and can be used in neuropathic cases (Lawrence & Thomas, 1987; Kato *et al.*, 1987).

A sophisticated and useful option to restore urethra competence and thus produce continence is by implantation of an artificial urinary sphincter (AUS; AMS Medical, UK Ltd). This device works by utilizing a compressive cuff implanted around either the bladder neck or the bulbar urethra, inflation of which is maintained at all times by connection to a pressure regulating reservoir, implanted suprapubically, and thus under the influence of abdominal pressure. Micturition can occur by deflation of the cuff by activating a small pump implanted in the scrotum in males and the labia in females. This allows fluid to be pumped out of the cuff and into the reservoir. Some 90 seconds later, the valvular mechanism automatically reverses, returning fluid from the reservoir to re-inflate the cuff. It is important always to be sure that detrusor pressure is never consistently elevated when an obstructing

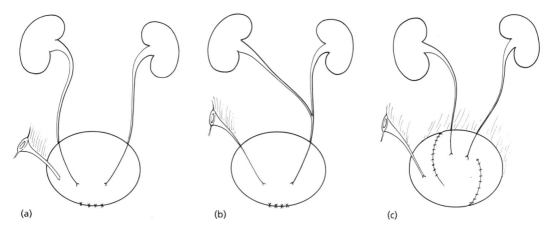

Fig. 25.11 (a) Mitrofanoff(1). Orthotopic low pressure bladder is used as the reservoir. The bladder neck is closed. 'Reversed' appendix as the catheterizable continent channel. (b) Mitrofanoff(2). Orthotopic low pressure bladder is used as the reservoir. The bladder neck is closed. Transuretero-ureterostomy. Distal ureteric continent catheterizable stoma. (c) Mitrofanoff(3). Ileocaecal pouch reservoir. Non-refluxing ureters. Appendix catheterizable continent stoma.

mechanism such as this is employed (Murray *et al.*, 1988).

The predominant use of the AUS in neuropathic incontinence is in cases of meningomyelocele where a prior sphincterotomy to abolish any dyssynergic urethral sphincteric activity may be needed, together with an interpositional cystoplasty if compliance is low (Stephenson & Mundy, 1985). Clean intermittent catheterization is used in those patients unable to empty the paralysed bladder by straining.

Cutaneous urinary diversion

Despite the application of a multitude of procedures designed to correct neuropathic vesico-urethral dysfunction occasionally it is necessary to divert the urine to the skin when all else fails. A classic ileal diversion can be performed remembering that the purpose of the procedure is to transmit urine to the collecting bag as efficiently and quickly as possible. The procedure therefore in no way is meant to construct an 'ileal bladder'.

Newer methods of urinary diversion, however, do set out to achieve just this aim by construction of an intra-abdominal urinary pouch which can be emptied by catheterization of a narrow tubed access pipe so that the diversion is continent. The principle of the surgery was first proposed by

Mitrofanoff (1980) who suggested that the atonic orthotopic bladder in which the bladder neck has been surgically closed should form the pouch. The catheterizable narrow tubed access was formed either by the appendix isolated on its mesentery, inverted with the distal end cut off, and implanted into the bladder by a non-refluxing submucosal tunnel with the caecal end brought to the skin as a catheterizable stoma, or, alternatively, a ureter transected and anastomosed to its contralateral mate to allow the proximal end of the distal third to be brought to the skin (Fig. 25.11a, b). The Mitrofanoff techniques prove particularly useful in congenital neuropathy due to spina bifida where spinal deformity and confinement to a wheelchair often makes urethral intermittent catheterization impossible. The catheterizable stoma may even be placed in the umbilicus (J.W. Duckett, personal communication) giving a cosmetically excellent result.

Adaptations of the Mitrofanoff principle have been suggested constructing an intra-abdominal pouch of bowel, usually an isolated, detubularized ileocaecal segment, to form the reservoir, and using similar techniques of construction of a catheterizable stoma (Fig. 25.11c).

These techniques are still in their infancy but no doubt will mean a greatly enhanced quality of life for patients who do require a cutaneous urinary diversion, and will be rid of the need for a collecting bag to be stuck to the skin.

Complications of the neuropathic bladder

The upper urinary tracts are always threatened by lower tract dysfunction. By the very nature of the neuropathy, these complications can be entirely asymptomatic and discovered by routine urological follow-up.

Chronic bacterial infection

Chronic bacterial infection is always a potential hazard and thus patients with vesico-urethral neuropathy should have regular bacteriological surveillance. By paralysing ureteric smooth muscle the infected neuropathic urinary tract is prone to upper tract dilatation, and compromised renal function.

Escherichia coli is the most frequent infecting organism, but *Proteus*, *Pseudomonas* and *Klebsiella* organisms are relatively common. There is now a wide range of antimicrobial agents available and it is advisable to choose one with the narrowest appropriate spectrum of activity for the initial treatment. It goes without saying that it is mandatory, wherever possible, to select antibacterial therapy on the basis of bacteriological cultures and to avoid 'blind therapy'. Recurrent relapse of infection is a major problem in which circumstance long-term antibacterial suppression should be considered, or as an alternative, rotating therapy in full doses with perhaps three agents.

When urinary tract infection occurs in the presence of obstruction, the risk of bacteraemia and renal impairment is increased. Any surgical intervention carries with it the risk of provoking bacteraemia and thus should always be covered by appropriate, preferably aminoglycoside, prophylaxis.

Vesico-ureteric reflux

Vesico-ureteric reflux may be transient or permanent and therefore more sinister, especially in the presence of chronic infection. It is commoner in higher lesions, and more prevalent the longer after the neurological lesion.

Reimplantation of a refluxing ureter into a grossly trabeculated neuropathic bladder is beset with difficulties, and it is mandatory before embarking on such surgery to ensure that there is no persistent midline bladder outflow obstruction. Nipple valve reimplantations are best avoided, because as the bladder distends the nipple is distracted and loses its anti-refluxing properties. Perhaps the easiest solution to the problem of vesico-ureteric reflux in a neuropathic bladder will be the use of submucosal teflon injected into the orifice (Puri & O'Donnell, 1984, 1987). This relatively simple technique is effective in correcting reflux without the risk of ureteric obstruction or the need for an open operation, and if unsuccessful at the first attempt may readily be repeated (Dewan & Guiney, 1990).

Intramural ureteric obstruction

Intramural ureteric obstruction may occur as the ureter passes through a grossly thickened detrusor, and is more likely in those cases with excessive fibrosis of the bladder wall. Scarring of the mucosal orifice itself as a result of chronic infection is a further cause of this type of upper tract obstruction in neuropathic bladder dysfunction. The condition surprisingly can occur rapidly and bilaterally producing acute renal failure and requiring decompression of the upper tracts by percutaneous nephrostomy. Ureteric reimplantation is required in those cases which do not respond to intensive antibacterial therapy after decompression.

Urinary calculi

Urinary calculi are more common in both the upper and lower tracts in neuropathic bladder dysfunction. Approximately 6% of patients with spinal injuries will form upper tract stone compared with 2% of the general population. The genesis of the stones relates to more than just recumbency as a result of the injury for over two-thirds will form after the first two years following injury. Intriguingly, though no correlation exists between the neurological level and the incidence of stones, they are never seen in spinal cord injured patients with a neurological level below L1, yet are depressingly common in congenital neuropathic patients, largely secondary to infection.

With the development of modern urological stone management, all calculi should be treated aggressively (Bush *et al.*, 1984; Brannen *et al.*, 1985; Marberger *et al.*, 1985; Mayo *et al.*, 1985). Modern percutaneous lithotriptors, whether electrohydraulic or ultrasonic, will disintegrate stones without significant morbidity (Wickham *et al.*, 1983) and rigid ureterorenoscopy allows access to the ureter endoscopically for intraureteric lithotripsy and stone retrieval (Ford *et al.*, 1983; Watson *et al.*, 1983).

External shock wave lithotripsy can also be employed provided that access is not hindered by spinal deformity.

Autonomic dysreflexia

Autonomic dysreflexia is seen in most patients with cervical and high dorsal spinal cord lesions, and consists of a hyperactive sympathetic response to stimuli below the lesion. Hypertension (sometimes fatal), sweating, piloerection and bradycardia occur, especially after bladder distension or contraction, during instrumentation, in detrusor—sphincter dyssynergia and after catheter blockage. Treatment involves avoiding or removing the cause if possible, or counteracting the sympathetic reaction with adrenoreceptor blockade (McGuire *et al.*, 1976). Indeed it is advisable always to have intravenous α-blocking drugs readily to hand when any urological manipulation is performed on a patient with significant neurological impairment.

Palliation of incontinence

Incontinence is a social disaster, and may be responsible for more misery than any other aspect of a particular neurological disorder. It still seems an unsavoury subject for discussion, sometimes even between patient and doctor, and perhaps doctors are not always aware of the options available. There has been little critical assessment of the various palliative methods and appliances, and still less effort expended on innovation. The number of advertisements in the national press suggests that many sufferers still seek advice through their pages. It is pleasing to note, however, that a continence advisary service is available in most health districts in the UK and that those nursing staff who have made this their area of expertise contribute greatly to the well-being of their incontinent patients.

Incontinence appliances

External appliances may be considered under the following headings: pants and pads, occlusive devices and drainage appliances.

Pants and pads

This is the commonest solution to the problem of incontinence used by more than 50% of sufferers. Indeed at present there still is no satisfactory alternative for the female patient. However, impervious plastic pants do not provide the best solution, and they lead to antisocial odour and skin problems. Often the effect is merely to keep the patients clothing dry whilst bathing the skin in urine. The development of marsupial pants (Wellington, 1976) has been an important contribution. They are made of hydrophobic material with an exterior pouch into which an absorbent pad can be placed. The skin is kept dry and the pad can absorb up to 300 ml before being changed.

Occlusive devices

These are of more use in the male though female urethral occlusive devices have been tried but withoutlasting success. None have yet survived the test of time. Penile clamps in men should be used only intermittently (Hall, 1965) and not at all in patients whose hygiene and intelligence is limited, because of the complications of penile swelling, urethral stricture and persistent urinary infection which may arise.

Drainage appliances

The condom sheath is the most commonly used device in the male paraplegic patient and can in fact be used with great benefit in other male patients, even those who are not neurologically compromised. A thin latex condom, perhaps coated with a silicone-based skin adhesive, is connected to tubing which drains into a leg-bag. There is complete freedom from retaining straps with this appliance which is a considerable advantage. The condom may be changed regularly but can often be left for 2–3 days without the need for it to be changed. In most cases it is an advantage for the patient to be circumcised to prevent inflammation and irritation of preputial skin left in constant contact with urine. The problem that may arise with this type of drainage is occasional splitting of the condom, usually as a result of the patient manoeuvring himself or exerting traction on the tubing. Penile retraction can hinder fitting a satisfactory condom urinal and in this case it may be necessary for a penile prosthesis to be implanted to enable a urinary collecting device to be used.

Inevitably, there is a temptation to seal the condom onto the penis with circumferential elastoplast, or in extreme cases with an elastic band. This practice is to be deprecated for the insensitive neuropathic penile shaft is vulnerable and autoamputation of the penis can result.

References

Anderson K.-E., Ek A., Hedlund H. & Mattiasson A. (1981) Effects of prazosin on isolated human urethra and in patients with lower motor neuron lesions. *Investigative Urology* **19**, 39–42.

Awad S.A., Downie J.W. & Kiruluta H.G. (1978) Alphaadrenergic agents in urinary disorders of the proximal urethra. II. Urethral obstruction due to 'sympathetic dyssynergia'. *British Journal of Urology* **50**, 336–339.

Barker A.T., Jalinous R. & Freeston I.L. (1985) Noninvasive magnetic stimulation of human motor cortex. *Lancet* **1**, 1106–1107.

Bary P.R., Day G., Lewis P., Chawla J., Evans C. & Stephenson T.P. (1982) Dynamic urethral function in the assessment of spinal injury patients. *British Journal of Urology* **54**, 39–44.

Bates C.P. (1971) Continence and incontinence, clinical study of the dynamics of voiding and of the sphincter mechanism. *Annals of the Royal College of Surgeons of England* **49**, 18–35.

Bertelsen S. & Pettinger W.A. (1977) A functional basis for classification of α-adrenergic receptors. *Life Sciences* **21**, 595.

Blacklock N.J. (1986) Catheters and urethral strictures. *British Journal of Urology* **58**, 475–478.

Blaivas J.G., Labib K.L., Bauer S.B. & Retik A.B. (1977) A new approach to electromyography of the external urethral sphincter. *Journal of Urology* **117**, 773–777.

Bors E. & Comarr E. (1971) *Neurologic Urology*. University Park Press, Baltimore.

Boyce W.H., Latham J.E. & Hunt L.D. (1964) Research related to the development of an artificial electrical stimulator for the paralysed human bladder. *Journal of Urology* **91**, 41–51.

Bradley W.E. & Sundin T. (1982) The physiology and pharmacology of urinary tract dysfunction. *Clinical Neuropharmacology* **5**, 131–158.

Bramble F.J. (1982) The treatment of adult enuresis and urge incontinence by enterocystoplasty. *British Journal of Urology* **54**, 693–696.

Bramble F.J. (1990) The clam cystoplasty. *British Journal of Urology* **66**, 337–341.

Brannen G.E., Bush W.H., Correa R.J., Gibbons R.P. & Elder J.S. (1985) Kidney stone removal: percutaneous versus surgical lithotomy. *Journal of Urology* **113**, 6–12.

Breithaupt D.J., Jousse A.T. & Wynne-Jones M. (1961) Late cause of death and life expectancy in paraplegia. *Canadian Medical Association Journal* **85**, 73–77.

Brindley G.S. (1973) Emptying the bladder by stimulating ventral sacral roots. *Journal of Physiology* **237**, 15–16P.

Brindley G.S. (1977) An implant to empty the bladder or close the urethra. *Journal of Neurology, Neurosurgery and Psychiatry* **40**, 358–369.

Brindley G.S., Polkey C.E., Rushton D.N. & Cardozo L. (1986) Sacral anterior root stimulation for bladder control in paraplegics – the first 50 cases. *Journal of Neurology, Neurosurgery and Psychiatry* **49**, 1104–1114.

Bush W.H., Brannen G.E., Gibbons R.P., Correa R.J. & Elder J.S. (1984) Radiation exposure to patient and urologist during percutaneous nephrostolithotomy. *Journal of Urology* **132**, 1148–1152.

Caine M. (1984) The autonomic pharmacology of the urinary tract. In Caine M. (ed.) *The Pharmacology of the Urinary Tract*. Springer-Verlag, Berlin.

Delaere K.P.J., Debruyne F.M.J. & Moonen W.A. (1983) Bladder neck incision in the female: a hazardous procedure. *British Journal of Urology* **55**, 283–286.

Deltenre P.F. & Thiry A.J. (1989) Urinary bladder cortical evoked potentials in man: suitable stimulation techniques. *British Journal of Urology* **64**, 381–384.

Desmond A.D. & Ramayya G.R. (1988) Comparison of pressure flow studies with micturitional urethral pressure profiles in the diagnosis of urinary outflow obstruction. *British Journal of Urology* **61**, 224–229.

Dewan P.A. & Guiney E.J. (1990) Endoscopic correction of vesico-ureteric reflux in children with spina bifida. *British Journal of Urology* **65**, 646–649.

Diokno A.C. & Sonda P. (1984) Pharmacological management of the neuropathic bladder and urethra. In Caine M. (ed.) *The Pharmacology of the Urinary Tract*. Springer-Verlag, Berlin.

Diokno A.C. & Taub M. (1975) Ephedrine in the treatment of urinary incontinence. *Urology* **5**, 624–625.

Donker P.J., Ivanovici F. & Noach E.L. (1972) Analyses of

the urethral pressure profile by means of electromyography and the administration of drugs. *British Journal of Urology* **44**, 180–193.

Ewing R., Bultitude M. & Shuttleworth K.E.D. (1983) Subtrigonal phenol therapy for incontinence in female patients with multiple sclerosis. *Lancet* **1**, 1304–1305.

Fall M. (1977) Thesis: Intravaginal electrical stimulation. *Scandinavian Journal of Urology and Nephrology* Supplement 44.

Fellows G.J., Cannell L.B. & Ravichandran G. (1987) Transrectal ultrasonography compared with voiding cystourethrography after spinal cord injury. *British Journal of Urology* **59**, 218–221.

Fenn N., Conn I.G., German K.A. & Stephenson T.P. (1992) Complications of clam enterocystoplasties with particular reference to urinary tract infection. *British Journal of Urology* **69**, 366–368.

Fidas A., MacDonald H.L., Elton R.A., McInnes A. & Chisholm G.D. (1989) Neurological defects of the voiding reflex arcs in chronic urinary retention and their relation to spina bifida occulta. *British Journal of Urology* **63**, 16–20.

Fletcher T.F. & Bradley W.B. (1978) Neuroanatomy of the bladder/urethra. *Journal of Urology* **119**, 153–160.

Ford T.F., Watson G.M. & Wickham J.E.A. (1983) Transurethral ureteroscopic removal of ureteric stones. *British Journal of Urology* **55**, 626–628.

Galloway N.T.M., Chisholm G.D. & McInnes A. (1985) Patterns and significance of sacral evoked responses (the urologist's knee jerk). *British Journal of Urology* **57**, 145–147.

Geisler W.O., Jousse A.T. & Wynne-Jones M. (1977) Survival in traumatic transverse myelitis. *Paraplegia* **14**, 262–275.

Geisler W.O., Jousse A.T., Wynne-Jones M. & Breithaupt D.J. (1983) Survival in traumatic spinal cord injury. *Paraplegia* **21**, 364–373.

Gibbon N.O.K. (1973) Division of the external sphincter. *British Journal of Urology* **45**, 110–115.

Gibbon N.O.K., Parsons K.F. & Woolfenden K.A. (1980) The neuropathic urethra. *Paraplegia* **18**, 221–225.

Glahn B.R. (1970) Neurogenic bladder diagnosed pharmacologically on the basis of denervation supersensitivity. *Scandinavian Journal of Urology and Nephrology* **4**, 13–24.

Godec C., Cass A.S. & Ayala G.F. (1976) Electrical stimulation for incontinence technique, selection and results. *Urology* **7**, 388–397.

Gosling J.A., Dixon J.S. & Lendon R.L. (1977) The autonomic innervation of the human male and female bladder neck and proximal urethra. *Journal of Urology* **118**, 302–305.

Gosling J.A. (1979) The structure of the bladder and urethra in relation to function. *Urological Clinics of North America* **6**, 31–38.

Guttman L. & Frankel H. (1966) The value of intermittent catheterisation in the early management of traumatic paraplegia and tetraplegia. *Paraplegia* **4**, 63–84.

Hall M.H. (1965) Appliances for the incontinent patient. *British Journal of Urology* **37**, 644–646.

Herr H.W. (1975) Intermittent catheterisation in neurogenic bladder dysfunction. *Journal of Urology* **113**, 477–479.

Hess C.W., Mills K.R. & Murray N.M.F. (1986) Measurement of central motor conduction in multiple sclerosis by magnetic brain stimulation. *Lancet* **ii**, 355–358.

Hitchcock E., Newsam D. & Salama M. (1974) The somatotrophic representation of the micturition pathways in the cervical cord of man. *British Journal of Surgery* **61**, 395–401.

Hunt G.M. & Whitaker R.H. (1990) A new device for self-catheterisation in wheelchair bound women. *British Journal of Urology* **66**, 162–163.

Jousse A.T., Wynne-Jones M. & Breithaupt D.J. (1968) A follow-up study of life expectancy and mortality in traumatic transverse myelitis. *Canadian Medical Association Journal* **98**, 770–772.

Kato K., Kondo A., Takita T., Gotoh M., Tanaka J. & Mitsuya H. (1987) Incontinence in female neurogenic bladders, resolution by endoscopic bladder neck suspension. *British Journal of Urology* **59**, 523–525.

Khanna O.P. (1976) Disorders of micturition: neuropharmacological basis and results of drug therapy. *Urology* **8**, 316–328.

Kock N.G. & Pompeius R. (1963) Inhibition of vesical motor activity induced by anal stimulation. *Acta Chirurgica Scandinavica* **126**, 244–250.

Kondo A., Kobayashi M., Otari T., Takita T. & Narita H. (1980) Supersensitivity to prostaglandin in chronic neurogenic bladders. *British Journal of Urology* **52**, 290–294.

Krane R.J. & Olsson C.A. (1973) Phenoxybenzamine in neurogenic bladder dysfunction. II. Clinical considerations. *Journal of Urology* **110**, 653–656.

Kunos G. & Nickerson M. (1976) Temperature-induced interconversion of α- and β-adrenoreceptors in the frog heart. *Journal of Physiology (Lond)* **256**, 23–40.

Kuru M. (1965) Nervous control of micturition. *Physiological Reviews* **45**, 425–494.

Lapides J., Friend C.R., Ajemian E.P. & Reus W.S. (1962) Denervation supersensitivity as a test of neurogenic bladder. *Surgery, Gynaecology and Obstetrics* **114**, 241–244.

Lapides J., Diokno A.C., Silber S.J. & Lowe B.S. (1972) Clean intermittent catheterisation in the treatment of urinary tract disease. *Journal of Urology* **107**, 458–461.

Lapides J., Diokno A.C. & Gould F.R. (1976) Further observations on self-catheterisation. *Journal of Urology* **116**, 169–171.

Laruelle L. (1948) Etude d'anatomie microscopique du nevraxe sur coupes longitudinales. *Acta Neurologica Belgica (Copenhagen)* **48**, 189–196.

Lawrence W.T. & Thomas D.G. (1987) The Stamey bladder neck suspension operation for stress incontinence and neurovesical dysfunction. *British Journal of Urology* **59**, 305–310.

Leyson J.F.J., Martin B.F. & Sporer A. (1980) Baclofen in the treatment of detrusor-sphincter dyssynergia in spinal cord injury patients. *Journal of Urology* **124**, 82–84.

Lucas M.G. & Thomas D.G. (1989) Lack of relationship of conus reflexes to bladder function after spinal cord injury. *British Journal of Urology* **63**, 24–27.

MacDonagh R.P., Forster D.M.C. & Thomas D.G. (1990) Urinary continence in spinal injury patients following complete sacral posterior rhizotomy. *British Journal of Urology* **66**, 618–622.

McGuire E.J., Wagner F.M. & Weiss R.M. (1976) Treatment of autonomic dysreflexia with phenoxybenzamine. *Journal of Urology* **115**, 53–55.

McGuire E.J. & Brady S. (1979) Detrusor sphincter dyssynergia. *Journal of Urology* **121**, 774–777.

McInerney P.D., Vanner T.F., Harris S.A.B. & Stephenson T.P. (1990) Permanent urethral stents for detrusor sphincter dyssynergia. *British Journal of Urology* **67**, 291–294.

McRae P., Murray K.H.A., Nurse D.E., Stephenson T.P. & Mundy A.R. (1987) Clam enterocystoplasty in the neuropathic bladder. *British Journal of Urology* **60**, 523–525.

Madersbacher H. & Scott F.B. (1976) The twelve o'clock sphincterotomy. Technique, indications, results. *Paraplegia* **13**, 261–267.

Marberger M., Stakl W., Hruby W. & Kroiss A. (1985) Late sequelae of ultrasonic lithotripsy of renal calculi. *Journal of Urology* **133**, 170–173.

Mayo M.E., Kriegger J.N. & Rudd T.G. (1985) Effect of percutaneous nephrostolithotomy on renal function. *Journal of Urology* **133**, 167–169.

Mitrofanoff P. (1980) Cystomie continente transappendiculaire dans le traitement des vessies neurologiques. *Chirurgurie Paediatrica* **21**, 297–305.

Mundy A.R., Shah P.J.R., Borzyskowski M. & Saxton H.M. (1985) Sphincter behaviour in meningomyelocele. *British Journal of Urology* **57**, 647–651.

Murray K.H.A., Nurse D.E. & Mundy A.R. (1988) Detrusor behaviour after implantation of the Brantley Scott artificial urinary sphincter for neuropathic incontinence. *British Journal of Urology* **61**, 122–128.

Nashold B.S., Friedman H., Glenn J.F., Grimes J.H., Barry W.F. & Avery R. (1972) Electromicturition in paraplegia. *Archives of Surgery* **104**, 195–202.

Nathan P.W. (1976) The central nervous connections of the bladder. In Williams D.I. & Chisholm G. (eds) *The Scientific Foundation of Urology*. Heinemann, London.

Nergardh A. (1975) Autonomic receptor function in the lower urinary tract. A survey of recent experimental results. *Journal of Urology* **113**, 180–185.

O'Flynn J.D. (1974) Neurogenic bladder in spinal cord injury. Management of patients in Dublin, Ireland. *Urologic Clinics of North America* **1**, 155–162.

Ohlsson B.L., Fall M. & Frankenberg-Sommar S. (1989) Effects of external and direct pudendal nerve maximal electrical stimulation in the treatment of the uninhibited overactive bladder. *British Journal of Urology* **64**, 374–380.

Parry J.R.W., Nurse D.E., Boucaut H.A.P., Murray K.H.A. & Mundy A.R. (1990) Surgical management of the congenital neuropathic bladder. *British Journal of Urology* **65**, 165–167.

Pedersen E., Harving H., Klemar B. & Torring J. (1978) Human anal reflexes. *Journal of Neurology, Neurosurgery and Psychiatry* **41**, 813–818.

Puri P. & O'Donnell B. (1984) Correction of experimentally produced vesicoureteric reflux in the piglet by intravesical injection of teflon. *British Medical Journal* **289**, 5–7.

Puri P. & O'Donnell B. (1987) Endoscopic correction of grades IV and V primary vesicoureteric reflux: six to 30 months follow-up in 42 ureters. *Journal of Pediatric Surgery* **22**, 1087–1091.

Rickwood A.K.M. (1982) Use of internal urethrotomy to reverse upper renal tract dilatation in children with neurogenic bladder dysfunction. *British Journal of Urology* **54**, 292–294.

Rickwood A.K.M., Thomas D.G., Philp N.H. & Spicer R.D. (1982) A system of management of the congenital neuropathic bladder based upon combined urodynamic and radiological assessment. *British Journal of Urology* **54**, 507–511.

Rockswold G.L. & Bradley W.E. (1977) The use of evoked electromyographic responses in diagnosing lesions of the cauda equina. *Journal of Urology* **118**, 629–631.

Rohner T.J. Jr, Hannigan J.D. & Sanford E.J. (1978) Altered in-vitro adrenergic responses of dog detrusor muscle after chronic bladder outlet obstruction. *Urology* **11**, 357–361.

Ross J.C., Gibbon N.O.K. & Damanski M. (1957) Resection of the external sphincter in the paraplegia – a preliminary report. *Transactions of the American Association of Genitourinary Surgeons* **69**, 193–198.

Sarica Y. & Karacan I. (1988) Electrophysiological correlates of sensory innervation of the vesico-urethral junction and urethra in man. *Neurology and Urodynamics* **6**, 477–484.

Shabsigh R., Fiskman I.J. & Krebs M. (1988) Combined transrectal sonography and urodynamics in the evaluation of detrusor-sphincter dyssynergia. *British Journal of Urology* **62**, 326–330.

Shaw P.J.R., Milroy E.J.G., Timoney A.G., El Din A. & Mitchell N. (1990) Permanent external striated urethral stents in patients with spinal injuries. *British Journal of Urology* **66**, 297–300.

Siroky M.B., Sax D.S. & Krane R.J. (1979) Sacral signal tracing: the electrophysiology of the bulbocavernosus reflex. *Journal of Urology* **122**, 661–664.

Stephenson T.P. & Mundy A.R. (1985) Treatment of the neuropathic bladder by enterocystoplasty and selective sphincterotomy or sphincter ablation and replacement. *British Journal of Urology* **57**, 27–31.

Sundin T. & Dahlstrom A. (1973) The sympathetic innervation of the urinary bladder and urethra in the normal state and after parasympathetic denervation at the spinal root level. *Scandinavian Journal of Urology and Nephrology* **7**, 131–149.

Thiry A.J. & Deltenre P.F. (1989) Neurophysiological assessment of the central motor pathway to the external urethral sphincter in man. *British Journal of Urology* **63**, 515–519.

Thomas D.G. (1979) Clinical urodynamics in neurogenic bladder dysfunction. *Urologic Clinics of North America* **6**, 237–253.

Torrens M.J. (1978) Urethral sphincter responses to stimulation of the sacral nerves in the human female. *Urology International* **33**, 22–26.

Torrens M.J. & Abrams P.H. (1979) Cystometry. *Urologic Clinics of North America* **6**, 79–85.

Vaidyanathan A., Rao M.S., Mapa M.K., Bapna B.C., Chary K.S.N. & Swamy R.P. (1981) Study of intravesical instillation of 15-(S)-15-methyl prostaglandin $F_{2\alpha}$ in patients with neurogenic bladder dysfunction. *Journal of Urology* **126**, 81–85.

Vinson R.K. & Diokno A.C. (1976) Uninhibited neurogenic bladder in adults. *Urology* **7**, 376–378.

Walsh P.C. & Donker P.J. (1982) Impotence following radical prostatectomy: insight into etiology and prevention. *Journal of Urology* **128**, 492–497.

Watson G.M., Wickham J.E.A., Mills T.N., Brown S.G., Swain P. & Salmon P.R. (1983) Laser fragmentation of renal calculi. *British Journal of Urology* **55**, 613–616.

Webb R.J., Styles R.A., Griffiths C.J., Ramsden P.D. & Neal D.E. (1989) Ambulatory monitoring of bladder pressure in patients with low compliance as a result of neurogenic bladder dysfunction. *British Journal of Urology* **64**, 150–154.

Wellington F.L. (1976) *Incontinence in the Elderly*, pp. 230–244. Academic Press, London.

Whitmore W.F. III, Fam B.A. & Yalla S.V. (1978) Experience with anteromedian [12 o'clock] external sphincterotomy in 100 male subjects with neuropathic bladder. *British Journal of Urology* **50**, 99–101.

Wickham J.E.A., Kellett M.J. & Miller R.A. (1983) Elective percutaneous nephrolithotomy in 50 patients: an analysis of the technique, results and complications. *Journal of Urology* **129**, 904–906.

Yeates W.K. (1972) Disorders of bladder function. *Annals of the Royal College of Surgeons of England* **50**, 335–353.

26: Rehabilitation of Faecal Incontinence

R.I. HALLAN, B.D. GEORGE
AND N.S. WILLIAMS

Prevalence of faecal incontinence, 382
Anatomy and physiology of the pelvic floor muscles, 382
Pathogenesis of faecal incontinence, 383
Idiopathic faecal incontinence (IFI), 384
    Muscle function in IFI, 384
    Rectal sensation, anorectal sampling and anal
        sphincter recruitment thresholds, 384
Global view of the maintenance of continence and the
        aetiology of IFI, 384
Treatment of faecal incontinence, 385
    Medical treatment, 385
    Surgical treatment, 386
    Electrical stimulation of the anal sphincter, 388

Prevalence of faecal incontinence

The true prevalence of faecal incontinence is un-known, as there have been few epidemiological studies. Brocklehurst (1972) estimated that it affected just under 1 per 1000 of the population. A study by Thomas et al. (1984) revealed the existence of many cases unknown to the health authorities. Their data show that the known prevalence of faecal or double incontinence is similar in males and females up to the age of 65 years (0.5 per 1000 population). They estimate, on the basis of a postal survey, that the true prevalence in the community may be 10 times as great. The known prevalence rises after the age of 65 years to 4.9 per 1000 population in males and 13.3 per 1000 population in females. Others have reported the incidence of faecal incontinence in elderly patients in hospitals. Incidences of 13%, 26%, 31% and 47% have been reported in patients of acute, geriatric, psychiatric (Clarke et al., 1979) and psychogeriatric wards (McClaren et al., 1981), and the proportion of doubly incontinent patients in local authority homes for the elderly varies from 10 to 14% (Gilleard, 1980), and indeed numerically this is the largest group of patients (Brocklehurst, 1975).

The stigma felt by patients with faecal incontinence is immense and results in reluctance in sufferers to seek advice. Clinical histories reveal that most patients have had symptoms for years before help is sought. It is now recognized that patients will 'disguise' their problem, complaining of diarrhoea when in reality they are incontinent (Read et al., 1979; Leigh & Turnberg, 1982).

There has been a marked improvement in the understanding of the physiological mechanisms responsible for the maintenance of continence in recent years. As a consequence the surgical treatment of faecal incontinence has also improved. A direct repair of the anal sphincter may restore continence in patients who have sustained segmental sphincter defects as a result of birth trauma (Browning & Motson, 1983). Postanal repair may improve continence in patients with idiopathic (neurogenic) faecal incontinence (IFI) (Browning & Parks, 1983).

Anatomy and physiology of the pelvic floor muscles

In order to understand the treatment of faecal incontinence, a basic knowledge of pelvic floor anatomy and physiology is required.

The rectum is the terminal portion of the colon and passes through the striated muscles of the pelvic floor (or diaphragm), at which level it becomes the anal canal. The middle part of the diaphragm, the puborectalis muscle, forms a sling behind the anorectal junction and causes an acute angulation, which is important in the maintenance of continence. The distal part of the anal canal is surrounded by the internal and external anal sphincters. The internal anal sphincter is the continuation of the rectal smooth-muscle wall and is surrounded by the external anal sphincter. The external sphincter consists of striated muscle and is closely related to the puborectalis muscle.

Continence is maintained by a combination of factors:

1 Basal tone in the smooth internal anal sphincter muscle.

2 Basal tone in the striated external anal sphincter, puborectalis and other muscles of the pelvic floor.

3 The tone in the striated muscles reflexly increases to maintain continence when intra-abdominal pressure is increased by coughing, carrying a heavy load, etc.

Further detailed information on pelvic floor anatomy and physiology can be found in an excellent review by Gordon (1987).

Pathogenesis of faecal incontinence

Incontinence may occur despite normal anorectal function in the presence of large quantities of liquid stool, which are able to overwhelm even the most normal anal sphincter. This can result from infestations or intoxications of the intestinal tract, e.g. *Salmonella* gastroenteritis. Autonomic neuropathy (e.g. diabetes mellitus) and inflammatory bowel disease (e.g. ulcerative colitis) may also be responsible for profound diarrhoea, and therefore present with incontinence of liquid stool.

Faecal incontinence presenting to coloproctologists, however, is usually due to abnormal anorectal function. The aetiology of faecal incontinence is classified in Table 26.1. In numerical terms the largest group is faecal impaction with overflow incontinence, usually occurring in elderly patients. The condition appears to develop in the presence of impaired rectal sensation (Bannister *et al.*, 1985); this finding could, however, be due to accommodation of the rectum to large volumes. In many cases of incontinence the cause of the abnormality in anorectal function can be identified. Rare congenital abnormalities can create severe problems: certain forms of anorectal atresia which are related to failure of pelvic floor development (Stephens & Smith, 1971) may cause incontinence. Trauma to the sphincters may be caused by surgery (e.g. fistula surgery), obstetric injury (third-degree tear), impalement injury or severe pelvic fractures. The majority of patients with rectal prolapse have a

Table 26.1 Classification of aetiological factors for faecal incontinence

Normal anal sphincters, rectum and pelvic floor
Diarrhoea
    Infective
    Inflammatory bowel disease
    Intestinal resection
    Metabolic (e.g. diabetes mellitus)
    Fistulae

Abnormal function of the anal sphincters, rectum and pelvic floor
Congenital anomalies of the anorectum
Trauma
    Iatrogenic
    Obstetric
    Fractures of the pelvis
    Impalement
Rectal prolapse, overt or occult rectal intussusception
Rectal and anal canal carcinoma
Anorectal infections (e.g. lymphogranuloma)
Faecal impaction
    Drugs
Neurological: upper motor neuron lesions
    Cerebral
        Dementia and other degenerative diseases
        Multiple strokes
        Multiple sclerosis
        Tumour
    Spinal
        Multiple sclerosis
        Degenerative disease, e.g. vitamin B_{12} deficiency
Neurological: lower motor neuron lesion
    Cauda equina syndrome
    Peripheral neuropathy (e.g. diabetes)
    Lumbar meningomyelocele (spina bifida)
    Tabes dorsalis

significant degree of faecal incontinence (Penfold & Hawley, 1972). This has been thought to be due to a dilatation effect on the internal anal sphincter, but there is evidence that incontinence in such patients is associated with neurogenic damage to the external sphincter apparatus (Neill *et al.*, 1981).

Neurological disorders affecting sphincter control can also result in faecal incontinence. In these patients the neurological deficit is widespread, and incontinence is only one component of their symptom complex. Deficient central control mechanisms of the anal sphincters can occur with dementia, strokes, multiple sclerosis and cerebral tumours. Nerve and nerve root lesions, including cauda equina injuries, peripheral neuropathy (e.g. diabetes), tabes dorsalis and spina bifida, may also result in faecal incontinence.

Idiopathic faecal incontinence (IFI)

A large number of patients presenting with faecal incontinence do not have any evidence of anorectal abnormality or generalized neurological disease, and Parks (1975) described this condition and called it idiopathic faecal incontinence.

Muscle function in IFI

Since the publication in 1975 of Parks's seminal paper, the cause of the weakness of the external anal sphincter has been extensively investigated. Parks *et al.* (1977) and Beersiek *et al.* (1979) reported on histological studies of biopsies from the striated sphincter apparatus of patients with IFI. There were changes of fibre type grouping in the less severely damaged biopsies, and atrophy and fatty replacement of muscle in the more severely diseased biopsies in patients with IFI. The changes were felt to be indicative of a neuropathic cause for the striated muscle weakness, associated with reinnervation. Studies of the puborectalis and superficial external anal sphincter muscles, involving both single-fibre (Neill & Swash, 1980; Neill *et al.*, 1981) and concentric needle (Bartolo *et al.*, 1983a, b) electromyography (EMG), detected abnormalities suggestive of neurogenic muscle damage.

The conclusion from these investigations is that there is damage to the innervation of the striated sphincter muscles in a high proportion of patients with IFI, and that abnormally excessive perineal descent during straining at stool may be one cause of such damage (Kiff & Swash, 1984). However, Womack *et al.* (1986) reported that, in a group of patients with abnormal perineal descent, there were no significant differences in the voluntary squeeze pressures and puborectalis fibre densities between the continent and incontinent patients. The only difference was a significant reduction in the basal pressure of the incontinent patients, suggesting that the incontinence was due to smooth internal anal sphincter muscle damage in patients who already had impaired striated sphincters.

Two recent publications have highlighted the importance of internal anal sphincter damage in neurogenic IFI (Lubowski *et al.*, 1988; Swash *et al.*, 1988). In four out of six patients with incontinence there was absence of smooth-muscle EMG activity. In all six patients there were abnormal responses of internal anal sphincter muscle strips to pharmacological manipulations and all showed ultrastructural abnormalities on electron microscopy.

Rectal sensation, anorectal sampling and anal sphincter recruitment thresholds

Investigators of faecal incontinence have reported defects in rectal sensation in faecal incontinence. Womack *et al.* (1986) reported increased thresholds of sensation to intrarectal balloon distension, which had previously been noted by Ihre (1974) and was more recently confirmed by Lubowski & Nicholls (1988). Mucosal electrosensitivity testing has demonstrated reduction in anal canal sensibility in IFI (Roe *et al.*, 1986; Rogers *et al.*, 1988a). Ambulatory anorectal manometry has shown a decreased frequency of sampling episodes in IFI compared with controls (Miller *et al.*, 1988a; Kumar *et al.*, 1989). Miller *et al.* (1987) have demonstrated a conscious awareness of temperature sensation in the upper anal canal, which they have suggested may be of importance in discrimination during anorectal sampling. Rogers *et al.* (1988b) suggested that the temperature gradient between the rectum and anal canal was too small to be detected by the anal canal mucosa, and that the mechanism of conscious appreciation of temperature differences of faeces passing from the rectum into the anal canal cannot take place during the anorectal sampling reflex. Womack *et al.* (1989) have investigated the recruitment threshold of the external anal sphincter and puborectalis in control subjects and incontinent patients, and have shown that recruitment of muscle EMG occurs at significantly higher intra-abdominal pressures in the incontinent group compared with controls.

Global view of the maintenance of continence and the aetiology of IFI

To summarize the discussion of the mechanism of the maintenance of anal continence and the aetiology of IFI, it must be said that neither is completely understood. It can, however, be said that a large number of factors are important in the maintenance of continence, including stool consistency, rectal motor activity and smooth internal anal sphincter activity, as well as striated external anal sphincter, puborectalis and pelvic floor muscle activity. The reflex control of these efferent continence mechanisms is via afferent sensory information from receptors in the pelvic muscles, rectal wall and anorectal mucosa, and these reflexes can be modulated by higher centres.

Faecal incontinence can occur if the damage to any one of these mechanisms is sufficiently severe. However, in the majority of patients with IFI, the incontinence is the result of subliminal damage to several mechanisms, each of which on its own is insufficient to cause incontinence, but which when the effects are summated causes sufficient impairment to the overall continence mechanism to result in incontinence.

Treatment of faecal incontinence

The management of faecal incontinence can be considered in terms of medical and surgical options.

Medical treatment

The principles of treating faecal incontinence conservatively are to minimize the threat to continence from the bowel contents and to use residual sphincter function to maximum efficiency. Hence all conditions that produce diarrhoea (e.g. diverticular disease, ulcerative colitis) should be treated appropriately. In patients in whom episodes of faecal incontinence are associated with liquid stools for which no specific condition is apparent, constipating drugs such as loperamide and codeine phosphate may be beneficial (Palmer et al., 1980; Read et al., 1982).

'Planned defaecation' can be an effective technique in patients with faecal incontinence and stools of normal consistency. Most patients will already have tried to determine when they become incontinent and have adjusted their daily pattern of activity accordingly. Bulk laxatives provide stools of predictable volume and consistency while making bowel actions more regular. Used in combination with glycerol suppositories in the morning, when the patient has ready access to the toilet, such a regime of planned defaecation may allow the patient to be continent for the remainder of the day.

Physiotherapy and pelvic floor exercises may improve residual sphincter function (Keighley & Fielding, 1983; Miller et al., 1988). They may be combined with techniques such as faradism or the use of implantable (Caldwell, 1963) or anal plug (Hopkinson & Lightwood, 1966; Hopkinson, 1972) electrodes to stimulate the sphincter muscles. These techniques rely on there being sufficient residual muscle to generate a useful force on contraction, and therefore the patients with the weakest muscles tend to do least well.

Biofeedback has been used successfully in the treatment of faecal incontinence (Schuster, 1977; Almy & Corson, 1979). The technique allows the patient to recognize rectal distension and in response to produce an improved sphincteric contraction. A balloon is inflated in the rectum and the subject watches a tracing of the intrarectal and intra-anal pressures and learns how to co-ordinate the sensation of rectal distension with a visible rise in intrarectal pressure and to produce a voluntary sphincter contraction. After a while the visual image of intrarectal pressure is removed and the subject has to rely on the renewed ability to discriminate rectal contents to control sphincteric function. Improvement of continence in 70–80% of patients has been reported using these techniques (Cerulli et al., 1979; MacLeod, 1987). The results are poor in conditions where there is impaired rectal sensation, and the best results have been obtained in patients with myogenic disorders and lesions of the sphincters secondary to surgery.

Continence aids

Continence aids are more appropriate for urinary incontinence, as there are few aids suitable for the collection of solid stool. The Incare drainable faecal collector (Hollister Inc., UK) is suitable for collecting liquid stool, e.g. ventilated patients in intensive care units. A wide range of disposable and reusable pads and sheets are available, and a number of continence advice centres in the UK are now providing a valuable service for incontinent patients.

Surgical treatment

The main principle involved in the surgical treatment of faecal incontinence is to remove any factors contributing to the cause of the incontinence and to repair or reinforce the sphincteric mechanism. As a last resort, if all such methods are unsuccessful, the surgeon can construct a permanent colostomy, which with modern stoma appliances is an easily controlled method of collecting faeces. However, it is not without social and psychological morbidity (Devlin *et al.*, 1971).

The factor associated with the development of faecal incontinence which is most amenable to surgical correction is rectal prolapse. When rectal prolapse and faecal incontinence coexist, repair of the rectal prolapse is the first step, as abdominal rectopexy restores continence in approximately half of such patients (Morgan *et al.*, 1972; Holmstrom *et al.*, 1978). Délorme's operation (Christenson & Kirkegaard, 1981) and rectosigmoidectomy (Theurkauf *et al.*, 1970; Friedman *et al.*, 1983) are less successful in improving continence, with success rates of only 20%. Rogers & Jeffery (1987) have introduced an intersphincteric Ivalon sponge rectopexy and combined this with a postanal repair for patients with rectal prolapse and faecal incontinence, with all 15 patients incontinent to solid stool preoperatively becoming continent. Brodén *et al.* (1988) recently reported that a successful outcome with improved faecal continence after abdominal rectopexy was associated with a significantly increased basal anal canal pressure.

The association between occult rectal prolapse (or 'internal procidentia') and faecal incontinence is less well recognized. However, Ihre & Seligson (1975) reported the results of the Ripstein procedure in 40 patients with internal procidentia demonstrated by proctography. Continence was restored by this procedure in 75% of the incontinent patients treated. Hallan *et al.* (1988) reported a correlation between the extent of rectal intussusception and impaired internal anal sphincter function. However, it was difficult to determine whether such a defect was the cause or the result of the incontinence.

Postanal repair

In the 1960s, as a result of investigations of the continence mechanisms (Phillips & Edwards, 1965;

Parks *et al.*, 1966), attention was focused away from the superficial part of the external anal sphincter and on to the function of the puborectalis muscle in patients with neurogenic IFI. Parks (1967) stated that in these patients incontinence resulted from loss of the angulation between the lower rectum and the anal canal. The loss of anorectal angulation was, in turn, ascribed to weakness of the puborectalis muscle. The angulation, Parks argued, was necessary to allow the functioning of a flap-valve mechanism at the anorectal junction. In order to treat such patients, he devised the operation of postanal perineorrhaphy, or postanal repair (Parks, 1967). This operation has the objectives of reconstruction of the anorectal angle (Parks, 1967), lengthening of the anal canal (Hardcastle & Parks, 1970) and increasing the efficiency of action of the external anal sphincter muscles (Parks & Percy, 1983).

There is general agreement that postanal repair initially restores continence in 70–80% of patients with IFI (Parks, 1975; Browning & Parks, 1983; Keighley & Fielding, 1983). There have been few reports of the long-term results of postanal repair. Yoshioka & Keighley (1989) in a series of 116 patients followed up for a median of 5 years after postanal repair suggest that 76% of the patients remain incontinent after surgery. Christianson & Skomorowska (1987) suggest that incontinence following a failed postanal repair can be successfully treated by an anterior perineoplasty.

Repair of divided anal sphincter

Surgical repair of the anal sphincter is indicated when the muscles of the sphincteric ring have been traumatically divided. Anterior division results most commonly from injury during childbirth. It does not involve the puborectalis sling and consequently produces incontinence that is less severe than that caused by injuries to the lateral and posterior aspects of the sphincter, which often involve the puborectalis muscle. These injuries are commonly the result of the surgical treatment of fistula in ano, and more rarely to direct penetrating injuries and severe pelvic fractures.

The early operative procedures employed direct end-to-end suture of the sphincteric muscles. Some good results have been reported using these techniques (Smith & Linton, 1929; Miller & Brown, 1937), but Goligher (1967) was more critical of the results and suggested that the muscle ends were difficult to identify and keep opposed by sutures during healing and maintained that this was the cause of some of the failures. Parks introduced the intraoperative use of muscle stimulation to identify the ends of the anal sphincter muscle, which were then overlapped (Parks & McPartlin, 1971). This led to some improvement in the results. In Parks's personal series (reported by Browning & Motson, 1983), full continence was restored in 92% of patients treated for obstetric and traumatic injuries of the sphincter and 66% of patients treated for injuries resulting from fistula surgery. Keighley & Fielding (1983) reported that 13 of 16 patients became continent or markedly improved by an overlapping sphincter repair.

Supplementation of weak anal sphincter

Thiersch procedure

The initial attempts to reinforce the anal sphincters were based on the hypothesis that the external anal sphincter, encircling the caudal part of the anal canal, was the most important part of the sphincteric apparatus. Thiersch's operation, which was reintroduced by Gabriel (1948), was the prototype for this type of procedure. Originally described as a treatment for rectal prolapse, it consists of encircling the anal orifice by silver or steel wire in order to constrict the anus in patients with laxity of the anal sphincter. In practice, the technique has several complications, which include recurrence of prolapse, faecal impaction and problems with the wire, such as breakage and erosion through the skin. The introduction of monofilament nylon (Plumley, 1966) reduced the incidence of breakage of the suture but the main problem with this procedure, the inelastic nature of the suture material, remained. Hunt et al. (1985) reported significant improvement of anal continence in poor-risk patients, whose rectal prolapse was controlled by using silastic rings to encircle the anal sphincters. Earnshaw & Hopkinson (1987) have used silicone rubber bands with similar results. Corman (1983) has used a Dacron-impregnated silastic sheet for the same purpose.

Dynamic sphincter supplementation

The logical step from static constriction of the anal canal by wire was to develop a 'dynamic' substitute for the anal sphincter. Such techniques make use of either biological tissues or implanted materials with physical characteristics better suited to the role of supporting the anal canal. Reinforcement by biological tissues was the first option to be explored, and Wreden (1929) and Stone (1929) described the use of fascial slings attached to the gluteus maximus muscle to create an artificial anal sphincter. Chittenden (1930) used gluteal muscle slips to reconstruct a sphincter for a perineal colostomy after a Kraske procedure. Later, Pickrell et al. (1952, 1954) used the transposed gracilis muscle, and Rappert (1952) and Fedorov & Shelygin (1989) the adductor longus muscle, for the same purpose. Corman (1980, 1983, 1985) has reported satisfactory long-term results using gracilis transposition in carefully selected patients.

The gracilis sling procedure

Pickrell described the gracilis sling procedure to improve faecal continence in four children with spina bifida and meningocoele in 1951 with encouraging results (Pickrell et al., 1952, 1954). By the time of a further publication in 1956 (Pickrell et al., 1956), the operation had been performed in 18 children and 16 adults. The children had all been incontinent since birth due to imperforate anus or a neurological abnormality affecting the anal sphincters. The results of the procedure were not fully discussed, but all of the patients were said to be continent to faeces and flatus.

The gracilis sling procedure in the treatment of adult faecal incontinence. Pickrell et al. (1956) also reported the use of the gracilis sling procedure for the treatment of 16 adults with faecal incontinence and claimed good results. The main recent proponent of the gracilis sling procedure in selected adults has been Corman (1979, 1980, 1983, 1985). His indication for performing the operation was that other surgical procedures such as direct muscle repair or a reefing procedure were considered impossible. Corman (1985) noted that the initial results were not so good and that there was a definite improvement with time. Of 14 patients, only three have required a colostomy on follow-up of 5 years. The remainder have a good or excellent function, defined as being continent at all times, not requiring the use of pads, and some patients using suppositories on a regular basis. Leguit *et al.* (1985) reported 10 cases of the gracilis sling procedure over a period of 17 years. Nine patients were markedly improved, good to excellent on Corman's criteria, and one patient remained incontinent. On manometric assessment in eight of these patients, two were found to have a scarred non-contractile neosphincter; the remainder had a relatively normal basal and squeeze anal canal pressure profile. The authors concluded that they were unable to determine the method by which the gracilis sling procedure produced continence.

The majority of colorectal surgeons perform the gracilis sling procedure for adult faecal incontinence very rarely. The operation is usually performed as a last-ditch procedure to attempt to avoid a permanent end colostomy and the results are generally felt to be unsatisfactory. Yoshioka & Keighley (1988) published an account of six cases of the gracilis sling procedure, where the operations were performed after other previously unsuccessful operations. The results were described as exceptionally disappointing and all of their patients were converted to a colostomy because of persisting incontinence.

Electrical stimulation of the anal sphincter

The concept of electrical stimulation to improve anal sphincter function was first used in Roman times to treat rectal prolapse (Kellaway, 1946). Caldwell (1963, 1965) implanted electrodes directly into the anal sphincter and used an implanted stimulator to treat rectal prolapse and faecal incontinence, and reported good results in several case reports. Hopkinson & Lightwood (1966) used an anal plug electrode to stimulate the anal sphincter transcutaneously in one patient with a good result and published a further report of nine cases (Hopkinson & Lightwood, 1967). Glen (1971) reported the use of the plug electrode in a series of 30 patients with a mixture of faecal and urinary incontinence. The overall results were described as

good. Of nine faecally incontinent patients, one was 'cured' and five 'controlled'. A report by Duthie's group (Collins *et al.*, 1969) was very critical of the results obtained in their hands by electrical stimulation of the anal sphincter with plug electrodes in faecal incontinence. Larpent *et al.* (1987) reported improvement in eight of 13 patients with faecal incontinence treated by electrical stimulation by anal plug electrodes. The use of anal sphincter stimulation to improve faecal continence has not become a generally accepted treatment as the results are inconsistent.

Direct stimulation of the anal sphincter in incontinent patients may perhaps fail as the end organ is already diseased. This problem could be avoided by stimulating healthy transposed muscle. In addition, it is now possible to transform fast-twitch fatiguable muscle to slow-twitch fatigue-resistant muscle by continuous low-frequency stimulation with an implanted pulse generator, leading to improvements in fatigue resistance (Salmons & Henriksson, 1981). After encouraging results from an electrically stimulated canine neosphincter model (Hallan *et al.*, 1990), we applied the concept of electrical stimulation to the gracilis sling procedure in patients with faecal incontinence, to activate the transposed muscle and to improve its fatigue resistance by fibre type transformation.

Electrically stimulated gracilis neoanal sphincter

Since 1988 32 patients have undergone this procedure, 20 of whom were incontinent due to a deficient sphincter mechanism (18 female, 2 male; median age 49.5 years, range 28–76; median follow-up 15 months, range 1–37). The remaining 12 patients have had the neoanal sphincter constructed as a part of a total reconstruction when the rectum and anal canal either had been removed by an abdominoperineal resection or was congenitally absent. Only the former group will be discussed in this chapter.

The aetiology of the incontinence in the 20 patients is shown in Table 26.2. Most (*n* = 11) of the patients in this group had undergone at least one conventional surgical procedure in an attempt to correct their incontinence (Table 26.3). In nine patients a conventional procedure was not indicated. All of the patients were severely incontinent

Table 26.2 Aetiology of incontinence of patients with faecal incontinence

Surgical trauma	3
Obstetric trauma	2
Rectal prolapse	3
Spina bifida	1
Idiopathic	9
Coloanal anastomosis	1
Ileal pouch−anal anastomosis	1
	$n = 20$

Table 26.3 Previous operations of patients

Postanal repair	9
Direct sphincter repair	1
Abdominal rectopexy	3
Gracilis sling	1

Table 26.4 Categorization of continence pre- and postoperatively in patients with a functioning neosphincter ($n = 12$)

	Preoperative	Postoperative
Category 1: Continent to solids, liquids and flatus	0	0
Category 2: Continent to solids and liquids but not flatus	0	9
Category 3: Continent to solids but occasional liquid incontinence	0	3
Category 4: Occasional incontinence of solids, frequent liquid incontinence	4	0
Category 5: Frequent episodes of incontinence of solids and liquids	8	0

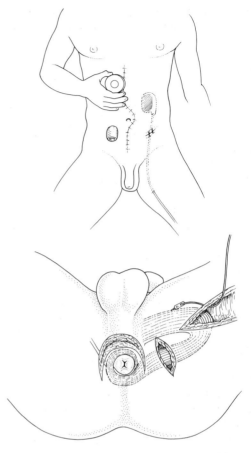

Fig. 26.1 The gracilis muscle is transposed around the anal or neoanal canal and its tendon sutured to the contralateral inferior pubic ramus. The electrode plate is sutured over the main nerve to the muscle, and the lead is connected to a totally implantable pulse generator, turned on and off with the magnet. The covering stoma is closed once muscle conversion is confirmed.

of solids and liquids (Table 26.4), and their only other option would have been a permanent colostomy.

The procedure has undergone various modifications since its inception but in essence consists of transposition of the gracilis around the deficient anal sphincter, implantation of an electrode on to the main nerve of the muscle and connection of the electrode to a totally implantable electrical pulse generator, which can be programmed by telemetry and is implanted on the chest wall (Fig. 26.1). The muscle is continually stimulated at a low frequency for a period of 8−10 weeks until evidence of transformation from fast-twitch to slow-twitch muscle has been achieved. At this stage the frequency of stimulation is increased so that the muscle contracts around the anal canal and occludes it continually. When the patient wishes to evacuate the stimulator can be switched off by passing a powerful magnet over the pulse generator, which contains a magnetic switch. Once evacuation is complete the stimulator can be turned on again by the magnet.

Of the 20 patients with incontinence treated by this technique, 12 have a functioning 'neo-sphincter'. All have been markedly improved and have avoided a permanent colostomy (Table 26.4). Of the remainder, six have failed and one is undergoing muscle transformation, and one patient died from an unrelated cause 8 months postoperation. The reasons for failure have most often been sepsis and ischaemia of the muscle. This problem occurred early in our experience. During this period, we frequently noticed that mobilization of the gracilis with division of the distal vascular pedicles resulted in ischaemia of the distal half of the gracilis muscle.

An anatomical study of the blood supply to the gracilis muscle was therefore carried out in 13 post-mortem and seven cadaveric specimens (Patel *et al.*, 1991). The results of this study demonstrated that, although the blood supply to the gracilis appeared segmental in distribution, there were intramuscular arterioarterial anastomoses between the segmental vessels. It was considered that, if the distal blood vessels were divided several weeks before transposition, these anastomotic vessels would open up and ensure viability of the distal part of the muscle.

Consequently we now delay the transposition of the gracilis for 4–6 weeks after first ligating the blood supply of the distal two-thirds of the muscle. Since we have adopted this modification, the problems of ischaemic necrosis and major sepsis have been eliminated.

The procedure is still in its infancy, and our results have recently been reported in the *Lancet* (Williams *et al.*, 1991). Baeten *et al.* (1991) have developed a similar technique in Holland and their results for the electrically stimulated gracilis neo-sphincter are similar to ours. We are cautiously optimistic that the results will continue to improve with the various modifications which have been introduced, and that the procedure will find a place in the therapy of faecal incontinence.

References

Almy T.P. & Corson J.A. (1979) Biofeedback – the light at the end of the tunnel? *Gastroenterology* **76**, 874–876.

Baeten C.G.M.I., Konsten J., Spaans F., Visser R., Habets A.M.M.C., Bourgeois I.M., Wagenmakers A.J.M. & Soeters P.B. (1991) Dynamic graciloplasty for treatment of faecal incontinence. *Lancet* **338**, 1163–1165.

Bannister J.J., Abouzerky L. & Read N.W. (1985) Overflow incontinence in the elderly faecally impacted patient. *British Journal of Surgery* **72** (Suppl.), S127.

Bartolo D.C.C., Jarratt J.A., Read M.G., Donnelly T.C. & Read N.W. (1983a) The role of partial denervation of the puborectalis in idiopathic faecal incontinence. *British Journal of Surgery* **70**, 664–667.

Bartolo D.C.C., Jarratt J.A. & Read N.W. (1983b) The use of conventional EMG to assess external sphincter neuropathy in man. *Journal of Neurology, Neurosurgery and Psychiatry* **46**, 1115–1118.

Beersiek F., Parks A.G. & Swash M. (1979) Pathogenesis of anorectal incontinence: a histometric study of the anal sphincter musculature. *Journal of the Neurological Sciences* **42**, 111–127.

Brocklehurst J.C. (1972) Bowel management in the neurologically disabled: the problems of old age. *Proceedings of the Royal Society of Medicine* **65**, 66–69.

Brocklehurst J.C. (1975) Management of anal incontinence. *Clinics in Gastroenterology* **4**, 479–487.

Brodén G., Dolk A. & Holström B. (1988) Recovery of the internal anal sphincter following rectopexy: a possible explanation for continence improvement. *International Journal of Colorectal Disease* **3**, 23–28.

Browning G.G.P. & Motson R.W. (1983) Results of Parks' operation for faecal incontinence after anal sphincter injury. *British Medical Journal* **286**, 1873–1875.

Browning G.G.P. & Parks A.G. (1983) Postanal repair for neuropathic faecal incontinence: correlation of clinical result and anal canal pressures. *British Journal of Surgery* **70**, 101–104.

Caldwell K.P.S. (1963) The electrical control of sphincter incompetence. *Lancet* **ii**, 174–175.

Caldwell K.P.S. (1965) A new treatment for rectal prolapse. *Proceedings of the Royal Society of Medicine* **58**, 12–13.

Cerulli M.A., Nikoomanesh P. & Schuster M.M. (1979) Progress in biofeedback conditioning for fecal incontinence. *Gastroenterology* **76**, 742–746.

Chittenden A.S. (1930) Reconstruction of anal sphincter by muscle slips from the glutei. *Annals of Surgery* **92**, 152–154.

Christenson J. & Kirkegaard P. (1981) Delorme's operation for complete rectal prolapse. *British Journal of Surgery* **68**, 537–538.

Christianson J. & Skomorowska E. (1987) Persisting incontinence after postanal repair treated by anterior perineoplasty. *International Journal of Colorectal Disease* **2**, 9–11.

Clarke N., Hughes A.O., Dodd K.J. *et al.* (1979) The elderly in residential care: patterns of disability. *Health Trends* **11**, 17.

Collins C.D., Brown B.H. & Duthie H.L. (1969) An assessment of intraluminal electrical stimulation for anal incontinence. *British Journal of Surgery* **56**, 542–546.

Corman M.L. (1979) Management of faecal incontinence by gracilis muscle transposition. *Diseases of the Colon and Rectum* **22**, 290–292.

Corman M.L. (1980) Follow-up evaluation of gracilis muscle transposition for fecal incontinence. *Diseases of the Colon and Rectum* **23**, 552–555.

Corman M.L. (1983) Management of anal incontinence. *Surgical Clinics of North America* **63**, 177–192.

Corman M.L. (1985) Gracilis muscle transposition for anal incontinence: late results. *British Journal of Surgery* **72** (Suppl.), 21–22.

Devlin H.B., Plant J.A. & Griffin M. (1971) Aftermath of surgery for anorectal cancer. *British Medical Journal* **3**, 413–418.

Earnshaw J.J. & Hopkinson B.R. (1987) Late results of silicone rubber perianal suture for rectal prolapse. *Diseases of the Colon and Rectum* **20**, 86–88.

Fedorov V.D. & Shelygin Y.A. (1989) Treatment of patients with rectal cancer. *Diseases of the Colon and Rectum* **32**, 138–145.

Friedman R., Muggia-Sulam J. & Freund H.R. (1983) Experience with one stage perineal repair of rectal prolapse. *Diseases of the Colon and Rectum* **26**, 789–791.

Gabriel W.B. (1948) Thiersch operation for anal incontinence. *Proceedings of the Royal Society of Medicine* **41**, 467–468.

Gilleard C.J. (1980) Prevalance of incontinence in local authority homes for the elderly. *Health Bulletin* **38** (6), 236–238.

Glen E.S. (1971) Effective and safe control of incontinence by the intra-anal plug electrode. *British Journal of Surgery* **58**, 249–252.

Goligher J.C. (1967) In *Surgery of the Anus, Rectum and Colon*, 2nd edn. Baillière, Tindall and Cassell, London.

Gordon P.H. (1987) The anorectum: anatomic and physiologic considerations in health and disease. *Gastroenterology Clinics of North America* **16**, 1–15.

Hallan R.I., Womack N.R., Waldron D.J., Morrison J.F.B. & Williams N.S. (1988) The role of rectal intussusception in the development of anal incontinence. *British Journal of Surgery* **75**, 1269.

Hallan R.I., Williams N.S., Hutton M.R.E. *et al.* (1990) Electrically stimulated sartorius neosphincter: canine model of activation and skeletal muscle transformation. *British Journal of Surgery* **77**, 208–213.

Hardcastle J.D. & Parks A.G. (1970) A study of anal incontinence and some principles of surgical management. *Proceedings of the Royal Society of Medicine* **63** (Suppl.), 116–118.

Holmstrom B., Ahlberg J., Bergstrand O., Goran B. &

Ewerth S. (1978) Results of the treatment of rectal prolapse operated according to Ripstein. *Acta Chirurgica Scandinavica Supplement* **482**, 51–52.

Hopkinson B.R. (1972) Electrical treatment of incontinence using an external stimulator with intra-anal electrodes. *Annals of the Royal College of Surgeons of England* **50**, 92–111.

Hopkinson B.R. & Lightwood R. (1966) Electrical treatment of anal incontinence. *Lancet* **i**, 297–298.

Hopkinson B.R. & Lightwood R. (1967) Electrical treatment of incontinence. *British Journal of Surgery* **54**, 802–805.

Hunt T.M., Fraser I.A. & Maybury N.K. (1985) Treatment of rectal prolapse by sphincteric support using silastic rods. *British Journal of Surgery* **72**, 491–492.

Ihre T. (1974) Studies on anal function in continent and incontinent patients. *Scandinavian Journal of Gastroenterology* **9** (Suppl. 25).

Ihre T. & Seligson U. (1975) Intussuseption of the rectum – internal procidentia: treatment and results in 90 patients. *Diseases of the Colon and Rectum* **18**, 391–396.

Keighley M.R.B. & Fielding J.W.L. (1983) Management of faecal incontinence and results of surgical treatment. *British Journal of Surgery* **70**, 463–468.

Kellaway P. (1946) The part played by electric fish in the early history of bioelectricity and electrotherapy. *Bulletin of the History of Medicine* **20**, 112–137.

Kiff E.S. & Swash M. (1984) Slowed conduction in the pudendal nerves in idiopathic (neurogenic) faecal incontinence. *British Journal of Surgery* **71**, 614–616.

Kumar D., Waldron D. & Williams N.S. (1989) Home assessment of anorectal motility and external sphincter EMG in idiopathic faecal incontinence. *British Journal of Surgery* **76**, 635–636.

Larpent J.L., Cuer J.C. & Da Poigny M. (1987) Clinical and manometric results of electrical stimulation in patients with anal incontinence. *Colo-Proctology* **9**, 183–184.

Leguit P., Van Baal J.G. & Brummelkamp W.H. (1985) Gracilis muscle transposition in the treatment of fecal incontinence. *Diseases of the Colon and Rectum* **28**, 1–4.

Leigh R.J. & Turnberg L.A. (1982) Faecal incontinence: the unvoiced symptom. *Lancet* **i**, 1349–1351.

Lubowski D.Z., Nicholls R.J., Burleigh D.R. & Swash M. (1988) Internal anal sphincter in neurogenic and faecal incontinence. *Gastroenterology* **95**, 997–1002.

McLaren S.M., McPherson F.M., Sinclair F. & Ballinger B.R. (1981) Prevalence and severity of incontinence among hospitalised female psychogeriatric patients. *Health Bulletin* **39** (3), 157–161.

MacLeod J. (1987) Management of anal incontinence by biofeedback. *Gastroenterology* **93**, 291–294.

Miller N.F. & Brown W. (1937) The surgical treatment of complete perineal tears in the female. *American Journal of Obstetrics and Gynecology* **34**, 196–209.

Miller R., Bartolo D.C.C., Cervero F. & Mortensen

N.J.McC. (1987) Anorectal temperature sensation: a comparison of normal and incontinent patients. *British Journal of Surgery* **74**, 511–515.

Miller R., Bartolo D.C.C., Locke-Edmunds J.C. & Mortensen N.J.McC. (1988) Prospective study of conservative and operative treatment for faecal incontinence. *British Journal of Surgery* **75**, 101–105.

Morgan C.N., Porter N.H. & Klugman D.J. (1972) Ivalon (polyvinyl alcohol) sponge in the repair of complete rectal prolapse. *British Journal of Surgery* **59**, 841–846.

Neill M.E. & Swash M. (1980) Increased motor unit fibre density in the external anal sphincter muscle in anorectal incontinence: a single fibre EMG study. *Journal of Neurology, Neurosurgery and Psychiatry* **43**, 343–347.

Neill M.E., Parks A.G. & Swash M. (1981) Physiological studies of the anal sphincter musculature in faecal incontinence and rectal prolapse. *British Journal of Surgery* **68**, 531–536.

Palmer K.R., Corbett C.L. & Holdsworth C.D. (1980) Double-blind cross-over study comparing loperamide, codeine and diphenoxylate in the treatment of chronic diarrhoea. *Gastroenterology* **79**, 1272–1275.

Parks A.G. (1967) Postanal perineorraphy for rectal prolapse. *Proceedings of the Royal Society of Medicine* **60**, 920–921.

Parks A.G. (1975) Anorectal incontinence. *Proceedings of the Royal Society of Medicine* **68**, 681–690.

Parks A.G. & McPartlin J.F. (1971) Late repairs of injuries of the anal sphincter. *Proceedings of the Royal Society of Medicine* **64**, 1187–1189.

Parks A.G. & Percy J.K. (1983) Postanal pelvic floor repair for anorectal incontinence. In Todd I.P. & Fielding L.P. (eds) *Rob and Smith's Operative Surgery – Alimentary Tract and Abdominal Wall, Vol. 3, Colon, Rectum and Anus*, pp. 433–438. Butterworths, London.

Parks A.G., Porter N.H. & Hardcastle J. (1966) The syndrome of the descending perineum. *Proceedings of the Royal Society of Medicine* **59**, 477–482.

Parks A.G., Swash M. & Urich H. (1977) Sphincter denervation in anorectal incontinence and rectal prolapse. *Gut* **18**, 656–665.

Patel J., Shanahan D., Riches D.J., Sinnatamby C.S., Williams N.S. & Watkins E.S. (1991) The arterial anatomy and surgical relevance of the human gracilis muscle. Abstract. *Journal of Anatomy* **176**, 270–272.

Penfold J.C.B. & Hawley P.R. (1972) Experiences with Ivalon sponge implant for complete rectal prolapse at St Mark's Hospital, 1960–1970. *British Journal of Surgery* **59**, 846–848.

Phillips S.F. & Edwards D.A.W. (1965) Some aspects of anal continence and defaecation. *Gut* **6**, 396–406.

Pickrell K.L., Broadbent T.R., Masters F.W. & Metzger J. (1952) Construction of a rectal sphincter and restoration of anal continence by transplanting the gracilis muscle:

report of four cases in children. *Annals of Surgery* **135**, 853–862.

Pickrell K., Masters F., Georgiade N. & Horton C. (1954) Rectal sphincter reconstruction using gracilis muscle transplant. *Plastic and Reconstructive Surgery* **13**, 46–55.

Pickrell K., Georgiade N., Maguire C., Crawford H. & Durham N.C. (1956) Gracilis muscle transplant for rectal incontinence. *Surgery* **40**, 349–363.

Plumley P. (1966) A modification to Thiersch's operation for rectal prolapse. *British Journal of Surgery* **53**, 624–625.

Rappert E. (1952) Plasticher Ersatz des Musculus sphincter ani. *Zentralblatt für Chirurgi* **77**, 579–581.

Read M.G., Read N.W., Barber D.C. & Duthie H.L. (1982) Effect of loperamide on anal sphincter function in patients complaining of chronic diarrhoea with faecal incontinence and urgency. *Digestive Diseases and Science* **27**, 807–813.

Read N.W., Harford W.V., Schmulen A.C., Read M.G., Santa Ana C. & Fordtran J.S. (1979) A clinical study of patients with fecal incontinence and diarrhea. *Gastroenterology* **76**, 747–756.

Roe A.M., Bartolo D.C.C. & Mortensen N.J.McC. (1986) New method for assessment of anal sensation in various anorectal disorders. *British Journal of Surgery* **73**, 310–312.

Rogers J. & Jeffery P.J. (1987) Postanal repair and intersphincteric Ivalon sponge rectopexy for the treatment of rectal prolapse. *British Journal of Surgery* **74**, 384–386.

Rogers J., Henry M.M. & Misiewicz J.J. (1988a) Combined sensory and motor deficit in primary neuropathic faecal incontinence. *Gut* **29**, 5–9.

Rogers J., Hayward M.P., Henry M.M. & Misiewicz J.J. (1988b) Temperature gradient between the rectum and anal canal: evidence against the role of temperature sensation as a sensory modality in the anal canal of normal subjects. *British Journal of Surgery* **75**, 1083–1085.

Salmons S. & Henriksson J. (1981) The adaptive response of skeletal muscle to increased use. *Muscle and Nerve* **4**, 94–105.

Schuster M.M. (1977) Biofeedback for fecal incontinence. *Journal of the American Medical Association* **238**, 2595–2596.

Smith G. & Linton J.R. (1929) Complete laceration of the perineum. *Surgery, Gynaecology and Obstetrics* **49**, 702–705.

Stephens F.D. & Smith E.D. (1971) *Anorectal Malformations in Children*. Year Book Medical Publishers, Chicago.

Stone H.B. (1929) Plastic operation for anal incontinence. *Archives of Surgery, Chicago* **18**, 845–851.

Swash M., Gray A., Lubowski D. & Nicholls R.J. (1988) Ultrastructural changes in internal anal sphincter in neurogenic faecal incontinence. *Gut* **29**, 1692–1698.

Theurkauf F.J., Beahrs O.H. & Hill J.R. (1970) Rectal prolapse: causation and surgical treatment. *Annals of Surgery* **171**, 819–835.

Thomas T.M., Egan M., Walgrove A. & Meade T.W. (1984) The prevalence of faecal and double incontinence. *Community Medicine* **6**, 216–220.

Williams N.S., Patel J., George B.D., Hallan R.I. & Watkins E.S. (1991) Development of an electrically stimulated neoanal sphincter. *Lancet* **338**, 1166–1169.

Womack N.R., Morrison J.F.B. & Williams N.S. (1986) The role of pelvic floor denervation in the aetiology of idiopathic faecal incontinence. *British Journal of Surgery* **73**, 404–407.

Womack N.R., Morrison J.F.B. & Williams N.S. (1989) Anal continence depends on sphincter recruitment by stress rather than absolute sphincter strength. *British Journal of Surgery* **76**, 636.

Wreden R.R. (1929) A method of reconstructing a voluntary sphincter ani. *Archives of Surgery, Chicago* **18**, 841–844.

Yoshioka K. & Keighley M.R.B. (1988) Clinical and manometric assessment of gracilis muscle transplant for fecal incontinence. *Diseases of the Colon and Rectum* **31**, 767–769.

Yoshioka K. & Keighley M.R.B. (1989) Critical evaluation of the quality of continence after postanal repair for faecal incontinence. *British Journal of Surgery* **76**, 1054–1057.

27: Rehabilitation of the Patient with Persistent Pain

D.M. LONG

The three views of chronic pain, 394
  The medical model, 394
  The behavioural approach to pain, 395
  The cognitive—affective concept of pain, 395
The chronic pain syndrome, 395
  The patients complaining of chronic pain, 396
  Clinical features of the chronic pain syndrome, 396
  Diagnostic and therapeutic individualization, 397
  Diagnosis of the pain-producing problem, 398
  Diagnostic testing, 399
  Use of diagnostic blocks, 399
  The diagnosis, 400
  The psychosocial examination, 400
  The final diagnosis and therapeutic plan, 401
  The in-patient programme, 402
  Reparative surgery and specific treatments for pain, 403
  The use of spinal cord stimulation, brain stimulation
    and intrathecal narcotics in otherwise intractable
    pain, 403
Discussion, 404

Evaluation and treatment of the patient complaining of pain has changed dramatically in the past 10 years. Ten years ago, the number of specialists interested in this frustrating field was small. There were few specialized centres for pain therapy. The principles of evaluation and treatment of these patients were relatively simple, but were not necessarily based upon a thorough understanding of pain as a medical problem (Crue *et al.*, 1976; Bonica, 1977; Addison, 1980; Crue & Pinsky, 1981; Booij, 1984).

The changes that have occurred in the past 10 years reflect both positive and negative influences in pain therapy. There have been enormous advances in diagnosis and specific treatments for some pain disorders (Long, 1987; Hardy, 1990). Psychiatric, socio-economic, and drug-related comorbidities are understood much better than they were at one time. There has been real dissemination of much of this information into the medical literature. On the other hand, pain has developed as an interest of many who are not necessarily expert in the field. There has been a proliferation of pain treatment programmes without much attention to the outcome of therapy from these units. While most experts hold the multidisciplinary approach to be the best, few true multispeciality programmes exist. Much is done in the name of the so-called 'pain treatment centre' which is narrowly based and ineffectual (East Central Michigan Health Systems Agency, 1978; Pepitone-Rockwell *et al.*, 1979; Long, 1981; Ghia & Sugioka, 1982; Ghia, 1983; Hannenberg & McArthur, 1983; Pernak, 1984; Gambone & Reiter, 1990).

The three views of chronic pain

In order to understand the changes that have occurred and determine which are salutary and which cannot be demonstrated to be of value, it is important to understand the three general concepts that underlie the major approaches to pain therapy.

The medical model

In this model pain is treated as a disease. The initial goal is to make an accurate diagnosis of the cause of the pain. Specific treatment is then instituted to relieve the pain. It is assumed that after relief of pain the patient will resume a normal, useful existence. If specific treatments are not available, then non-specific techniques may be employed. Co-morbidities are generally ignored. Virtually all general medical care based upon the complaint of pain naturally follows the medical model. In the best pain treatment programmes, which utilize accurate diagnosis as the foundation for therapy, the co-morbidities are not ignored. Depression, anxiety and other psychiatric problems are recognized and diagnosed. Drug misuse or abuse is corrected. The social and economic consequences of the patient's personality and behaviour and the illness are all recognized and treated. Unfortunately, this comprehensive approach is rarely evident in the general medical care these patients receive. Furthermore, a substantial number of units that style themselves pain treatment centres utilize only the medical model in one form or another (International Association for the Study of Pain, 1986; Andy, 1987; Horenstein, 1989).

The behavioural approach to pain

In this model the actual pain-producing process is less important than the consequent behaviour (Anderson et al., 1977; Keefe & Gil, 1986). Pain therapy generally consists of an attempt to reduce negative pain behaviour which has detrimental side-effects for the patient. Behaviour which is at least more acceptable to the therapist is encouraged. Behavioural therapy is an important part of virtually every major multidisciplinary pain programme. It is the only focus of some.

The cognitive–affective concept of pain

In this theory of pain the relevant variables in the pain equation are the person's personality, reactions to stress, coping styles and similar specific attributes. Dealing with pain is primarily an attempt to alter these factors rather than treat the pain process (Houpt et al., 1984).

Competent pain treatment centres generally emphasize one of these three approaches and the best use elements of all. Unfortunately, in the United States at least, there has been a proliferation of self-styled pain treatment centres in which these philosophical and practical bases are not recognized or not realized. Some emphasize only a few, even one, treatment modality. Outcome studies are few, costs are high, and there is significant disenchantment with the concept of specialized therapy for pain because of the number of therapists who do

not utilize what has been learned about pain as a medical problem in the past 20 years (Perl et al., 1985).

The chronic pain syndrome

The appellation 'pain patient' is odious throughout the world. Health professionals everywhere recognize the description of an unpleasant complaining patient who fails to improve, manipulates the therapists and rarely goes away. When such patients do leave, they generally do so in anger and a series of complaints, even lawsuits, then occur (Stieg, 1987). These patients are miserable themselves, frustrating to therapists who like to see patients improve and extremely costly both in terms of medical care and the costs of disability.

It is equally clear that there are many patients with painful states who do not develop this syndrome. These individuals with similar diseases seem to function in spite of their pain and respond well to treatment (Long et al., 1988).

There is a broad spectrum of patients presenting with the complaint of pain. On one end of this continuum is the patient with a straightforward pain-producing problem who needs only pain relief to be completely functional again. On the other end is the patient whose complaint of pain is an expression of psychiatric disease without any organic basis. Between lie a diverse group of patients, alike only in that they have a complaint of pain, but who have many different levels of co-morbidity. It is the business of the pain treatment centre to provide a medical diagnosis for these patients and assess co-morbidities and individualized treatments according to individual needs (Black, 1975; Addison, 1984; Crook et al., 1986).

The day of the stereotyped programme applying a set of rules for the management of all pain problems is now past (Long, 1981). Such programmes were useful during the time we were learning about chronic pain, but no longer represent the best that pain treatment has to offer. No doubt the kind of programme that I describe now will suffer the same fate as our knowledge of chronic pain states increases (East Central Michigan Health Systems Agency, 1978; Ghia & Sugioka, 1982; Ghia, 1983; Hannenberg & McArthur, 1983; Gambone & Reiter, 1990).

The patients complaining of chronic pain

In this discussion I will not consider the patient suffering pain of neoplastic disease. They represent very different management problems. It is the patient who complains of incapacitating pain complicating non-lethal disease and is unresponsive to standard medical therapies that presents the major problem.

In the United States the preponderance of patients incapacitated by persistent pain of non-neoplastic disease suffer from pain of spinal origin (Ritterhoff, 1975; Long, 1984; Carron *et al.*, 1985; Archer & Awwad, 1986; Tollison *et al.*, 1989). Another very large group have pain from peripheral nerve injury. There are other patients with highly specific complaints who do not come to pain programmes routinely, but who also represent large categories of pain-sufferers. Patients with known generalized arthritis are one such group. Patients suffering from chronic headache are almost as numerous as those complaining of back or neck pain. Women complaining of pelvic pain are another sizeable group. Such patients are usually managed in specialized programmes, but, when they develop the chronic pain syndrome, they may require comprehensive management. (The diagnoses made in a sequential group of patients referred to our chronic pain treatment programme are found in Table 27.1.)

Clinical features of the chronic pain syndrome

It is worth stressing the clinical features of the chronic pain syndrome (Reuler *et al.*, 1980; Erskine & Melvill, 1981; Evans, 1984; Lipowski, 1990). The first unifying symptom is a complaint of incapacitating pain. Most of these patients are seriously limited in vocational and self-care areas. This incapacitation is based upon the complaint of pain, not demonstrable physical impairment, in most patients. In our evaluation of more than 1500 such patients, there was no relationship between physical impairment and the vocational status of the patient.

These patients also exhibit predictable patterns of prescription drug utilization. In the United States the majority take substantial amounts of narcotics.

Table 27.1 Patients by diagnostic category

	Patients
Total admissions (1977–1982)	1541
Principal diagnoses	
Pain of Spinal Origin – 67% of total	1032
Low back and leg pain with multiple operations	826
Low back and leg pain without multiple operations	52
Neck and arm pain with multiple operations	102
Neck and arm pain without multiple operations	31
Other spinal pain	21
Pain of non-spinal origin – 33% of total	509
Pain of peripheral nerve origin	77
Pain of central nervous system origin	30
Cancer	15
Abdominal pain	16
Other physical cause	63
Apparent psychiatric origin	231
Unknown	77

Clear addiction with drug-seeking behaviour is relatively rare, occurring in no more than 10–15%. However, the majority of patients take narcotics in amounts beyond those usually prescribed for acute pain relief. The side-effects of narcotic administration, particularly inanition, are common. An equal number of patients utilize psychotropic drugs. Diazepam or its relatives are the most common. The side-effects of prolonged diazepam ingestion are commonly seen. Withdrawal symptoms occur in the majority of patients when both of these drugs are eliminated. It is increasingly unusual for patients to be intoxicated on these medications, but dependence is common (Hendler *et al.*, 1980).

Anxiety and depression are common concomitants of chronic pain. The patients exhibit typical vegetative signs of depression, particularly insomnia.

Patients also exhibit the typical stages of chronic disease in varying degrees. Some present in the phase of desperately seeking help, no matter how unlikely the proposed therapy may be. Some are angry and in the rejecting phase. Most are depressed and in the helpless, hopeless phase. Only a small number present with a rational understanding of their problem and its potentials for treatment.

Of course, not all patients develop this full-blown symptomatology. Many sustain chronic pain for long periods of time without developing the chronic pain syndrome. It has been popular to state that pain lasting longer than some specific period of time, 6 months to 1 year being the average, results in the chronic pain syndrome. Our studies of more than 5000 patients with low back pain suggests that this is not true at all. There was no evidence that pain lasting years produced this syndrome. Nor does the evidence suggest that the severity of the pain is related. In an examination of 1541 patients presenting with the chronic pain syndrome, the most serious disabilities were found among those complaining of back or neck pain without demonstrable physical impairments.

What are the characteristics that seem to be correlated with the development of the problem (Pilowsky et al., 1977; Pinsky, 1978; deFigueiredo et al., 1980; Pelz & Merskey, 1982; Muse, 1985, 1986; Burloux et al., 1989)? It is my belief that personality vulnerabilities are more important than the pain itself. This concept has developed from extensive studies done on more than 2500 patients with the chronic pain syndrome who were admitted to an in-patient programme for examination and therapy. All of these patients were examined by a psychiatrist, a clinical psychologist, an experimental psychologist, social workers, vocational specialists and psychiatric nurses. All underwent a thorough physical examination as well. In addition to the psychosocial interviews, the patients took an extensive battery of psychological tests, which included, as a minimum, intelligence testing, the McGill pain questionnaire, the California personality inventory and the Beck, Eysenck and Pilowsky tests. The Minnesota multiphasic examination was given to many and the Folstein minimental examination and the Hendler pain questionnaire were also employed with a large number.

Collation of these extensive psychological evaluations with complete physical examination overseen by a neurosurgeon, with appropriate consultants, produced four separate categories of patients. Remember, all of these patients exhibited the symptoms of the chronic pain syndrome in greater or lesser degree.

The first group comprised 15–20% of the total. These patients were given a psychiatric diagnosis and had no apparent physical reason for their pain complaint. Endogenous depression, somatiform disorder and manic–depressive disease were the most common diagnoses. Anxiety disorders, schizophrenia and agoraphobia were all identified less frequently. A broad spectrum of other individual diagnoses were made infrequently.

Approximately 30% of the patients were found to have a straightforward, diagnosable physical condition, reasonably associated with incapacitating pain and significant physical impairment. The spectrum of this disease was equally large. It included peripheral nerve injury, spinal cord injury, brain injury, trigeminal neuralgia, previously undiagnosed cancer, metabolic arthropathy and cardiac and visceral disease. Of this group of patients, 85% suffered from back or neck problems. In the majority, demonstrable abnormalities such as spondylolisthesis or complications of previous surgery correlated with the complaints of pain. This group of patients was further characterized by the absence of any premorbid psychological abnormalities. Depression and anxiety as a part of the chronic pain syndrome were present routinely.

The third major group represented 55% of the total. These were patients who had historical evidence for personality disorder or personality dysfunction which antedated the pain-producing illness. These patients were characterized by disturbance of function in virtually all spheres of their life, incapacitation by a complaint of pain and the lack of significant demonstrable physical impairment. The diagnoses in these patients were restricted to complaints of spinal pain and diagnoses such as headache, temporomandibular joint syndrome, myositis and other non-specific descriptive diagnoses. The group as a whole had pain complaints and disability out of proportion to diagnoses and impairment.

A small group of patients (5%) had pain complaints without demonstrable physical or psychiatric abnormalities.

Diagnostic and therapeutic individualization

Characterization of these broad groups of patients helps understand the problem of chronic pain as presented to a comprehensive pain treatment programme. The data have completely changed our approach. We have moved from an in-patient unit, where all patients complaining of chronic pain were grouped together, to a programme which is primarily out-patient (Carron & Rowlingson, 1980; Wang *et al.*, 1980; Arakawa, 1981). Only the need for detoxification and/or indications for psychiatric hospitalization are considered reasons for admission now. Instead of a relatively stereotyped programme based upon group therapy, group exercise and peer and staff pressure for behavioural modification, we have moved to an individualized programme based upon the complete characterization of each patient.

Diagnosis of the pain-producing problem

The key to appropriate therapy is an appropriate diagnosis (Long, 1979, 1984; Tollinson, 1984; International Association for the Study of Pain, 1986; Andy, 1987; Horenstein, 1989). The current diagnostic team includes neurologists and neurosurgeons for the initial evaluation. Consultants are used for all specialized systems, depending upon the nature of the complaints. The multidisciplinary group includes over 40 people, representing nine departments and divisions. Chief among these are neurosurgery, anaesthesiology, neurology, psychiatry, orthopaedics, general surgery, gynaecology, oral surgery, clinical psychology and experimental psychology. Physical and rehabilitative medicine plays an important role. Social services are available and psychiatric nursing liaison is a part of the resources for the programme.

Our first step in the evaluation of a patient complaining of persistent pain is to review those records of previous care which we can obtain. Review of all X-rays and imaging studies, as well as the results of other diagnostic tests, is also undertaken. We try to have these sent in advance so that the patient can be prepared for the first visit. The initial evaluation is undertaken according to the apparent needs of the patient. Various members of the team have specialized interests and the patients will be assigned according to those interests. Most commonly, patients are initially seen by a neurosurgeon or a neurologist, though specialists from other disciplines who have had primary care experience may also carry out the initial evaluation. Several of our anaesthesiologists are trained in pri-

mary diagnostic specialities as well and serve on the initial diagnostic team. If the records indicate a strong psychiatric component to the problem or there is evidence of major drug misuse, early psychiatric consultation is also planned. It may be possible to plan diagnostic testing in advance, although these tests are always modified as necessary at the time of the initial visit.

Since the majority of patients in the United States complain of low back pain or neck pain, the evaluation of these patients will be described in more detail. The principles remain the same for any other disease.

The history is more important that the physical examination. It is frequently complex and more often a psychosocial recitation than anything that relates to the actual origins of the pain. This kind of approach by the patient is the first clue to the importance of co-morbidity factors. The examiner must decide if the history is believable, consistent and commensurate with the pain process described and previously diagnosed. Exaggerated complaints and the use of emotion-laden words are important clues to the chronic pain syndrome. The history should include an evaluation of the patient's personal and vocational history. It is also important to remember that the initial history obtained may well be erroneous. Of the patients admitted to our pain treatment programme, over 60% provided major changes in the history over the course of a 2-week hospitalization. Important questions should be repeated in different form and the history retaken periodically to look for these inconsistencies and changes.

The physical examination is only marginally helpful from the diagnostic standpoint. However, it is important to determine the physical impairments which exist. General physical examination may or may not have any relevance. This must be decided on the basis of the pain complaint. The specific examination related to the pain complaint will vary according to that complaint. In some situations, such as peripheral nerve injury, the examination may be highly specific and very valuable. The typical syndrome of sympathetically dependent hyperalgesia is a good example where the history and physical examination together are virtually diagnostic of the condition. In the chronic low back syndrome it is unlikely that the examination will give the diagnosis, but the presence or absence of signs of nerve root compression or injury can be validated. The presence or absence of muscle spasm is helpful. Atrophy may help substantiate the complaint of disability. It is also important that the patient's behaviour during the examination be assessed. The signs described by Waddell are very useful. These include excessive pain behaviour, exaggerated loss of function, and excessive pain or tenderness following minor palpation or manipulation. Inconsistencies in the physical examination from one position to another or one time to another are very useful in assessing the overall patient.

At the end of the physical examination, you should have an understanding of the patient's physical abnormalities for comparison with claimed dysfunction. However, the presence of a normal examination does not mean the patient does not have pain.

Diagnostic testing

The diagnostics employed will depend entirely on the pain problem (Hoyt *et al.*, 1981; Uematsu *et al.*, 1981; Archer & Awwad, 1986; Ashburn & Fine, 1990). The basic principle should be a parsimonious examination which has the best possibility to determine potential causes for the pain complaint. Two serious errors are consistently made in the evaluation of these patients. One is failure to employ the straightforward tests which are available to evaluate the patient's complaint. The more common error is to do far more than is indicated. If enough studies are done, surely something will be abnormal. Whether the abnormalities discovered relate to the generation of pain in any significant way is a matter for expert interpretation. While it is important not to miss diagnoses which are relevant, it is equally important not to overdiagnose and to substantiate claimed pain and disability on the basis of studies whose relations to both are not certain.

Another important question is how far to carry a new diagnostic protocol on the basis of ongoing or new complaints. Repeatedly we see patients who have been evaluated over and over again. The first question concerning diagnostics is, 'Are the existing studies adequate?' If they are, there is no reason for them to be repeated. If they are not, a logical sequential evaluation should be performed. The

related question is how often should procedures be repeated when patients fail to improve. In general, there is no reason to repeat previously adequate studies simply because the patient does not improve. The question of how new complaints should be treated is more difficult. Not every new complaint deserves complete restudy with expensive imaging examinations. In general, those associated with objective physical findings or a typical constellation of symptoms can be pursued. A great deal of clinical judgement is required in making these decisions, but it is important to stress that complaints of pain alone, particularly new or different pain, do not constitute a valid reason for repeating exhaustive diagnostic studies. It is not unusual for us to see patients who have had 10 or more computerized tomography (CT), magnetic resonance imaging (MRI) and CT myelogram evaluations of the lumbar spine. All have been done for the same complaint and all have failed to show any significant cause.

The matter of how much to do in terms of diagnosis is a difficult one. Patients and frequently referring doctors press for extensive studies. Patients are particularly reassured by new studies done on new machines. Most come convinced that one more study interpreted by a different physician will undoubtedly give an answer. Part of the therapy begins with helping patients understand what evaluations are necessary, what the studies are likely to show and that no studies show pain.

With these caveats, it is important to proceed with a diagnostic programme adequate to exhaust a reasonable differential diagnosis. The high-quality imaging studies now give virtually anatomical details of the lumbar spine. Cranial and skull base imaging is equally good. Electrodiagnostics have limited utility except for peripheral nerve injury. Imaging of other organ systems, while not quite as good as with spine and head, has greatly improved and may be useful. The key to diagnosis is the exploration of important complaints by experts, who can choose the diagnostic studies appropriately. There is no excuse for a stereotyped diagnostic battery based only on complaints.

Use of diagnostic blocks

Diagnostic blockade of peripheral nerves has utility, but like many other diagnostics can be overdone.

We utilize diagnostic blocks in the following way. First, there must be a specific clinical diagnosis which constitutes a reason for the block. Haphazard application of blocks in the hopes that something may be discovered is of no use. The blocks have specific purposes. Sympathetic blockade is utilized when it appears there is a strong probability that the diagnosis is sympathetic-maintained hyperalgesia. Individual peripheral nerves are blocked when the pain distribution indicates that they may be involved. Individual roots are blocked when root injury or root compression needs to be proved. Blockade of zygapophyseal joints and pseudoar-throses may help in determining pain originating in instability.

It must be stressed that these blocks have never been proved to be of value by prospective studies. It is logical to assume they are useful, but blocks have never been shown to be predictors for therapy.

Provocative anaesthetic discography is also in vogue again. The concept is that some patients have pain secondary to disc disease. These abnormal discs can be identified by the fact that injections into them both produce pain initially and relieve pain eventually. This is an attractive logical sup-position, but has not yet been proved. Our use of these blocks currently is within an investigative framework.

There are a number of other interventional tests that can be employed. Sympathetic blockade with specific antagonists may be used instead of the traditional anaesthetic block. Intravenous local anaesthetics and intrathecal narcotics or other drugs have been employed. These are interesting studies, but have not yet been proved to be of utility in the evaluation of the typical patient with chronic pain.

The diagnosis

Our concept for rehabilitation of the patient with chronic pain, which is individualization of therapy according to the specific needs of that patient, re-quires an accurate set of diagnoses. The first step is a comprehensive physical diagnosis. This process has two phases. The first is to identify the physical abnormalities which potentially are causing the pain complaint. The second step is to determine the relationship of these physical abnormalities to the complaint of pain. It is quite possible to find a number of abnormalities which will not be different from those found in an uncomplaining general population. The simple discovery of a physical problem does not mean it is pain-producing or that it is sufficient to explain that patient's disability.

The psychosocial examination

It is clear that, whatever the physical abnormalities, psychosocial co-morbidity may be important. These aspects of the pain complaint deserve attention in all patients and require therapy in many. In my experience the key factors to be examined are drug use, illness-related disability and anxiety, the pres-ence or absence of psychiatric disease, characteris-tics of personality dysfunction, spousal relationships and vocational status (Carron et al., 1985; Gaston-Johansson et al., 1985; Hendler et al., 1985; Pilow-sky, 1986; Poulsen et al., 1987).

In our experience the best way to get at these features is through the interview process. There is a vast literature on psychological testing and pain, but no algorithm has yet been forthcoming from that literature which allows the clinician to depend upon it to characterize the patient. Rather, we use the tests to validate clinical impressions. We have found the California personality inventory, the sick-ness impact test, the McGill pain questionnaire, the Beck depression score and the Eysenck test all par-ticularly useful. However, there are many others and all have value. The use of these tests is really going to be a matter of choice for those employing them.

The psychiatric examination is more important in our formulation of a therapeutic plan. Obtaining the important information from the interview re-quires skill and understanding of the factors which are important. Acquiring these skills is fundamental to psychiatric training, but not emphasized in most of the rest of medicine. Those coming from other backgrounds will need to read the relevant literature and have an opportunity to learn how these inter-views are conducted with someone skilled in their use.

The first aspect of the interview is observing the patient. Is the patient's behaviour appropriate to the complaint? Does there appear to be wilful exaggeration? Is pain behaviour exaggerated? Are the complaints commensurate with anatomical and physiological reality? Look for the vegetative signs of depression. Is there evidence for drug intoxication? Determine what drugs the patient is taking and on what schedule. Remember that many patients will not give honest answers concerning the drugs they take or the sources from which they get them. Over 50% of our patients obtain the same drugs from multiple physicians and take significantly more of these drugs than they admit on first examination. Ask about educational background and experience. Spousal relationships are very important. Detailed vocational questions need to include whether the patient is employed or not, the presence of litigation which may influence the situation, job satisfaction and relationships with employer and fellow employees. A few questions will usually lead the patient into a spontaneous description of problems in all these areas. However, remember that many patients are well guarded and often those with the most striking dysfunction will tell the first examiner that there are no difficulties with any of the relationships.

Clues for the diagnosis of overt psychiatric illness are important. In our series of patients, endogenous depression, somatiform disorder, dipolar disease and schizophrenia are the most common psychiatric problems presenting with a complaint of pain. A true personality disorder is not unusual. We utilize psychiatric consultation regularly for patients with chronic pain. Only the most straightforward do not have the benefit of psychiatric opinion for psychosocial problems related to the pain complaint.

At the end of the combination of interview, consultation and testing, it should be possible to define the patient's premorbid and current status.

The final diagnosis and therapeutic plan

In our programme we combine the physical abnormalities and the psychosocial characteristics of the patient to identify all of the areas in which that particular patient needs help and so individualize a treatment plan for each patient. There are some fundamental principles which apply to most patients, but no aspect of the plan is stereotyped.

Once this list of physical and psychosocial problems is produced, the first step is to determine if the physical pain-producing problem is amenable to treatment. Is there a reparative surgery which will correct the spinal or peripheral nerve pathology? Is there a specific treatment, such as radiofrequency neurotomy for trigeminal neuralgia, which can relieve the pain? Are there medications, specific or non-specific, that may affect the patient's pain? Our general approach is to be as conservative as possible, but these questions need to be answered at the outset of therapy for, if straightforward, specific procedures do exist, they can be employed promptly.

It is more likely that non-specific symptomatic treatments will be utilized before any major intervention is contemplated. This programme consists of a specific treatment plan to reduce the consequences of the incapacitation and multiple operations that these patients have frequently experienced. It consists of physical measures to reduce pain from myositis and fasciitis; joint range of motion and tendon stretching are frequently important; strengthening little used muscles and improving general physical function is vital (Wyant, 1979; Hendler et al., 1983; Long, 1988; McCain & Scudds, 1988; Reilly & Littlejohn, 1990).

Our first step generally is the assessment of physical impairments and a conservative therapy and exercise programme designed to correct them over a period of time. Patients need to be encouraged by assuring them that the increased pain these programmes often produce is transient and will not worsen them.

At the same time, we begin a programme to bring order into the medical drug intake of the patients. Useless drugs without withdrawal potential are eliminated immediately. Then the drugs that are addictive and have negative side-effects which impede the patient's therapy are reduced. Narcotics and a variety of psychotropics are in this category. Diazepam and its derivatives are the most common psychotropic drugs which need control. We arbitrarily withdraw these drugs over a 10–14 day period. A reasonable rule is 10% per day, but the speed with which the withdrawal proceeds must be judged by the patient's symptomatology. Patients who have taken these drugs for long periods of time often require a much slower withdrawal (Spector, 1981; Egbunike & Chaffee, 1990).

Narcotics are treated in the same way. Injectables are changed to oral medications, usually methadone, in equivalent doses. Otherwise, patients are withdrawn from whatever drug they are taking. The issue of narcotic use for pain control in these patients is a difficult one to settle, based upon data currently available (Brodner & Taub, 1978; Hendler *et al.*, 1980). Our experience is that these patients are not relieved of pain by their narcotic ingestion. All continue to seek help and come to the pain treatment centre for pain control. Our experience with these withdrawal programmes now extends over 20 years. Withdrawal has been accomplished in 90% of patients. Approximately 10% sign themselves out of the programme upon learning they would have to withdraw from their medications. Less than 10% of those withdrawn from narcotics believe their pain to be worse after withdrawal than it was with the drug. An almost equivalent number discovered their pain was better after withdrawal. These two figures are commensurate with long-term placebo and nocebo effect. For these reasons we insist upon withdrawal from narcotics as a part of the initial programme. This does not mean that narcotic maintenance may not be chosen as the best treatment for the pain eventually.

Patients who are intoxicated or who show obvious drug-seeking behaviour are more difficult to manage. Withdrawal should always be undertaken on an in-patient basis for those with obvious signs of intoxication. Those truly addicted who demonstrate drug-seeking behaviour are a minority, but a difficult one. They are managed on an in-patient basis and have referral for follow-up to one of the organized drug withdrawal programmes in the area.

At the same time that drug withdrawal and physical rehabilitation begin, we also treat the depression and anxiety which are ubiquitous in this syndrome. Tricyclic antidepressants have been shown to have pain-relieving potential and therefore we still use them in many patients. There are a number of other excellent antidepressants and the choice is really left to the preference of the therapist and the side-effect produced in the patients. Anxiety rarely requires separate therapy. Patients learn to manage anxiety through relaxation techniques and biofeedback. A small number of patients can actually control pain through these modalities.

A key decision is whether this early therapy needs to be done on an in-patient basis or not. We use out-patient programmes for most patients.

However, those taking large amounts of drugs, those who exhibit either intoxication or drug-seeking behaviour and those with serious depression are all admitted for intensive treatment.

In-patient care is still useful for patients with significant behavioural abnormalities, particularly those who are distressed by their pain to the point of an incapacitation which is out of character with the demonstrated findings.

The in-patient programme

Patients are hospitalized as a group to take advantage of the opportunities for group therapy and group process (Houpt *et al.*, 1984). Drug withdrawal is begun immediately. The patients are withdrawn from the potentially harmful drugs they are taking. The programme is discussed in detail, the schedule is discussed with the patient and the reasons for the elimination of certain classes of drugs is presented. The usual withdrawal programme requires 10–14 days and includes elimination of habituating psychotropics as well as narcotics.

Depression and anxiety, when present, are treated immediately. Utilizing antidepressants at bedtime takes advantage of the sedative effect of some of these drugs and helps restore a normal sleep pattern. Insomnia is often a serious problem for these patients.

A physical therapy assessment is undertaken and a group exercise programme begun. Individual exercises are also prescribed.

Transcutaneous electrical stimulation and passive measures, such as heat massage, stretching and ultrasound, are used for relief of muscle spasm, myositis and fasciitis.

The patient's ability to perform activities of daily living is assessed and help given so that these patients can be more effective in caring for themselves and doing the things they need to do for support.

Nursing support is limited. The patients are expected to engage in self-care and the programme is specifically designed to have them do such things as make their own bed, get meal trays, eat together as a group, dress themselves and take responsibility for attendance at activities.

Selected patients are taught biofeedback and relaxation techniques to help them both tolerate and control their pain. Educational programmes in the anatomy and physiology of pain, spinal anatomy and physiology, the theory of exercise, dietetics, weight control and drug use are provided.

Physician rounds are made daily and the patients meet at least once weekly with the entire treatment team. The pain group meets weekly and selected patients are presented for discussion and decision-making.

Diagnostic procedures are limited during this in-patient stay. Whenever possible, most diagnostics are done on an out-patient basis before the programme begins so that the patient will not be deflected from the goals of the programme.

There is a problem inherent in a single in-patient facility which needs to be addressed. Some of the patients are potentially candidates for specific or non-specific surgical therapies, but have drug, personality and behavioural issues which need attention before a procedure. Other patients have no procedures available to them and, in some of these, the only issues are those of drugs and psychosocial factors. It has been our experience that, when these patients are combined, it is counter-productive. Those who know they may have a procedure planned do not participate fully in the programme. Those who have no procedures participate less well because they become convinced that something will be found that can be done. Both groups of patients do less well than they should if they focus only upon the comprehensive programme. For that reason, we generally do not make decisions concerning treatment until after the patients who require this type of intensive in-patient care have completed it. Once they have reached maximum benefit, consideration can be given to a procedure. Therefore, we do not discuss reparative surgery or spinal cord stimulation until after the response to the pain treatment programme is seen.

Reparative surgery and specific treatments for pain

For some patients with spinal and peripheral nerve problems, there will be direct surgery which may be useful (Long *et al.*, 1988). Specific pain-relieving procedures are also indicated for a small number of patients. The recent book by Gybels & Sweet provides an up-to-date review of those procedures and their indications. It is a basic precept of our programme to utilize these procedures when it appears that the benefit to the patient will warrant the risks. There is no reason to put a patient through the multidisciplinary comprehensive programme when they do not exhibit the features of the chronic pain syndrome which require that approach. When pain alone is the problem, it should be treated directly. When minor degrees of the various aspects of the chronic pain treatment syndrome exist, they can be managed in the course of definitive therapy. It is important not to waste time and resources on therapies that are unnecessary. It is equally important not to proceed with these specific treatments in the face of serious co-morbidity. In my experience, performing indicated surgery in patients with the full-blown pain syndrome is usually ineffective. The patients continue to be incapacitated by their co-morbidities and little is accomplished by the procedures. These procedures should be carried out when the patient's drug intake is appropriately ordered, depression and anxiety are treated, the behavioural consequences of the problem have been addressed and a thorough physical rehabilitation programme has been undertaken. If the patient's pain still needs treatment, this is the time to proceed.

The use of spinal cord stimulation, brain stimulation and intrathecal narcotics in otherwise intractable pain

Spinal cord stimulation plays an important role in the chronic pain programme (Long *et al.*, 1981; Siegfried & Lazorthes, 1982). In the United States the majority of pain-sufferers have low back pain and a substantial percentage of these have the residuals of multiple failed operations. We have recently compared the results of indicated reparative surgery and spinal cord stimulation. While our study was not prospective, the comparison suggests that spinal cord stimulation is as effective or more effective in pain control and has fewer side-effects. We utilize spinal cord stimulation as an alternative therapy for all those with the postlaminectomy syndrome who have failed the multidisciplinary approach. The patients are given a thorough trial of temporary stimulation with an implanted electrode before permanent implantation is undertaken. Only those who respond well are given the complete implant.

Experience has taught us several things which we incorporate into the overall programme. Patients who continue to take narcotics during the stimulation period cannot be assessed appropriately. We require withdrawal for several months before the stimulator is tried. Patients who do not co-operate with the multidisciplinary programme are poor candidates for any form of therapy. Some patients cannot learn what is required to make the stimulator function and they should not be considered as candidates. This is usually not a matter of intelligence, but rather personality. Patients with psychiatric diagnoses other than reactive depression are poor candidates for stimulation.

Brain stimulation is also useful in a select number of patients, principally those with central pain states. We use the same criteria for patient selection for this specialized modality.

Intrathecal pumps for the delivery of morphine and other drugs have been employed extensively with cancer pain, but sparingly for pain of benign disease. At present, our experience is limited to two patients. The technique is cumbersome, but pain relief has been satisfactory and tolerance has not been the problem that we expected. At present, the technique plays virtually no role in our comprehensive pain programme.

Discussion

Chronic pain is not synonymous with the chronic pain syndrome. Many of our patients suffer pain for many years and develop none of the drug-related or psychosocial disabilities exhibited by the patients with the chronic pain syndrome. The medical model suits them very well. They can be treated by direct or indirect methods immediately. Some patients who come complaining of chronic pain apparently have this complaint only as a symptom of psychiatric disease. Others have an underlying abnormality competent to produce a complaint of pain, but seem to be disabled beyond what seems warranted by the physical diagnoses made. All of these patients may have been given potentially harmful drugs by well-intentioned physicians. Many have undergone ineffectual direct therapies. Reactive depression and anxiety are common. Job-related stresses are common.

All of these factors must be considered in outlining a therapeutic regimen for the patient incapacitated by pain. Pain is not a diagnosis. The chronic pain syndrome is a constellation of symptoms that a group of diverse patients share, but is descriptive only. To make the diagnosis of chronic pain syndrome means nothing except a shorthand for describing patients who share some features of an otherwise heterogeneous group of complaints.

Since pain cannot be considered a diagnosis, it is impossible to treat generically. Stereotyped programmes applied only for the relief of this symptom are unlikely to be effective.

The therapeutic approach we now use for problems of persistent pain is sequential. The first step is the best diagnosis possible. Care must be taken not to emphasize diagnoses which may be true, but which are not important in the patient's overall complaint and disability. Concomitantly, a psychiatric and psychosocial evaluation is important. These patients need help in many spheres of their life and function. The contribution of drug use, depression and anxiety must considered. This can all be accomplished on an out-patient basis and rarely requires hospitalization except for specific procedures which have risks, drug withdrawal or psychiatric therapy.

The therapeutic programme should be individualized to deal with the needs of the specific patient. Virtually all these patients need an active rehabilitation programme. This programme includes the treatment of local dysfunction, such as the myositis and fasciitis which so often complicate multiple operations and prolonged disability. It also includes an exercise and educational programme to improve tolerance. For some it may be extended to work-hardening and vocational rehabilitation. The harmful effect of drug intake must be eliminated and appropriate medications chosen when indicated. These patients may need much help with personal troubles. They are often embroiled in interpersonal, social and vocational problems which they do not understand and cannot control.

It is important to recognize that depression is not pain; that psychiatric disease is not pain; that personality dysfunction is not pain. There are a few other general observations that are important.

While we focus upon an accurate physical and psychiatric diagnostic programme, we must always recognize that the fact that we do not make a diagnosis today does not mean that there is not an underlying problem which will be diagnosable in the future. The point of the physical diagnosis is not to judge whether a patient's pain complaint is real or not. We cannot determine that except by inference. The purpose is to find a disease that can be treated and to restrict hopeful treatments given for pain without anatomical or pathological cause.

It is also important to recognize how manipulative and how distressed many of these patients are. They can be extremely disruptive to any medical system. It is not unusual for individual patients to call the office and various members of the pain team many times per day. Many seem to derive satisfaction from manipulating one member of the pain team against another. It is very important that the therapeutic programme be organized in such a way that it cannot be manipulated. Clinic schedules must be maintained. Specific times for reporting and discussing results and plans are important, as are specific times for telephone contact. Drug instructions must be clear, concise and enforced in spite of patients' non-compliance. Patients who exhibit true drug-seeking behaviour and who are not controlled within the pain programme easily should be referred to addiction programmes.

One of the greatest problems is the demand of some of the patients for more and more evaluation. The physician in charge and the pain team need to know when to stop. Once everything has been done to make or exclude important physical diagnoses, it serves no useful purpose to repeat the test based simply upon new complaints. It is not unusual to see patients who have had literally dozens of MRI and CT scans. It is easy for the physician to fall into the trap of abdicating responsibility for the evaluation and simply refer the patient interminably for yet another consultation or study. One of the most important therapeutic manoeuvres for the patients who would pursue this course is to stop the evaluation when it is complete and reinstitute study only for clear medical indications. This presupposes that the study is comprehensive and skilled diagnosticians are secure in their opinions.

As long as pain is treated as a complaint, pain therapy will be ineffectual. It may be possible to modify behaviour by non-specific methods and that can have real value. Still, the lack of insistence upon accurate diagnosis serves only to continue our lack of understanding of chronic pain. Satisfactory therapy depends upon accurate diagnosis and specific reparative or symptomatic treatments. We must have thorough assessment of the patient's impairments and corrective measures to restore function are necessary. The co-morbidities must be examined. The effects of inappropriate drug use are very important and must be considered. Psychiatric and personality dysfunctions require separate evaluation and treatment. Assistance with psychosocial and vocational problems are essential for many patients, at least in the United States. There is a group of people who reject this approach and do not desire to be treated appropriately. This rejection usually relates to significant psychiatric disease.

When all of these things have been done, there remains a small group of patients who are apparently made functional by reasonable doses of narcotics and for whom no other treatment exists. It is not clear whether the narcotics truly relieve pain or simply maintain an addiction. However, the doses of drug are small; the drugs used do not have significant abuse potential (codeine and oxycodone); and the patients continue taking small doses, ranging from 15 mg to 120 mg of codeine and 15 mg to 30 mg of oxycodone per day. At present, we choose patients for narcotic maintenance by group meeting. The decision is not made by an individual. Patients are carefully monitored to be certain that there are no abuses. Our criteria are an obvious, untreatable cause of pain, failure of a comprehensive multidisciplinary evaluation and treatment plan, and function maintained by the drugs which is not possible without it. The patients are asked to sign an informed consent that they understand the ramifications of long-lasting narcotic use and they must agree to follow the directions for drug use exactly. Under these circumstances a small number are chosen for narcotic maintenance.

The past 10 years have brought an enormous increase in our understanding of the various chronic pain syndromes (Devoghel, 1980; Aronoff & Evans, 1982; Aronoff *et al.*, 1983; Fitzpatrick *et al.*, 1987). We are well past the time when stereotyped programmes which are the same for all patients complaining of pain are acceptable (Pinsky *et al.*, 1979; Hallett & Pilowsky, 1982; Kleinke & Spangler, 1988). Given our current understanding, exhaustive diagnosis followed by specific therapies as indicated by the patient's particular needs form the basis for our approach to chronic pain. Because of the complexity of the chronic pain programme, this approach, of necessity, requires a multidisciplinary unit to provide these unfortunate patients all they require for treatment (Anon., 1978; Swerdlow, 1978; Editorial, 1982; Welch, 1983; Roy, 1984; Sturgis *et al.*, 1984; Simmons *et al.*, 1988).

References

Addison R.G. (1980) Treatment of chronic pain: the Center for Pain Studies, Rehabilitation Institute of Chicago. *NIDA Research Monographs* **36**, 12–32.

Addison R.G. (1984) Chronic pain syndrome. *American Journal of Medicine* **77** (3A), 54–58.

Anderson T.P., Cole T.M., Gullickson G., Hudgens A. & Roberts A.H. (1977) Behavior modification of chronic pain: a treatment program by a multidisciplinary team. *Clinical Orthopaedics* **129**, 96–100.

Andy O.J. (1987) Chronic pain syndromes. *Applied Neurophysiology* **50** (1–6), 434–435.

Anon. (1978) The pain clinic: boon or boondoggle? *Patient Care* **12** (15), 188, 193–194, 196–197 passim.

Arakawa K. (1981) Outpatient pain clinic: review of a two-year experience. *Journal of the Kansas Medical Society* **82** (6), 292–294.

Archer C.R. & Awwad E.E. (1986) Computed tomography in the evaluation of acute and chronic low back pain syndromes commonly seen. *Seminars in Neurology* **6** (4), 350–371.

Aronoff G.M. & Evans W.O. (1982) The prediction of treatment outcome at a multidisciplinary pain center. *Pain* **14** (1), 67–73.

Aronoff G.M., Evans W.O. & Enders P.L. (1983) A review of follow-up studies of multidisciplinary pain units. *Pain* **16** (1), 1–11.

Ashburn M.A. & Fine P.G. (1990) Evaluation and treatment of chronic pain syndromes. *Comprehensive Therapy* **16** (2), 37–42.

Black R.G. (1975) The chronic pain syndrome. *Surgical Clinics of North America* **55** (4), 999–1011.

Bonica J.J. (1977) Basic principles in managing chronic pain. *Archives of Surgery* **112** (6), 783–788.

Booij L.H. (1984) Organization of a university pain centre in Amsterdam. *Applied Neurophysiology* **47** (4–6), 171–175.

Brodner R.A. & Taub A. (1978) Chronic pain exacerbated by long-term narcotic use in patients with nonmalignant disease: clinical syndrome and treatment. *Mount Sinai Journal of Medicine* **45** (2), 233–237.

Burloux G., Forestier P., Dalery J. & Guyotat J. (1989) Chronic pain and posttraumatic stress disorders. *Psychotherapy and Psychosomatics* **52** (1–3), 119–124.

Carron H. & Rowlingson J.C. (1980) Coordinated outpatient management of chronic pain at the University of Virginia Pain Clinic. *NIDA Research Monographs* **36**, 84–91.

Carron H., DeGood D.E. & Tait R. (1985) A comparison of low back pain patients in the United States and New Zealand: psychosocial and economic factors affecting severity of disability. *Pain* **21** (1), 77–89.

Crook J., Tunks E., Rideout E. & Browne G. (1986) Epidemiologic comparison of persistent pain sufferers in a specialty pain clinic and in the community. *Archives of Physical and Medical Rehabilitation* **67** (7), 451–455.

Crue B.L. & Pinsky J.J. (1981) Chronic pain syndrome four aspects of the problem: New Hope Pain Center and Pain Research Foundation. *NIDA Research Monographs* **36**, 137–168.

Crue B.L., Pinsky J.J., Agnew D.C. *et al.* (1976) What is a pain center? *Bulletin of the Los Angeles Neurological Society* **41** (4), 160–167.

deFigueiredo J.M., Baiardi J.J. & Long D.M. (1980) Briquet syndrome in a man with chronic intractable pain. *The Johns Hopkins Medical Journal* **147**, 102–106.

Devoghel J.C. (1980) A pain clinic: the first thousand cases. *Acta Anaesthesiologica Belgica* **31** (Suppl.), 197–202.

East Central Michigan Health Systems Agency (1978) *Report of the Task Force on 'Pain Centers'*, p. 32. East Central Michigan Health Systems Agency, Inc., Saginaw.

Editorial (1982) The work of a pain clinic. *Lancet* **i** (8270), 486–487.

Egbunike I.G. & Chaffee B.J. (1990) Antidepressants in the management of chronic pain syndromes. *Pharmacotherapy* **10** (4), 262–270.

Erskine W.A. & Melvill R.L. (1981) Chronic pain problems: experience in a pain clinic. *South African Medical Journal* **59** (24), 859–860.

Evans W.O. (1984) The chronic pain syndrome: its evaluation and treatment. *PRN Forum* **3** (5), 1–3.

Fitzpatrick R.M., Bury M., Frank A.O. & Donnelly T. (1987) Problems in the assessment of outcome in a back pain clinic. *International Disabilities Studies* **9** (4), 161–165.

Gambone J.C. & Reiter R.C. (1990) Nonsurgical management of chronic pelvic pain: a multidisciplinary approach. *Clinical Obstetrics and Gynecology* **33** (1), 205–211.

Gaston-Johansson F., Johansson G., Felldin R. & Sanne H. (1985) A comparative study of pain description, emotional discomfort and health perception in patients with chronic pain syndrome and rheumatoid arthritis. *Scandinavian Journal of Rehabilitation Medicine* **17** (3), 109–119.

Ghia J.N. (1983) The organization of a pain center. *Journal of Ambulatory Care Management* **6** (3), 66–77.

Ghia J.N. & Sugioka K. (1982) Are pain centers viable? *North Carolina Medical Journal* **43** (7), 493–495.

Hallett E.C. & Pilowski I. (1982) The response to treatment in a multidisciplinary pain clinic. *Pain* **12** (4), 365–374.

Hannenberg A.A. & McArthur J.D. (1983) Establishing a pain clinic. *International Anesthesiology Clinics* **21** (4), 1–10.

Hardy P.A. (1990) The role of the pain clinic in the management of the terminally ill. *British Journal of Hospital Medicine* **43** (2), 142–146.

Hendler N., Cimini C., Ma T. & Long D.M. (1980) A comparison of cognitive impairment due to benzodiazepines and to narcotics. *American Journal of Psychiatry* **137**, 828–830.

Hendler N., Fink H. & Long D. (1983) Myofascial syndrome: response to trigger-point injections. *Psychosomatics* **24** (11), 990–999.

Hendler N.H., Mollett A., Viernstein M. *et al.* (1985) A comparison between the MMPI and the 'Hendler Back Pain Test' for validating the complaint of chronic back pain in men. *Journal of Neurological and Orthopaedic Medicine and Surgery* **6** (4), 333–337.

Horenstein S. (1989) Chronic low back pain and the failed low back syndrome. *Neurological Clinics* **7** (2), 361–385.

Houpt J.L., Keefe F.J. & Snipes M.T. (1984) The Clinical Specialty Unit: the use of the psychiatry inpatient unit to treat chronic pain syndromes. *General Hospital Psychiatry* **6** (1), 65–70.

Hoyt W.H., Hunt H.H. Jr, DePauw M.A. *et al.* (1981) Electromyographic assessment of chronic low back pain syndrome. *Journal of the American Osteopathic Association* **80** (11), 728–730.

International Association for the Study of Pain, Subcommittee on Taxonomy (1986) Classification of chronic pain: Descriptions of chronic pain syndromes and definitions of pain terms. *Pain* Suppl. 3, S1–S226.

Keefe F.J. & Gil K.M. (1986) Behavioral concepts in the analysis of chronic pain syndromes. *Journal of Consultative and Clinical Psychology* **54** (6), 776–783.

Kleinke C.L. & Spangler A.S. Jr (1988) Predicting treatment outcome of chronic back pain patients in a multidisciplinary pain clinic: methodological issues and treatment implications. *Pain* **33** (1), 41–48.

Lipowski Z.J. (1990) Chronic idiopathic pain syndrome. *Annals of Medicine* **22** (4), 213–217.

Long D.M. (1979) Evaluation and treatment of the 'multiple surgery' low-back cripple. *Contemporary Neurosurgery* **17**, 1–6.

Long D.M. (1981) A comprehensive model for the study of therapy of pain: Johns Hopkins Pain Research and Treatment Program. In Ng L.K.Y. (ed.) *New Approaches to Treatment of Chronic Pain: a Review of Multidisciplinary Pain Clinics and Pain Centers*, pp. 66–75.

Long D.M. (1984) The chronic low back cripple. In Scheinberg P. (ed.) *Neurology and Neurosurgery Update Series*, Vol. 5 (10).

Long D.M. (1987) Acute and chronic pain. In Davis J.H., Drucker W.R., Foster R.S. *et al.* (eds) *Clinical Surgery*, Vol. 1, Chapter 17, pp. 509–534. C.V. Mosby, St Louis, Missouri.

Long D.M. (1988) Nonsurgical therapy for low back pain and sciatica. *Clinical Neurosurgery* **35** (18), 351–359.

Long D.M., Erickson D., Campbell J. & North R. (1981) Electrical stimulation of the spinal cord and peripheral nerves for pain control: a 10-year experience. *Applied Neurophysiology* **44**, 207–217.

Long D.M., Filtzer D.L., BenDebba M. & Hendler N.H. (1988) Clinical features of the failed-back syndrome. *Journal of Neurosurgery* **69**, 61–71.

McCain G.A. & Scudds R.A. (1988) The concept of primary fibromyalgia (fibrositis): clinical value, relation and significance to other chronic musculoskeletal pain syndromes. *Pain* **33** (3), 273–287.

Muse M. (1985) Stress-related, posttraumatic chronic pain syndrome: criteria for diagnosis, and preliminary report on prevalence. *Pain* **23** (3), 295–300.

Muse M. (1986) Stress-related, posttraumatic chronic pain syndrome: behavioral treatment approach. *Pain* **25** (3), 389–394.

Pelz M. & Merskey H. (1982) A description of the psychological effects of chronic painful lesions. *Pain* **14** (3), 293–301.

Pepitone-Rockwell F, Rosenblatt R. & Corkill G. (1979) Pain clinic model for community practice. *Western Journal of Medicine* **131** (2), 166–170.

Perl E.R., Covino B.G., Fields H.L. *et al.* (1985) *Report of the Research Briefing Panel on Pain and Pain Management*, Research Briefings 1985, pp. 20–32. National Academy of Sciences, National Academy of Engineering, Institute of Medicine, National Academy Press, Washington, DC.

Pernak J.M. (1984) A pain clinic in a small regional hospital – yes or no? *Applied Neurophysiology* **47** (4–6), 188–194.

Pilowsky I. (1986) Abnormal illness behaviour (dysnosognosia). *Psychotherapy and Psychosomatics* **46** (1–2), 76–84.

Pilowsky I., Chapman C.R. & Bonica J.J. (1977) Pain, depression, and illness behavior in a pain clinic population. *Pain* **4** (2), 183–192.

Pinsky J.J. (1978) Chronic, intractable, benign pain: a syndrome and its treatment with intensive short-term group psychotherapy. *Journal of Human Stress* **4** (3), 17–21.

Pinsky J.J., Griffin S.E., Agnew D.C., Kamdar M.D., Crue B.L. & Pinsky L.H. (1979) Aspects of long-term evaluation of pain unit treatment program for patients with chronic intractable benign pain syndrome: treatment outcome. *Bulletin of the Los Angeles Neurological Society* **44** (1–4 Spec. Ed.), 53–69.

Poulsen D.L., Hansen H.J., Langemark M., Olesen J. & Bech P. (1987) Discomfort or disability in patients with chronic pain syndrome. *Psychotherapy and Psychosomatics* **48** (1–4), 60–62.

Reilly P.A. & Littlejohn G.O. (1990) Fibrositis/fibromyalgia syndrome: the key to the puzzle of chronic pain. *Medical Journal of Australia* **152** (5), 226–228.

Reuler J.B., Girard D.E. & Nardone D.A. (1980) The chronic pain syndrome: misconceptions and management. *Annals of Internal Medicine* **93** (4), 588–596.

Ritterhoff E. (1975) A symposium on the chronic pain syndrome in problem low back cases: psychiatric evaluation and feasibility of psychiatric therapy. *Journal of Occupational Medicine* **17** (10), 656–657.

Roy R. (1984) Pain clinics: reassessment of objectives and outcomes. *Archives of Physical and Medical Rehabilitation* **65** (8), 448–451.

Siegfried J. & Lazorthes Y. (1982) Long-term follow-up of dorsal cord stimulation for chronic pain syndrome after multiple lumbar operations. *Applied Neurophysiology* **45** (1–2), 201–204.

Simmons J.W., Avant W.S. Jr, Demski J. & Parisher D. (1988) Determining successful pain clinic treatment through validation of cost effectiveness. *Spine* **13** (3), 342–344.

Spector R. (1981) Treatment of moderate and severe chronic pain syndromes with morphine and adjunctive drugs. *Journal of the Iowa Medical Society* **71** (2), 72, 74, 76.

Stieg R.L. (1987) Why be concerned with chronic pain treatment? *Risk Management* **34** (1), 28–30.

Sturgis E. T., Schaefer C.A. & Sikora T.L. (1984) Pain center follow-up study of treated and untreated patients. *Archives of Physical and Medical Rehabilitation* **65** (6), 301–303.

Swerdlow M. (1978) The value of clinics for the relief of chronic pain. *Journal of Medical Ethics* **4** (3), 117–118.

Tollison C.D. (1984) Diagnosing and managing chronic pain syndrome. *Journal of the South Carolina Medical Association* **80** (9), 449–452.

Tollison C.D., Kriegel M.L., Satterthwaite J.R., Hinnant D.W. & Turner K.P. (1989) Pain clinic No. 13. Comprehensive pain center treatment of low back workers' compensation injuries: an industrial medicine clinical outcome follow-up comparison. *Orthopaedics Review* **18** (10), 1115–1117, 1121–1122, 1125–1126.

Turk D.C. & Rudy T.E. (1987) IASP taxonomy of chronic pain syndromes: preliminary assessment of reliability. *Pain* **30** (2), 177–189.

Uematsu S., Hendler N., Hungerford D., Long D. & Ono N. (1981) Thermography and electromyography in the differential diagnosis of chronic pain syndromes and reflex sympathetic dystrophy. *Electromyographic and Clinical Neurophysiology* **21** (2–3), 165–182.

Wang J.K., Ilstrup D.M., Nauss L.A., Nelson D.O. & Wilson P.R. (1980) Outpatient pain clinic – a long-term follow-up study. *Minnesota Medicine* **63** (9), 663–666.

Welch G.T. (1983) Cost effectiveness of pain clinics. *Proceedings of the Annual Meeting of the Medical Section of the American Council of Life Insurers*, pp. 119–123.

Wyant G.M. (1979) Chronic pain syndromes and their treatment. II. Trigger points. *Canadian Anaesthetists Society Journal* **26** (3), 216–219.

28: Management of Communication and Swallowing Disorders

D.P. FULLER, D.B. PUGH AND W.M. LANDAU

Language disorders, 409
　　Communication evaluation – diagnosis, 411
　　Management of aphasia, 412
　　Effect of treatment, 415
Rehabilitative management of swallowing disorders, 420
　　Muscular and neural control, 420
　　Evaluation and treatment, 423
Summary, 424
Motor speech disorders, 425

The act of communication is the basis of most patient treatment strategies, involving both diagnosis and treatment. The use of speech to elicit, receive and decode language is the core of the communication process. Thus, a disorder of the communication process represents a significant hurdle that can, at a minimum, impede the treatment and recovery of any of the disorders addressed in this book.

Hand in hand with disorders of communication are disorders of swallowing. Speech pathologists have added significant knowledge to the diagnosis and treatment of dysphagia. Our task of rehabilitation is to provide instruction and compensatory tools that will return that individual to the mainstream of life as quickly as possible.

This chapter is designed to provide the reader with a practical guide for individualized problem-solving, using the varieties of diagnostic and treatment approaches that we have found useful. The expectation is that the reader will use this outline as a springboard and reference.

Language disorders

Rosenbek *et al.* (1989) suggest that 'people with aphasia are to be helped, not handled!' We hold that the optimal process of diagnosis and treatment includes the clinician, the patient and patient's family. This process should:

1 Identify those receptive and expressive skills that remain, regardless of how fragmented they may be.
2 Help the patient and family to recognize those remaining skills.
3 Develop strategies to utilize those remaining skills to their fullest potential.
4 Provide a 'safe environment' to pursue these strategies.

Each patient with aphasia is unique. Some symptoms present themselves obviously, some we must discover through tools such as standardized tests, while others are realized and expressed by the patient. The diagnosis and treatment process is dependent upon multiple sources of information rather than individual tests. The best opportunity for analyisis may not be at the time when the standardized evaluation is being administered. Rather, it is diverse information collected by a number of professionals that may provide the most accurate picture.

The neuroscientific enquiries of the last century and a half provide an array of definitions which mirror the evolution of descriptive verbiage for the encoding and decoding process that we use to communicate. Table 28.1 is a historical review of these definitions.

No matter how simple or sophisticated the definition,

> Almost everyone agrees that aphasic patients differ. Some talk a lot, others speak very little, some understand more than others and so on. But, disagreement begins when one suggests these differences can be used to sort aphasic patients into specific types. Some hold that aphasia is aphasia while others specify aphasia

Table 28.1 Definitions

1861	Broca (Eisenson, 1973)	'A loss of speech consequent to a lesion of the frontal lobe of the brain'
1879	Jackson (Eisenson, 1973)	'An impairment of linguistic formulation and expression'
1891	Freud (Eisenson, 1973)	Aphasic disturbances 'represent instances of functional retrogression of a highly organized apparatus, and therefore correspond to earlier states of its functional development. This means that under all circumstances an arrangement of associations, which, having been acquired later, belongs to a higher level of functioning, will be lost, while an earlier and simpler one will be preserved'
1906	Pierre Marie (Eisenson, 1973)	'True aphasia is a combination of impairment in the comprehension of language and associated mental decrement'
1926	Head (Eisenson, 1973)	Disturbances of 'symbolic formulation and expression'
1959	Penfield & Roberts (Eisenson, 1973)	'That state in which one has difficulty in speech comprehension of speech, naming, reading and writing, or any one or more of them; and it is associated with misuse and/or preservation of words, but is not due to disturbance in the mechanism of articulation or involvement of peripheral nerves, nor due to general mental insufficiency'
1963	Osgood & Miron (Eisenson, 1973)	'Aphasia is a nonfunctional impairment in the reception, manipulation, and/or expression of symbolic content whose basis is to be found in organic damage to relatively central brain structures. Such a definition would include all modalities and forms of linguistic signs, but would exclude such things as perceptual disorganization, disturbance in learning, in abstracting and problem-solving, and purely sensory or motor impairments – except as they specifically involve language symbols. This clinical distinction, of course, does not mean that aphasia should be studied without reference to simultaneous non-aphasic symptomatology or that language behavior is in any sense separable from behavior in general'
1964	Schuell *et al.* (1964)	'A general language deficit that crosses all language modalities and may be complicated by other sequelae of brain damage'
1967	Bay (Eisenson, 1973)	'Aphasia should be limited to troubles which primarily and immediately concern language as a specific human property. Such troubles are revealed by erroneous interpretations of verbal message, and on the expressive side, by faulty use of language as demonstrated, for instance, by the appearance of verbal paraphasias'
1973	Eisenson (1973)	'An impairment of language fundamentally of persons who have incurred cerebral damage that results in a reduced likelihood that an individual involved in a communicative situation will understand or appropriate verbal formulations'
1973	Brookshire (1973)	'As a deficit in the ability to process symbolic materials which exists in all stimulus modalities (auditory, visual, tactile) and in all response modalities (speaking, writing and gesturing)'
1981	Chapey (1986)	'An acquired impairment of language and the cognitive process which underlies language caused by organic damage to the brain. It is characterized by a reduction in and dysfunction of language content or meaning, language form or structure, and language use or function and the cognitive processes which underlie language such as memory and thinking. This impairment is manifested in listening, speaking, reading and writing, although not necessarily to the same degree in each'
1982	Darley (1982)	'Impairment, as a result of brain damage, of the capacity for interpretation and formulation of language symbols; multi-modality loss or reduction in efficiency of the ability to decode and encode conventional–meaningful linguistic elements (morphemes and larger syntactic units); disproportional to impairment of other intellectual functions; not attributable to dementia, confusion sensory loss, or motor dysfunction, and manifest in reduced availability of vocabulary, reduced efficiency in application of syntactic rules, reduced auditory retention span and impaired efficiency in input and output channel selection'

may be Broca's aphasia, Wernicke's aphasia, conduction aphasia etc. (Rosenbek *et al.*, 1989)

Communication evaluation – diagnosis

Evaluation is the process of information-gathering from the patient, the physician and affiliated medical specialities, friends and family, and data from a standardized evaluation. We (therapists) thoroughly review the medical chart to note the results of all ancillary testing and lab work, initiate an informal bedside evaluation with the patient and a parallel family/friend interview, and complete an in-depth communication evaluation with a standardized test protocol.

The communication evaluation is the basis from which the clinician plans and organizes the treatment, thus setting goals and giving the patient and family an accurate picture. This exercise relieves anxiety and begins the process of helping to compensate for/cope with lost and impaired skills. It is the bench-mark that determines which remaining skills should be strengthened and which will need to be compensated for. In the future this is the reference point to determine progress and goal attainment, or failure.

The medical chart facilitates communication to and from the physician regarding history, diagnosis and prognosis of the patient. This review should provide the language clinician with the aetiology, site and size of lesion, and an order to provide the patient with an evaluation and treatment programme. The physician is the primary caregiver and should act as the focal point of care for the patient, the patient's family and all other professionals.

The informal bedside communication evaluation should achieve two goals:
1 An introduction of the therapist and what the therapist is going to do.
2 A brief inventory of the type and level of the encoding and decoding communication skills.
We use two items per subtest of a standardized test, the Boston aphasia scale (Boston) (Goodglass & Kaplan, 1987) and plus/minus scoring. Used for screening, this tool reliably and quickly indicates whether the patient is fluent or non-fluent, gives a rough estimate of severity and indicates the level of

the patient's coping mechanisms in dealing with the disability.

We use the interview of family and friends to find out what the patient was like before the lesion in terms of personality, occupation, habits, routines, educational level and communication habits. This information is invaluable when planning treatment and when to terminate treatment. This is also an excellent opportunity to educate the family and group of friends about what treatment will and will not accomplish; the groundwork is laid for the 'treatment' programme to follow. The screening provides the rough picture of the communication disorder while the standardized evaluation provides the detail.

Table 28.2 is a list of standardized systems currently used in the evaluation process and found in most literature discussions. Use of a standardized test goes beyond detecting the presence of aphasia by providing an in-depth sampling across all communication modalities. In general, the more complex the evaluation the more thorough the evaluation sampling. Being more complex also means more lengthy to administer. Usually a Boston can be administered in $1\frac{1}{2}$ hours, while the Minnesota test for differential diagnosis of aphasia (MTDDA) may require up to 3 hours. The preference in our practice is the former.

This standardized evaluation provides the most complete and uniform measure of the patient's remaining communication skills and, implicitly, a comparison with other individuals who have had a similar condition. Some evaluations, such as the Boston and the Porch index of communicative abilities (PICA), allow the scores to be profiled. Thus generalized predictions can be made as to what skill levels can be expected with treatment over a specific period of time. A word of caution should be extended: patient motivation, family support and individual speech–language clinician skills are variables that cannot be easily measured or predicted.

We extend the following 'rules of the road' for selection and use of an evaluation tool:
1 Use a test that profiles the patient, using terms that one's own team uses. The Boston, for example, uses a classic neurological classification while the PICA profiles the patient in terms of expressive and receptive coding.

Table 28.2 Standardized tests

Test	Author	Scoring	No. of subtests
Boston aphasia scale (Boston)	Goodglass & Kaplan (1983)	Z profile of raw scores	31
Porch index of communicative abilities (PICA)	Porch (1967)	16-Point multidimensional	18 of 10 items each
Minnesota test for differential diagnosis of aphasia (MTDDA)	Schuell (1973)	7-Point (0–6)	47
Western aphasia Battery	Kertesz (1982)	Raw score AQ, PQ & CQ*	11
Language modalities test for aphasia	Wepman & Jones (1961)	6-Point	26
Sklar aphasia scale (SKLAR)	Sklar (1966)	4 Categories	4
Neurosensory Center comprehensive examination for aphasia	Spreen & Benton (1977)	Profile of percentile scores correlated for age and education	24
Aphasia language performance scale (ALPS)	Keenan & Brassell (1975)	1–10 Within modality	4 ten-part
Functional communication profile (FCP)	Sarno (1969)	9-Point scale	45 activities
Communicative abilities in daily living (CADL)	Holland (1980)	3-Point scale (0–2)	68 tasks

* AQ (Aphasia Quotient) is the total score of the oral language sub-tests multiplied by 2; CQ (Cortical Quotient) is the summation of the total raw scores.

2 Attempt to evaluate the patient in one sitting and select a tool that will accommodate this goal.

3 Use the evaluation test's scoring and plotting tables for standardized record-keeping.

4 Use a scheduled retest in reference to the initial study as the primary tool for re-evaluation.

5 Organize goals and treatment to address the areas shown to need and likely to benefit from treatment. Do not 'teach the test' as a strategy for treatment.

6 Be willing to redesign and address goals in either a positive or negative direction.

7 Recognize goal attainment.

8 Set discharge criteria at the time of the initial evaluation and plan concretely toward the schedule for termination.

We propose an evaluation programme that uses the following:

1 A brief review of the patient's medical chart, paying attention to the pathological nature, site, size and date of the lesion.

2 A brief bedside evaluation to sample the encoding and decoding process.

3 An evaluation utilizing a tool that is standardized for similar patients. We suggest either the Boston, PICA or MTDDA due to their standardized format, understandable plotting formats for patient and family, test–retest reliability and communication skill projects.

4 A supplementary inventory of 'everyday communication skills'. We use the communication abilities in daily living (CADL) because of its 'everyday' items and format.

5 A scheduled re-evaluation using the same tests. We suggest a 6-week re-evaluation schedule.

Management of aphasia

We submit the premise that successful rehabilitation of the aphasic patient is not a treatment process but, rather, a management process. 'Treatment' sends the message that the patient will recover! We do not wish to enter the highly and emotionally debated question as to whether 'treatment' really cures in the sense that penicillin cures pneumonia. We believe that there are no convincing, well-controlled data to support 'cure' as an effect. Management means that the patient and his/her support system of friends, family and/or co-workers will experiment and educate with various strategies that will best utilize the remaining communication skills. The management process, to use an old adage, will teach the patient to 'change those things that s/he can change and accept those things that s/he can't change'. Thus successful management should produce an individual who has learned successfully to cope with his/her retained abilities. So as not to misquote sources, 'treatment' will be used as quoted. However, the reader should view our meaning to be 'management'.

Many authorities have addressed this management vs. cure concept. Rosenbek *et al.* (1989) suggest that three goals of treatment are:

1 To assist people to regain as much communication as their brain damage allows and their needs to drive them to.

2 To help them learn how to compensate for residual deficits.

3 To help them learn to live in harmony with the differences between the way they were and they way they are.

Brookshire (1973) provides four essential assumptions:

1 Aphasia is the deficit in the ability to process language stimuli.

2 Many of the aberrant learning patterns exhibited by aphasic patients in reacquiring speech and language represent exaggerations of patterns exhibited by non-aphasic individuals in many kinds common learning situations.

3 Treatment procedures, in order to remain efficient and effective, must be regularly evaluated and revised when the evidence suggests that they are either inefficient or ineffective.

4 Treatment, in order to be effective, must be directed towards the patient's current levels of abilities and disabilities.

All management programmes must be individualized. Each session builds upon the previous session, with all sessions aimed at easing the difficulty of communication. We suggest that more than one modality be the target of the management session. This is where the interview with the family and friends becomes invaluable. Rehabilitation sessions with pictures of meaningful family members, including pets, using pet and family members' names,

meaningful items of clothing and memorabilia, important past events and current newsworthy items all contribute to motivation and interest. The task at hand is to name, describe and respond effectively. We follow Brookshire's (1973) eight principles of treatment:

1 Structure the programme so that most patients' experiences are with tasks at levels of difficulties such that performance is slightly deficient but not completely erroneous. [Motivation to continue a task is contingent upon level of success. The wise clinician will design the programme and its individual steps with this in mind.]

2 Keep stimulus materials used in treatment simple and relevant to the patient's areas of deficit. [This is the point where the family interview to probe the patient's premorbid interests and education is valuable.]

3 Elicit large numbers of responses from the patient. [The patient should be in the act of communication at least 60% of the session time or more. The clinician must provide time for the patient to respond.]

4 Begin the session with familiar tasks in which the patient is generally successful. [This is where the family photo album and a naming task might be an easy 'warm-up' session.]

5 Introduce new materials and procedures as extensions of familiar materials and procedures.

6 Provide feedback regarding accuracy and appropriateness of the patient's responses where such feedback appears to be beneficial. [This can range from an oral 'well done' to a system of charting progress by the patient.]

7 Show the patient his progress.

8 Direct treatment toward key areas of deficit whenever possible. [The patient should participate in the direction s/he wants to go. He/she should have the opportunity on a regular basis to select an area or areas that he/she has particular interest in improving, e.g. remembering and saying the names of family members.]

The management process is a constant tailoring of experiences and stimuli that will influence, stimulate and, if possible, elicit responses that compensate for the damaged encoding and/or decoding modality function. We recommend a programme that provides a minimum of 120 minutes of one-to-one effort per week with a modest amount of 'homework' as a means of encouraging 'carry-over' from one session to the next. The home treatment programme must also conform to the reasonable limits of the patient's family time and resources. A successful home programme will reflect the regular treatment sessions. An occasional 'vacation' is as refreshing for the patient as it was before from his/her regular job. We cannot over-emphasize the importance of regular evaluation probes to adjust and, if necessary, to set new goals. As the patient approaches the long-range goals, preparation for termination of the programme must be made. Knowing when to terminate and discharge the patient is perhaps the most undeveloped skill in current aphasia management. This concept of attaining a plateau of performance must be built into the programme from the beginning. Then it is reasonable and acceptable for the patient to 'graduate'. Of course, such a goal-orientated management programme must be feasible within the limitations of the patient's health-care support system.

It is virtually impossible to pick and choose specific commercially available programmes or parts of programmes that are best for any given patient. These readily available programmes, stimulus materials and exercises make it far too easy for the clinician to fall into using them without really looking at the base strategy of individualized treatment. Sarno (1981) and Chapey (1986) offer chapters of remediation strategies in great detail from many authors. Eisenson (1973), Darley (1982), Johns (1978) and Rosenbek et al. (1989) also provide multifaceted treatment strategies and programmes.

Every treatment programme has two basic components that continue to act upon each other: the clinician and the patient. Both must work in harmony to achieve the goals of treatment. At the same time, each individual brings pre-existing baggage to the situation that can successfully or adversely influence treatment. Although stated before, we review these concepts from the clinician–patient perspective.

The clinician

Far too often the clinician does not bring the enthusiasm and the self-direction to the clinical situation that set the standard for the patient's expectations. We suggest that the patient be viewed

as though he/she were a member of the family. Foremost, the clinician must be a professional. This means being prepared with appropriate materials and stimuli for every session and being realistic about the expectations based upon the patient's performance on the evaluation and in previous treatment sessions. The clinician needs to be excited and motivated about the task. Motivation is difficult to measure but easy to detect. The patient will be no more enthusiastic about the task than the clinician! Goal-orientated material must be relevant to the patient's interest and education level. The task of the clinician is to design treatment that allows for success and at the same time challenges the affected modality. The successful clinician is quick to indicate that patients who realize success try for more.

The patient

The patient brings to the treatment session his/her experiential background as well as the environment where s/he existed prior to his/her disability. As part of the original evaluation process, it is important to find out specific details, such as occupation, premorbid education level and type of personality from supportive persons such as friends, family, work peers, etc. As Brookshire (1973) indicated, patients exhibit behaviour that is an amplification of their pre-existing condition. If they were doing their best before, they will set about doing the best they can to adjust to their disability (Rosenbek et al., 1989). Rosenbek et al. (1989) also view the future with: 'The patient and family need to begin the process of preparing for a lifetime of aphasia.' It is important in the early stages to indicate what treatment is about and why we are doing it. We are not returning the patient to his/her former state, but rather helping him/her achieve those skills that are possible. A realistic goal from the very beginning will set the stage for the patient and the patient's family's positive attitude toward the treatment process.

The patient and the clinician together need to explore and set realistic goals. They also need to explore those areas for which the clinician may need other professional help. Good speech pathologists are resource people for other professionals.

'The good aphasiologist must resist being all things to all people' (Rosenbek *et al.*, 1989). Attempting to be vocational counsellors/therapists and social workers as well as speech pathologists is not a service to the patient but rather a detriment. The speech pathologist cannot set him/herself as an intermediary in all of these situations. The effective clinician is an effective referral source!

Effect of treatment

No subject in aphasia causes more heated discussion among professionals than does the subject of effect of treatment. What does treatment really do? Is the patient really better off having received a complex course of treatment? Does the cost in time, effort and money justify the results? Is the strategy of treatment to help the patient realize his/her remaining skills and build upon them? Is every patient, considering age, medical prognosis, type of aphasia and severity, a candidate?

All authorities agree that spontaneous improvement of acutely acquired aphasia due to 'stroke' requires 6 months to a year, assuming that there are no new lesions. All concur that every patient should receive humane encouragement and motivational support to deal with the disability. Whether any specific mode of language instruction and exercise will reliably deliver additional and significant long-term language accomplishment is the unresolved controversy.

Over a period of more than seven decades (Darley, 1982), various reports have dealt largely with patients affected by military wounds or by strokes. Many management strategies have been developed and advocated. These studies compared with what may be considered to be spontaneous recovery have led investigators to line up on either side of the issue. Darley (1982) cautions that

> No single study reviewed has proved to be so comprehensive and so creatively and rigorously designed and executed as to provide by itself the unequivocal answer to questions about the efficacy of aphasia treatment. Therefore, to hold any single study to the light as the answer to our dilemma of efficacy would be foolish.

Yet it is interesting, when reviewing studies, to compare and contrast differences of research design.

Table 28.3 summarizes our review of ten representative studies regarding the effect of aphasia treatment. These comprise less than one-fifth of the best-known reports now extant.

Some investigations that make an effort to provide controls conclude that the 'treatment' under study was ineffective or that professional speech therapists were not essential to the clinical course. 'Conventional therapy' has never been a standardized delivery of care. Statistical success in different studies varies widely in relation to reference standards, management techniques and intensity of treatment. The bottom line is that many of the patients treated by the therapeutic enthusiasts improve very little, and none improve more than a few percentage points on an aphasia scale. None of these advocates has claimed that aphasia 'treatment' has brought patients back to a linguistically 'normal' status. It is obvious that there are no definitive data to answer the key question: 'Is this specific type of therapy with this specific type of population for this specific period of time effective?'

The challenge of the decade and the century should be:

1 What patients should be treated?
2 What are the most effective treatment techniques?
3 When has maximum gain been achieved?

To answer these questions standardized selection, evaluation, treatment and termination criteria must be used. If we continue to debate using a cluttered set of data results, we will also continue to utilize questionable techniques with patients that may or may not be the most favourable. An ideal study of 'treatment' should provide:

1 Large numbers of patients matched for general similarity of age, educational status, aetiology, size and location of lesion, duration post-onset, general medical condition, handedness and major descriptive variety of aphasia must be randomized prospectively for competitive modes of treatment. Thus a 'non-treatment' mode of treatment must somehow provide equivalent motivational and emotional support for the patient and family.
2 The agents and tools of measurement must be independent of the therapeutic programmes and have sufficient dimension and linearity so that floor and ceiling effects may be minimized. Tests should

Table 28.3 Review of ten studies

Variables	Basso *et al.* (1979)
1 Evaluation tool(s) used	1 Basso-Vignola (unpublished) disinterested persons?
2 Were tests administered by disinterested persons?	2 no
3 Total number in study	3 281
4 Individual or group treatment?	4 Individual
5 Nature of reference group(s).	5 Non-treatment; patients unable to attend treatment
6 Number treated	6 162
7 Number in reference group(s)	7 119

8 Screening criteria for inclusion in study:
  A Age
  B Sex
  C Hearing
  D Vision
  E Education
  F Severity of primary affliction
  G Lesion site
	8
	  A Yes
	  B Yes
	  C No
	  D No
	  E Yes
	  F Yes
	  G Yes

9 Were non-stroke patients included in the study?	9 Yes
10 Were left-handed patients included?	10 Yes
11 Were reference patients randomly selected?	11 No
12 Were reference patients matched to treatment patients for clinical features, lesions, age, etc.?	12 No
13 Did reference patients receive support management?	13 No
14 Average time (weeks) post-stroke upon entering study.	14 'Recent' (less than 2 months): 137; 'Intermediate' (2–6 months): 86; 'Long-standing' (6 months or more): 58
15 Amount of treatment received per week in minutes.	15 150 to 250
16 Number of treatment sessions per week.	16 3 to 5
17 Duration of treatment in weeks.	17 22 minimum
18 Was there improvement in those treated by 'professionals'?	18 Yes
19 Was treatment effective for those treated by 'non-professionals'?	19 NA
20 Was there difference between treated and reference groups?	20 Yes
21 Statistical significance of 20.	21 $P = 0.02$ to 0.001
22 Was long-term follow-up/functional status ascertained?	22 No

continued

Table 28.3 *Continued*

David *et al.* (1982)	Hartman & Landau (1987)	Lincoln *et al.* (1984)
1 Functional Comunication profile	1 Porch index of communicative abilities (PICA)	1 PICA, Boston and functional communication profile
2 Yes	2 Yes	2 Yes
3 96 at completion; 155 at onset of study	3 60	3 161
4 Individual at 14 multicentres	4 Individual	4 Individual
5 Volunteers; 1 to 1 general support	5 Non-treatment; counselling	5 Non-treatment
6 48	6 30	6 87
7 48	7 30	7 74
8	8	8
A Yes	A No	A No
B No	B No	B No
C Yes	C Yes	C No
D Yes	D Yes	D No
E No	E No	E No
F Yes	F No	F Yes
G No	G Yes	G No
9 No	9 No	9 No
10 Yes	10 No	10 Yes
11 Yes	11 Yes	11 Yes
12 No	12 No	12 No
13 Yes	13 Yes	13 No
14 3 to 145 (median 4 weeks for speech therapy group and median 5 weeks for volunteer group)	14 4	14 6
15 Approx. 120 (30 hours over 15–20 weeks)	15 120	15 120
16 2	16 2	16 2
17 15 to 20	17 26	17 28
18 Yes	18 Yes	18 Yes
19 Yes	19 NA	19 NA
20 No	20 No	20 No
21 NS	21 NS	21 NS
22 No	22 No	22 No

Table 28.3 continued overleaf

Table 28.3 *Continued*

Poeck *et al.* (1989)	Sarno *et al.* (1970)	Sarno & Levita (1979)
1 Aachen aphasia test	1 Functional Communication Profile	1 Function communication profile, visual naming, sentence repetition, word fluency, token test and subtests of Neurosensory Centre comprehensive examination for aphasia
2 No	2 No	2 No
3 160	3 31	3 34
4 Both	4 Individual: A programmed instruction B non-programmed speech therapy	4 Individual
5 Multicentre, non-treatment, non-contemporaneous	5 Non-treatment	5 None
6 68	6 A = 16, B = 7	6 34: 14 global, 8 fluent, 12 non-fluent
7 68 (excluding 23 of original 92 who 'completely recovered between first and second examination')	7 8	7 None
8	8	8
A No	A Yes	A No
B No	B No	B No
C No	C Yes	C Yes
D No	D Yes	D No
E No	E No	E No
F No	F Yes, all were severe	F No
G Yes	G Yes	G Yes
9 No	9 No	9 No
10 No	10 No	10 No
11 No	11 No	11 NA
12 No	12 No	12 NA
13 No	13 No	13 NA
14 4 to 1186	14 12 to 624	14 4 (?)
15 540	15 98 average	15 Not stated, estimate 90 to 300
16 9	16 3.1 (mean)	16 3 to 5
17 6 to 8	17 4 to 36 (17.1 mean)	17 48
18 Yes	18 Yes	18 Yes
19 NA	19 NA	19 NA
20 Yes	20 No	20 NA
21 $P = 0.007$ to 0.980	21 NS	21 NA
22 No	22 No	22 No

	Treated	Untreated
Early (1 to 4 months)	23	92
Late (4 to 12 months)	26	69
Chronic (>12 months)	19	0

continued

Table 28.3 *Continued*

Shewan & Kertesz (1984)	Wertz *et al.* (1981)	Wertz *et al.* (1986)
1 Western aphasia battery and auditory comprehension test for sentences	1 PICA, Token test and Boston severity Scale	1 PICA, Token test & Boston Severity Scale
2 Yes	2 Yes	2 Yes
3 100	3 34 at completion; 67 at onset	3 94
4 Individual: (A) Language-orientated, (B) Stimulation–facilitation, (C) Nurse provided stimulation therapy	4 Individual; stimulus–response	4 Individual: (A) Clinic treatment administered, by speech pathologist (B) Home treatment prepared by speech pathologist and administered by family member
5 Non-treatment	5 Group; interaction–discussion	5 Non-treatment for 12 weeks; clinic treatment during weeks 12 to 24
6 66 at conclusion; 77 at onset	6 18 at completion; 35 at onset	6 A 29 at week 24 B 36 at week 24 A 31 at week 12 B 37 at week 12 A 38 at onset B 43 at onset
7 15 at conclusion; 23 at onset	7 16 at completion; 32 at onset	7 29 at week 24 35 at week 12 40 at onset
8 A No B No C Yes D No E No F Yes G Yes	8 A Yes B Yes C Yes D Yes E Yes F Yes G Yes	8 A Yes B Yes C Yes D Yes E Yes F Yes G Yes
9 No	9 No	9 No
10 Yes	10 Yes	10 Yes
11 Yes	11 Yes	11 Yes
12 Yes	12 No	12 No
13 No	13 Yes	13 No
14 $1\frac{1}{2}$ to 7 (mean $4\frac{1}{2}$)	14 4	14 2 to 24 (mean 7)
15 180	15 480	15 480 to 600
16 2 to 3	16 8	16 8 to 10
17 48	17 44	17 12
18 Yes	18 Yes	18 Yes
19 Possibly ($P < 0.06$)	19 NA	19 Yes
20 Yes	20 Yes (borderline)	20 Yes at 12 weeks; No at 24 weeks
21 A $P = 0.05$, B $P = 0.05$ C $P = 0.06$	21 $P = 0.05$ only as measured by PICA	21 $P = 0.05$ at 12 weeks; NS at 24 weeks
22 No	22 No	22 No

be administered by disinterested personnel who are blind to the 'treatment' modality.

3 Measurement devices of real-life performance are necessary. These must be independently validated and correlated to the performance needed in the real world.

It is reasonable to hope that statistically valid effects favouring one teaching and support modality over another may lead by approximation to better techniques than we now know. We now believe that patients and family should be offered an individualized, time-limited effort to help them understand and cope with residual disability.

Rehabilitative management of swallowing disorders

Oral–pharyngeal swallowing disorders occur in a wide variety of chronic and acute neurological diseases, most frequently associated with bilateral lesions (Donner & Silbiger, 1966; Silbiger *et al.*, 1967; Meadows, 1973; Donner, 1974; Veis & Logemann, 1985; Gordon *et al.*, 1987; Horner *et al.*, 1988; Robbins & Levine, 1988; Bushmann *et al.*, 1989; Kirshner, 1989; Jones & Donner, 1991). Lesions may range from involvement of the upper motor neuron at any level, basal ganglia, cerebellum, brain stem, including both the upper and lower motor neuron and sensory structures, to the neuromuscular junction and myopathic disease processes (Table 28.4). Although most swallowing dysfunctions result from bilateral involvement, current research is beginning to identify disorders resulting from unilateral hemispheric damage. Robbins & Levine (1988) conducted a preliminary study on patients with unilateral cerebral stroke. Their findings suggested that left cortical stroke dysphagia was characterized primarily by impaired oral stage function and difficulty initiating coordinated motor activity. Right cerebral stroke patients demonstrated pharyngeal pooling, entry of the bolus into the laryngeal vestibule above the level of the vocal cords and tracheal aspiration. This study is well defined as 'preliminary'. Further research is needed to define not only the quality but also the incidence and prognosis of dysphagia from unilateral lesions.

Dysfunctions of the swallowing mechanism may include any one or combination of the following:

impaired range of motion, strength and/or control of the lips, tongue, cheeks and soft palate; delayed or absent swallowing reflex; impaired lingual peristalsis; reduced pharyngeal peristalsis; insufficient or absent laryngeal closure; cricopharyngeal dysfunction; vestibular penetration and tracheal aspiration, including 'silent' aspiration. Silent aspiration is a term used to describe tracheal aspiration in the absence of a cough reflex. Because many neurological disease processes affect sensory feedback and attention regarding the position of the food in the vocal tract, and entry of the food into the airway, the neurologically impaired patient must be carefully assessed for this potential phenomenon (Logemann, 1983). The multiplicity of disorders in the neurologically impaired population requires objective evaluation of the physiology of the oral–pharyngeal swallowing mechanism safely and reliably to determine appropriate nutritional maintenance, and in order to establish treatment programmes.

Muscular and neural control

Swallowing occurs as an orderly physiological process that transports saliva or ingested material from the mouth to the stomach (Dodds, 1989). This process normally occurs without conscious effort at a rate of approximately once per minute in awake individuals, and occurs in response to salivation which must be either swallowed or expectorated (Dodds, 1989). Salivation during eating acts as a lubricant and facilitates the initiation of the swallow, and the transport of the bolus through the pharynx. The oral–pharyngeal swallow is divided into four phases:

1 The oral preparatory phase which involves mastication, manipulation and positioning of the bolus on the tongue in preparation for the swallow.

2 The oral phase in which the tongue propels the bolus posteriorly from the oral cavity into the pharynx.

3 The pharyngeal phase which transmits the bolus into the oesophagus.

4 The oesophageal phase which transports the bolus through the length of the oesophagus into the stomach.

The act of swallowing begins with movements of the tongue. As the swallowing reflex is triggered,

Table 28.4 Neurodegenerative and vascular disorders associated with dysphagia prevalent in the elderly

Disorders	Radiological observations
Diseases of the brain and brain stem	
Vascular disorders	
Bilateral cortical stroke	Aphagia
Unilateral cortical stroke (preliminary data)	Swallow may be preserved (brain stem receives input from opposite hemisphere)
	Unilateral tongue weakness and poor oral bolus control may be observed
	Impairment may not be characteristic
Left-sided cerebrovascular accident	Impaired oral-stage function
	Difficulty initiating co-ordinated swallows (apraxia)
Right-sided cerebrovascular accident	Pharyngeal pooling
	Airway penetration and aspiration
Brain stem stroke	
Pseudobulbar palsy (upper motor neurons) (corticobulbar tract, upper motoneuron disease in upper brain stem)	Swallow abnormal in bilateral involvement
	Oral phase most affected
Bulbar palsy (lower motor neurons) (lower brain stem nuclei, cranial nerves, neuromuscular junction, muscles, lower motoneuron disease)	Weakness and atrophy
	Pharyngeal phase most impaired
	Complete swallowing incoordination
	Pharyngo-oesophageal segment does not relax on time
	Often no swallow at all
Wallenberg's syndrome (unilateral vertebral artery occlusion)	
Intracranial haemorrhage	
Subdural, subarachnoid, intraparenchymal	Findings in oropharynx depend on location and extent of bleeding, and complications (e.g. mass effect, raised intramural pressure)
Amyotrophic lateral sclerosis	
Commonest form of motoneuron disease	
Upper and lower motor neurons in brain stem affected	Considerable oropharyngeal muscle atrophy, cricopharyngeal segment relaxation maintained
Common cause of insidious dysphagia in the elderly	Signs of compensation may be present
Multiple sclerosis	
Multifocal white matter lesions, course relapsing and remitting, may be steadily progressive	Findings as in bilateral corticobulbar lower brain stem lesions
	Severity of dysphagia varies with disease remission or exacerbation
Movement disorders and neurodegenerative diseases	
Parkinson's disease	Primarily difficulty with oral initiation
(Degeneration of dopamine-producing neurons in substantia nigra)	
May represent example of premature ageing	
Less common:	
Spinocerebellar degeneration	Oral-phase impairment
Progressive supranuclear palsy	Feeding and swallowing impairment depending on facial, oral, ligual or palatopharyngeal muscle involvement
Huntington's disease	
Alzheimer's disease	
Dystonia and dyskinesia	

Table 28.4 continued overleaf

Table 28.4 *Continued*

Disorders	Radiological observations
Infections	
Poliomyelitis	Residual dysphagia following acute infection of motor neurons
	Pharyngeal dysfunction may slowly worsen due to progressive post-polio muscle atrophy
Neurosyphilis	Dysphagia and swallowing impairment depending on site of central nervous system involvement
Encephalitis, meningitis	
Medication effects	
Antibiotics, immuno- and central nervous system-suppressive drugs	May mimic or worsen underlying neurological impairment
	Pharyngeal constriction frequently affected
Diseases of cranial nerves	
Involving muscles of cranial nerves V (jaw), VII (face), IX/X (palate, pharynx and larynx) and XII (tongue)	Oropharyngeal impairment (nerve palsies) depending on selection and degree of nerve involvement by trauma or disease process
Nerves may be interrupted along their course by trauma, neoplasms, infections and inflammatory and immune-mediated disorders	
Diseases of the neuromuscular junction	
Myasthenia gravis	Various degrees of generalized pharyngeal muscle weakness with features of increasing fatigue during swallowing
Eaton−Lambert syndrome (in setting of malignancy)	Generalized pharyngeal impairment
	Sluggish contractions during swallowing
Familial dysautonomia (Riley−Day syndrome)	Delay in cricopharyngeal sphincter relaxation with airway penetration
Diseases of the muscle	
Polymyositis, dermatomyositis	Sluggish pharyngeal contraction
Myopathies	Tongue/palate usually involved
Sarcoid myopathy	Pharyngo-oesophageal segment relaxes on time, closes early
Metabolic myopathy	
Cortisone myopathy	
Mitochondrial myopathy (ragged red fibre disease)	
Dysthyroid myopathy	
Muscular dystrophy	
Myotonic dystrophy	Oropharyngeal muscles usually uniformly involved
	Sluggish pharyngeal contractions
Duchenne's muscular dystrophy	Pharyngeal retention
	Aspiration likely
Oculopharyngeal dystrophy	In myotonic dystrophy, chilled barium aggravates changes

Taken from Donner & Jones (1991) with permission of authors and publisher.

the mylohyoid, geniohyoid and digastric muscles move the tongue toward the hard palate. The base of the tongue is then forced against the soft palate and posterior pharyngeal wall by action of the styloglossus and hyoglossus muscles. The soft palate elevates and retracts by way of the levator and tensor veli palatini muscles and acts to seal the nasopharyngeal cavity from nasal regurgitation. Simultaneously, the larynx is elevated and the hypopharynx is narrowed by the action of the middle and inferior constrictors. The pharyngeal contractions act to propel the bolus toward the cricopharyngeal sphincter. Lastly, the downward tilt of the epiglottis and the closure of the aryepiglottic folds and the true and false vocal cords produce sufficient laryngeal closure to prevent entry of the bolus into the laryngeal vestibule or trachea.

There are currently two major hypotheses, although not mutually exclusive, which describe the neural control of the oral and pharyngeal phases of swallowing:

1 The reflex chain hypothesis, which suggests that stimulation of sensory receptors sequentially triggers the next step in the swallowing sequence.

2 The central pattern generator hypothesis, which concludes that, once swallowing is initiated, it is programmed in a stereotyped manner by the network of nerves in the brain stem swallowing centres, which function independently of any sensory feedback (Dodds *et al.*, 1990). Most investigators believe that neural control results from integration of the two hypotheses.

Primary neural control resides in paired swallowing centres in the hindbrain. These are not discrete focal areas, but rather ill-defined broad zones (Dodds, 1989), which incorporate the nucleus tractus solitarius (NTS) and the ventromedial reticular formation (VMRF). Each centre consists of an array of interneurons (not well understood), which process incoming information, generate an integrated swallow response and distribute signals to the appropriate cranial nerve motor nuclei. There are also data to suggest that cerebral input, such as the intent to swallow, or wetting of the lips and face, facilitates swallowing by augmenting the input from existing background pharyngeal stimuli (Dodds, 1989). The sensory cranial nerve input is provided mainly by the glossopharyngeal and vagus nerves, with some participation by the tri-

geminal, facial and superior laryngeal nerve (O'Gara, 1990). The optimal stimuli to elicit swallowing show regional variation with origination within the oral cavity, pharynx and larynx. There is also variation with changes in volume and consistency of the bolus. The motor function is carried through cranial nerves IX, X and XII to the many muscles mentioned above.

Evaluation and treatment

Videofluoroscopic evaluation of the oral–pharyngeal swallow has earned attention in recent years because it 'captures' the rapid and dynamic process of the swallowing mechanism during the act of swallowing. An evaluation termed the 'modified barium swallow' (MBS), but also known as the 'cookie swallow', was first described by a number of authors in the late 1970s (Logemann, 1983). The assessment includes evaluation of the anatomy and physiology of the oral and pharyngeal cavities, the cricopharyngeal sphincter and the cervical oesophagus. The primary purpose of this examination is to identify normal and abnormal physiology and the presence of tracheal aspiration, and to introduce compensatory modifications. Modifications may include changes in bolus placement, consistency and amount of food, head or body position, using different food consistencies, multiple swallows, etc. These are implemented during the videofluoroscopic evaluation.

For example, a patient identified with a delayed swallowing reflex, who aspirates before the swallowing reflex triggers, may be asked to modify his/her position by tilting the chin toward the chest. This change alters the physiology of the vallecular space, creating a larger pocket secondary to the anterior displacement of the tongue and the posterior tilt of the epiglottis. The larger the vallecular space, the more the bolus can be retained above the level of the open larynx. As the bolus increases in volume, it creates greater pressure, thus eliciting the swallowing reflex. In addition, the slight posterior tilt of the epiglottis contributes to greater protection for the open larynx. Another example would be a head turn to the affected side, as in the patient with a unilateral vocal cord paralysis who aspirates during the swallow. The head turn to the affected side closes off that side, and directs the bolus to the stronger unaffected side. Thus, the MBS evaluation provides the examiner with objective evidence to support the prescribed treatment programme.

During the MBS study, thin and thick liquid barium, puréed barium and a 'cookie' (biscuit or cake) coated in barium are administered systematically. Viewing is typically performed from the side. An anterior–posterior view is important, however, in assessing symmetry of movement of the pharyngeal walls and vocal cords. The bolus sizes vary from 3, 5 or 10 ml to uncontrolled amounts which are more representative of the amounts individuals may take during a meal. Following the radiological evaluation, the swallowing therapist and radiologist confer on the nature and type of swallowing disturbance and the appropriate diet or means of nutritional maintenance. As appropriate, they establish a rehabilitative care plan, including direct and indirect swallowing therapy approaches.

Therapy approaches are defined in terms of direct and indirect treatment. *Direct* treatment refers to the modifications implemented during the videofluoroscopic examination and have been described previously. An additional focus during direct treatment is to ensure that the patient receives adequate nutritional support and maintenance of hydration (O'Gara, 1990). The team, including the patient, family, swallowing therapist, physician, nursing and dietitian must work together to ensure proper management of oral intake. It may be necessary to provide alternate nutritional support through the use of such methods as a gastrostomy tube or nasogastric tube. Alternative feeding may be indicated if a patient demonstrates reduced caloric/nutritional intake or unmodifiable aspiration on liquids or solid foods.

Indirect treatment typically involves one of three types of exercises (Logemann, 1983):
1 Exercises to improve oral motor control, range of motion and strength required during the voluntary phase of the swallow.
2 Stimulation of the swallowing reflex to heighten the sensitivity of the reflex.
3 Exercises to increase vocal cord adduction to improve airway protection during the swallow. Indirect treatment programmes are designed by the swallowing therapist based upon the dysphagic symptoms resulting in aspiration, or the risk of aspiration. Oral exercise programmes are individu-

ally planned to improve strength and range of motion, bolus control, manipulation of food and liquid boluses, and oral propulsion. The recommended treatment approach for a delayed swallowing reflex is a technique known as thermal stimulation. Application of light strokes with a cold size 00 laryngeal mirror to the anterior faucial arches is intended to heighten the sensitivity of the reflex. The anterior portion of the faucial arches and cold contact have been found to be the most sensitive area and temperature for the triggering of the swallow reflex (Pommerenke, 1928; Lazzar *et al.*, 1986). Exercises to improve laryngeal competence may be implemented if impaired closure exists. These exercises can involve laryngeal adduction exercises, which contribute to improved muscle activity of the larynx, and glottal adduction exercises, which improve vocal cord closure.

Kasprisin *et al.* (1989) demonstrated that rehabilitative management of swallowing problems in patients with various medical aetiologies can be extremely effective, even in patients with previous histories of aspiration pneumonia. Three of 48 treated dysphagic patients without prior history of aspiration pneumonia experienced aspiration pneumonia within 1 year after treatment. Two of 13 treated patients with a prior history of aspiration pneumonia experienced recurrent pneumonia within 1 year. All patients (eight of eight) who were untreated developed pneumonia within 1 year of diagnosis. There is, however, no well-controlled research to support the impact of indirect treatment approaches on the recovery process.

Lazzar *et al.* (1986) conducted a study of the impact of thermal stimulation on the triggering of swallow reflex in neurologically impaired patients. They found that 23 of the 25 patients receiving cold stimulation to the anterior faucial arches (thermal stimulation) demonstrated improved triggering of the swallow reflex immediately following sensitization. This study, however, did not account for the improvement normally seen during neurophysiological recovery, or provide data that would account for the influence that repeated tactile sensation has on eliciting a more timely reflex.

Summary

Rehabilitative management of oral pharyngeal swallowing disorders has gained popularity in recent years. Videofluoroscopic evaluations are an objective means of distinguishing normal vs. abnormal anatomy and physiology, identifying tracheal aspiration and determining whether modifications prevent or reduce the risk of aspiration with various food consistencies. This provides the physician with data to manage nutritional support and determine the most appropriate and safe means of nutritional maintenance. Although additional research is needed regarding the efficacy of rehabilitative management of dysphagia in the neurologically impaired population, little doubt exists that rehabilitative management has enhanced the quality of life for many patients, and can alleviate the cost of multiple hospitalizations associated with recurrent aspiration pneumonia.

Motor speech disorders

Motor execution difficulties are often the result of brain lesions. These disorders may or may not be associated with language or dysphagia problems. Most of the aphasia evaluation batteries in Table 28.1 suggest specific testing procedures to differentiate the motor speech disorders from aphasia. Using the Darley *et al.* (1975) classification, the motor disorders of dysarthria and apraxia affect the verbal output modality through disturbed co-ordination of movement and respiratory support. Thus, these symptoms comprise both articulation and/or voice disturbances. Dysarthria is a collective name for a group of related speech disorders that may be considered to be lower-level disorders of movement execution. Apraxia of speech is a higher order of *variable* clumsy performance, a disturbance of speech movement co-ordination due to central nervous system lesion(s), i.e. cerebral cortex, basal ganglia, brain stem or the cerebellar system.

Dysarthric swallowing and speech disorders result from lesions at the lower levels of motor neuron, cranial nerve, neuromuscular junction or striated muscle Some degree of weakness, slowness, incoordination or altered muscle tone characterizes the activity of the speech mechanism. The resultant articulation is weak and results in *consistent* error pattern for the same phoneme. Communication treatment of the dysarthric patient, like the aphasic, requires individual design and structure on a co-operative basis between the therapist and the patient. Emphasis in the communication treatment

process for the dysarthric is upon adaptation of the systems used to produce and articulate phonation, i.e. tongue, vocal cords, diaphragm and articulators. Rosenbek & LaPoint (Johns, 1978) suggest three major considerations for dysarthria treatment:
1 Every attempt is made to restore lost function (e.g. medication, surgery, prostheses).
2 The dysarthric patient's life is structured to eliminate the need for lost function.
3 Efficient use of residual function is maximized.
They also suggest that management be 'designed to achieve specific goals in speech. These include improving posture, strength, and tone; improving respiration; improving phonation; improving resonance; improving articulation; improving prosody and improving communication through the use of alternative modes.' Helping the patient to realize specific goals may require a change of lifestyle. What is important to address on the part of the patient may not be the communication skills but rather the physical mobility. Thus, planning the treatment goal with the patient is truly a team concern, which must include the patient, physician, family and other professionals.

When forebrain or cerebellar structures are impaired, the resulting articulation disorder is called apraxia of speech. 'Apraxia of speech is a sensorimotor disorder of articulation and prosody' (Johns, 1978). The patient's ability to make consistent volitional articulatory movements is so disrupted that repeated attempts result in an inconsistent error pattern. Thus, apraxic errors of articulation are usually variable for the same phoneme. This articulation is not weak but rather consists of movements that are off target. The patient with Parkinson's disease, in the later stages, typically presents a monotone, low-intensity voice which may increase with emotional excitement. An aggressive programme to address these variables and expect positive change is unreasonable. Rather, a programme to maximize and concentrate energy while speaking may be more on target. This may also require a prioritization of treatment. Rosenbek (Johns, 1978) points out that severe apraxia of speech is harder to describe because severely apraxic patients often have severe aphasia across all modalities (encoding and decoding), making test interpretations extremely difficult. Apraxia is most often classified by site affected. Thus, 'oral apraxia' is differentiated from 'verbal apraxia' as follows:

1 Oral apraxia involves those movements in the oral cavity that are used to articulate laryngeal sounds or those movements in the oral cavity that serve to masticate, organize a bolus and pass the bolus to the rear of oral cavity in preparation to swallow.

2 Verbal apraxia involves those laryngeal movements necessary voluntarily to produce a voice.

Treatment for apraxia begins with an in-depth evaluation of the patient's output problems and moves into treatment with a hierarchy from easiest movement to the most complicated. The goal of therapy is to help the apraxic patient regain voluntary, accurate control in programming the position of his/her articulators to produce phonemes and phoneme sequences (Darley *et al.*, 1975). Rosenbek (Johns, 1978) suggests, 'the methods to achieve this goal can include the following therapies: imitation, melodic intonation therapy, phonetic derivation, phonetic placement, visual reorganization, gestures, contrastive stress drills as well as instrumentation'. Again, tailoring the treatment to the specific needs and performance of the patient is fundamental.

Of greatest benefit to the motor speech patient is the area of augmentative and computer-driven communication. The last decade has seen this area explode from simple pretaped communication boards to synthetic communication with sentences and inflection. Computer programming can be prescribed to match individual needs and skills. The patient needs encouragement to approach this idea since many see this approach to be an admission of defeat rather than a new and effective mode of communication.

In either dysarthria or apraxia, it is most important to consider the aetiology and severity of the disorder before setting the goals of treatment. It goes without saying that the design for the terminal or preterminal patient will have different considerations from those of the patient with a post-stroke or longer-term degenerative neurological disease. As with language disorders, having a definite goal and terminating treatment when the goals have been met are essential. Since there has been no controlled research in this field, the onus is upon the therapist to provide ascertainable improvement, not just busy work!

References

Basso A., Capitani E. & Vignolo L. (1979) Influence of rehabilitation of language skills in aphasic patients. *Archives of Neurology* **36**, 190–196.

Brookshire R. (1973) *An Introduction to Aphasia*. BRK Publishing, Minneapolis.

Bushmann M., Dobmeyer S.M., Leeker L. & Perlmutter J.S. (1989) Swallowing abnormalities and their response to Parkinson's disease. *Neurology* **39**, 1309–1314.

Chapey R. (ed.) (1986) *Language Intervention Strategies in Adult Aphasia*. 2nd edn. Williams & Wilkins, Baltimore.

Darley F. (1982) *Aphasia*. W.B. Saunders, Philadelphia.

Darley F.L., Aronson A.E. & Brown J.R. (1975) *Motor Speech Disorders*. W.B. Saunders, Philadelphia.

David R., Enderby P. & Bainton D. (1982) Treatment of acquired aphasia: speech therapists and volunteers compared. *Journal of Neurology, Neurosurgery and Psychiatry* **45**, 957–961.

Dodds W.J. (1989) The physiology of swallowing. *Dysphagia* **3**, 171–178.

Dodds W.J., Steward E.T. & Logemann J.A. (1990) Physiology and radiology of the normal oral and pharyngeal phases of swallowing. *American Journal of Radiology* **154**, 953–963.

Donner M.W. (1974) Swallowing mechanism and neuromuscular disorders. *Seminars in Roentgenology* **9** (4), 273–282.

Donner M.W. & Johns B. (1991) Aging and neurological disease. In Donner M.W. & Jones B. (eds) *Normal and Abnormal Swallowing: Imaging in Diagnosis and Therapy*, pp. 196–197. Springer-Verlag, New York.

Donner M.W. & Silbiger M.L. (1966) Cinefluorographic analysis of pharyngeal swallowing disorders in neuromuscular disorders. *American Journal of the Medical Sciences* May.

Eisenson J. (1973) *Adult Aphasia: Assessment and Treatment*. Appleton-Century-Crofts, San Francisco.

Goodglass H. & Kaplan E. (1987) *The Assessment of Aphasia and Related Disorders*, 2nd edn. Lea & Febiger, Philadelphia.

Gordon C., Hewer R.L. & Wade D.T. (1987) Dysphagia in acute stroke. *British Medical Journal* **295**, 411–414.

Hartman J. & Landau W. (1987) Comparison of formal language therapy with supportive counseling for aphasia due to acute vascular accident. *Archives of Neurology* **44**, 646–649.

Horner J., Massey E.W., Riski J.E., Lathrop D.L. & Chase K.N. (1988) Aspiration following stroke: clinical correlates and outcome. *Neurology* **38**, 1359–1362.

Johns D. (ed.) (1978) *Clinical Management of Neurogenic Communicative Disorders*. Little, Brown & Co., Boston.

Jones B. & Donner M.W. (eds) (1991) *Normal and Abnormal Swallowing: Imaging and Diagnosis and Therapy*, pp. 189–202. Springer-Verlag, New York.

Kasprisin A.T., Clumeck H. & NinoNurcia M. (1989) The

efficacy of rehabilitative management of dysphagia. *Dysphagia* **4**, 48–52.

Kertesz A. (1983) *Western Aphasia Battery*. Grune & Stratton, New York.

Kirshner H.S. (1989) Causes of neurogenic dysphagia. *Dysphagia* **3**, 184–188.

Lazzar G., Lazarus C. & Logemann J.A. (1986) Impact of thermal stimulation on the triggering of the swallow reflex. *Dysphagia* **1**, 73–77.

Lincoln N., McGuirk E., Mulley G., Lendrem W., Jones A. & Mitchell J. (1984) Effectiveness of speech therapy for aphasic stroke patients. *Lancet* June 8388, 1197–1200.

Logemann J. (1983) *Evaluation and Treatment of Swallowing Disorders*, pp. 213–227. College Hill Press, Austin, Texas.

Meadows J.C. (1973) Dysphagia in unilateral cerebral lesions. *Journal of Neurology, Neurosurgery and Psychiatry* **36**, 853–860.

O'Gara J.A. (1990) Dietary adjustments and nutritional therapy during treatment for oral–pharyngeal dysphagia. *Dysphagia* **4**, 209–212.

Poeck K., Huber W. & Willmes K. (1989) Outcome of intensive language treatment in aphasia, *Journal of Speech and Hearing Disorders* **54**, 471–479.

Pommerenke W. (1928) A study of sensory areas eliciting the swallow reflex. *American Journal of Physiology* **84**, 36–41.

Robbins J. & Levine R.L. (1988) Swallowing after unilateral stroke of the cerebral cortex: preliminary experience. *Dysphagia* **3**, 11–17.

Rosenbek J.C., LaPointe L.C. & Wertz R.T. (1989) *Aphasia: a Clinical Approach*. Little, Brown & Co., Boston.

Sarno M. (1969) *Functional Communication Profile*. Rehabilitation Monograph 42, New York University Medical Center, Institute of Rehabilitation Medicine, New York.

Sarno M. (1981) *Aphasia Treatment*. Academic Press, London.

Sarno M. & Levita E. (1979) Recovery in treated aphasia in the first year post-stroke. *Stroke* **10** (6), 663–669.

Sarno M., Silverman M. & Sands E. (1970) Speech therapy and language recovery in severe aphasia. *Journal of Speech and Hearing Research* **13**, 607–623.

Schuell H. (1973) *Differential Diagnosis of Aphasia with the Minnesota Test*, revised by Sefer J. University of Minnesota Press, Minneapolis.

Schuell H., Jenkins J. & Jimenez P. (1964) *Aphasia in Adults: Diagnosis, Prognosis and Treatment*. Harper & Row, New York.

Shewan C. & Kertesz A. (1984) Effects of speech and language treatment on recovery from aphasia. *Brain and Language* **23**, 272–299.

Silbiger M.L., Pikielney R. & Donner M.W. (1976) Neuromuscular disorder affecting the pharynx. *Investigative Radiology* **2**, 442–448.

Veis S. & Logemann J. (1985) Swallowing disorders in persons with cerebrovascular accident. *Archives of Physical Medicine Rehabilitation* **66**, 372–375.

Wertz R., Collins M., Weiss D. *et al.* (1981) Veterans Administration cooperative study on aphasia: a comparison of individual and group treatment. *Journal of Speech and Hearing Research* **24**, 580–594.

Wertz R., Weiss D., Aten J. *et al.* (1986) Comparison of clinic, home, and deferred language treatment for aphasia. *Archives of Neurology* **43**, 653–658.

29: Management of Sexual Disability

M.A. JAMOUS

Anatomy and physiology, 428
Clinical conditions, 430
    Head injury, 431
    Stroke, 431
    Multiple sclerosis, 432
    Peripheral neuropathies, 432
    Parkinson's disease, 433
    Spinal cord injury, 433
Management of specific difficulties, 433
    Erection, 433
    Sexual intercourse, 434
    Fertility, 434

Physical difficulties such as hand or leg paralysis might alter sexual athletics, but they do not alter orgasmic potential. (C.C. Dahlberg, a psychiatrist who had suffered a stroke (Dahlberg & Jaffe, 1977))

Sexual disability has for too long been neglected and is still not considered an important goal that a patient is expected to achieve before being discharged from a large number of rehabilitation centres where patients with different neurological disabilities are treated. This is a major error, as physical disability neither brings functional castration nor necessitates sexual sublimation. Sex has been a taboo, and remains so despite society's claims to the contrary. Discussing the patient's premorbid sexual function and how to manage in the future having sustained neurological trauma or disease with physical and sexual disability is thought to be a private matter which is best left to the individual to sort out with his/her partner. Whilst it is understandable that in discussing the patient's sexual disability, the attending physician is not only invading the patient's privacy but also that of the healthy partner, leaving the subject to the patient and partner might well result, not unexpectedly, in disasters and irreparable damage. The aim of rehab-ilitation is to return the patient to some form of 'normality', and this task cannot be complete without frank discussion and guidance regarding the future management of the patient's future sexual function.

The approach adopted should also take into account the type of society that the physician is dealing with; what is possible in a Western society, for example, cannot be applied in a culturally different society. This does not imply that the subject of sex should not be addressed in such a society, but merely that the approach has to be different.

The psychological effect of the physical disability has a major implication with regard to sexual dysfunction. Therefore, addressing a patient's sexual disability not only entails assessing his/her ability to take part in the sexual act as well as the fertility aspect of his/her sexual disability, but also addressing the behavioural problems. Whilst it may be an easier task to enable the patient to continue to practise and enjoy the act of sex in whatever appropriate form suits that particular individual within the limitations of the physical disability, the issue of fertility, especially of male patients, is more complex. Fertility depends on a variety of factors, such as the gender and the age of the patient at the time of sustaining the disability, the fertility status of the partner, the long-term prognosis of the disease and whether or not there are any biological contraindications if the disability has been caused by an illness rather than the result of trauma, and finally whether or not the couple have had any children prior to the onset of the disability.

Anatomy and physiology

Sexual disability can result from many disorders of either the central or the peripheral nervous systems; the sexual function can be impaired by traumatic or non-traumatic peripheral, spinal cord or cerebral lesions. Sexual dysfunction can be acute in onset following traumatic lesions, or it can be gradual as is the case in many neurological diseases. In addition, the disability sustained as a result of trauma is usually static in contrast to the progressive nature of many disabilities resulting from various neurological conditions.

Although a good deal is known of the anatomy and physiology of the spinal cord and the peripheral nervous system controlling the sexual functions, very little is known about the equivalent centres and pathways in the higher centres of the central nervous system. It appears that although the sexual organs receive sensory and motor somatic innervation, the autonomic nervous system provides the main nerve supply of these organs.

The *male* sexual organs are innervated by parasympathetic fibres originating in the intermediolateral cells of S2–S4 spinal segments and pass via the pelvic nerves to form the perivesicular, prostatic and cavernous plexuses. These fibres are thought to be primarily responsible for reflexogenic erection; this is a purely spinal reflex produced by direct physical stimulation of the glans penis. The sympathetic fibres, on the other hand, arise from the lower thoracic and upper lumbar spinal segments (T10–L2) and pass via the hypogastric nerves. They supply the vas deferens, seminal vesicles, prostate and testes; they are thought to play a role in seminal fluid emission as well as in the so-called psychogenic erection, i.e. erection produced by mental stimuli. The somatic innervation of the male sexual organs originates from the anterior horn cells of S2–S4 spinal segments and travels via the pudendal nerves to supply the bulbocavernous and ischiocavernous muscles, which are concerned with erection and ejaculation; the pudendal nerves also carry sensory fibres responsible for skin sensation in the S2–S5 dermatomes, including the anal region, the scrotum and the penis.

It is generally agreed that erection results from parasympathetic stimulation, which produces dilatation of the arteries and vasoconstriction of the veins within the erectile tissue of the corpora cavernosa and the corpus spongiosum of the penis (Weiss, 1972). Although it is generally believed that the sympathetic system is responsible for the relaxation of the penis following ejaculation by contracting the smooth muscle of the corpora cavernosa, it is also possible that this system can produce erection (Bors & Turner, 1967). Ejaculation, on the other hand, is a more complex event; it involves reflex patterns starting with stimulation of the glans of the penis. Impulses enter the sacral spinal segments via the somatic sensory dorsal nerve of the penis and the pudendal nerves, and travel in part to the lumbar spinal cord, from where they pass via the hypogastric sympathetic nerves, causing semen to be expelled into the prostatic urethra; at the same time contraction of the bulbocavernous and ischiocavernous muscles, mediated by the motor somatic fibres of the pudendal nerves, leads to emission and ejaculation. Erections without spinal cord or higher centre involvement but on a purely hormonal basis can occur; nocturnal ejaculation, on the other hand, is felt not to require the same stimulation of the spinal cord segments. It seems that sleep removes the inhibitory effects of the higher centres on spinal cord reflexes (Chusid, 1985).

The *female* sexual organs are also innervated by parasympathetic fibres, originating in the intermediolateral cells of the S2–S4 spinal segments, which pass via the pelvic nerves; this is thought to be responsible for the swelling of the clitoris and to lead to increase in vaginal secretion. Nerves of the sympathetic system whose preganglionic fibres originate in the intermediolateral cells of T10–T11 spinal segments pass via the splanchnic nerves and supply the ovaries, the fallopian tubes and the broad ligaments. The tubes, the ligaments and the uterus are thought to receive parasympathetic fibres from the hypogastric and uterine plexuses, although the parasympathetic supply of the uterus is disputed; this is thought to play a role in the contraction of the smooth muscles of the tubes and uterus. In addition to the autonomic nervous system, the female sexual organs are supplied by somatic fibres originating in the anterior horn cells of S2–S4 spinal segments, which pass via the pudendal nerves. This includes sensory fibres to the vulva, motor fibres to the superficial perineal muscles, the anal and vaginal sphincters and the levatores ani, and sensory fibres in the form of the dorsal nerve of the clitoris. The motor somatic fibres cause contractions of the pelvic floor as well as the vaginal sphincter.

The role of the autonomic nervous supply to the clitoris and external genitals of the female is obviously clear, but the same could not be said for its role in the physiology of the ovaries, the fallopian tubes or the uterus (Brodal, 1981); women with neurological lesions leading to complete denervation can still menstruate, become pregnant and deliver. Although swelling of the clitoris was thought to be the equivalent of erection of the penis, the general opinion is that the clitoris is a unique organ with no equivalent in the male and that there is no counterpart in the female sexual function to male ejaculation (Masters & Johnson, 1966).

It is suggested that the sexual pathways, from the lower part of the spinal cord to the higher centres, are located in the anterolateral column in close association with the spinothalamic tracts (Olive-crona, 1947). Although they continue in the lateral portion of the medulla, nothing is known as to whether this arrangement continues in the pons or the midbrain; there have been some animal studies suggesting that stimulation of some parts of the thalamus can produce erection and ejaculation (MacLean, 1973). The role of the hypothalamus, and in particular a centre in the preoptic area and a centre in the area of the median eminence, has been controversial (Lisk, 1967); it is thought that the hypothalamus influences the sexual functions by affecting the level of sex hormones, although it is worth mentioning that, once normal sexual function is established in males, only severe deficiency of androgens can lead to sexual impairment (Martin et al., 1977). The limbic lobe, the amygdala as well as the septal region, has been reported to have an influence on human sexual function, whereas in the cerebral hemispheres the main areas thought to be related to sexual behaviour are the frontal and temporal lobes (Boller & Frank, 1982).

Clinical conditions

It is apparent from the foregoing that normal sexual function depends on the co-ordinated activity of cerebral, spinal and peripheral components of the nervous system. Although it is possible to discuss the major conditions which can cause physical and sexual disabilities along these anatomical divisions, it should be remembered that, except in cases of traumatic origin, many neurological conditions affect several different systems. It is therefore best to discuss these major conditions as entities, remembering that various neurological conditions have common adverse effects on the sexuality of a patient.

Furthermore, sexual dysfunction is not necessarily related only to the inability to participate in the sexual act or to procreate. It is the reduction, distortion or loss of many aspects. The patient may not be able to establish a sexual impression because of problems in his/her appearance or behaviour. Sexual drive or libido, which determines the frequency and intensity of sexual activity, might be depressed by many diseases or the medication used to treat these diseases. The ability to express the sexual feelings through physical contact could be diminished or lost if the neurologically disabled patient is unable to get physically close to his/her sexual partner, unable to move his/her body or communicate, or unable to exert sufficient control over his/her various bodily functions (Hamilton, 1980).

Different disabilities may also adversely affect the various stages of arousal, erection, ejaculation and orgasm in the male or the equivalent in the female. Arousal may be diminished due to many disabling diseases or their treatment. The inability to get erection or to maintain an erection sufficient for sexual intercourse can result from a variety of psychological or physical diseases; multiple sclerosis, Parkinson's disease, spinal cord lesions and diabetes are among the large array of conditions which can cause impotence. The loss of ability to ejaculate even when erection is present can occur in patients with brain or spinal cord injuries (stroke, head injury, spinal cord injuries, multiple sclerosis). On the other hand, patients who lose perineal sensation due to trauma or disease of the spinal cord can no longer experience orgasm. Finally, the degree of sexual dysfunction of a neurologically disabled person is related to his or her ability and freedom to meet members of the opposite sex and establish relationships. The more dependent the patient is, the less likely it is for him or her to have the opportunity of meeting a prospective partner and engage in any sexual activity.

Head injury

Patients sustaining head injury of varying severity are commonly young males who are otherwise sexually active. This suggested that sexual dysfunction after head injury rarely has a physical basis. Although residual physical disabilities may impose some limitations on the sexual expression of the patient, it is the cognitive and behavioural sequelae that have more profound effects (Ducharme, 1987).

Patients after head injury are regarded generally as sexually competent in that they can experience the intact neurophysiological sequence of sexual activity. The frontal and temporal lobes are the most common areas of the brain susceptible to contusion, due to the ragged nature of the floors of the anterior and middle fossae. Patients sustaining closed head injuries resulting in frontal or temporal lobe contusion exhibit sexual behaviours similar to those exhibited by patients who have undergone frontal or temporal lobectomies or those suffering from temporal lobe epilepsy (Blumer & Walker, 1967).

Sexual drive is usually decreased in the early recovery phase; subsequently the level of sexual drive of the individual is dependent upon the location of the areas of the brain which were irreversibly damaged as a result of the injury as well as the degree of damage sustained. Although patients left with temporal deficit commonly become impotent, there has been some suggestion that they may exhibit an increase in libido (Evans, 1981). Disinhibition is often one of the greatest problems, and is sometimes more obvious in male patients. Much of the disinhibition is thought to be due to frontal lobe involvement. The behavioural changes can be mild and no more than the usual backchat toward the nursing staff, or they can be more serious when the patient makes determined attempts to force nursing staff to have some form of sexual intercourse; masturbation in public is common among these patients, and can be very disturbing to those giving care, whether they are staff or relatives (Evans, 1981).

The physical disability of the head-injured patient rarely leads to serious sexual dysfunction, but the behavioural changes have more far-reaching consequences. Several strategies have been advanced to address the neuropsychological and emotional factors. Wood (1984) suggested two strategies: one involves overlearning, where patients learn to monitor their bodily contact, and the second involves punishment in response to undesirable behaviour. This is certainly counterproductive and gives rise to serious ethical concern. Careful explanation of the nature and cause of the disinhibited sexual behaviour is very important to both staff and families. If a patient starts to masturbate in public, he/she should then be taken to a side-room and the reasons for the move explained to him/her. Any attempts to be intimate with members of staff should be corrected immediately, unnecessary peripheral stimulation should be avoided and a non-provocative form of behaviour should be adopted by both nursing staff and carers.

Stroke

The degree of sexual disability after a stroke depends on the age of the patient, the severity of the stroke and the premorbid sexual function. Cerebrovascular accidents frequently affect middle-aged people who still experience strong sexual desire. On the other hand, in some reported series, the average age of the patient was 74 years with very low or non-existent premorbid sexual activity (Wade et al., 1985).

Following a cerebrovascular accident, in the majority of cases the sexual drive and competence are initially lost. If the stroke is unilateral and mild, they usually return within 3 weeks; this period can be as long as 3 months, or the sexual drive and competence may not return if the stroke is severe and bilateral. Furthermore, libido is commonly more severely diminished after strokes affecting the dominant hemisphere than after those affecting the non-dominant hemisphere (Heilman et al., 1975).

Although in general patients continue to have the desire for sexual activity and their libido remains consistent with their premorbid levels, several factors contribute to their sexual dysfunction. The physical sequelae can significantly affect the sexual function and create severe sexual problems, although some authors felt that motor paralysis was not a factor contributing to sexual dysfunction.

Other factors contributing to sexual dysfunction are fear that the physical stress of the sexual activity might be a health risk, as well as associated diseases or drugs taken by the patient for the stroke or the associated diseases. Nevertheless, as with head injury, the behavioural changes or reaction to the physical disability represent an important contributing factor to sexual dysfunction following cerebrovascular accidents. Careful enquiry about patients' sexual function after stroke is essential. Premorbid sexual history and level of activity is an excellent predictor of post-stroke activity. Those who were inactive before the stroke tend to remain so; the couples with a low premorbid sexual drive will not be interested in establishing a new sexual pattern, particularly considering the additional limitations resulting from the disability. Those who were active before the stroke and whose decreased motor function is a hindrance should be counselled in adopting different positions from previously to accommodate the loss of agility of the disabled partner. Finally, supportive psychological counselling is important, as it is felt that sexual dysfunction after a stroke is most often due to poor coping rather than physiological problems (Hamilton, 1980).

Multiple sclerosis

Multiple sclerosis affects mainly young adults. Sexual dysfunction in patients suffering from multiple sclerosis depends on the sites of neurological involvement, whether in the brain, brain stem or spinal cord. If the main lesion is in the spinal cord, the pattern might be similar to that after spinal cord injury, with one notable difference in that it might remit and relapse. There is a high percentage of males suffering from multiple sclerosis with impaired sexual function, while Lundberg (1978) found that 52% of females studied were experiencing sexual problems despite being at an early stage of multiple sclerosis, and had little or no physical disability. Impotence occurred in 26% of patients and was the presenting symptom in 7% of patients studied at the Mayo Clinic (Ivers & Goldstein, 1963). This is thought to be due to lesions in the thoracolumbar segments of the spinal cord.

Despite the loss of erection in the male suffering from multiple sclerosis, libido is often increased;

ejaculation and orgasm may also be infrequent or absent.

In the female patient, there is a decrease in sexual drive, difficulty with orgasmic response, dyspareunia and in some patients lack of vaginal lubrication (Lundberg, 1978). Fertility in the male patient is considerably reduced but apparently unimpaired in the female patient. Opinions differ regarding the effect of pregnancy and lactation on the disease. Some authors think that it will exacerbate the disease (McAlpine et al., 1972). The oscillating nature of the sexual dysfunction should be taken into consideration when counselling such patients; they should be advised that their impotence might not be permanent, and that their sexual function may return, albeit on a temporary basis.

Peripheral neuropathies

Diabetic neuropathy is the most common of all the peripheral neuropathies. Male diabetics frequently suffer from sexual difficulties, and occasionally this might be the presenting symptom. Erectile dysfunction is present in 25–50% of male diabetics (Rubin & Babbott, 1958); although this is often due to the peripheral neuropathy, some of the sexual problems in diabetic patients may be related to the vascular changes that they acquire. Some authors reported some indirect evidence that impotence may be due to neuropathy of the autonomic nervous system or even due to hormonal disorders (Ewing et al., 1973).

In female diabetics, the main sexual dysfunction is loss of orgasmic response (Kolodny, 1971). This seems to be related to the duration of the disease and is often associated with a decrease in vaginal lubrication, chronic vaginitis and dyspareunia. The possibility that sexual dysfunction is psychogenic should always be considered. General medical management will restore sexual function if impotence is due, as it is occasionally in acute diabetes, to malnutrition and weakness. Unfortunately, in most instances, when the cause of impotence is neurogenic, proper control of the diabetes fails to restore sexual function. Careful evaluation and counselling for both male and female patients is essential, taking into account that these patients tend to have a normal sex drive.

Parkinson's disease

The decreased sexual function of patients suffering from Parkinson's disease is thought to be related to depression and impaired movements. It is not known whether it is related to a decrease in dopamine levels (Barbeau *et al.*, 1971). There have been anecdotal reports of increased sexual drive and sexual performance following treatment with levodopa and other adrenergic drugs. Bowers & Van Woert (1972) showed some improvement in sexual function after treatment with levodopa. However, it is thought that the increase in libido is probably the result of improved motor activity and affect, rather than the direct effect of restoring dopamine levels.

Spinal cord injury

Sexual dysfunction after spinal cord injury has attracted far more interest compared with dysfunction after other physical disabilities, and therefore there have been many reports in the literature on the sexual consequences of spinal cord injury. This has been in part due to the fact that trauma to the spinal cord is usually a tragedy which befalls young, active and otherwise healthy people. In addition, the injury is usually non-progressive and the neurological outcome is static unless the patient develops the uncommon complication of post-traumatic syringomyelia. In the spinal shock phase, all reflex activities below the level of the lesion are abolished; these include reflex penile erection, bulbocavernous and scrotal reflexes in the male and the anal reflex in both sexes. These reflexes return over a variable period, depending on the length of spinal shock. Thereafter the degree of sexual dysfunction is determined by the level of the spinal cord lesion as well as whether the lesion is complete or incomplete. Tarabulcy (1972) showed that the injuries to the spinal cord affect sexual function more than bladder function, which is more common than disturbance of bowel function.

In the *male* spinal cord-injured patient, sexual drive or libido is not affected; sexual competence, or the ability to experience the sequence of arousal, erection, ejaculation and orgasm, is seriously affected, whereas sexual expression, or the ability of the patient to express his sexual feelings through bodily movements, is frequently hindered by the paralysed limbs and spasticity, which in turn hinder the act of sexual intercourse in its traditional form. Erection in this group of patients is still preserved in 77%, ejaculation in 10% and the ability to procreate in 3.4% (Tarabulcy, 1972), although with modern techniques it could be 10–20%.

In the *female* spinal cord-injured patient, on the other hand, sexual drive is not affected and sexual competence, inasmuch as it concerns the patient's ability to have intercourse in the traditional form, is preserved. Although orgasm during intercourse is absent, Guttmann (1969) suggested that arousal can still be achieved from tactile stimulation of certain parts of the body innervated by the spinal cord above the level of the lesion, e.g. the region around the breast for women with a lesion below T4. After a period of temporary amenorrhoea soon after injury, menstruation and fertility return to normal (Comarr, 1985).

Management of specific difficulties

Although the principles discussed in this section apply mainly to spinal cord-injured patients, some, especially those concerned with the management of erectile dysfunction, can be used to help patients with stroke, multiple sclerosis and peripheral neuropathies.

Erection

Psychogenic erection is lost in all complete spinal cord lesions above the second lumbar spinal cord segment; nevertheless, reflex as well as spontaneous erections are still possible. However, psychogenic erection is still possible in incomplete lesions involving the T11–L2 spinal cord segments. In lesions of the conus or the cauda equina, there is a complete loss of reflex erection (Donovan, 1985).

In assessing sexual function, it is important to assess the type of erection that the patient is capable of achieving, the fullness of the erection and whether or not it is adequate for penetration, as well as its duration. The reports on the percentage of the male spinal cord-injured patients who can obtain erections good enough for sexual intercourse and for long enough vary considerably (48% in Jocheim

& Wahle (1970) to 92% in Fitzpatrick (1974)). Although the technique of stuffing the flaccid penis into the vagina is often used, and some couples find it pleasurable and exciting, for those patients who were unable to have erection or in whom the quality or the duration of the erection is not satisfactory, there are several ways to improve the situation:

1 *Local injection of drugs.* Several drugs have been used with good results. The most commonly used drugs to date are papaverine (Wyndaele *et al.*, 1986) and prostaglandin E (Virag & Adaikan, 1987). This can be done by the patient after the dose has been established by the physician and after the patient has been trained, or it can be done by the partner. If the patient failed to respond to a maximum dose of 80 mg of papaverine, then a mixture of 40 mg of papaverine and 0.5 mg of phentolamine can be used (Earle *et al.*, 1992). The commonest side-effect is priapism and the long-term side-effect is fibrosis (Hu *et al.*, 1987), which gradually diminishes the effect of the drug, although it has been claimed that prostaglandin E causes less local reaction than papaverine.

2 *Vacuum tumescence with constriction/retention bands.* There are several makes of such devices on the market. This option is equally efficient in the patients who do not respond to the local injections of the above-mentioned drugs or were unable to carry out the procedure, or who are no longer getting good results from the local injections, having obtained good erections earlier (Lloyd *et al.*, 1989).

3 *Penile implants.* In recent years a variety of penile prostheses have been developed. They have to be implanted surgically; mechanical failure, infections and erosions continue to be common problems, making their use rather limited (Collins & Hackler, 1988).

Lubrication of the female genitalia is thought to be controlled by the same neurophysiological mechanisms which control erection in the male (Stien, 1992). Although the effect of spinal cord injuries on the motor reflexes involved in intercourse is unclear, it has been suggested that vaginal secretions remain active as part of the genital reflex (Griffith & Trieschmann, 1975). If vaginal secretions have been reduced as part of the spinal cord injury, the patient should be instructed to use lubricants such as KY jelly to make intercourse easier. Lubricants should be rather more acidic than neutral so that they do not disturb the natural vaginal environment and put the patient at risk of vaginal infections.

Sexual intercourse

The ability to achieve genital intercourse in the superior/inferior position is usually complicated by the presence of spasticity and weakness or loss of voluntary movements. It may be necessary for the patient to assume alternative positions allowing his/her partner to take a more active role. It is important that the patient feels free to experiment with any position he/she and his/her partner think would enhance their sexual relationship. In addition to difficulty with positioning for sexual intercourse, the commonest problems encountered by spinal cord-injured patients are those related to their bladder management, and whether the patient uses a condom sheath urinal (in the male), intermittent catheterization or suprapubic or urethral indwelling catheters. Normally, there is no problem when the patient has a suprapubic catheter, as it is away from the genitalia, and in fact it is one of the reasons why the male patient opts for this form of bladder management. The advice that should be given to the patient using a condom sheath urinal or intermittent catheterization is to empty his/her bladder immediately prior to attempting sexual intercourse with his/her partner. As for patients with an indwelling urethral catheter, they can either opt to remove the catheter, or the catheter can be folded over and back along the shaft of the penis and held in place with a tape or by placing a condom over it in the case of the male, or taping it to the abdomen or thigh in the case of the female. In addition, if pelvic floor spasticity or adductor spasms make penetration difficult, then a dose of benzodiazepine as an adjuvant therapy can be very useful.

Fertility

The inability of the male spinal cord-injured patients to procreate is due to their inability to ejaculate and the abnormal features of the semen when obtained by various methods. Ejaculation is rarely achieved spontaneously. It occurs in less than 10%, as reported by many authors. Various methods to stimulate the ejaculatory reflex have been proposed. If masturbation is not sufficient, and providing that the reflex arc is present as demonstrated by the presence of the sole scratch reflex, then a vibrator should be used. The application of strong vibration (80 Hz) to the frenulum of the penis will provoke ejaculation in 60–70% of spinal cord-injured males (Comarr, 1970). If this method fails, then rectal electroejaculation can be attempted (Francois *et al.*, 1978). According to Brindley (1984), electroejaculation is the induction of seminal emission by elecrical stimulation through the rectum and is rarely or never a true ejaculation. Of spinal cord-injured males, 70–80% will produce an ejaculate through this method. The use of drugs such as intrathecal Prostigmine (Guttmann & Walsh, 1971) or subcutaneous physostigmine has been abandoned due to their side-effects. New techniques such as semen capsules implanted into the vas and hypogastric plexus stimulator have been introduced. Unfortunately, the quality of the semen specimens obtained from the former has not been good (Brindley, 1986) and there has been an increasing rate of device infection, whereas the experience in the latter technique has been rather limited (Brindley *et al.*, 1989). Patients with a neurological level at T6 or above run the risk of autonomic dysreflexia at the time of ejaculation, which means that they can only be ejaculated under medical supervision and occasionally under general anaesthetic. This adds to the difficulties and reduces their chances of procreation.

There are numerous characteristics which make a semen specimen of a spinal cord-injured man less likely to achieve procreation. Prominent among these is the percentage of fully active sperms. The method used to obtain the semen seems to influence the volume and the number of sperms. Providing there are no gynaecological reasons in the female partners which preclude their use, intravaginal insemination, intrauterine insemination with or without ovarian stimulation and assisted reproductive techniques, including *in vitro* fertilization, are all methods employed to achieve fatherhood. Francois *et al.* (1983) reported a 38% success by those wanting a child.

In contrast, spinal cord injury in the female, whether complete or incomplete, and providing that the lesion is above the sacral segments, does not interfere with fertility. Couples should be made aware of the fact that, even during the period of post-traumatic amenorrhoea, pregnancy is still possible, and precautions should be taken if this is not desirable. As pregnancy advances, there is an increased tendency for urinary incontinence, which can be distressing for the mother-to-be. Whether the female feels the movements of the child depends on her neurological level. Patients with a lesion above T10 do not feel the movements of the child, between T10 and T12 the movements are felt inconsistently, whereas females with lesions below T12 feel the movements normally (Francois & Maury, 1987). The same problem is encountered during labour. The most troublesome cases are the patients with a neurological lesion between T6 and T10. They may not feel the uteric contractions, neither will they suffer from the autonomic dysreflexia which patients with a lesion above T6 will commonly experience. This can be extremely dangerous, and therefore the delivery of such patients should be undertaken only in centres with experience, where the blood-pressure is monitored continuously and the sympathetic discharge blocked by epidural anaesthesia (Hughes *et al.*, 1991).

References

Barbeau A., Mars H. & Gillo-Joffrey L. (1971) Adverse clinical side-effects of levodopa therapy. In McDowell F.H. & Markham C.H. (eds) *Recent Advances in Parkinson's Disease*. Davis, Philadelphia.

Blumer D. & Walker A.E. (1967) Sexual behavior in temporal lobe epilepsy. *Archives of Neurology* **16**, 7–43.

Boller F. & Frank E. (1982) *Sexual Dysfunction in Neurological Disorders: Diagnosis, Management and Rehabilitation*. Raven Press, New York.

Bors E. & Turner R.D. (1967) History and physical examination in neurologic urology. In Boyarsky S. (ed.) *The Neurogenic Bladder*, pp. 64–74. Williams & Wilkins, Baltimore.

Bowers M.B. & Van Woert M.H. (1972) Sexual behavior during L-dopa treatment of Parkinson's disease. *Medical Aspects of Human Sexuality* **1**, 88–98.

Brindley G.S. (1984) The fertility of men with spinal injuries. *Paraplegia* **22**, 337–348.

Brindley G.S. (1986) Sexual and reproductive problems of paraplegic men. *Oxford Reviews and Reproductive Biology* **8**, 214–222.

Brindley G.S., Sauerwein D. & Hendry W.F. (1989) Hypogastric plexus stimulators for obtaining semen from paraplegic men. *British Journal of Urology* **64**, 72–77.

Brodal A. (1981) *Neurological Anatomy*, 3rd edn. Oxford University Press, New York.

Chusid J.G. (1985) *Correlative Neuroanatomy and Functional Neurology*, 19th edn. Lange Medical Publications, Los Angeles.

Collins K.P. & Hackler R.H. (1988) Complications of penile prostheses in the spinal cord injury population. *Journal of Urology* **140**, 984–985.

Comarr A.E. (1970) Sexual function among patients with spinal cord injury. *Urologia Internationalis* **23**, 134–168.

Comarr A.E. (1985) Sexuality and fertility among spinal cord and/or cauda equina injuries. *Journal of the American Paraplegia Society* **8** (4), 67–75.

Dahlberg C.C. & Jaffe J. (1977) *Stroke: a Doctor's Personal Story of His Recovery*. Norton, New York.

Donovan W.H. (1985) Sexuality and sexual function. In Bedbrook G.M. (ed.) *Life Time Care of the Paraplegic Patient*, pp. 149–161. Churchill Livingstone, Edinburgh.

Ducharme S. (1987) Sexuality and physical disability. In Caplan B. (ed.) *Rehabilitation*, Vol. 4, pp. 419–435. Aspen, Baltimore.

Earle C.M., Keogh E.J., Ker J.K., Cherry D.J., Tulloch A.G.S. & Lord D.J. (1992) The role of intracavernosal vasoactive agents to overcome impotence due to spinal cord injury. *Paraplegia* **30**, 273–276.

Evans C.D. (1981) *Rehabilitation after Severe Head Injury*. Churchill Livingstone, Edinburgh.

Ewing O.J., Campbell I.W., Burt A.A. *et al.* (1973) Vascular reflexes in diabetic autonomic neuropathy. *Lancet* **ii**, 1353–1356.

Fitzpatrick W.F. (1974) Sexual functioning in the paraplegia patient. *Archives of Physical Medicine and Rehabilitation* **55**, 221–227.

Francois N. & Maury M. (1987) Sexual aspects in paraplegic patients. *Paraplegia* **25**, 289–292.

Francois N., Maury M., Jouannet D., David G. & Vacant J. (1978) Electroejaculation of a complete paraplegic followed by pregnancy. *Paraplegia* **16**, 248–251.

Francois N., Jouannet P. & Maury M. (1983) La fonction génitosexuelle des paraplégiques. *Journal de l'Urologie – Néphrologie* **89**, 159–166.

Griffith E.R. & Trieschmann R.B. (1975) Sexual functioning in women with spinal cord injury. *Archives of Physical and Medical Rehabilitation* **56**, 18–21.

Guttmann L. (1969) Clinical symptomatology of spinal cord lesions. In Vinken P.J. & Bruyn G.W. (eds) *Handbook of Clinical Neurology*, Vol. 2, pp. 178–216. North Holland, Amsterdam.

Guttmann L. & Walsh J.J. (1971) Prostigmine assessment test of fertility in spinal man. *Paraplegia* **1**, 39–50.

Hamilton A. (1980) Sexual problems of the disabled. In Nichols P.J.R. (ed.) *Rehabilitation Medicine: the Management of Physical Disabilities*, 2nd edn. Butterworths, London.

Heilman K.M., Scholes R. & Watson R.T. (1975) Auditory affective agnosia. *Journal of Neurology, Neurosurgery and Psychiatry* **38**, 69–72.

Hu K.N., Burks C. & Christy W.C. (1987) Fibrosis of tunica albuginea: complication of long-term intracavernous pharmacological self-injection. *Journal of Neurology* **138**, 404–405.

Hughes S.J., Short D.J., Usherwood M.M. & Tebbutt H. (1991) Management of the pregnant woman with spinal cord injuries. *British Journal of Obstetrics and Gynaecology* **98** (6), 513–518.

Ivers R.R. & Goldstein N.P. (1963) Multiple sclerosis: a current appraisal of symptoms and signs. *Mayo Clinical Procedures* **38**, 457–466.

Jocheim K.A. & Wahle H. (1970) A study of sexual function in 56 male patients with complete irreversible lesions of the spinal cord and cauda equina. *Paraplegia* **8**, 166–172.

Kolodny R.C. (1971) Sexual dysfunction in diabetic females. *Diabetes* **20**, 557–559.

Lisk R. (1967) Sexual behavior: hormonal control. In Martini L. & Ganong W.F. (eds) *Neuroendocrinology*, Vol. 2, pp. 197–239. Academic Press, New York.

Lloyd E.E., Toth L.L. & Perkash I. (1989) Vacuum tumescence: an option for spinal cord injured males with erectile dysfunction. *SCI Nursing* **6** (2), 25–28.

Lundberg P.O. (1978) Sexual dysfunction in multiple sclerosis. *Sexual Disability* **1**, 218–222.

McAlpine D., Lumsden C.E. & Acheson E.D. (1972) *Multiple sclerosis: a reappraisal*, 2nd edn. Churchill Livingstone, Edinburgh.

MacLean P.D. (1973) New findings on brain function and sociosexual behavior. In Zubin J. & Money J. (eds) *Contemporary Sexual Behavior*, pp. 53–74. Johns Hopkins University Press, Baltimore.

Martin J.B., Reichlin S. & Brown G.M. (1977) *Clinical Neuroendocrinology*. Davis, Philadelphia.

Masters W.H. & Johnson V.E. (1966) *Human Sexual Response*. Little, Brown & Co., Boston.

Olivecrona H. (1947) The surgery of pain. *Acta Neurologica Scandinavica (Suppl.)* **46**, 268–280.

Rubin A. & Babbott D. (1958) Impotence and diabetes mellitus. *Journal of the American Medical Association* **168**, 498–500.

Stien R. (1992) Sexual dysfunctions in the spinal cord injured. *Paraplegia* **30**, 54–57.

Tarabulcy E. (1972) Sexual function in the normal and in paraplegia. *Paraplegia* **10**, 201–208.

Virag R. & Adaikan P.G. (1987) Effects of prostaglandin E_1 on penile erection and erectile failure. Letter to the editor. *Journal of Urology* **140**, 1417–1419.

Wade D.T., Langton Hewer R., Skilbeck C.E. & Davis R.M. (1985) *Stroke: a Critical Approach to Diagnosis, Treatment and Management*. Chapman and Hall Medical, London.

Weiss H.D. (1972) The physiology of human penile erection. *Annals of Internal Medicine* **76**, 793–799.

Wood R.L. (1984) Behavior disorders following severe

brain injury: their presentation and psychological management. In Brooks N. (ed.) *Closed Head Injury: Psychological, Social and Family Consequences*, pp. 195–219. Oxford University Press, Oxford.

Wyndaele J.J., De Meyer J.M., De Sy W.A. & Claessens H. (1986) Intracavernous injection of vasoactive drugs, an alternative for treating impotence in spinal cord injury patients. *Paraplegia* **24** (5), 271–275.

30: Genetic Management in Chronic Neurological Disorders

N.R. DENNIS

Basic genetics, 439
Testing for single-gene defects by DNA analysis, 440
The genetic management of specific conditions, 443
    Huntington's disease, 444
    Myotonic dystrophy, 446
    Charcot–Marie–Tooth disease, 447
    Dementias, 448
    Inherited ataxias, 448
    Hereditary spastic paraplegia, 449
    Duchenne and Becker muscular dystrophies, 449
    Other dystrophies, 451
    Mitochondrial disorders, 451
    Prion disease, 452
    Multiple sclerosis, 453

A high proportion of our complement of genes is expressed in the central nervous system (CNS), with the result that its function is affected by almost any microscopically visible chromosome abnormality and by many single-gene disorders. Several inherited neurological disorders have provided paradigms for the genetic approach to a disease, and can be used to illustrate the way in which genetics may clarify familial risks and, when the gene is identified, mutational mechanisms and pathogenesis. In addition, the CNS is the prime target for two recently discovered disease mechanisms showing novel patterns of transmission: prion diseases and mitochondrial deoxyribonucleic acid (DNA) defects.

This chapter is about genetic management in those situations where a significant familial dimension arises. Most doctors are used to concentrating on the problems of the individual patient. Leaving aside the question of expertise and genetic knowledge, it calls for an additional investment of time and energy to address questions such as risks to close relatives and prenatal or presymptomatic testing. It is rarely possible to do so adequately as part of a routine clinic appointment. The atmosphere required for genetic counselling is quite different from that normally associated with management of the affected patient.

Many clinicians will want to deal with the commoner genetic problems within their own speciality, and one of the clinical geneticist's roles is to facilitate this process. On the other hand, the rapid pace of research and its application over the last few years have led to changes in the genetic management of many diseases as new tests have been developed. Some of these may become part of the routine clinical armamentarium; however, the heterogeneity of many genetic disorders and the speed of progress make it difficult for anyone not in close daily contact with the field to be sure of giving up-to-date advice.

Regional genetic services, including clinical genetics and the related laboratory services of cytogenetics and molecular genetics, are now well established in most parts of the UK. An established genetic diagnosis is not a prerequisite for a referral, as the geneticist can often help in the recognition or exclusion of high-risk situations. Nor should every genetic diagnosis lead automatically to a genetic referral. It is wise to find out whether the patient and family have questions to which they want answers before suggesting that they attend another clinic whose purpose may not be clear to them.

The typical agenda of a genetic counselling consultation may be summarized as follows. The term 'client' rather than 'patient' is used deliberately because the person requiring genetic advice is often unaffected by the condition in the family.
1 Establish the diagnosis.
2 Record a detailed family history.
3 Estimate the recurrence risk and convey it to the clients.

4 Discuss the nature, treatment and prognosis of the condition.

5 Discuss the various reproductive options, including prenatal diagnosis if applicable.

6 Assess the client's emotional state, understanding of the information given and need for follow-up appointments or additional help from other sources.

In most cases, non-medical genetic associates, who are usually nurses but may be social workers, are closely involved in genetic counselling. Although the main clinic session will usually be taken by the clinical geneticist, the genetic associate provides continuity by means of pre- and post-clinic contacts, and may keep in touch with families over many years to assess the need for follow-up.

It is generally agreed by clinical geneticists that, to be effective, genetic counselling must be non-directive. The aim is to give information which clients may use in reaching their own decisions. Any hint that the counsellor 'knows what is best for them' is likely to interfere with this process.

Basic genetics

A very brief outline of genetic mechanisms is given here, which can be skipped or supplemented by several introductory texts, such as Connor & Ferguson Smith (1991) or Weatherall (1991).

It is estimated that 50 000–100 000 separate genes are carried by the 23 pairs of human chromosomes. Chromosomes contain a single, very long, much coiled and folded, double-helical DNA molecule, whose main function is to encode the amino acid sequence of proteins. A gene can be defined as a section of the DNA molecule coding for a single protein or peptide. Although DNA can be replicated so that the genetic complement (genome) is handed on largely unchanged during cell division, changes in genes, called mutations, sometimes occur. They may or may not cause a loss of function in the corresponding protein.

Some genes can be disabled by mutation without a clinical effect being produced, as long as only one of an individual's pair of genes is affected and one normal one remains. If both parents transmit the defective gene, a clinical disorder results, which is then said to show recessive inheritance. Recessively inherited disorders tend to recur in brothers and sisters of patients, with a 1-in-4 risk, and are rare in other branches of the family because of the need for both parents to be carriers of the same gene defect in order to have an affected child.

When a single dose of a defective gene is enough to cause a clinical disorder despite the presence of a normally functioning gene on the other paired chromosome, the condition is said to be dominant. Such conditions show a 50% risk of transmission from an affected parent to each child, and often therefore produce pedigrees showing generation-to-generation transmission. If a dominant disorder for any reason severely impairs reproduction, it will tend to disappear from the population, unless the gene concerned has a relatively high mutation rate, which means that one can expect to meet cases with unaffected parents.

Sometimes the same clinical condition can be inherited as a recessive in some families and a dominant in others, for example Charcot–Marie–Tooth disease (CMT) or hereditary spastic paraplegia (HSP). Presumably, either different genes are involved or the same gene has mutated in different ways in the different families. An apparently sporadic case could then be a result of a fresh dominant mutation or of recessive inheritance acting, as is usually the case, in the presence of a clear family history. Genetic counselling for such sporadic cases can be very difficult in the absence of a direct test for the mutant gene, and has to depend on estimates of the relative frequency of dominant and recessive cases.

Of the 23 pairs of chromosomes, numbers 1–22 are inherited identically in males and females. They are known as autosomes. The genes on them show autosomal inheritance, either dominant or recessive, meaning that the probability of inheriting a particular gene is independent of the sex of the parent or offspring. Recently, it has been shown that the effects (but not the probability of transmission) of some genes differ according to whether they are transmitted by the mother or father, a phenomenon known as imprinting.

Genes carried on the sex chromosomes, the X and Y, are transmitted by a father according to the sex of his offspring, since a man transmits his X chromosome to all his daughters and his Y chromosome to all his sons. In males there is only a single copy of the genes on the X and Y, so X-linked defects which are recessive in females are expressed

in males. There are very few Y-linked disorders
and even fewer that are familial, since most cause
infertility. The characteristic pattern of X-linked
recessive inheritance, where affected males are born
to carrier mothers and have sisters half of whom
are also carriers, is easily recognized in large
families; however, conditions which severely reduce fertility in affected males, such as Duchenne
muscular dystrophy (DMD), tend not to persist in
families for many generations and are more often
caused by a recent mutation, so large pedigrees are
rare.

Testing for single-gene defects by DNA analysis

The use of recombinant DNA techniques has been
the most far-reaching biomedical development of
the second half of the twentieth century, and its
full potential has not yet been realized in the field
of inherited disease. A knowledge of DNA structure
and function is now as important to general medical
understanding as, for example, cardiovascular physiology. The application of DNA analysis to testing
and prediction in families depends on a few basic
genetic principles which are not widely understood
by doctors. A very brief summary of these principles
is given here. A fuller explanation is available from
introductory texts, such as Weatherall (1991) or
Connor & Ferguson Smith (1991).

Human chromosomes contain a great deal more
DNA – perhaps 100 times more – than is needed to
encode the amino acid sequences of all the proteins
that humans produce. Most DNA does not have a
coding function and non-coding DNA lies between
genes or within them, for, surprisingly, the coding
regions (exons) of most genes are interrupted by
non-coding segments called introns.

Whether or not it is coding, DNA has the same
basic structure: a long thread-like molecule bearing
a sequence of purine and pyrimidine bases. The
bases are of four types. Within coding regions their
sequence determines the amino acid sequence of a
protein, and changes that alter this in functionally
significant ways are likely to be both rare and
clinically important. Within non-coding regions,
far more variation in DNA sequence can exist between chromosomes in the population.

Genetic variants, whether of non-coding DNA

sequences or of coding DNA and its derived protein,
which are relatively common in the population
(arbitrarily, present in one individual in 100 or
more) are known as polymorphisms. Well-known
protein polymorphisms include blood groups, serum
protein electrophoretic variants and human
leucocyte antigen (HLA) types.

The power of DNA analysis in human genetics
depends on its ability to 'read' the DNA sequence
at specific points in the genome. Most of the difficulties are related to focusing on the right region
to analyse. Finding a gene of some tens of thousands
of bases in size in a genome of 3 000 000 000
bases can be very difficult unless a lucky short cut
presents itself.

DNA analysis depends on a number of essentially
simple properties of DNA and related enzymes.
Some of these are listed below.

1 Restriction endonuclease enzymes cut the DNA
strand wherever they encounter a specific sequence
of bases. Each enzyme has its own recognition
sequence. The same enzyme acting on different
DNA samples will therefore produce different patterns of DNA fragments if the samples differ, even
by a single base, at one of the enzyme's cutting
sites.

2 DNA fragments can be separated by size on an
electrophoretic gel.

3 DNA in its normal double-stranded form can be
denatured, separating the paired strands, which
can then be made to reassociate by adjusting the
physical or chemical conditions. The reassociation
process depends on the correctness of the match
between the base sequences on the single strands
involved (normally, bases on paired strands are
matched so that each of the four bases on one
strand always has the same partner on the opposite
strand). This property can be used to identify
sequences of interest among a large collection of
heterogeneous DNA fragments by introducing a
short, radioactively or chemically labelled, single-
stranded DNA fragment, known as a probe, to the
reassociation process.

4 DNA can be replicated *in vitro*, using polymerase
enzymes which may use as a template either
genomic (chromosomal) DNA or messenger
ribonucleic acid (RNA); the latter produces a copy
of the gene without the introns, known as complementary DNA (cDNA).

The polymerase chain reaction is a phenomenally accurate way of targeting DNA replication, so that a tiny segment of the genome is repetitively amplified to produce analysable amounts from a minute initial sample.

The aim of DNA analysis in single-gene disorders is to identify the defective gene and show how it differs from the normal gene. One should then have a definitive test for the condition and a start to determining its pathogenesis by defining the protein defect. An important complication is that few single-gene disorders are caused by a single mutation: the gene will have mutated in different ways in different families, especially if the condition is maintained in the population by recurrent mutation rather than by transmission of mutations from earlier generations. In the case of dominant and X-linked conditions, this means that those reducing fertility are likely to be heterogeneous at the DNA level. Autosomal recessive conditions are sometimes homogeneous at the DNA level even when effectively lethal, because recessive inheritance shields mutations from selection.

The pattern of mutations in a condition, if it is known, will dictate tactics when families request testing. The ideal is to know which mutation to look for in each family, but it is sometimes impracticable to screen a whole gene for mutations. An alternative approach is to use the principle of linkage, sometimes known as 'gene tracking'. If the position of the gene on a chromosome is known but the gene has not been precisely identified, linkage is the only approach possible. Table 30.1 shows the usual stages in the identification of a disease gene and their clinical implications.

By linkage one follows a gene through a family

Table 30.1 Stages in the identification of disease genes

State of knowledge	How established	Application	Examples
Known Mendelian condition	Family studies	Genetic counselling, risk estimation	Dominant ataxias (some), CMT (some), HSP
Chromosome location identified	Linkage studies, disease-associated translocations	(i) Linkage homogeneity: refined risk estimates and prenatal diagnosis	HD, Friedreich, FSH dystrophy, acute/ subacute SMA
		(ii) Heterogeneity: above only possible in large families and/or with reduced accuracy	Tuberous sclerosis, dominant ataxias
Gene identified	Chromosome walking and jumping, protein product known so cDNA can be identified, cloning of translocation breaks	Highly accurate testing using intragenic polymorphisms (locus heterogeneity may still be a problem)	DMD, BMD cases where no mutation identified
Mutations identified	Screen exons for deletions/ duplications, techniques for identification of single-base changes	(i) One or a small number of mutations: gives a highly specific test for condition in families and in general population	Myotonic dystrophy, CMT 1 (most)
		(ii) Many different mutations: accurate testing usually possible in families with preparatory work; less helpful as diagnostic test in new case	DMD, BMD

BMD = Becker muscular dystrophy; CMT = Charcot−Marie−Tooth disease; DMD = Duchenne muscular dystrophy; FSH = facioscapulohumeral dystrophy; HD = Huntington's disease; HSP = hereditary spastic paraplegia; SMA = spinal muscular atrophy.

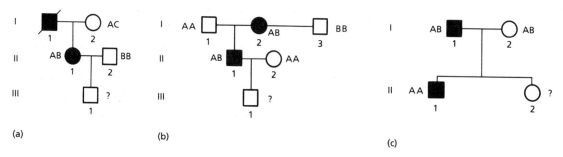

Fig. 30.1 Pedigree showing the use of linkage analysis in diagnosis.

(a) A genetic marker (usually a DNA polymorphism) can exist, on different chromosomes, as A, B or C, and is known to be closely linked to the disease gene in which we are interested. Person III,1 is at 50% risk of a late onset dominant disorder such as Huntington's disease and wants to know whether he has inherited the condition from his mother. The family study shows that person II,1 must have inherited B from her father, therefore, in her, B is linked to the disease gene and A to the normal gene. III,1 will either be BB (high risk) or AB (low risk).

(b) In this example, the interpretation of linkage phase depends on paternity. If I,1 was the father of II,1 AA would be a low risk result for III,1 and AB a high risk result, but if I,3 was the father, this would be reversed.

(c) In this example note (i) the reliability of a result on II,2 is approximately half what it is in the previous 2 examples because linkage phase in I,1 has been deduced from his son II,1, so that there are two opportunities for recombination (see text), (ii) if II,2 has the genotype AB, the test will be uninformative for this marker.

by following the inheritance of genetic polymorphisms, usually DNA sequence polymorphisms, known to be located within or very close to the gene of interest and therefore almost always transmitted with it. One must first have established the linkage phase, which means finding out which version (or 'allele') of the polymorphism is linked to the disease gene and which ones are linked to the normal genes in that particular family. Some form of family study is always necessary before a linkage-based test can be used. Usually, two or three close relatives of known affected, unaffected or carrier status must be tested before results on the unknown can be interpreted. Some examples are given in Fig. 30.1.

Recombination (crossing over) takes place between homologous chromosomes when they become associated during early meiosis (Fig. 30.2). The effect of this process is that whole grandmaternal or grandpaternal chromosomes are not transmitted to the offspring intact; instead, composite chromosomes are formed containing blocks of the grandmother's and grandfather's genes.

The probability that two loci on a chromosome will be separated by a crossover between them increases with their physical separation. Gene tracking is thus most reliable when the genetic markers used are very close to or even within the gene of interest. When a gene is first mapped, the closest known polymorphisms may give 10–20% recombination at meiosis, which would be of limited value for a clinical test. Rapid progress can usually then be made in detecting more tightly linked markers. Any linkage-based test will have an error rate attributable to crossing over, although, if the region around the gene is well mapped, the error rate may be less than 1%.

There is usually no significance in which allele of a polymorphism is linked to the disease allele of a particular gene. It differs between families, and typing for the polymorphism would tell one nothing about the likelihood of an unrelated person having the disease gene.

Another prerequisite for a linkage-based test is a correct diagnosis, for the assumption is made that the disease gene in the family being tested is in the same chromosomal location as it was in the families used for the original gene-mapping studies. Linkage studies are difficult when different genes can mutate and cause a similar clinical disorder. For example, it is clear that at least two different genes on the short arm of the X chromosome can cause retinitis pigmentosa. In a large family, it may be possible to establish which gene is responsible, but in a small

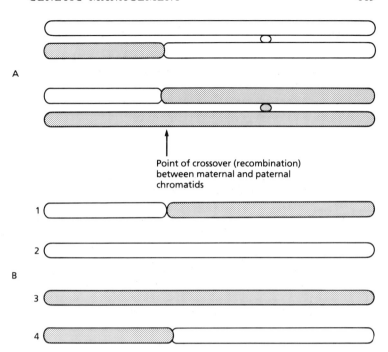

Point of crossover (recombination) between maternal and paternal chromatids

Fig. 30.2 Chromosome diagram showing crossing over at meiosis. (A) Maternal and paternal chromosomes at meiosis. (B) Chromosomes received by different gametes.

family the contribution of DNA testing may be limited.

It follows from the above discussion that, whether mutational testing or linkage is used, the availability of DNA from an affected person may determine whether testing can be offered to relatives. Enough DNA for most purposes can be extracted from 20 ml of blood, and clinical geneticists will advise on local procedures. One may therefore need to consider storing DNA from an affected person in case relatives request testing years later, after the affected person has died. If the relevant analysis can be done by the polymerase chain reaction, it may be possible to extract enough DNA from minute tissue samples, such as neonatal screening blood spots or fixed tissue in paraffin blocks.

The genetic management of specific conditions

The pace of research in human genetics is such that significant advances in some of the diseases discussed here will certainly be made while this book is in press. The discoveries of mutations causing CMT (Lupski *et al.*, 1992) and myotonic

dystrophy (Harley *et al.*, 1992) are very recent, but they are already being used in clinical practice.

This chapter uses the genetics of some of the better-known chronic neurological disorders to illustrate the principles of genetic counselling. It is not intended to substitute for the excellent and far more exhaustive reviews of neurological genetics by Bundey (1992) and Baraitser (1990). They cover the highly important area of differential diagnosis, including rare conditions. Decisions on what to include in this chapter have been somewhat arbitrary. MacMillan & Harper (1991) review the epidemiology of the more important neurological single-gene disorders: hereditary motor and sensory neuropathy, myotonic dystrophy, DMD and Becker muscular dystrophy (BMD), facioscapulohumeral dystrophy, spinal muscular atrophy, Huntington's disease (HD), tuberous sclerosis, von Hippel–Lindau disease, HSP and neurofibromatosis. They show that, in aggregate, these 11 disorders have a prevalence (in South Wales) of 58.6 per 100 000, half that of multiple sclerosis. Four disorders in this list, spinal muscular atrophy, tuberous sclerosis, neurofibromatosis and von Hippel–Lindau disease, are not covered here.

The importance of establishing the correct diagnosis cannot be overstated in genetic counselling for neurological disorders. Hearsay diagnoses should never be accepted. A precise diagnosis is often the key to the genetics, especially when the family history is unhelpful. For this reason, the *London Neurogenetics Database* (Baraitser & Winter, 1992) is indispensable for anyone involved in neurological genetics. It contains details of over 2000 neurological conditions, which can be retrieved using combinations of clinical and genetic features.

The second essential of genetic counselling is a correct family history. Given the variability of many genetic neurological conditions, this often means not only accurate history-taking but examining and testing relatives to determine their status. Even when a precise diagnosis cannot be made, the family history often shows the inheritance pattern.

Huntington's disease

HD has a prevalence of between 5 and 10 per 10 000, but, given that a gene carrier is asymptomatic for around three-fifths of his/her life, it follows that between 1 in 4000 and 1 in 5000 people are born with the gene for the condition. At least twice this number of people are identifiably at risk and, if their spouses are included, up to 1 in 1000 people may potentially be concerned with the condition and require genetic advice – 300 people in a medium-sized health district.

The diagnosis of HD is usually made with knowledge of a positive family history. The dangers of a false diagnosis are such that the features of the index case must be critically reviewed, and clinical and pathological confirmation of affected relatives must be sought whenever possible. In an apparently sporadic case, the correctness of genetic advice rests on the clinical assessment of a single patient, something that most clinical geneticists will not be happy to undertake without help from a neurologist. The differential diagnosis is reviewed by Quarrell & Harper (1991). Other possible explanations for a sporadic case should be considered when taking the family history: false paternity, death of a parent while still presymptomatic or undiagnosed (which cannot be completely excluded up to the late 70s), and fresh mutation, which is very rare.

Family breakdown and illegitimacy are common in HD families. Occasionally it is justifiable to carry out paternity testing, using hypervariable DNA polymorphisms in the course of genetic counselling or predictive testing. If so, it is obviously desirable that all those involved should know about and consent to this type of testing. When false paternity is inadvertently discovered in the course of family studies, most clinical geneticists will simply tell the client that the test was 'uninformative' or 'low risk' without giving the reason (see Fig. 30.1).

HD illustrates more clearly than any other condition the intimate connection between a client's reaction to risk information and his or her experience of the condition. For that reason, genetic counselling needs to take place in the context of a review of the disease in the client's family, and to be somehow allied to the prospect of planning care for those already affected, and, by implication, those possibly to be affected in the future. In practice, time spent discussing the memories of an affected relative, the client's role as carer, and the resulting image he or she has of the condition is valuable and important. It often releases reactions of sadness and guilt that have been repressed for years. Misconceptions about the nature and inheritance of HD can be noted and corrected.

Some people who come requesting risk information or predictive testing are already clinically affected. Others are responsible for the care of an affected parent, and need advice on management and sources of help in the community. It is therefore helpful to offer genetic counselling for HD as a joint consultation with a specialist in neurological rehabilitation. A third member of the team is the genetic associate, whose role is to maintain contact with the family, providing support and reinforcement of information given in the clinic, by means of telephone calls and home visits. Each HD family represents an open-ended commitment for the genetic service, to provide information and help whenever the family needs it, in the light of its changing circumstances and scientific advances. A genetic register, usually run by the genetic associate, is the means by which help can be offered.

We have found at Southampton that, although the genetic associate, the rehabilitation specialist and the clinical geneticist form the core of the HD service, the genetic clinic provides a natural focus for other disciplines, such as social work, psychiatry, occupational and speech therapy and dietetics. We recommend anyone providing a service for HD to foster such contacts, and to hold regular multidisciplinary meetings to discuss general issues and individual patient problems.

The genetic facts of HD are relatively straightforward. The offspring of an affected parent has a 50% risk of inheriting the defective gene, and those who do will eventually develop symptoms, but the age of onset varies widely, from childhood to the 70s, and little is known of the factors governing this variability. The offspring of affected fathers tend to have earlier onset than those of affected mothers, so that cases with juvenile onset are almost all in the former group. The mechanism of this effect is not yet known. Ages of onset are also positively correlated within families, and may be related to other genes controlling longevity (Farrer & Conneally, 1985) but the correlation is not enough to make a great difference to genetic counselling. A cumulative frequency curve of onset against age shows that 50% of those with the gene are symptomatic by their late 40s (Harper & Newcombe, 1992). This means that an asymptomatic person who was at 50% risk has become at 33% risk by his or her late 40s, and this figure can be halved for the risk to his or her children. The family must understand that if the at-risk person becomes affected (or is shown to be at high risk by a predictive test) the risk to the children will rise to 50% (or almost, depending on their age).

The HD gene was shown by linkage studies by Gusella et al. in 1983 to be on chromosome 4 and no family has yet been reported in which linkage data have been inconsistent with this localization. When the gene is identified, it will become clear whether all affected families have the same type of gene defect (mutation). The lack of selection against the disorder, shown by its long persistence in the population and its geographical distribution as a European gene, suggest that derivation of all or most HD genes from a single ancestral mutation is a possibility. If so, the diagnosis may be confirmed or virtually excluded by a simple blood test. If not, the mutation will need to be identified by testing a blood sample from an affected person in each family.

Presymptomatic testing for HD has a long history, dating back to various clinical and pharmacological manoeuvres that were tried before the DNA era. The uptake of predictive testing, since it became technically possible in 1983, has been lower than many people expected. A common response to learning of one's at-risk status seems to be to request testing in order to resolve some of the uncertainty of the situation; however, during the 'cooling-off period' imposed by counselling protocols and the need to obtain family samples and check informativeness, some candidates for testing change their minds (Craufurd et al., 1989). This appears to validate the offering of predictive testing only as part of a protocol, which includes two or three pre-test counselling sessions. At present, all centres in the UK undertaking presymptomatic testing belong to a consortium which encourages adherence to the agreed protocol and facilitates the collection of national data on referrals and completed tests (Tyler et al., 1992). It remains to be seen whether, if 'free-standing' mutational testing becomes available, the consortium will be able to prevent its being offered as a laboratory service without clinical back-up. See Fig. 30.1 for an explanation of the use of linked genetic markers in diagnosis.

The principles of predictive testing embodied in the protocol will be relevant to other late-onset genetic disorders, many of which are neurological, as presymptomatic testing becomes available for them.

During the pre-test counselling sessions it seems appropriate to encourage the client to think about his or her reasons for requesting predictive testing and how it would feel to receive a high- or a low-risk result. It is important to identify the pressure which relatives often apply to at-risk people towards predictive testing and to make as certain as possible that the decision to proceed is the client's own. Sources of support for the period of testing, which will inevitably generate anxiety, need to be identified. There are no hard-and-fast rules, but it is desirable that a partner or close friend be involved and that the general practitioner is fully aware of the procedure (a few clients wish to keep their general practitioner in ignorance of their at-risk status). It is helpful if an interested professional (who could be a social worker, community nurse or the general practitioner) can be nominated as a first-line contact in crisis. Pre-test counselling should also help the client to understand the technical basis of the test, including the error rate. At present, the most closely linked probes used for HD testing show a crossover rate of 2% or less with the HD gene (Harper *et al.*, 1991). The resulting error rate in clinical testing will vary with the structure of the pedigree as well as with the probes used in a particular family. Candidates for predictive testing should be asked whether, if a definitive test becomes available in the future, they would like their DNA retested, understanding that there will be a (usually small) chance that the original predictive test result will be reversed. The ability to provide definitive testing may, as pointed out above, depend on the availability of DNA from one affected person in the family.

Those at-risk people who decide against predictive testing may still wish to know whether they show any clinical signs of HD, and they may wish to attend yearly or 2-yearly follow-up to have this confirmed. If signs then develop, the doctor may face a difficult problem of how much to tell. It will help if there has been prior discussion of how much the client wants to know, and also of the fact that clinical certainty is unlikely to be instant but may require repeated examinations over months or years.

It is sometimes possible to test the pregnancy of an at-risk parent to show whether the fetus has inherited a high-risk genetic marker from its affected grandparent or a low-risk marker from its unaffected grandparent, so-called prenatal exclusion. This approach is likely to appeal to those who have a strong wish not to pass on the condition to the next generation. It requires the couple to consider termination when the fetus is at essentially the same risk of HD (usually 50%) as the at-risk parent. If a high-risk pregnancy is continued, the resulting child will be at close to 100% risk if the at-risk parent later becomes affected, and this is ethically questionable. In practice, there has been little demand for prenatal exclusion. Its existence is a by-product of gene tracking by linkage and it will be difficult to sustain when mutational testing becomes available.

In March 1993, the discovery was announced of a convincing candidate for the HD gene (Huntington's Disease Collaborative Research Group, 1993), which appears to be mutated in all

or the great majority of HD patients and not in controls. The mutation is a trinucleotide (CAG) repeat sequence expansion, similar to the fragile X and myotonic dystrophy mutations. It therefore seems likely that predictive testing will be freed from the necessity for linkage studies. Whenever possible, however, one index patient in each family should be tested, to confirm that the family has the usual mutation, before testing at-risk individuals. The predictive testing counselling protocol should still be followed. The test may also be used diagnostically in patients who have a clinical presentation suggestive of HD.

Myotonic dystrophy

A prominent feature of myotonic dystrophy which has made genetic counselling difficult is its variability. Although it shows regular autosomal dominant inheritance, severely affected patients often have parents and grandparents who are mildly or minimally affected, leading to the appearance of anticipation – the increasing severity of a genetic disorder in successive generations. Geneticists have traditionally regarded anticipation as an artefact of ascertainment: those families showing earlier onset in succeeding generations are more likely to be recognized as having a dominant disorder.

The gene defect causing myotonic dystrophy has recently been identified (Harley *et al.*, 1992a, b), linkage to chromosome 19 having first been detected in 1982. The mutation has been found to consist of amplification of a trinucleotide (CTG) repeat in the non-coding part of the gene at its 'downstream' end. The degree of amplification tends to increase in successive generations and correlates with, but does not entirely explain, the degree of severity. In the general population there are between 5 and 40 copies of the three-base repeat, and in almost all patients with myotonic dystrophy so far tested there are over 50 and up to 2000 or more. Experience with the new molecular test is reviewed by Suthers *et al.* (1992) and by several other authors in the November 1992 issue of the *Journal of Medical Genetics*. They knew of only three out of several hundred myotonic dystrophy patients tested who did not show the CTG repeat amplification.

Clinical evaluation of at-risk relatives will still be

important in genetic counselling, firstly to clarify the degree of correlation between the mutational pattern and clinical severity, and secondly to help in discussing the significance of the diagnosis to a particular family. The most important features to look for are the characteristic distribution of weakness and wasting, clinical and electrical myotonia, and cataracts on slit-lamp examination of the eyes. It seems likely, however, that the new molecular test will allow definitive identification of gene carriers in a family, and will probably provide a diagnostic test that can be used on patients with no family history.

It is clearly appropriate to offer presymptomatic testing to at-risk adults who may be concerned about the risks to their children. Some of the considerations discussed above in testing for HD also apply here. Presymptomatic testing of children is, in this condition and others where no treatment or preventive measures are available, ethically controversial and probably unjustified, unless there is a clinical indication, such as symptoms that may be related to the disease.

The greatest problem in genetic counselling in myotonic dystrophy arises over prenatal diagnosis and prediction of congenital involvement, which is the most severe form of the disease. Congenitally affected infants, who suffer from neonatal hypotonia and have a significant early mortality rate, are always born to affected mothers (not fathers), who are themselves at least moderately affected. A mother who has had one congenitally affected infant faces an increased risk that other affected infants will be congenitally affected; however, it is not yet clear whether molecular testing will be able to identify fetuses destined for congenital onset. In this condition, as in many others, a family's response to genetic counselling will depend largely on its own experience of what it means to be affected.

Charcot–Marie–Tooth disease (CMT, hereditary motor and sensory neuropathy)

In this group of conditions inheritance is autosomal dominant in most families but autosomal recessive in a minority. Motor nerve conduction velocity is severely reduced (<30 m/sec) in neuronal (type 1)

CMT, but normal or mildly reduced in the axonal type (type 2). There are pathological differences between the two types, and they tend to breed true within families (Vance, 1991). Genetically, therefore, pedigree pattern and nerve conduction velocity allow four different autosomal varieties of CMT to be recognized. There is also a well-documented but rare X-linked recessive variety. Diagnostic confusion between CMT and the inherited ataxias and spastic paraplegias may occur because of the occasional occurrence of pyramidal and cerebellar signs in CMT.

Often, the pedigree will indicate the mode of inheritance in a particular family, but an apparently sporadically affected person with a negative family history could have either a fresh mutation to dominant CMT, with a 50% risk to offspring, or recessive CMT with a very low risk. Before accepting that the patient's parents are unaffected, one should examine them for distal weakness, high-arched feet and absent ankle jerks, or request examination by a competent observer, and consider referring them for neurophysiological tests. These are particularly helpful in type 1 families with severely slowed nerve conduction.

Genetic counselling concerning risks to the offspring of affected or at-risk clients is often made difficult by variation in severity which can occur within families. Prospective parents will want to know the risk of severe involvement rather than the risk of transmitting the gene, and this is unpredictable. In some families, males tend to be more severely affected than females, but not dependably so. Although CMT does not seem to doctors to be among the most severe of neurological disorders, in the author's experience affected families often take the risk of transmission very seriously, and some are likely to request prenatal diagnosis when it is available.

Linkage to chromosome 17 was shown in type 1 CMT families in 1989, and recently a chromosomal duplication of at least 1 million base pairs at 17p11.2 was shown to be the basis of the mutation in the majority of type 1 dominant CMT families (Lupski et al., 1992). The presence of this duplication can therefore be used as a highly specific diagnostic test for one variety of CMT, now known as CMT1A, which appears to account for the majority of cases of dominantly inherited type 1 CMT. It is likely to be helpful in confirming the diagnosis in at-risk members of families known to be segregating this particular mutation, and in prenatal diagnosis. It will also identify some sporadic cases as new dominant mutations.

The minority of type 1 dominant CMT families which do not show linkage to chromosome 17 include some families with linkage to the Duffy blood group on chromosome 1. The mapping of other CMT genes (apart from the X-linked type, which has been mapped to Xq13) remains an important task for the future.

Dementias

Genetic counselling in the dementias is made difficult by late onset and heterogeneity. Dementia is of course a feature of HD (and is sometimes the presenting feature), and of some of the hereditary ataxias, spongiform encephalopathies and mitochondrial disorders, as well as occurring secondarily in a wide range of medical conditions.

In an isolated, apparently primary, dementia, close relatives may request genetic counselling, especially if onset is early. Unfortunately, two of the main neuropathological entities, Alzheimer's and Pick's disease, cannot be reliably clinically distinguished. Both show increased risks to first-degree relatives of between 3 and 10%, higher for Pick's disease than for Alzheimer's (Baraitser, 1990). Both are sometimes familial, with a pattern suggesting autosomal dominant inheritance, and in such families the risk faced by the offspring of affected persons of developing the condition by old age is higher and may approach 50% in some families.

The occurrence of an Alzheimer-like dementia in Down syndrome led to the discovery of linkage in some familial Alzheimer pedigrees to chromosome 21. In other families a gene or genes elsewhere appear to be responsible. In some of the chromosome 21-linked families, mutations have been found in the amyloid protein precursor gene at 21q21. This was regarded as a candidate gene because its product includes the protein that accumulates in Alzheimer's disease (Kosick, 1992).

The practical implications of these findings are that presymptomatic testing can only be offered in families where either a causative mutation has been identified or linkage studies within the family are able to indicate with a fair degree of reliability that the responsible gene in that family maps to the site of a known Alzheimer gene. At present these requirements exclude all but a small minority of at-risk people from presymptomatic testing, but that will change if more Alzheimer mutations are discovered over the next few years. The guidelines described above for HD testing should be applied to Alzheimer testing and in any other late-onset, chronic, progressive condition.

Mutation in the amyloid protein precursor gene is also responsible for Dutch-type hereditary cerebral haemorrhage with amyloidosis. It is not unexpected that different mutations in the same gene should cause different diseases, and other examples, such as DMD and BMD, are well known. More speculatively, one may wonder whether polymorphic variations in the amyloid protein precursor gene and other genes implicated in familial Alzheimer's disease affect susceptibility to the sporadic disease. If so, population typing for dementia risk factors could follow, but would probably not be popular unless there were preventive measures.

Inherited ataxias

Friedreich's ataxia

The main division is between Friedreich's ataxia and the rest. Friedreich's is defined (Harding, 1984) as having onset before the age of 25, cerebellar ataxia and dysarthria, absent tendon reflexes in the lower limbs, extensor plantar responses and abnormalities of peripheral nerve conduction. Other features may include sensory loss, optic atrophy and cardiomyopathy, but not dementia. When defined in this way, Friedreich's ataxia consistently follows an autosomal recessive inheritance pattern.

Many cases of familial ataxia have in the past been wrongly labelled as Friedreich's, leading to confusion about the genetics. It is particularly important with familial ataxias not to accept diagnosis at face value.

The gene responsible was mapped to the long arm of chromosome 9 by linkage studies in 1988 and no discrepant families have been reported, suggesting that only a single gene locus is involved

(Chamberlain *et al.*, 1989). Although at the time of writing the gene has not been identified, very closely linked DNA markers are available, allowing accurate prenatal diagnosis in the siblings of affected cases. The diagnosis is rarely made early enough, however, for parents to be warned of the 25% sibling recurrence risk or to be offered prenatal diagnosis.

Although a frequent cause for concern in affected families, the recurrence risk in the offspring of patients and of their unaffected siblings is low. Occasional recurrences in the next generation can be accounted for by an unrelated partner being a gene carrier. With a birth incidence of the disease around 1 in 40 000, 1 in 100 of the general population are expected to be carriers, which means that the risk to the offspring of an affected person is 1 in 200. If a person with Friedreich's ataxia marries a first cousin, their risk of an affected child is 1 in 8.

Other ataxias

Ataxia can be a presenting feature of many important but rare genetic disorders such as Refsum disease, abetalipoproteinaemia, ataxia telangiectasia, late-onset lysosomal storage disorders, mitochondrial enzyme defects with both nuclear and mitochondrial mutations, and Gerstmann–Straussler syndrome. Cerebellar ataxia with adult onset and no identifiable underlying cause is often genetic and usually autosomal dominant. The wide range of associated features such as optic atrophy, ophthalmoplegia, dementia, spasticity and deafness in such cases has led to terminological confusion. The writings of Harding (1984) are recommended as an antidote.

The presence of a dominant family history will often confirm the inheritance pattern. A pitfall may be to fail to recognize mitochondrial inheritance where transmission is only by females, but the pattern of associated features will usually alert one to a mitochondrial defect.

Genetic counselling in late-onset dominantly inherited ataxias is difficult because of their variability. Within a single family, one person may be affected in the teens and another may remain asymptomatic until middle age. Many of the associated features are also inconsistent within families.

So far, only one form of dominant ataxia has been mapped, that linked to the HLA region on chromosome 6, and the mutation has recently been shown to be another trinucleotide repeat amplification (Orr *et al.*, 1993). This could be used for presymptomatic or prenatal testing in families showing the mutation.

Hereditary spastic paraplegia (HSP)

Harding (1984) gives an excellent summary of the genetics of this group of disorders. 'Pure' HSP excludes the many conditions where HSP is associated with mental retardation, dementia, visual abnormalities, ataxia or other major neurological features; however, even in 'pure' HSP there may be clinical and pathological evidence of posterior column involvement.

Harding found that inheritance was dominant in the majority of families with familial HSP, and autosomal recessive in a minority. Because there is no definitive test, however, recessive HSP can only be diagnosed with reasonable certainty in the presence of affected sibs or parental consanguinity. Single cases may be difficult to separate from cerebral palsy from non-genetic causes.

Family studies suggest that autosomal dominant HSP exists in at least two genetically distinct varieties, one with an early onset (infancy up to the 30s) and slow progression, and one with later onset (15 years to old age) and more rapid progression. Within each type there is wide variation in severity, but all adult gene carriers show clinical signs (brisk tendon jerks, extensor plantars, spastic gait) on examination. Relatives cannot be assumed to be unaffected on the basis of history alone. So far, genes for HSP have not been mapped, except that there does appear to be a rare X-linked variety caused by a mutation on the long arm of the X chromosome (Keppen *et al.*, 1987). Caution is needed in interpreting a pedigree as X-linked because females have tended to be more mildly affected than males in some of the autosomal dominant HSP families.

Duchenne and Becker muscular dystrophies (DMD, BMD)

These were among the first diseases to be tackled by the molecular genetic techniques which came into

HIS OLD MUM WAS RED HOT	The normal message
HIS OLD GUM WAS RED HOT	Single base substitution alters one amino acid (missense)
HIS MUM WAS RED HOT	Three base (in phase) deletion removes one amino acid
HIS OLD ASR EDH OT	Four base (frameshift) deletion which alters the message downstream and is likely to generate a 'stop' codon
HIS OLD MUM WAS RED HOT BOO WAA YAA	Mutation of a splice site or 'stop' codon which extends the message into parts of the gene not normally translated
H	Large deletion affecting most or all of the coding sequence

Fig. 30.3 Illustration of different types of gene mutations using a written language analogy. Like the DNA message, this message consists of three-letter words. In DNA each 'word' would represent an amino acid or a 'stop' codon and the whole language would contain only four 'letters' (bases), and therefore 64 'words' (triplets or codons). Note that the reading frame (the grouping of bases in threes) is determined only by the starting-point and not by any intrinsic property of DNA structure.

use in the early 1980s. It is remarkable that only 10 years ago there was uncertainty whether DMD and BMD resulted from mutations in the same gene or different genes. Kingston *et al.* (1983) showed that they mapped to the same part of the X chromosome, and later both were shown to be sometimes associated with deletion of the same DNA markers. In general, DMD mutations render undetectable the gene's protein product (dystrophin), whereas BMD mutations cause a less severe deficiency.

The dystrophin gene is located at Xp21.2 on the short arm of the X chromosome. It is 2.7 mb (2.7×10^6 bases) in size but its messenger RNA, which contains the translated sequences, is only 16 000 bases in length. There are about 70 exons (coding sequences), which can be screened for molecular deletions by a multiple polymerase chain reaction procedure. About two-thirds of DMD and BMD patients show deletions, or, more rarely, duplications, of part of the dystrophin gene by this procedure. Most of the variation in severity is determined by whether the deletion is in frame (affecting a multiple of three bases) or not. If not, its effects will extend beyond the 3' ('downstream') end of the deletion by disrupting the reading frame of the gene, a so-called frame-shift mutation, which often truncates the protein by producing a 'stop' codon (see Fig. 30.3).

If a dystrophin gene deletion or duplication is found in a patient with a muscle disorder, it can reasonably be assumed to be causative, although a few dystrophin deletions with very mild effects such as muscle cramps have been described, and the range of normal variation in dystrophin is not yet known. The detection of dystrophin mutations has allowed patients previously labelled as limb-girdle muscular dystrophy and as spinal muscular atrophy to be assigned to BMD.

The birth prevalence of BMD is thought to be about 1 in 20 000 males. There is considerable between-family variation in the age of onset, rate of progression of weakness and presence or absence of learning difficulties, as might be expected with the great variety of mutations (Bushby, 1992).

The occurrence of mental retardation in DMD and BMD is not fully explained; the dystrophin gene is expressed in the brain but its function there is not known.

In the 30–40% of BMD and DMD cases where no mutation is detected in the index patient, it is assumed that small deletions, duplications and point mutations exist. Newer techniques will be able to demonstrate these in some cases, although they may remain too labour-intensive for routine use in the near future. The detection of a mutation makes possible definitive prenatal and carrier testing in families. Where no mutation has been detected, considerable uncertainty may remain, especially if no affected males are available for linkage studies, or an affected male is apparently the first case in the family. In these cases the probability of a woman being a carrier must be calculated by combining information from the pedigree, creatine kinase levels and linked marker studies, using Bayes' theorem. The daughters of affected males are all carriers, as in any X-linked disorder, and the risk to the offspring of a woman of uncertain carrier status is her carrier risk times one-quarter, or times one-half if she is known to have a male fetus.

BMD and DMD families should be known to the regional genetics service and included on a genetic register so that genetic counselling and testing can be offered to at-risk women at the appropriate times.

Other dystrophies

Limb-girdle dystrophy

Limb-girdle dystrophy, once a commonly used diagnosis, is now regarded as an unsatisfactory label (Walton & Gardner-Medwin, 1988). Cases thus classified might have a histologically specific myopathy, including a mitochondrial myopathy, a spinal muscular atrophy or BMD, or, in the case of females, could be manifesting carriers of DMD or BMD. A search for dystrophin gene mutations should therefore be considered in the investigation of both limb-girdle dystrophy and 'spinal muscular atrophy' showing a limb-girdle distribution.

Facioscapulohumeral dystrophy

Typically, the pattern is of facial and shoulder-girdle weakness coming on in the teens or early 20s, sometimes in childhood. There may be lower limb weakness, giving a facioscapuloperoneal pattern. Inheritance is usually clearly autosomal dominant. Family studies (Lunt & Harper, 1991) show that gene carriers are very likely to have clinical signs of weakness and wasting by the age of 20, but it is unwise to rely for genetic counselling on a statement that a given relative is asymptomatic, since one-third of gene carriers remain mildly affected. A small proportion of cases are isolated, with parents who are normal on examination. Most of these probably represent fresh mutations of the gene; a few may have a gene carrier parent who shows non-penetrance, but Lunt & Harper found non-penetrance in adults to be rare. In either event, there will be a 50% risk to the offspring of the affected person.

Linkage to chromosome 4 (reviewed in Sarfarazi et al., 1992) was established in 1990, but the available markers may still be unreliable for prenatal or presymptomatic diagnosis. A recent observation by Wijmenga et al. (1992) suggests that identification of the gene may be imminent.

So far, there has been little or no demand for prenatal diagnosis, probably because in most families the condition is not perceived as being severe enough. There may be a role for presymptomatic DNA diagnosis where a young at-risk adult is considering having children.

Mitochondrial disorders

A good summary of current knowledge can be found in Brenton (1992).

Oxidative phosphorylation, the main source of energy in the cell, takes place in mitochondria. Most mitochondrial proteins are coded for by nuclear genes, so that deficiencies of some respiratory chain enzymes, such as pyruvate dehydrogenase and fumarase, are inherited in a Mendelian fashion. Thirteen enzyme subunits necessary for oxidative phosphorylation are determined by the mitochondrial genome, a 16 500 base pair, circular, double-stranded DNA molecule. Some components of the protein synthesis machinery within the mitochondria are coded for by the mitochondrial DNA, but others, plus the replication mechanism for mitochondrial DNA, are specified in the nucleus.

Mitochondrial disorders are typically multisystem and progressive, but may be sufficiently slowly progressive to be included in this chapter. Although the CNS and skeletal and cardiac muscle are their prime targets, other organs such as the liver, kidney, pancreas and bone marrow may also be affected. The diagnosis is often suggested by the clinical picture, muscle biopsy findings and lactic acidaemia, but a more specific diagnosis requires biochemical assays of the oxidative phosphorylation enzyme complexes and/or analysis of mitochondrial DNA.

Mutations in mitochondrial DNA have been identified in a wide range of clinical conditions, including Leber's optic atrophy, myoclonic epilepsy with ragged red fibres (MERRF), mitochondrial myopathy, encephalopathy, lactic acidosis and stroke-like episodes (MELAS), Kearns–Sayre syndrome and Leigh's disease; however, many cases do not fit neatly into these categories. Both point mutations (base substitutions) and deletions have been observed, affecting both the genes for respiratory enzymes and those for transfer RNA molecules, part of the protein-synthesizing machinery.

Mitochondrial mutations may be homoplasmic, that is, present in all mitochondria, or heteroplasmic, when a mixture of defective and normal mitochondria is present in proportions that may differ between tissues and between relatives in a family.

Homoplasmic mutations, which include those associated with Leber's optic atrophy, are likely to be familial. Heteroplasmic mutations, which are associated with the Kearns–Sayre syndrome, mitochondrial myopathy, MELAS and MERRF, may be either sporadic or familial. Whereas only a single copy of nuclear genes is transmitted by a parent, a mother transmits many mitochondrial genomes to each egg cell. At each cell division, daughter cells receive a sample of the parent cell's mitochondria. Therefore, heteroplasmy, with varying proportions of normal and abnormal mitochondria, can persist from generation to generation and from tissue to tissue in an individual. This explains why the familial heteroplasmic disorders are so highly variable.

The genetic hallmark of mitochondrial disorders is maternal transmission, and an absence of paternal transmission. Prenatal diagnosis is unlikely to be helpful even if a defect has been defined at the DNA level, because the abnormality is likely to be detected in fetal tissue if the mother is affected, but the proportions of affected and normal mitochondria in the trophoblast cells obtained by chorionic villus sampling will convey little about the child's eventual clinical status.

In a few families, Mendelian inheritance of mitochondrial DNA defects has been reported, mostly with autosomal dominant inheritance. This is thought to arise from mutations in nuclear genes which encode proteins necessary for mitochondrial DNA replication.

The possibility that the accumulation of somatic mutations in mitochondrial DNA could account for some non-inherited age-related disorders, in particular Parkinson's disease, is discussed by Harding (in Brenton, 1992).

Prion diseases

These conditions, although rare, are important in drawing attention to new molecular mechanisms in disease. They enter the differential diagnosis of several of the conditions discussed in this chapter, and may be readily diagnosable, in their inherited forms, by direct gene analysis. For further details see Brown *et al.* (1991).

Mutations in the prion protein gene on the short arm of chromosome 20 have been identified in familial Gerstmann–Straussler syndrome and familial Creutzfeldt–Jakob disease, which are associated with the accumulation of a protease-resistant form of the gene product in the brain. The normal function of prion protein, which contains approximately 245 amino acids, is unknown.

Prion diseases occur in sporadic, infective and inherited forms. The sporadic and infective forms include various spongiform encephalopathies of animals, and most cases of Creutzfeldt–Jakob disease in humans. Some of these are transmissible by ingestion or inoculation of infected CNS material. It is not clear whether sporadic cases where no route of infection has been identified will turn out to be infective, or whether some result from somatic mutations. The infective agent appears to be an altered form of the normal prion protein.

Brain material from patients with inherited prion diseases is infective in experimental systems and can cause spongiform encephalopathy when injected into animals. There thus seem to be genetic and epigenetic mechanisms of protein structure modification, either of which can result in disease by the accumulation of a protease-resistant form of prion protein in the brain.

Susceptibility to sporadic, infective and inherited prion diseases is influenced by normal genetic variation within the prion protein gene. Amino acid 129 is methionine in around two-thirds of normal Caucasian prion protein molecules and valine in the remainder. Patients with all forms of prion disease are more likely to be homozygous for one or other variant than to be heterozygous, with one prion gene expressing the methionine variant and one the valine.

Because the clinical spectrum of prion diseases is still expanding, mutations in the prion protein gene should be looked for in patients with dominantly inherited syndromes, including dementia and ataxia, which do not fit into other well-recognized clinical categories. At present, there is no definitive diagnostic test for sporadic or infective cases short of neuropathology. In families where a pathogenetic prion protein gene mutation has been identified, presymptomatic testing can be offered to at-risk relatives, but the protocol outlined above for Huntington's disease should be followed.

Multiple sclerosis

This is an example of a familial, non-Mendelian disorder. The relevant family data and risks for genetic counselling are well reviewed by Baraitser (1990). First-degree relatives of affected patients face a risk of developing the condition which is about 20 times the population risk, but which is still relatively low in absolute terms (2% or less). It is likely that more than one susceptibility gene is involved, plus environmental factors. One or more of the susceptibility genes may be in the HLA region on chromosome 6, but the nature of the HLA association or linkage is still not sufficiently clear to make typing helpful in advising families.

One strategy for research in diseases of this type is to look for 'candidate genes' and see whether variation in these genes is correlated with disease

susceptibility – for example, apolipoprotein genes in coronary heart disease. In the case of multiple sclerosis, proteins that are expressed in the CNS and whose function may be related to myelination are of obvious interest (Tienari et al., 1992).

References

Baraitser M. (1990) *The Genetics of Neurological Disorders.* Oxford Medical Publications, Oxford.

Baraitser M. & Winter R.M. (1992) *London Neurogenetics Database.* Oxford Medical Databases, Oxford.

Brenton D. (ed.) (1992) Review issue. Mitochondrial DNA and associated disorders. *Journal of Inherited Metabolic Diseases* **15**, 437–498.

Brown P., Goldfarb L.G. & Gajdusek D.C. (1991) The new biology of spongiform encephalopathy: infectious amyloidoses with a genetic twist. *Lancet* **337**, 1019–1022.

Bundey S. (1992) *Genetics and Neurology.* Churchill Livingstone, Edinburgh.

Bushby K. (1992) Genetic and clinical correlations of Xp21 muscular dystrophy. *Journal of Inherited Metabolic Diseases* **15**, 551–564.

Chamberlain S., Shaw J., Wallis J. et al. (1989) Genetic homogeneity at the Friedreich ataxia locus on chromosome 9. *American Journal of Human Genetics* **44**, 518–521.

Connor J.M. & Ferguson Smith M.A. (1991) *Essential Medical Genetics.* Blackwell Scientific Publications, Oxford.

Craufurd D., Dodge A., Kerzin-Storrar L. & Harris R. (1989) Uptake of presymptomatic predictive testing for Huntington's disease. *Lancet* **ii**, 603–605.

Farrer L.A. & Conneally P.M. (1985) A genetic model for age at onset in Huntington's disease. *American Journal of Human Genetics* **37**, 350–357.

Gusella J.F., Wexler N.S., Conneally P.M. et al. (1983) A polymorphic DNA marker genetically linked to Huntington's disease. *Nature* **306**, 234–238.

Harding A.E. (1984) *The Hereditary Ataxias and Related Disorders.* Churchill Livingstone, Edinburgh.

Harley H.G., Brook J.D., Rundle S.A. et al. (1992a) Expansion of an unstable region and phenotypic variation in myotonic dystrophy. *Nature* **355**, 545–546.

Harley H.G., Rundle S.A., Reardon W. et al. (1992b) Unstable DNA sequence in myotonic dystrophy. *Lancet* **339**, 1125–1128.

Harper P.S. & Newcombe R.G. (1992) Age at onset and life table risks in genetic counselling for Huntington's disease. *Journal of Medical Genetics* **29**, 239–242.

Harper P.S., Morris M.R. & Tyler A. (1991) Predictive tests in Huntington's disease. In Harper P.S. (ed.) *Huntington's Disease*, pp. 337–372. Saunders, London.

Huntington's Disease Collaborative Research Group

(1993) A novel gene containing a trinucleotide repeat that is expanded and unstable in Huntington's disease chromosomes. *Cell* **72**, 1–20.

Keppen L.D., Leppert M.F., O'Connell P. *et al.* (1987) Etiological heterogeneity in X-linked spastic paraplegia. *American Journal of Human Genetics* **41**, 933–943.

Kingston H.M., Thomas N.S.T., Sarfarazi M. & Harper P.S. (1983) Genetic linkage between Becker muscular dystrophy and a polymorphic DNA sequence on the short arm of the X chromosome. *Journal of Medical Genetics* **20**, 255–258.

Kosick K.S. (1992) Alzheimer's disease: a cell biological perspective. *Science* **256**, 780–783.

Lunt P.W. & Harper P.S. (1991) Genetic counselling in facioscapulohumeral muscular dystrophy. *Journal of Medical Genetics* **28**, 655–664.

Lupski J.R., Wise C.A., Kuwano A. *et al.* (1992) Gene dosage is a mechanism for Charcot–Marie–Tooth disease type 1A. *Nature Genetics* **1**, 29–33.

MacMillan J.C. & Harper P.S. (1991) Single gene neurological disorders in South Wales: an epidemiological survey. *Annals of Neurology* **30**, 411–414.

Orr H.T., Chung M.-Y., Banfi S. *et al.* (1993) Expansion of an unstable trinucleotide CAG repeat in spinocerebellar ataxia type 1. *Nature Genetics* **4**, 221–226.

Quarrell O.W.J. & Harper P.S. (1991) The clinical neurology of Huntington's disease. In Harper P.S. (ed.) *Huntington's Disease*, pp. 61–75. Saunders, London.

Sarfarazi M., Wijmenga C., Uphadyaya M. *et al.* (1992) Regional mapping of facioscapulohumeral muscular dystrophy gene on 4q35: combined analysis of an international consortium. *American Journal of Human Genetics* **51**, 396–403.

Spadaro M., Giunti P., Lulli P. *et al.* (1992) HLA-linked spinocerebellar ataxia: a clinical and genetic study of large Italian kindreds. *Acta Neurologica Scandinavica* **85**, 257–265.

Suthers G.K., Huson S.M. & Davies K.E. (1992) Instability versus predictability: the molecular diagnosis of myotonic dystrophy. *Journal of Medical Genetics* **29**, 761–765.

Tienari P.J., Wilkstrom J., Sajantila A., Palo J. & Peltonen L. (1992) Genetic susceptibility to multiple sclerosis linked to myelin basic protein gene. *Lancet* **340**, 978–991.

Tyler A., Ball D. & Craufurd D. (1992) Presymptomatic testing for Huntington's disease in the United Kingdom. *British Medical Journal* **304**, 1593–1596.

Vance J.M. (1991) Hereditary motor and sensory neuropathies. *Journal of Medical Genetics* **28**, 1–5.

Walton J. & Gardner-Medwin D. (1988) The muscular dystrophies. In Walton J. (ed.) *Disorders of Voluntary Muscle*, pp. 519–568. Churchill Livingstone, Edinburgh.

Weatherall D.J. (1991) *The New Genetics and Clinical Practice*, 3rd edn. Oxford University Press, Oxford.

Wijmenga C., Brouwer O.F., Padberg G.W. & Frants R.R. (1992) Transmission of *de-novo* mutation associated with myotonic dystrophy. *Lancet* **340**, 985–986.

Part 6
New Concepts in
Neurological Rehabilitation

31: Sensory Substitution, Volume Transmission and Rehabilitation: Emerging Concepts

P. BACH-Y-RITA

Volume transmission in the brain, 457
Sensory substitution, 459
   Tactile vision substitution system (TVSS), 459
   Cutaneous sensory substitution in leprosy patients, 463
   Comments on sensory substitution, 463
Home stroke rehabilitation, 464
Conclusion, 466

Until recently, neurological rehabilitation has not been in the mainstream of medical science, and theory has not played an important role in determining neurological rehabilitation protocols. The historical factors that have led to the exclusion have been discussed elsewhere (Bach-y-Rita, 1988a, 1990a). Among the factors is the more than century-long domination of the neurosciences by localizationist concepts, following the demonstration by Broca in 1861 of the cerebral localization of the motor control of speech in the third convolution of the left frontal lobe. During that time, concepts of brain plasticity and the possibility of reorganizing function after brain lesions did not fit into the 'conceptual substance' (Frank, 1986) of the neurological sciences. Thus, the development of rehabilitation methodologies was left to the fringes of medicine, and the result was the proliferation of approaches bearing the names of the developers, with poor or non-existent theoretical foundations and virtually no validation.

Now that brain plasticity has entered the mainstream of neuroscience, scientifically based neurological rehabilitation is an accepted research subject. One result is the emerging field of pharmacological treatment combined with appropriate physical rehabilitation (Feeney *et al.*, 1982; Crisostomo *et al.*, 1988; Boyeson & Bach-y-Rita, 1989; Bach-y-Rita & Bjelke, 1991). Studies related to biological and psychosocial factors in functional recovery following brain damage have been discussed elsewhere (Bach-y-Rita, 1980a, 1981a,b; Cotman & Nieto-Sampedro, 1985; Bach-y-Rita & Wicab Bach-y-Rita, 1990a,b). In this chapter, I shall discuss three brain plasticity-related emerging research areas: (i) volume transmission in the brain and its possible relevance to functional reorganization following brain damage; (ii) sensory substitution following sensory loss; and (iii) home stroke rehabilitation programmes based on demonstrated biological and psychosocial factors. This chapter includes material from the articles cited here.

Volume transmission in the brain

Recovery of function is possible after brain damage; it can proceed over a period of years, and specific rehabilitation is necessary to obtain maximum return of function. This has stimulated research in recent years to uncover the neural mechanisms of the recovery, and several have been identified (see Bach-y-Rita, 1980a, 1981a, 1988a; Finger & Stein, 1982; Kaplan, 1988; Bach-y-Rita & Wicab Bach-y-Rita, 1990a). Recently, an extrasynaptic mechanism of cell-to-cell communication has been identified, and the studies have been summarized in a volume entitled *Volume Transmission in the Brain: Novel Mechanisms for Neural Transmission* (Fuxe & Agnati, 1991). In a speculative synthesis, the possible relevance of volume transmission to neurological rehabilitation has been discussed (Bach-y-Rita, in press, a, c); it may also have a role in normal mass, sustained, functions (such as sleep and wakefulness, attention, mood and brain 'tone') and in abnormal mass functions (such as epilepsy, spasticity, mood changes and cocaine addition) (Bach-y-Rita, 1991).

458 CHAPTER 31

Fuxe & Agnati (1991) consider that wiring transmission and volume transmission are separate but complementary modes of electrochemical communication in the brain. In the classical wiring transmission, communication between cells is confined to the synaptic cleft. Changeux (1991) also considers that volume transmission may be a 'complementary, if not alternative, mechanism to classical chemical synaptic transmission'. He notes that the concept proposes that, in the nervous system, signalling may also efficiently take place via the extracellular spaces as well as via synapses. This means of extrasynaptic communication had previously been proposed following an analysis of the mechanisms of production of late cellular responses in brain stem reticular formation cells, in which the recorded responses were considered to have been produced by local neurohumoral diffusion in the extracellular space (Bach-y-Rita, 1964).

Receptors for specific neuroactive substances are located not only on the postsynaptic membrane, but elsewhere on the cell membrane and even on glia (see Fuxe & Agnati, 1991). Injury can produce marked changes in the distribution of receptors (receptor plasticity). For a long time, it has been known to occur in the muscle fibre membrane (see receptor plasticity review by Bach-y-Rita, 1990c, 1993), in which an up-regulation of nicotinic acetylcholine receptors occurs in the whole muscle fibre membrane following destruction of the corresponding motor nerve. Furthermore, the up-regulation of dopamine receptors following unilateral brain stem stroke has recently been shown to occur in humans (De Keyser et al., 1989).

Laboratory studies have also revealed receptor plasticity in the brain. Following 10 minutes of ischaemia induced by common carotid occlusion combined with hypotension, Westerberg et al. (1989) studied changes in excitatory amino acid receptor–ligand binding in rat hippocampal subfields. They demonstrated long-lasting receptor changes, even in areas considered resistant to ischaemic insult. Some receptors were down-regulated while others appeared to be up-regulated on the surviving cells. Preliminary results from work in progress shows the up-regulation of dopamine receptors in the rat nucleus accumbens following the selective destruction of dopamine pathways to the accumbens (Bjelke et al., in preparation).

Bach-y-Rita (1993) has recently proposed a conceptual model of neurotransmitter receptor responses (plasticity) to brain damage. Following cell loss from brain damage, surviving cells that have been totally or partially denervated may have one or more of three responses: (i) the 'strengthening' of synapses from secondary connections; (ii) the development of extrasynaptic receptors on the membrane of the surviving cells; or (iii) receptor development related to the new synapses formed by the sprouting of processes from surviving cells. A postulated example of the first mechanism, unmasking, may occur following the loss of visual input to visual cortical cells. Murata et al. (1965) showed that many visual cortical cells in normal cats also have auditory and/or somatosensory inputs, although the non-visual inputs are 'weaker', with longer latencies. In blind persons, the visual cortex is metabolically very active (Wanet-Defalgue et al., 1988): such activity may represent the unmasking of non-visual inputs, with receptor up-regulation at the synapses of those inputs.

A postulated example of the second class of responses is the dopamine receptor up-regulation that De Keyser et al. (1989) have demonstrated in human stroke patients following the destruction of dopamine pathways. Bach-y-Rita (1991) has suggested the possibility that the up-regulation of receptors may occur on the extrasynaptic membrane (comparable to the response noted on the denervated muscle fibre (see above)). This may lead to supersensitivity to the neurotransmitters in the extracellular fluid, with activation by volume transmission, resulting in adaptive and maladaptative responses.

The third class of responses to damage, sprouting, has been discussed elsewhere (e.g. Bach-y-Rita, 1981b; Bach-y-Rita & Wicab Bach-y-Rita, 1990a). Such responses may be comparable to the sprouting from surviving motoneurons to denervated muscle fibres in polio.

In addition to the possible role of volume transmission in functional changes following rehabilitation, the possible effects of receptor up- and down-regulation on drug (therapeutic and recreational, such as alcohol) actions must be considered, since the drugs may reach extrasynaptic receptors via the extracellular fluid. Future studies will determine the importance to neurological rehabilitation of volume transmission and receptor plasticity.

Sensory substitution

Sensory substitution is the provision to the brain of information that is usually in one sensory domain (e.g. visual information via the eyes and visual pathways) by means of the receptors, pathways and brain projection areas of another sensory system (e.g. visual information via the skin). In this section, sensory substitution will be discussed primarily in regard to tactile sensory substitution for the blind, which is a neurological rehabilitation method for a sensory loss (blindness); blindness can be considered to result in 'brain damage', since the loss of a major sensory input, such as vision, markedly alters cortical activity (Bach-y-Rita, 1988b).

Tactile vision substitution system (TVSS)

A person who becomes blind does not necessarily lose the capacity to 'see'. Rather, the use of the sensory end organ (the eye) is lost. The eye is normally capable of transducing optical signals into patterns of neural activity, which are sent to the central nervous system for processing into a visual percept. However, a substitute end organ, such as a miniature television camera, can be placed under the motor control of the blind person, and the optical signals received by the camera can be transduced into stimuli applied to another sensory system (such as the tactile sensory system) for relay to the brain (Fig. 31.1). Under these conditions a blind person can be trained to use the information as 'visual'. In fact, even congenitally blind persons develop the ability to use visual means of analysis for adequate processing of the information.

Systems designed to relay optical information to the brain through the skin of blind persons have been developed in several laboratories. Each of these systems utilizes a matrix of artificial photoreceptors connected point-to-point with a matrix of skin stimulators, generally placed on the skin of the trunk or forehead (see Bach-y-Rita, 1972; Collins & Bach-y-Rita, 1973). One of the most sensitive areas of skin is found on the fingertips; Bliss (1971) has utilized this sensitivity in developing a reading aid, the Optacon, for the blind, and we are studying the development of real-time displays of two- and three-dimensional computer graphics by means of a haptic display (Bach-y-Rita, 1990b).

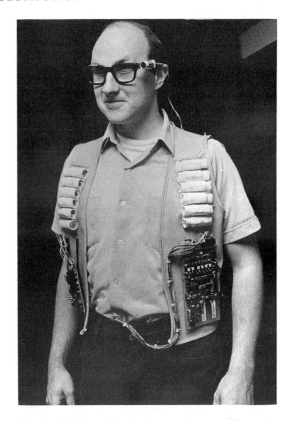

Fig. 31.1 A blind subject is shown using a portable tactile vision substitution system. The television camera is mounted on the frame of a pair of spectacles. The image is led to an electronic commutator (mounted on his vest) which converts it into a tactile image delivered to the skin of his abdomen by an array of electrical stimulators (under his shirt). The batteries are mounted bandolier-style on the vest.

The ability of one sensory system to convey information normally mediated by another (lost) sensory system is dependent on the existence of plastic neural mechanisms. Evidence that brain pathways are not fixed and immutable is available from many sources. These include studies of recovery of function following brain lesions, of changes in individual neurons during learning, of alterations in evoked potentials, and of assessment of cortical structure and chemistry during sensory deprivation or enrichment (reviewed elsewhere, including Bach-y-Rita, 1972; Bach-y-Rita & Wicab Bach-y-Rita, 1990a). With advances in modern technology, the plastic mechanisms which permit the brain to respond to new functional requirements, and to training, may provide the adaptability necessary for compensation for sensory losses.

With training, the blind subjects using the TVSS have been able to identify, and correctly locate in space, complex forms, objects, figures and faces. Perspective, parallax and size constancy, including looming and zooming and depth cues, are correctly utilized. The subjective localization of the information obtained through the television camera is not on the skin; it is accurately located in the three-dimensional space in front of the camera, whether the skin stimulation matrix is placed on the back, on the abdomen or on the thigh, or changed from one of these body locations to another.

The equipment developed for these studies and the sensory substitution experiments have been extensively reported elsewhere (e.g. Bach-y-Rita, 1967, 1971, 1972, 1979; Bach-y-Rita et al., 1969; White et al., 1970; Collins & Bach-y-Rita, 1973; Scadden, 1974; Jansson, 1983; Bach-y-Rita & Hughes, 1985; Miletic et al., 1988). An extended extract (seven pages) of a first-person account by a congenitally blind subject (Guarniero, 1974, 1977) was included in the first edition of this book (Bach-y-Rita, 1982).

Theoretical aspects of the TVSS studies

One of the major goals of the TVSS project was to study brain plasticity, the capacity of the brain to reorganize following injury and to restore function. Our principal work was with congenitally blind persons. These were considered to be 'natural' experiments; the major source of afferent information had been eliminated before they had the opportunity to develop the mechanisms for the analysis of visual information. A discussion of brain plasticity is beyond the scope of this chapter. It has been extensively discussed elsewhere (Bach-y-Rita, 1967, 1971, 1972, 1975a, b, 1980a, 1981a, 1988a, 1989; Bach-y-Rita & Wicab Bach-y-Rita, 1990a).

There is evidence that the brain is capable of incorporating the substitute sensory information into daily life. Braille and sign language are practical for many people with sensory losses. In sign language for the deaf, information usually coded in high frequencies and low simultaneous (parallel)

presentation are translated into hand movements, which present the information in a manner the visual system can transmit to the brain: the hand sign changes are of very low frequency, but with a relatively high parallel content. American sign language has been discussed elsewhere as a sensory substitute strategy (Bach-y-Rita, 1981a), and in the context of sensory substitution for space gloves and space robotics (Bach-y-Rita et al., 1987).

Practical applications of vision substitution devices

A number of factors must be considered in the development of a practical sensory substitution system. In the first place, it is necessary for the device to have a sound physiological basis. This sometimes occurs, either by chance or by appropriate interaction with physiologists and other members of a development team. Often, however, the devices have no sound physiological basis and, although a great amount of money is expended, no practical device can be developed. Even when a physiologically sound device is developed, the chances of it ever becoming practical are limited. Some factors involved include: per unit cost, cost of developing a product from the successful prototype, limited potential market, availability of other approaches to the problem that may be well established or less costly, maintenance and reliability problems and cosmetic and acceptability problems (Bach-y-Rita, 1979, 1980b). The enthusiasm of the research team is thus rarely crowned by the success of a product that is actually used by handicapped persons.

Our TVSS system is an example of a rehabilitation instrumentation development project that has not yet been translated into practice. We were certain that this crude prototype would quickly lead to the development of practical visual substitution systems for the blind, for school, vocational, mobility and general adaptation. Furthermore, it seemed feasible to apply the same principles to other sensory losses (e.g. an auditory substitution system for deaf persons and tactile and kinaesthetic substitution systems for amputees). We seemed to be in a particularly favourable environment for substitution system development, and our research team included psychologists and consumers to complement our professional qualifications.

The 5 years following the appearance of the first

prototype were full of theoretical and instrumentation development successes (summarized in Bach-y-Rita, 1972). However, the practical device eluded us. The technical problems are enormous, since normal sight is such a highly complex function and is so difficult to reproduce with present-day machines. The interface between machine and man is another major problem. Developing devices that are physiologically acceptable and that take advantage of receptor and transmission capacities of the substitute sensory system (e.g. the skin of the abdomen and its receptors and pathways for parallel input of information from a television camera, the fingertips for haptic exploration of a surface, or the cochlea and the highly sequential nature of the auditory system for the reception of spatial information translated into auditory signals) is a major challenge.

Experimental subjects for the development projects have generally been highly intelligent, well-adapted blind persons – in other words, unusual persons who may not reflect the capabilities of the great majority of the blind. The technical problems of developing research prototypes are great, but those of developing a useful product from a successful prototype are even greater and at least 10 times as costly. If a successful system is developed, future problems would include: unit cost and distribution, maintenance and reliability, cosmesis and acceptability. And, on top of all of these problems, the psychological factors involved in the transition from a blind person to one who had acquired some degree of 'sight' would have to be carefully considered.

One limitation of sensory substitution systems is the result of differing properties of the individual sensory systems. For example, the visual system is able to receive a great deal of information simultaneously: a brief flash (or tachistoscopic presentation) is sufficient to recognize a face. However, it is very poor at resolving high frequencies. The ear, on the contrary, has a very high frequencies response; it is excellent for resolving sequential information, but poor at simultaneous information. The skin is in between: it resolves more simultaneous information than the ear, but less than the eye, and higher frequencies than the eye, but less than the ear. Thus, blind subjects using the TVSS do not perceive objects instantaneously. They scan

the object, which consumes considerable time. Furthermore, receptor density and two-point discrimination are important factors (although less so than could have been predicted). The nervous system extracts information from dynamic patterns of stimulation more than from static unpatterned stimuli; for example, while the maximal visual (grating) acuity is approximately $\frac{1}{2}$ minute of arc, vernier acuity is only 2 seconds of arc (discussed in Bach-y-Rita, 1972). However, one of the limitations of a sensory substitution system is that the receptors and pathways of the substitute normal system may not be capable of adequately carrying the information required to provide a practical sensory substitute.

At present, no blind or deaf person is using our tactile sensory substitution devices on a regular basis, although the studies supported the conclusion that the brain is a highly plastic organ and that the perceptual mechanisms are sufficiently malleable to enable a congenitally blind person to interpret the information from a tactile sensory substitution system in visual terms. We considered a teaching device for blind children to be feasible, especially in the classroom setting, where time constraints are manageable, where portability is not a concern, where focal length and lighting can be easily controlled and where specific training can take place: for example, to teach geometry and graphical material, to train the blind children in three-dimensional spatial perception, to allow them to observe moving animals, to teach microscopic information (such as the structure of a fly wing, or of a red blood cell). Yet even such a relatively simple form of the TVSS is a long way from practicability. We developed a programme with a modified Optacon, and, although there were severe instrumentation limitations, interesting results were obtained (Miletic et al., 1988). The programme was evaluated with 30 congenitally blind children ranging in age from 8 to 14 years. Following 15–24 hours of training in camera control, object identification, and phenomena related to spatial perception (relative size, linear perspective, interposition, recovery of structure from motion), the children acquired the ability to make three-dimensional spatial judgements based on the tactile input from a head-mounted camera (Fig. 31.2). In addition to research data, the children made observations and

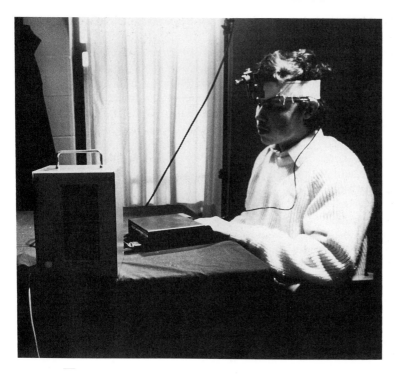

Fig. 31.2 Blind child using the modified Optacon with headband camera. The image is transduced into vibrotactile stimuli delivered to the index fingertip by an array of 144 vibrotactors. (Reprinted with permission from Miletic *et al.*, 1988.)

remarks that provided interesting anecdotal evidence of the acquisition of visual spatial concepts.

A vocational test of the TVSS revealed its potential application to jobs presently reserved for sighted workers. A person totally blind since 2 months after birth spent 3 months on the miniature diode assembly line of an electronic manufacturer. During the assembly process, he received a frame containing 100 small glass cylinders with attached wires as the frame emerged from an automatic filling machine that filled the cylinders with a small piece of lead solder (Figs 31.3 and 31.4). The automatic process was 95% efficient, and so approximately 5% of the cylinders remained unfilled. His first task after receiving each frame was to inspect each of the cylinders and to fill by hand those (5%) that remained unfilled. This was accomplished with a small television camera mounted in the ocular of a dissecting microscope under which the blind person passed the frame containing the cylinders. The information from the television camera was passed through an electronic commutator in order to transform it into a tactile image and was delivered to the skin of the abdomen of the blind worker by

means of 100 small vibrating rods in an array clipped to the work-bench. In order to receive the image, the worker had only to lean his abdomen against the array (without removing his shirt). The blind worker did not wear any special apparatus and his hands were left free to perform the assembly task under the microscope. He filled the empty cylinders by means of a modified injection needle attached to a vacuum: he placed the needle into a dish filled with small pieces of solder. The needle picked up only one piece, and was blocked when the tip of the needle was covered by a piece of solder. He then brought the needle with the piece of solder into the 'visual' field under the microscope and by hand–'eye' co-ordination placed the needle in an empty cylinder. When the needle was in the cylinder, he released the vacuum, allowing the piece of solder to fall into the cylinder.

The blind worker repeated the process for each of the empty cylinders encountered. When all 100 were filled, the frame passed to another loading machine, where it was automatically filled with the diode wafers. Again, the task was to identify the unfilled cylinders (5%) and to fill them by hand as

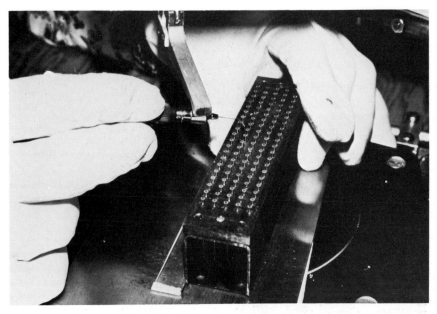

Fig. 31.3 A blind worker on an assembly line for diode construction in an electronics firm. The metal frame ('boat') contains 100 glass cylinders. The blind assembler is in the process of filling one of the cylinders, which he found to be empty by moving the boat into his 'field of view' under a television camera. (Photo courtesy of Al Alden.)

described above. However, this stage offered two extra problems: the wafers were very thin and light and they did not always fall flat into the cylinders. Sometimes they landed on edge. Furthermore, the wafers were gold on one side and silver on the other, and they had to be correctly orientated: the worker had the additional task of turning over the 50% of wafers that were incorrectly orientated. This task was accomplished by identifying the colour (silver or gold) on the basis of light reflectance, since the silver reflected more light.

The blind worker was not able to come into the criterion established for the sighted workers in regard to velocity of performing the assembly task and in regard to errors, but in the time spent on the assembly line he approximated the performance of a beginning untrained worker. With the prototype device used for this task, the blind worker became fatigued more often from the effort of concentration and required more frequent rests than other workers. However, we considered that the feasibility of the rather primitive vocational device was established, but further practical development did not occur.

Cutaneous sensory substitution in leprosy patients

A preliminary study of sensory substitution of touch, pressure and temperature in leprosy patients with absence of these sensations has provided valuable information for the development of a sensory substitution system for amputees. Figure 31.5 shows a leprosy patient with absent cutaneous sensation in the hands wearing a glove containing strain gauges providing information on touch and pressure. The skin stimulation site was the forehead, since his sensation there was intact. Within a few hours he could accurately locate the sensations to his fingers, and could gain pleasure from perceiving textures.

Comments on sensory substitution

Evidence from our laboratories and from other laboratories has shown that sensory substitution devices can, at least in the laboratory, provide information that the brain can learn to integrate with information from intact sensory systems. Technical

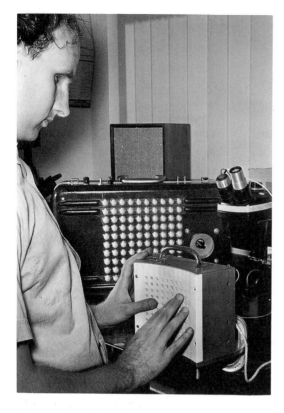

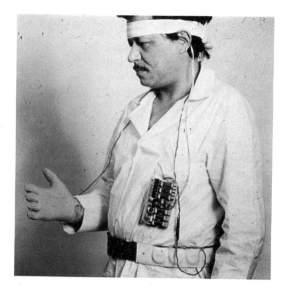

Fig. 31.5 A leprosy patient is shown wearing a glove fitted with strain gauges. The signals are converted to tactile stimuli by the commutator clipped to his shirt pocket, and delivered to the skin of his forehead. He is wearing a belt containing batteries.

Fig. 31.4 A blind subject is shown examining a laboratory version of the system used in Fig. 31.3. The array of vibratory stimulators is clipped to the workbench (the subject has his right hand on the array). A TV camera is shown in a microscope, substituting for an ocular. The array of lights (middle background) provides a visual display corresponding point-for-point to the tactile display, thus allowing the instructor to monitor the blind subject's activities.

difficulties and expense will continue to be major barriers to common usage of these devices even if they do become available. At present, the most successful sensory substitution systems continue to be braille for blind persons and sign language for deaf persons; neither system requires high-tech instrumentation. The research findings discussed above, and the success of braille and sign language, demonstrate that the brain is capable of incorporating substitute information to modify concepts and function. This justifies the serious efforts that are now under way to harness recent technological

advances to the development of flexible, efficient and practical sensory substitution systems.

Home stroke rehabilitation

Present stroke rehabilitation programmes are primarily hospital-based. Through custom, certain criteria have evolved that have never been validated scientifically. For example the use of the term 'plateau' in neurological rehabilitation implies a final level of function. However, in other areas, a plateau is considered to be a stage of consolidation between two acquisition phases. For example, Kuhn (1970) has considered scientific development as a succession of tradition-bound periods punctuated by non-cumulative breaks, and Bach-y-Rita & Balliet (1987) have discussed the possibility that stroke patients may reach plateaux (consolidation phases) between phases of acquisition. However, acquisition–consolidation alternating phases in neurological rehabilitation have not been evaluated; in most stroke rehabilitation programmes, patients are discharged when they reach a plateau, and little further recovery is obtained. Thus, two recent studies (Lindmark, 1988; Kelly-Hayes *et al.*, 1989) revealed that usually only minimal recovery is gained beyond 3 months after a stroke. Intensive in-patient rehabilitation by multispeciality teams of therapists is often provided during the first 3 months, with little further therapy provided after discharge and little expectation by the research team for further recovery. The expectations of the therapists (which are conveyed directly or indirectly to the patient) may have an effect on the outcome: this has been discussed (Bach-y-Rita & Wicab Bach-y-Rita, 1990a, b) in the context of the disparity between the demonstrated capacity for long-term recovery and the limited recovery obtained after 3 months in traditional programmes, as exemplified by the Lindmark (1988) and Kelly-Hayes *et al.* (1989) studies noted above.

The importance of the intervention of each of the various therapies, such as speech, occupational, physical and others, has not been demonstrated. A case could be made for providing virtually all the therapy by a single 'rehabilitation therapist' (Bach-y-Rita, 1992), and in fact training programmes combining occupational and physical therapy have been established (Tarditi, 1989).

Since there is strong evidence that the brain is capable of reorganization for years after brain insults, we have been exploring the development of long-term stroke rehabilitation programmes that incorporate the biological and psychosocial factors that have been discussed elsewhere (Bach-y-Rita & Wicab Bach-y-Rita, 1990a, b; Bach-y-Rita & de Pedro-Cuesta, 1991). Such programmes must take into consideration the desirability of returning persons who have had an illness or disability to the home environment as soon as possible. Thus, we have concentrated our efforts in two areas: (i) late rehabilitation programmes, starting 1 or more years after the brain-damaging event, based on infrequent out-patient therapy sessions and extensive self-administered home therapy (Bach-y-Rita & Balliet, 1987); and (ii) integrated hospital–home stroke rehabilitation, with the primary emphasis on the early discharge from the hospital and the selection of individual programmes from therapist-developed modules for home therapy, which are to be undertaken primarily without the presence of a therapist. Only the latter will be discussed here.

Physiological, psychosocial and even economic factors suggest that the patient and the support system involvement and home and community settings should play important roles in such programmes. It may be particularly effective to consider activities that are of considerable interest to the patients. Examples of this are:

1 Real-life therapeutic activities based on the interests of each patient (Bach-y-Rita, 1980a; Bach-y-Rita & de Pedro-Cuesta, 1991).

2 Devices based on computer games that can be prescribed for specific motor rehabilitation needs (e.g. upper extremity), such as the device we developed, using a Herring track to drive the paddle of an electronic pong game so that the movements of a hemiplegic upper extremity are included in an interesting activity (Cogan *et al.*, 1977); the patient ceases to think of 'arm exercises' and perceives paddle movement rather than arm movements. The psychosocial factors in this approach, as well as neurophysiological and neurochemical factors, have been discussed elsewhere (Bach-y-Rita & Wicab Bach-y-Rita, 1990b).

The development of individualized programmes of stroke rehabilitation, planned with the co-operating hospitals and rehabilitation centres and carried out primarily at home, constitutes an effort to create interfaces between institutional and home care and between formal and informal rehabilitation. Up to the present, the rationale for the timing of rehabilitation or for the optimal facilities for it has not been based on scientific studies (Bach-y-Rita, 1992). We have recently reviewed the few existing randomized, controlled, stroke rehabilitation studies (de Pedro-Cuesta *et al.*, in preparation); it is evident that stroke rehabilitation as practised today is not based on scientific evidence.

A stroke rehabilitation programme is under development in Stockholm, with the goals of developing a conceptually based, hospital–home, function-orientated long-term stroke rehabilitation programme, taking advantage of the biological and psychosocial factors related to recovery from brain damage, using informal care-givers to provide guidance; detecting differences between two comparison groups in outcomes, attributable to a function-orientated stroke rehabilitation programme; and evaluating related health economic and health policy issues (Bach-y-Rita & de Pedro-Cuesta, 1991). Rehabilitation, leading to functional improvement in the areas of most importance to the individual patient, has significant educational as well as psychosocial requirements. We plan to reduce the hospital-based specialized services while providing increased individually determined home services in those cases (estimated from Swedish records to be approximately 25% of all stroke patients) that are determined to be appropriate for this research project.

The entire programme includes many components. A number of professionals with diverse interests, such as basic science related to recovery of function, delivery of rehabilitation services, epidemiology, health policy and health economics, are collaborating on it. Preliminary results have been very positive, including an important reduction in costs. The programme is expected to be in development for a considerable period of time (Bach-y-Rita & de Pedro-Cuesta, 1991).

Conclusion

The entry of neurological rehabilitation into the mainstream of clinical neuroscience has already led to the initiation of studies that should bring the level of rehabilitation services up to the level of other clinical services. Three emerging areas of neurological rehabilitation have been briefly discussed here. As noted elsewhere (Bach-y-Rita et al., 1988), to be successful, the scientific bases of these three areas (as well as all other areas of neurological rehabilitation) must be developed without losing the humanism and strong patient service orientation that has been the hallmark of rehabilitation medicine.

References

Bach-y-Rita P. (1964) Convergent and long latency unit responses in the reticular formation of the cat. *Experimental Neurology* **9**, 327–344.

Bach-y-Rita P. (1967) Sensory plasticity: applications to a vision substitution system. *Acta Neurologica Scandinavica* **43**, 417–426.

Bach-y-Rita P. (1971) Neural substrates of sensory substitution. In Klinke R. & Grusser O.J. (eds) *Pattern Recognition in Biological and Technical Systems*, pp. 130–142. Springer-Verlag, Berlin.

Bach-y-Rita P. (1972) *Brain Mechanisms in Sensory Substitution*. Academic Press, New York.

Bach-y-Rita P. (1975a) Plasticity of the nervous system. In Zulch K.J., Creutzfeldt O. & Galbraith G.C. (eds) *Cerebral Localization*, pp. 203–216. Springer-Verlag, Berlin.

Bach-y-Rita P. (1975b) Plastic brain mechanisms in sensory substitution. In Zulch K.J. (ed.) *Cerebral Localization*, pp. 313–327. Springer-Verlag, Berlin.

Bach-y-Rita P. (1979) The practicality of sensory aids. *International Rehabilitation Medicine* **1**, 87–89.

Bach-y-Rita P. (1980a) Brain plasticity as a basis for therapeutic procedures. In Bach-y-Rita P. (ed.) *Recovery of Function: Theoretical Considerations for Brain Injury Rehabilitation*, pp. 225–263. H. Huber, Berne, Switzerland.

Bach-y-Rita P. (1980b) Outlook. In Gloor P. & Bruckner R. (eds) *Rehabilitation of the Visually Disabled and the Blind at Different Ages*, pp. 136–143. H. Huber, Berne, Switzerland.

Bach-y-Rita P. (1981a) Brain plasticity as a basis of the development of rehabilitation procedures for hemiplegia. *Scandinavian Journal of Rehabilitation Medicine* **13**, 73–83.

Bach-y-Rita P. (1981b) Central nervous system lesions: sprouting and unmasking in rehabilitation. *Archives of Physical Medicine and Rehabilitation* **62**, 413–417.

Bach-y-Rita P. (1982) Sensory substitution in rehabilitation. In Illis L., Sedgwick M. & Granville H. (eds) *Rehabilitation of the Neurological Patient*, pp. 361–383. Blackwell Scientific Publications, Oxford.

Bach-y-Rita P. (1988a) Brain plasticity. In Goodgold J. (ed.) *Rehabilitation Medicine*, pp. 113–118. C.V. Mosby, St Louis.

Bach-y-Rita P. (1988b) Sensory substitution and recovery from 'brain damage'. In Finger S., LeVere T.E., Almi C.R. & Stein D.G. (eds) *Brain Injury and Recovery: Theoretical and Controversial Issues*, pp. 323–334. Plenum Press, New York.

Bach-y-Rita P. (1989) Physiological considerations in sensory enhancement and substitution. *Europa Medicophysica* **25**, 107–128.

Bach-y-Rita P. (1990a) Paul Broca: aphasia and cerebral localization. *Current Contents* **22** (38), 18.

Bach-y-Rita P. (1990b) Three-dimensional spatial graphics for blind computer users. In Fellbaum K. (ed.) *Access to Visual Computer Information by Blind Persons*, pp. 81–85. Technical University of Berlin, Berlin.

Bach-y-Rita P. (1990c) Receptor plasticity and volume transmission in the brain: emerging concepts with relevance to neurologic rehabilitation. *Journal of Neurological Rehabilitation* **4**, 121–128.

Bach-y-Rita P. (1991) Thoughts on the role of volume transmission in normal and abnormal mass sustained functions. In Fuxe K. & Agnati L.F. (eds) *Volume Transmission in the Brain*, pp. 489–496. Raven Press, New York.

Bach-y-Rita P. (1992) Applications of principles of brain plasticity and training to restore function. In Young

R.R. & Delwaide P.J. (eds) *Principles and Practice of Restorative Neurology*, pp. 54–64. Butterworth, London.

Bach-y-Rita P. (1993) Nonsynaptic diffusion neurotransmission (NDN) in the brain. *Neurochemistry International* **23**, 297–318.

Bach-y-Rita P. & Balliet R. (1987) Recovery from stroke. In Duncan P.W. & Badke M. (eds) *Stroke Rehabilitation: the Recovery of Motor Control*, pp. 79–107. Year Book Publishers, New York.

Bach-y-Rita P. & Bjelke B. (1991) Lasting recovery of motor function, following brain damage, with a single dose of amphetamine combined with physical therapy: changes in gene expression? *Scandinavian Journal of Rehabilitation Medicine* **23**, 219–220.

Bach-y-Rita P. & de Pedro-Cuesta J. (1991) Neuroplasticity in the aging brain: development of conceptually based neurologic rehabilitation. In Molina A., Parreño J., Martin J.S., Robles E. & Moret A. (eds) *Rehabilitation Medicine*, pp. 5–12. Excerpta Medica, Amsterdam.

Bach-y-Rita P. & Hughes B. (1985) Tactile vision substitution: some instrumentation and perceptual considerations. In Warren D. & Strelow E. (eds) *Electronic Spatial Sensing for the Blind*, pp. 171–186. Martinus-Nijhoff, Dordrecht, The Netherlands.

Bach-y-Rita P. & Wicab Bach-y-Rita E. (1990a) Biological and psychosocial factors in recovery from brain damage in humans. *Canadian Journal of Psychology* **44**, 148–165.

Bach-y-Rita P. & Wicab Bach-y-Rita E. (1990b) Hope and active patient participation in the rehabilitation environment. *Archives of Physical Medicine Rehabilitation* **71**, 1084–1085.

Bach-y-Rita P., Collins C.C., Saunders F., White B. & Scadden L. (1969) Vision substitution by tactile image projection. *Nature* **221**, 963–964.

Bach-y-Rita P., Webster J., Tompkins W. & Crabb T. (1987) *Sensory Substitution for Space Gloves and for Space Robots*, pp. 51–57. Jet Propulsion Laboratories, Pasadena, CA.

Bach-y-Rita P., Lazarus J., Boyeson M., Balliet R. & Myers T. (1988) Neural aspects of motor function as a basis of early and post-acute rehabilitation. In DeLisa J.A. (ed.) *Principles and Practice of Rehabilitation Medicine*, pp. 175–195. J.P. Lippincott, Philadelphia.

Bliss J.C. (1971) A reading machine with tactile display. In Sterling T.D. (ed.) *Visual Prosthesis: the Interdisciplinary Dialogue*, pp. 259–263. Academic Press, New York.

Boyeson M.G. & Bach-y-Rita P. (1989) Determinants of brain plasticity. *Journal of Neurological Rehabilitation* **3**, 35–57.

Broca P. (1861) Remarques sur le siège de la faculté du langage articule; suivies d'une observation d'aphémie (perte de la parole). *Bulletin Société Anatomie de Paris* **6**, 330–357.

Changeux J.-P. (1991) Concluding remarks. In Fuxe K. & Agnati L.F. (eds) *Volume Transmission in the Brain: Novel Mechanisms for Neural Transmission*, pp. 569–585. Raven Press, New York.

Cogan A., Madey J., Kaufman W., Holmlund G. & Bach-y-Rita P. (1977) Pong game as a rehabilitation device. *Proceedings of the Fourth Annual Conference on Systems and Devices for the Disabled*, F3–F4. Seattle, WA.

Collins C.C. & Bach-y-Rita P. (1973) Transmission of pictorial information through the skin. *Advances in Biological and Medical Physics* **14**, 285–315.

Cotman C.W. & Nieto-Sampedro M. (1985) Progress in facilitating the recovery of function after central nervous system trauma. In Nottebohm F. (ed.) *Hope For a New Neurology*, pp. 83–104. New York Academy of Sciences, New York.

Crisostomo E.A., Duncan P.W., Propst M., Dawson D.V. & Davis J.N. (1988) Evidence that amphetamine with physical activity promotes recovery of motor function in stroke patients. *Annals of Neurology* **23**, 94–97.

De Keyser J.D., Ebinger G. & Vauquelin G. (1989) Evidence for a widespread dopaminergic innervation of the human cerebral cortex. *Neuroscience Letters* **104**, 281–285.

Feeney D.M., Gonzalez A. & Law W.A. (1982) Amphetamine, haloperidol and experience interact to affect rate of recovery after motor cortex injury. *Science* **217**, 855–857.

Finger S. & Stein D.G. (1982) *Brain Damage and Recovery: Research and Clinical Perspectives*. Academic Press, Orlando, FL.

Frank R.G. (1986) The Columbian exchange: American physiologists and neuroscience techniques. *Federation Proceedings* **45**, 2665–2672.

Fuxe K. & Agnati L.F. (1991) *Volume Transmission in the Brain: Novel Mechanisms for Neural Transmission*. Raven, New York.

Guarniero G. (1974) Experience of tactile vision. *Perception* **3**, 101–104.

Guarniero G. (1977) Tactile vision: a personal view. *Journal of Visual Impairment and Blindness* March, 125–130.

Jansson G. (1983) Tactile guidance of movement. *International Journal of Neuroscience* **19**, 37–46.

Kaplan M.S. (1988) Plasticity after brain lesions. *Contemporary Archives of Physical Medicine and Rehabilitation* **67**, 984–991.

Kelly-Hayes M., Wolf P.A., Kase C.S., Gresham G.E., Kannel W.B. & D'Agostino R.B. (1989) Time course of functional recovery after stroke: the Framingham study. *Journal of Neurological Rehabilitation* **3**, 65–70.

Kuhn T.S. (1970) *The Structure of Scientific Revolutions*, 2nd edn. University of Chicago Press, Chicago.

Lindmark B. (1988) Evaluation of functional capacity after stroke, with special emphasis on motor function and activities of daily living. *Scandinavian Journal of Rehabilitation Medicine, Suppl.* **21**, 1–40.

Miletic G., Hughes B. & Bach-y-Rita P. (1988) Vibrotactile stimulation: an educational program for spatial concept development. *Journal of Visual Impairment and Blindness* November, 336–370.

Murata K., Cramer H. & Bach-y-Rita P. (1965) Neuronal convergence of noxious, acoustic and visual stimuli in the visual cortex of the cat. *Journal of Neurophysiology* **28**, 1223–1239.

Scadden L. (1974) The tactile vision substitution system: applications in education and employment. *New Outlook for the Blind* **68**, 394–397.

Tarditi G. (1989) La scuola per terapisti della rihabilitazione dell'USSL VIII Torino. *Europa Medicophysica* **25**, 143–146.

Wanet-Defalgue M.C., Veraart C., DeVolder A. *et al.* (1988) High metabolic activity in the visual cortex of early blind human subjects. *Brain Research* **446**, 369–373.

Westerberg E., Monaghan D.T., Kalimo H., Cotman C.W. & Wieloch T.W. (1989) Dynamic changes of excitatory amino acid receptors in the rat hippocampus. *Journal of Neurosciences* **9**, 798–805.

White B.W., Saunders F.A., Scadden L., Bach-y-Rita P. & Collins C.C. (1970) Seeing with the skin. *Perception and Psychophysics* **7**, 23–27.

32: Pharmacological Approaches to Rehabilitation: Noradrenergic Pharmacotherapy and Functional Recovery after Cortical Injury

R.L. SUTTON AND D.M. FEENEY

Pharmacotherapy in animal models of brain damage, 469
    Sensorimotor functions, 469
    Visual functions, 473
    Noradrenergic mediation of recovery, 473
Pharmacotherapy in brain-damaged humans, 475
    Motivation, 475
    Agitation and cognition, 475
    Sensorimotor function, 476
    Aphasia, 477
Mechanisms underlying beneficial pharmacotherapies, 478

The need for developing rational, empirically based pharmacotherapies and rehabilitation strategies for promoting functional recovery after central nervous system injury cannot be overemphasized. In the US alone there are over half a million new cases of brain damage from stroke and trauma every year. The economic and emotional costs resulting from these injuries place an enormous burden and strain on patients, families and the health care system. The traditional indirect approach to the treatment of brain injury after trauma or stroke, including attempts to limit the spread of cerebral damage by improving cerebral blood flow or reducing metabolic demands in ischaemic tissue, has not been successful in improving outcome. For patients with completed injuries, only physical and/or cognitive therapy is generally used and, while beneficial, these rehabilitation efforts may not promote functional recovery. This approach to the treatment of brain injury is changing due to compelling basic science and clinical data indicating that pharmacological interventions can markedly alter recovery of function.

This review focuses on results of laboratory experiments on the effects of the acute administration of drugs affecting central catecholaminergic, particularly noradrenergic, transmission on behavioural recovery after cortical injury. Other pharmacological interventions or experiments examining only physiological variables are briefly mentioned because of their theoretical relevance. Some clinical studies and case reports using similar pharmacological agents to treat symptoms in brain-damaged humans are also discussed. Since many of these drug effects have been interpreted as altering diaschisis, this concept is briefly described in relation to an evolving hypothesis of the response to cerebral injury (see Feeney, 1991).

Pharmacotherapy in animal models of brain damage

Sensorimotor functions

Several studies published between 1946 and 1977 reported that administration of amphetamine compounds could temporarily reinstate 'permanently' lost behaviours such as righting or placing (tactile and visual) reflexes in decerebrate or cortically injured animals (see Feeney & Sutton, 1987, 1988, for reviews). Additionally, Donald and Patricia Meyer and their colleagues conducted numerous experiments on the use of amphetamine to produce temporary or enduring recovery after cortical injuries, often noting that a combination of drug plus appropriate behavioural training/testing was required for promoting recovery and that drug-induced recovery implied that a diaschisis-like state ensued after cortical injury. In their pioneering work, the Meyers repeatedly showed that amphetamine treatment after brain injury could reveal 'the existence of latent capacities that will never be expressed unless active steps are taken to induce their expressions' (Meyer & Meyer, 1982, p. 204).

Our research has primarily dealt with short-term administration of drugs affecting catecholaminergic (or noradrenergic) synaptic transmission, which, when combined with 'physical therapy' (symptom-relevant experience), promotes functional recovery, even when treatment is initiated as long as 12 days after injury (for reviews, see Feeney, 1991; Feeney & Sutton, 1987, 1988). To determine if drug therapy would be efficacious in altering recovery of sensorimotor behaviour after cortical injury, we have investigated the effect of D-amphetamine and related compounds on recovery from hemiplegia after unilateral sensorimotor cortex injury in rats and cats. In these studies the symptoms of hemiplegia are assessed using a beam-walking task where the animals' ability to utilize their hemiplegic limb(s) while traversing a narrow, elevated beam is quantified using a rating scale, with the highest score representing normal paw placements during beam-walking and the lowest score indicating inability to balance on the beam (see Feeney et al., 1982; Hovda & Feeney, 1984). The animals are trained on the beam-walking task prior to surgery and then retested after unilateral sensorimotor cortical injury to establish measures of postsurgical deficits. Following these baseline trials, animals are injected with drug or saline, given several tests during the period of drug action, and beam-walking is assessed every other day for several weeks.

Results using this experimental model in several laboratories indicate the potential usefulness of the model for screening drugs which may exert beneficial or harmful effects on functional recovery. Specifically, a renewed interest in catecholamines and brain injury followed our report that recovery from hemiplegia, measured by beam-walking, after unilateral sensorimotor cortical ablation was accelerated by administration of a single low dose of D-amphetamine 24 hours after injury, if symptom-relevant experience (sensory feedback?) was provided during the period of drug action (Feeney et al., 1982). In subsequent work we (Sutton & Feeney, 1992) and others (Goldstein, 1988; Goldstein & Davis, 1990a) have confirmed that D-amphetamine improved recovery from hemiplegia after cortical ablation and also facilitated beam-walking recovery in rats with traumatic sensorimotor cortical contusion injury (Sutton et al., 1987).

The D-amphetamine-induced acceleration of recovery from hemiplegia is blocked by haloperidol, implicating the catecholamines in recovery of motor function after cortical damage (Feeney et al., 1982).

Since the effects of D-amphetamine endure after a single injection given 24 hours after injury, we hypothesized that the drugs enable structures involved in locomotion to be permanently modified by an interaction with experience (beam-walk testing during drug action, or symptom-relevant experience). This interpretation is supported by the observation that placing rats in a small box to reduce locomotor movements (for 8 hours after drug administration) blocks the D-amphetamine-induced acceleration of recovery (Feeney et al., 1982). This necessity for symptom-relevant experience during D-amphetamine intoxication for acceleration of recovery from hemiplegia in the rat has been independently replicated (Goldstein & Davis, 1990a).

In a study of recovery of function in hemiplegic cats (Hovda & Feeney, 1984), the benefits of D-amphetamine were extended to another species, which provided information that has implications for the rehabilitation of the brain-injured human. For example, it was demonstrated that D-amphetamine could produce a higher level of functional recovery than would occur spontaneously, treatment could be delayed for several days after injury, and multiple treatments produced a more rapid recovery. Cats with unilateral sensorimotor cortical lesions that received the drug combined with beam-walking experience 10 days after surgery recovered significantly faster than saline-treated controls, who remained significantly disabled for at least 2 months post-injury. Multiple injections (four injections spaced at 4-day intervals, beginning 10 days after injury) combined with beam-walking experience were more effective for inducing recovery than was a single treatment. Four D-amphetamine plus symptom-relevant experience treatment sessions produced complete recovery on the beam-walking task by 24 days post-surgery.

The important role of symptom-relevant experience combined with D-amphetamine treatment in promoting recovery from hemiplegia was clearly illustrated in this study with cats. One group of

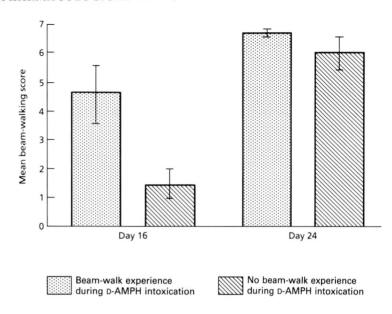

Fig. 32.1 Mean (±SEM) beam-walking scores illustrating the interaction of drug treatment and symptom-relevant experience (SRE) on recovery from hemiplegia in cats with unilateral sensorimotor cortex ablations. By day 16 post-surgery animals given SRE during the period of D-amphetamine action (on days 10 and 14) showed significantly better beam-walking recovery than animals given the same experience prior to drug treatment. By 24 days post-surgery, following two additional drug treatments (on days 18 and 22), the 'experience' and 'no experience' groups did not differ significantly in degree of beam-walking recovery.

animals received multiple drug treatments but, rather than experiencing beam-walking during the 6 hours after injection, tests were conducted at 6, 5, 4 and 1 hour *before* injection and the cats were returned to a large (group) home cage after each injection. These injured animals not tested during drug action showed no promotion of recovery after two injections of amphetamine (see Fig. 32.1). However, after four injections the cats not given physical therapy during intoxication had recovered to levels attained by D-amphetamine-treated cats given symptom-relevant experience (Fig. 32.1). It was hypothesized that locomotor experience gained by walking in the home cage during D-amphetamine intoxication may have generalized to the beam-walk task, since multiple drug treatments overrode the necessity for physical therapy.

When recovery occurs following unilateral cortical injury, it is often suggested that recovery is mediated by spared remnants of adjacent tissue or that the contralateral homotypical cortex 'vicariously' assumes the functions of the injured area. We tested this hypothesis and found that extension of the ablation to include the contralateral sensorimotor cortex, or much larger frontal cortex ablations, did not greatly alter the effects of D-amphetamine on recovery of beam-walking (Sutton *et al.*, 1989b). In this experiment three

injections of D-amphetamine (given at 4-day intervals beginning 12 days after injury) significantly accelerated beam-walking recovery in cats with bilateral frontal cortex ablations (see Fig. 32.2). This drug-enhanced recovery was evident in cats with extensive bilateral frontal cortex ablations as well as those with bilateral lesions restricted to the sensorimotor cortex. Thus, neither the contralateral homotopic cortex nor spared remnants of cortex immediately adjacent to the primary sensorimotor cortex are mediating the effects of D-amphetamine on recovery of beam-walking after unilateral sensorimotor cortex injury. The results of this study led us to suggest that subcortical motor regions (e.g. the basal ganglia, brain stem nuclei and/or cerebellum) provide sufficient anatomical substrates to mediate recovery of beam-walking after unilateral or bilateral sensorimotor cortex injury and that D-amphetamine may act on these regions to promote functional recovery.

The effect of low-dose D-amphetamine treatment has also been evaluated using an embolic stroke model in rats (Salo & Feeney, submitted), which produces more severe and enduring motor deficits than sensorimotor cortex ablation or contusion. In this model a single injection had little effect. However, animals given continuous infusion of a low dose of D-amphetamine (for 7 days beginning

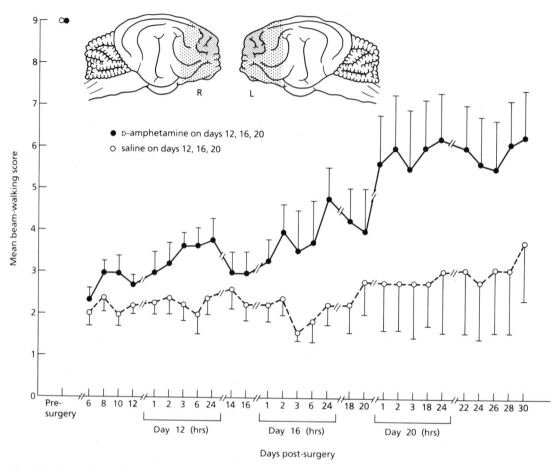

Fig. 32.2 Mean (±SEM) beam-walking scores for saline- and D-amphetamine-treated cats with bilateral frontal cortex ablations, illustrating the effect of three injections of D-amphetamine on recovery. Note that accelerated recovery in D-amphetamine-treated cats endures after the third injection. The inset depicts the smallest (stippled regions) and largest (shaded area) of the ablations. (Copyright 1989 by the American Psychological Association. Reprinted from Sutton *et al.*, 1989b, with permission.)

24 hours post-stroke) recovered to functional levels not attained by saline controls. This treatment regimen also significantly reduced both mortality and the volume of cortical necrosis.

In addition to D-amphetamine, other sympathomimetics have been shown to accelerate recovery in the hemiplegic rat and cat (Feeney & Sutton, 1987; Sutton *et al.*, in preparation). A single injection of the D-amphetamine analogue phentermine or the over-the-counter diet aid phenylpropanol-

amine, administered 24 hours after unilateral sensorimotor cortex ablation in the rat, was found to promote beam-walking recovery. Phentermine, administered at 10, 14, 18 and 22 days after surgery, was also found to significantly improve recovery from hemiplegia in cats with unilateral sensorimotor cortex ablation. Although less effective than either D-amphetamine or phentermine in the cat model, phenylpropanolamine (six injections spaced at 4-day intervals, beginning 10 days after injury) improved beamwalking recovery compared with saline-treated cats with sensorimotor cortical injury.

Visual functions

Additional work in our laboratory demonstrated that D-amphetamine plus sensory-relevant experience will induce recovery from visual deficits which, if untreated, are permanent, and this behavioural recovery also endures after drug therapy is terminated. This was shown in experiments measuring binocular depth perception, using a visual cliff task, in cats with bilateral visual cortex ablations. On this task cats with bilateral ablations of the primary visual cortex show a permanent deficit in stepping down on to the closer of two shelves which are of varying depth from a start box. However, if these animals are given four drug treatments and tested during the period of drug action there is a rapid, and in some cases complete, restoration of accurate visual cliff performance. This D-amphetamine-induced recovery of depth perception is completely blocked if the animals are housed in darkness, even when as many as seven injections are given. Furthermore, the effect of D-amphetamine is also blocked by co-administration of haloperidol (Feeney & Hovda, 1985; Hovda & Feeney, 1985; Hovda et al., 1989). Therefore, like the promotion of recovery from hemiplegia after a sensorimotor cortical lesion, this effect also requires symptom-relevant experience during intoxication and the D-amphetamine effect on recovery is mediated by the catecholamines.

Some aspects of this work in cats with visual cortex ablation deserve special emphasis. First, the restoration of what had seemed to be a permanently lost behaviour after brain injury by treatments with amphetamine is dependent on symptom-relevant experience during intoxication and additional drug treatments will not override the need for physical therapy (sensory feedback?) in this model of brain injury as they do in the cat hemiplegia model of brain injury and recovery. Second, the restored ability of cats to respond to binocular depth cues endures for months after discontinuation of treatment. Finally, recovery occurred when treatments were begun 10 days after surgery but not when

D-amphetamine treatment was delayed until 3 months. These data suggest that a therapeutic window exists after visual cortex ablation during which D-amphetamine plus sensory-relevant experience treatments can restore binocular depth perception.

Noradrenergic mediation of recovery

Although D-amphetamine exhibits a complex pharmacological profile, affecting neurons producing dopamine, noradrenaline and serotonin, several studies indicate that facilitation of beamwalk recovery by D-amphetamine is most probably mediated through actions on central noradrenergic neurons of the nucleus locus ceruleus (i.e. via a direct releasing action on noradrenergic nerve terminals and inhibition of noradrenaline reuptake). The effects of D-amphetamine on behavioural recovery after cortical ablation are blocked by the co-administration of haloperidol (Feeney et al., 1982; Hovda & Feeney, 1985) or phenoxybenzamine (Feeney & Sutton, 1987), suggesting that catecholaminergic systems, particularly the alpha-noradrenergic receptors, are mediating the effects of D-amphetamine on recovery.

Intraventricular infusion of noradrenaline enhances recovery of beam-walking in rats with unilateral sensorimotor cortex ablation, whereas intraventricular dopamine does not improve recovery (Boyeson & Feeney, 1990). Administration of the alpha$_2$-noradrenaline receptor antagonist yohimbine, which increases noradrenaline release, 24 hours after unilateral sensorimotor cortex ablation also enhances beam-walking recovery in rats (Sutton & Feeney, 1992). Yohimbine did not significantly improve beam-walking recovery in rats with unilateral sensorimotor cortical contusion, perhaps due to the additional subcortical damage induced by cortical impact trauma compared with ablation (Feeney & Westerberg, 1990). The cerebellum has been suggested as the site of action of noradrenaline-facilitated recovery of beam-walking ability, since infusion of noradrenaline into the cerebellar hemisphere contralateral, but not ipsilateral, to sensorimotor cortical ablation in rats produces a significantly improved rate of beam-walking recovery relative to

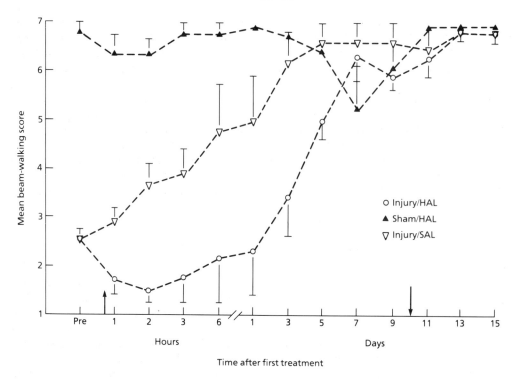

Fig. 32.3 Mean (±SEM) ratings of beam-walking in rats with unilateral contusion injury to the sensorimotor cortex, illustrating the retarding effect of 10 daily doses of haloperidol (HAL; begun at upward arrow and ending at downward arrow) on recovery from hemiplegia. Administration of HAL early after injury produced an initial worsening of beam-walking ability compared with rates of spontaneous recovery shown by animals treated with saline (SAL). Chronic treatment with HAL to rats without brain damage (Sham/HAL) did not effect initial beam-walking, but slightly impaired performance after the seventh dose. (Copyright 1990 by the Canadian Psychological Association. Adapted from Feeney & Westerberg, 1990, with permission.)

saline-treated control animals (Boyeson & Krobert, 1992). However, the particular noradrenaline receptor subtype(s) mediating D-amphetamine or noradrenaline effects on beam-walking recovery have remained elusive. A single administration of the alpha$_1$-noradrenaline agonists l-phenylephrine and methoxamine or the non-specific beta-noradrenaline antagonist propranolol did not significantly affect beam-walking recovery after sensorimotor cortical injury in the rat (Feeney & Westerberg, 1990; Sutton & Feeney, 1992).

Conversely, drugs that reduce noradrenaline release or block specific postsynaptic alpha-noradrenaline receptors may adversely affect functional recovery. For example, a single dose of haloperidol (Feeney *et al.*, 1982) or clonidine (Goldstein & Davis, 1990b; but see also Sutton &

Feeney, 1992) administered 24 hours after sensorimotor cortical ablation retards beam-walking recovery in rats. Chronic treatment with haloperidol (see Fig. 32.3) was also found to significantly retard beam-walking recovery in rats with unilateral sensorimotor cortex contusion (Feeney & Westerberg, 1990). Although haloperidol is most often considered a dopamine receptor blocker, its adverse effects on recovery may be due to its potent blockade of postsynaptic alpha$_1$-noradrenaline receptors. Clonidine produces a reduction of noradrenaline release as a result of its alpha$_2$-noradrenergic agonist properties. The alpha$_1$-noradrenergic antagonist prazosin and the alpha$_{1,2}$-noradrenergic antagonist phenoxybenzamine have been found to retard recovery of beam-walking ability in rats with unilateral sensorimotor cortical injury if they are administered 24 hours after injury (Feeney & Sutton, 1988; Feeney & Westerberg, 1990). Finally, noradrenaline has also been shown to play a crucial role in the maintenance of recovery in cortically injured animals. Clonidine, prazosin and phenoxybenzamine have all been found to reinstate symptoms of hemiplegia in rats and cats that have recovered beam-walking ability after sensorimotor cortical injury (Feeney & Sutton, 1987, 1988; Sutton & Feeney, 1992). These studies indicate that spontaneous recovery of beam-walking is mediated by noradrenaline, most probably via actions on alpha$_1$-noradrenergic receptors, and that the state of functional recovery after injury is vulnerable to pharmacological challenge from drugs that either reduce noradrenaline or block alpha$_1$-noradrenergic receptors.

Pharmacotherapy in brain-damaged humans

Many of the clinical reports on the use and efficacy of psychostimulant treatment in brain-damaged subjects have been confounded by lack of objective measures and/or appropriate control procedures. In addition, it is likely that improvements reported in many of these investigations are due to drug effects on complex psychological processes rather than effects on neurological functions. However, the available clinical studies and case reports provide ample evidence that drugs increasing catecholamine activity after brain injury can benefit patient outcome and facilitate rehabilitation efforts. Details from some of these studies, including the drugs utilized, noted side-effects and functions improved, are given below.

Motivation

Clark & Mankikar (1979) initiated a 3-week treatment with D-amphetamine (increasing doses weekly from 2.5 mg twice/day to a maximum of 10 mg twice/day) in 88 elderly patients, 28 with stroke, who exhibited features of 'poor motivation syndrome'. These patients showed lack of self-care, complaints of chronic tiredness and lower limb weakness. Forty-eight patients were reported to show improvement during and after D-amphetamine treatment, becoming more alert,

communicative, independent and co-operative with their therapists. Failure to respond or show improvement after treatment was significantly increased with age. Treatment was terminated in 23 patients after appearance of side-effects, including uncooperative behaviour (10 cases), confusion or delusion (seven cases) or hypomania, vomiting or constipation (one case each). Importantly, no cardiac side-effects were noted, with the exception of one case where a pre-existing multifocal atrial rhythm became more irregular. Side-effects rapidly disappeared when drug treatment was stopped.

Agitation and cognition

Lipper & Tuchman (1976) described beneficial effects of D-amphetamine treatment in a 25-year-old patient with behavioural and cognitive disturbances subsequent to closed head injury suffered in an automobile accident. This patient was hospitalized 16 months post-injury (a large, transverse right frontal laceration and possible brain stem contusion), after a suicide attempt. The patient was confused and depressed and had blunted affect and a persistent deficit in short-term memory. Within 1 week after beginning D-amphetamine treatment (5 mg, orally, twice/day initially and increased to 15 mg twice/day over 5 days) the patient exhibited lessened confusion and paranoid ideation as well as improved affect and short-term memory. Vital signs, weight and sleep patterns were unchanged. When placebo capsules were substituted for D-amphetamine, the patient relapsed and showed increasing paranoia, confusion and agitation. Subsequent therapy with D-amphetamine (15 mg twice/day) combined with amitriptyline (a catecholamine reuptake blocker; 300 mg/day) resulted in improved affect as well as reduced paranoia and delusional thoughts.

Jackson et al. (1985) used amitriptyline (50 mg/day) to treat agitation in a 32-year-old patient after frontal lobe closed head injury. Amitriptyline therapy was begun 6.5 months after injury, when the patient's continued aggressive behaviour was obstructing rehabilitation efforts. Within 2 weeks of initiating treatment, the patient exhibited improved mood, co-operation with staff, increased attention span and concentration and enhanced cognitive ability. These behavioural and cognitive gains persisted after tapering of drug therapy 1 year after its initiation. Since haloperidol is often utilized to control agitation in brain-injured patients, and this drug can adversely affect recovery (see animal studies reviewed above and human data below), the positive results obtained with amitriptyline suggest that tricyclic antidepressants (or other catecholamine reuptake blockers) are worthy of further investigation in patients with agitation after brain trauma.

In a controlled case study, Evans et al. (1987) reported that both methylphenidate (0.15 mg/kg and 0.30 mg/kg, twice/day) and D-amphetamine (0.10 and 0.20 mg/kg, twice/day) improved outcome in a young man who had sustained a severe head injury 2 years prior to treatment. Both psychostimulants were shown to improve verbal learning and memory skills, sustain attentional set and improve overall behavioural performance on a wide range of neuropsychological tests.

Sensorimotor function

Based on the data from treatment of hemiplegia in rats and cats using the combination of D-amphetamine and symptom-relevant experience, a double-blind, placebo-controlled study using objective measures of recovery has recently been performed to evaluate the effect of D-amphetamine on recovery in stroke patients (Davis et al., 1987). Within 10 days of stroke, eight highly selected patients with clinically stable motor deficits were assigned to receive either a single oral dose of D-amphetamine (10 mg) or placebo. Baseline (pretreatment) motor deficits were established by administering the Fugl-Meyer scale of motor performance on the evening and morning before treatment. Drug and placebo patients were given at least 45 minutes of intensive physical therapy after treatment, to provide appropriate symptom-relevant experience during drug intoxication, and motor performance was re-evaluated the following morning. Compared with placebo controls, patients receiving D-amphetamine showed significant improvement in motor performance when retested the day after treatment (see Fig. 32.4).

In agreement with the data gleaned from animal research (reviewed above and by Feeney & Sutton,

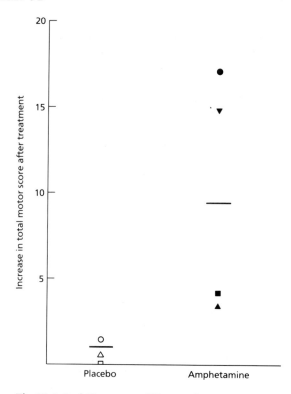

Fig. 32.4 Fugl-Meyer score differences between baseline and after receiving either D-amphetamine or placebo and physical therapy for eight stroke patients. Each symbol represents a single patient and the horizontal bars are the means of each group. (Copyright 1987 by Raven Press, Ltd. Reprinted from Davis et al., 1987, with permission.)

1987, 1988), some drugs given to patients with brain injury may exert detrimental effects on recovery. Goldstein et al. (1990) conducted a prospective study of stroke outcome in 58 patients, utilizing the Fugl-Meyer scale to assess sensorimotor function within 48 hours of admission and 5 and 30 days thereafter, and the Barthel index to assess independence in activities of daily living. Upon completion of this prospective phase, patients were divided into two groups for retrospective analysis of the effects of drugs administered before onset of neurological symptoms or during hospitalization. One group consisted of patients receiving drugs hypothesized to be detrimental (based on animal data), including antihypertensives (clonidine or prazosin), neuroleptics (haloperidol, chlorpromazine, prochlorperazine), benzodiazepines (triazolam, alprazolam, chlordiazepoxide) or phenytoin. Patients in the 'neutral drug' group received other (unspecified) medications. Although the groups were similar with regard to functional deficits at admission, prognostic factors and stroke risk factors, data analysis indicated that patients in the 'detrimental drug' group had significantly lower Fugl-Meyer scores than 'neutral drug' patients at 5 and 30 days after stroke. At 30 days post-stroke the median Barthel index for patients in the 'detrimental drug' group was also significantly lower than that of patients in the 'neutral drug' group. While these results must be interpreted cautiously, they indicate that medications shown to slow recovery in laboratory studies may produce detrimental effects on functional recovery when administered to stroke or head trauma patients.

Aphasia

In a double-blind case study, Homan *et al.* (1990) reported benefits of D-amphetamine treatment in a 53-year-old patient with transcortical motor aphasia and hemiplegia subsequent to (1.5 years post) a left internal carotid endarterectomy. Oral drug (15 mg) or placebo was administered using a single-dose crossover design followed by a chronic phase (six consecutive daily doses) of D-amphetamine or placebo treatment. The drug treatment was reported to transiently improve several behaviours, exerting greatest effects on measures of language performance (e.g. naming, morphemes per second, pauses per utterance) and motor performance assessed using a simulated driving test. Additionally, IQ and signal detection improvements were noted after D-amphetamine treatment.

Walker-Batson *et al.* (1992) have recently reported beneficial effects of D-amphetamine treatment on recovery from aphasia in six patients with a left middle cerebral artery occlusion. Patients were admitted to the study between 10 and 30 days after stroke and received an oral dose of D-amphetamine (10 to 15 mg) followed in 30 minutes by 1 hour of intensive speech/language therapy. The drug treatment/therapy combination was administered for 10 sessions, separated by 4-day intervals. Severity of aphasia was measured using the Porch index of communicative ability (PICA) and expected recovery levels were calculated using

Table 32.1 Initial aphasia severity (PICA overall percentile), 3 months post-onset (MPO) PICA percentile score, and the percentage of 6 MPO predicted outcome that was achieved at 3 MPO of stroke for six patients treated with D-amphetamine. (Copyright 1992 by Elsevier Press. Adapted from Walker-Batson *et al.*, 1992, with permission.)

Subject	Initial PICA percentile	3 MPO PICA percentile score	Percentage of 6 MPO prediction
S1	19	40	80
S2	42	80	105
S3	23	66	114
S4	42	83	109
S5	46	82	104
S6	17	53	126
Means	31	67	106

a mathematical model that reliably predicts recovery from aphasia using PICA scores. As shown in Table 32.1, by 3 months post-stroke five patients obtained a level of recovery from aphasia that was in excess of 100% of their 6-month predicted recovery score and the other patient had scored 80% of his 6-month predicted recovery. Thus, rates of recovery from aphasia were accelerated well above those predicted (using a reliable, quantitative recovery scale) by the combination of D-amphetamine treatment and speech/language therapy. Importantly, no significant fluctuations of heart rate or blood pressure were noted, even with the repeated D-amphetamine treatment regimen used in this study. Two patients who received treatment during afternoon sessions had sleep disturbances on the day of drug administration.

The effects of catecholamine antagonists on recovery of function after brain injury have only recently received attention in human studies. As mentioned above, haloperidol is often the drug of choice for the control of post-traumatic agitation and, in animal studies, this drug has been shown to retard recovery from hemiplegia when given early after sensorimotor injury (Feeney *et al.*, 1982; Feeney & Westerberg, 1990; see Fig. 32.3). During a study on recovery from aphasia following stroke, in which patients received speech therapy and monthly aphasia testing, haloperidol treatment was found to exert negative effects on recovery in one

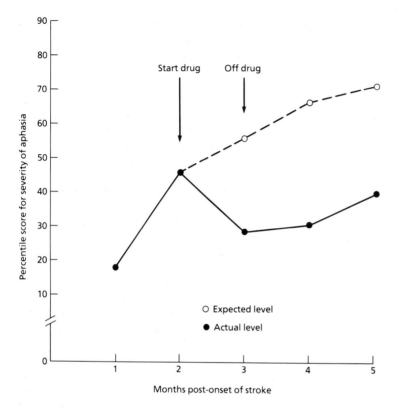

Fig. 32.5 Severity of aphasia as measured monthly using the Porch index of communicative ability (PICA) in a 60-year-old man with a left hemisphere infarct. Haloperidol (5 mg/day) treatment was begun the day following the second PICA test, producing a worsening of PICA scores, mental status and attentional deficits which could not be accounted for by neurological and computerized tomography evaluations. Haloperidol was discontinued 1 week after the third PICA evaluation and, while the patient did not recover to predrug language ability at 5 months post-onset of stroke, some improvement was observed over the next 2 months. The expected level of recovery is based on mathematical modelling for prediction of recovery from aphasia, using PICA scores. (Copyright CRC Press, Inc., Boca Raton, FL. Redrawn with permission from Feeney & Sutton, 1987.)

patient (see Fig. 32.5). This patient showed a marked loss of function after haloperidol treatment was begun 2 months following stroke. Although some recovery resumed when haloperidol was discontinued in the third month post-stroke, a persisting effect of the drug on recovery from aphasia was apparent. In retrospective studies on recovery from aphasia in stroke patients, both thiazides and antihypertensives (clonidine and Aldomet) were found to significantly lower patients' predicted recovery, and this group of patients also exhibited lower recovery levels than did patients not on medications (Porch & Feeney, 1986).

Mechanisms underlying beneficial pharmacotherapies

As is illustrated by the work reviewed above, drug treatments after brain injury can improve rates of spontaneous recovery and reinstate some behavioural functions that have frequently been presumed to be lost due to damage of 'essential'

neural circuits. Conversely, other drug interventions after brain injury can worsen impairments or slow behavioural recovery. These laboratory and clinical studies (see also Feeney & Baron, 1986; Feeney & Sutton, 1987, 1988; Feeney, 1991) suggest that cerebral dysfunctional states, related to the concept of diaschisis, are important therapeutic targets for enhancing recovery of function after brain injury. As stated by Teuber (1975);

> diaschisis-like processes will have to be identified . . . by appropriate histological and histochemical means since the phenomena of recovery seem to demand it. Such an understanding of mechanisms is all the more important since . . . external stimulation of internal states (e.g. pharmacological influences on the internal environment) might hasten or retard such recovery, or limit or enlarge its ultimate extent. (p. 475)

It has been suggested (Feeney *et al.*, 1985; Feeney & Sutton, 1987, 1988; Feeney, 1991) that the more descriptive phrase 'remote functional depression', often used by others, should replace the older concept of diaschisis.

Work in our laboratories has shown that there is a widespread depression of metabolic function, as indicated by the local cerebral metabolic rate of glucose utilization (LCMRGlu), cytochrome oxidase activity and intensity of histochemical staining for the oxidative enzyme alpha-glycerophosphate dehydrogenase (α-GPDH), after unilateral sensorimotor cortex lesions in the rat (Feeney et al., 1985; Sutton et al., 1986, 1989a). Consistent with the behavioural data presented above, D-amphetamine alleviates the widespread depression of glucose metabolism or cytochrome oxidase activity seen after sensorimotor cortex ablation (Feeney et al., 1985; Sutton et al., 1986), and LCMRGlu depression is worsened by haloperidol (Feeney et al., 1985). Likewise, treatment with D-amphetamine after cortical injury blocks the reduced staining for α-GPDH and, similar to its lack of effect in improving behavioural recovery (Feeney & Sutton, 1988), apomorphine did not alter α-GPDH staining after cortical injury. The effects of D-amphetamine on α-GPDH staining is blocked by co-administration of haloperidol and the injury-induced depression of α-GPDH is worsened by prior lesion of the locus ceruleus. These findings support the hypothesis that noradrenaline from the locus ceruleus plays an important role in spontaneous recovery and imply that the locus ceruleus–noradrenaline system may mediate the effects of D-amphetamine on attenuation of injury-induced metabolic disturbances and acceleration of behavioural recovery.

The mechanisms by which D-amphetamine and drugs affecting noradrenaline alter behavioural recovery after cortical injury are uncertain. We have proposed that D-amphetamine may benefit functional recovery after stroke or cortical injury by preventing or reversing an injury-induced remote functional depression of catecholamine levels and turnover in brain tissue (Hovda & Feeney, 1984; Feeney & Sutton, 1987, 1988). In addition, experimental data indicate that the alleviation of a metabolic remote functional depression, either spontaneously (Colle et al., 1986) or by pharmacotherapy combined with symptom relevant experience (see above), may induce recovery of function after brain injury, perhaps by increasing

responsivity of remaining (alternate, or unmasked) neuronal pathways (Dietrich et al., 1990). Preliminary work also suggests that drugs disrupting behavioural outcome may produce their effects by worsening or prolonging a metabolic remote functional depression (Feeney et al., 1985).

In preliminary clinical studies it has been reported that spontaneous recovery from neurological or language deficits is correlated with the magnitude of impaired cerebral perfusion and/or metabolism (Vallar et al., 1988; Bushnell et al., 1989). A recent double-blind study of a small sample of ischaemic stroke patients reported that the calcium channel blocker nimodipine, which has been shown to significantly improve clinical outcome if treatment is initiated within 48 hours of infarct, was capable of significantly alleviating the widespread depression of cortical LCMRGlu in patients (Heiss et al., 1990). These studies illustrate the feasibility of using positron emission tomography (PET) and/or single-photon emission computerized tomography (SPECT) to monitor functional disturbances in brain regions remote from the primary injury and their potential alleviation by drug, physical or speech therapies. Additional work with these and other non-invasive monitoring methods will further our understanding of remote functional depression after brain injury and the hypothesized mechanisms by which drug therapies can alleviate dysfunctional states.

Acknowledgements

Preparation of this manuscript was supported by DHHS Grant S06-RRO-08139-18 and the US Army Medical Research and Development Command under Grant No. DAMD-17-91-Z-1006. Opinions, interpretations, conclusions and recommendations are those of the authors and are not necessarily endorsed by the US Army. In conducting research using animals, the investigators adhered to the laws of the United States and regulations of the Department of Agriculture.

References

Boyeson M.G. & Feeney D.M. (1990) Intraventricular norepinephrine facilitates motor recovery following sensorimotor cortex injury. *Pharmacology, Biochemistry and Behaviour* **35**, 497–501.

Boyeson M.G. & Krobert K.A. (1992) Cerebellar nor-epinephrine infusions facilitate recovery after sensori-motor cortex injury. *Brain Research Bulletin* **29**, 435–439.

Bushnell D.L., Gupta S., Mlcoch A.G. & Barnes W.E. (1989) Prediction of language and neurologic recovery after cerebral infarction with SPECT imaging using *N*-isopropyl-*P*-(^{123}I)iodoamphetamine. *Archives of Neurology* **46**, 665–669.

Clark A.N.G. & Mankikar G.D. (1979) D-Amphetamine in elderly patients refractory to rehabilitation procedures. *Journal of the American Geriatric Society* **27**, 174–177.

Colle L.M., Holmes L.J. & Pappius H.M. (1986) Correlation between behavioral status and cerebral glucose utiliz-ation in rats following freezing lesion. *Brain Research* **397**, 27–36.

Davis J.N., Crisostomo E.A., Duncan P., Propst M. & Feeney D.M. (1987) Amphetamine and physical therapy facilitate recovery of function from stroke: cor-relative animal and human studies. In Raichle M.E. & Powers W.J. (eds) *Cerebrovascular Diseases*, pp. 297–304. Raven Press, New York.

Dietrich W.D., Alonso O., Busto R. & Ginsberg M.D. (1990) The effect of amphetamine on functional brain activation in normal and post-infarcted rat. *Stroke* **21** (Suppl. 3), 147–150.

Evans R.W., Gualtieri C.T. & Patterson D. (1987) Treat-ment of chronic closed head injury with psychostimu-lant drugs: a controlled case study and an appropriate evaluation procedure. *Journal of Nervous and Mental Diseases* **175**, 106–110.

Feeney D.M. (1991) Pharmacological modulation of re-covery after brain injury: a reconsideration of diaschisis. *Journal of Neurological Rehabilitation* **5**, 113–128.

Feeney D.M. & Baron J.-C. (1986) Diaschisis. *Stroke* **17**, 817–830.

Feeney D.M. & Hovda D.A. (1985) Reinstatement of binocular depth perception by amphetamine and visual experience after visual cortex ablation. *Brain Research* **342**, 352–356.

Feeney D.M. & Sutton R.L. (1987) Pharmacotherapy for recovery of function after brain injury. *CRC Critical Reviews in Neurobiology* **3**, 135–197.

Feeney D.M. & Sutton R.L. (1988) Catecholamines and recovery of function after brain damage. In Stein D.G. & Sabel B.A. (eds) *Pharmacological Approaches to the Treat-ment of Central Nervous System Injury*, pp. 121–142. Plenum Press, New York.

Feeney D.M. & Westerberg V.S. (1990) Norepinephrine and brain damage: alpha noradrenergic pharmaco-logy alters functional recovery after cortical trauma. *Canadian Journal of Psychiatry* **44**, 34–252.

Feeney D.M. & Westerberg V.S. (1990) Norepinephrine and brain damage: alpha noradrenergic pharmaco-logy alters functional recovery after cortical trauma. *Canadian Journal of Psychology* **44**, 233–252.

Feeney D.M., Sutton R.L., Boyeson M.G., Hovda D.A. & Dail W.G. (1985) The locus coeruleus and cerebral metabolism: recovery of function after cortical injury. *Physiological Psychology* **13**, 197–203.

Goldstein L.B. (1988) Amphetamine-facilitated func-tional recovery after stroke. In Ginsberg M.D. & Dietrich W.D. (eds) *The 16th Princeton Conference on Cerebral Vascular Diseases*, pp. 303–308. Raven Press, New York.

Goldstein L.B. & Davis J.N. (1990a) Post-lesion practice and amphetamine-facilitated recovery of beam-walking in the rat. *Restorative Neurology and Neuroscience* **1**, 311–314.

Goldstein L.B. & Davis J.N. (1990b) Clonidine impairs recovery of beam-walking after a sensorimotor cortex lesion in the rat. *Brain Research* **508**, 305–309.

Goldstein L.B., Matchar D.B., Morgenlander J.C. & Davis J.N. (1990) Influence of drugs on the recovery of sen-sorimotor function after stroke. *Journal of Neurological Rehabilitation* **4**, 137–144.

Heiss W.D., Holthoff V., Pawlik R.G. & Neveling M. (1990) Effect of nimodipine on regional cerebral glucose metabolism in patients with acute ischemic stroke as measured by positron emission tomography. *Journal of Cerebral Blood Flow and Metabolism* **10**, 127–132.

Homan R., Panksepp J., McSweeny J. *et al.* (1990) D-Amphetamine effects on language and motor behavior in a chronic stroke patient. *Society for Neuroscience Abstracts* **16**, 439.

Hovda D.A. & Feeney D.M. (1984) Amphetamine with experience promotes recovery of locomotor function after unilateral frontal cortex injury in the cat. *Brain Research* **298**, 358–361.

Hovda D.A. & Feeney D.M. (1985) Haloperidol blocks amphetamine induced recovery of binocular depth per-ception after bilateral visual cortex ablation in cat. *Proceedings of the Western Pharmacological Society* **28**, 209–211.

Hovda D.A., Sutton R.L. & Feeney D.M. (1989) Amphetamine-induced recovery of visual cliff per-formance after bilateral visual cortex ablation in cats: measurements of depth perception thresholds. *Behavi-oural Neuroscience* **103**, 574–584.

Jackson R.D., Corrigan J.D. & Arnett J.A. (1985) Amitriptyline for agitation in head injury. *Archives of Physical and Medical Rehabilitation* **66**, 180–181.

Lipper S. & Tuchman M.M. (1976) Treatment of chronic post-traumatic organic brain syndrome with dextro-amphetamine: first reported case. *Journal of Nervous and Mental Diseases* **162**, 366–371.

Meyer P.M. & Meyer D.R. (1982) Memory, remembering, and amnesia. In Isaacson R.L. and Spear N.E. (eds) *The Expression of Knowledge*, pp. 179–211. Plenum, New York.

Porch B.E. & Feeney D.M. (1986) Effects of antihyper-tensive drugs on recovery from aphasia. *Clinical Aphasiology* **16**, 309–314.

Salo A.A. & Feeney D.M. (submitted) Amphetamine reduces morbidity and mortality after embolic stroke in the rat.

Sutton R.L. & Feeney D.M. (1992) α-Noradrenergic agonists and antagonists affect recovery and maintenance of beam-walking ability after sensorimotor cortex ablation in the rat. *Restoration Neurology and Neuroscience* **4**, 1–11.

Sutton R.L., Chen M.J., Hovda D.A. & Feeney D.M. (1986) Effects of amphetamine on cerebral metabolism following brain damage as revealed by quantitative cytochrome oxidase histochemistry. *Society for Neuroscience Abstracts* **12**, 1404.

Sutton R.L., Weaver M.S. & Feeney D.M. (1987) Drug-induced modifications of behavioral recovery following cortical trauma. *Journal of Head Trauma Rehabilitation* **2**, 50–58.

Sutton R.L., Hovda D.A. & Chugani H.T. (1989a) Time course of local cerebral glucose utilization (LCGU) alterations after motor cortex ablation in the rat. *Society for Neuroscience Abstracts* **15**, 128.

Sutton R.L., Hovda D.A. & Feeney D.M. (1989b) Amphetamine accelerates recovery of locomotor function following bilateral frontal cortex ablation in cat. *Behavioural Neuroscience* **103**, 837–841.

Sutton R.L., Hovda D.A., Chen M.J. & Feeney D.M. (in preparation) Recovery of function after cortical injury in rats and cats: lack of effects with dopamine agonists and beneficial effects of sympathomimetics.

Teuber H.L. (1975) Recovery of function after brain injury in man. In *Outcome of Severe Damage to the Nervous System*, pp. 159–190. Ciba Foundation Symposium 34, Elsevier North Holland, New York.

Vallar G., Perani D., Cappa S.F., Messa C., Lenzi G.L. & Fazio F. (1988) Recovery from aphasia and neglect after subcortical stroke: neuropsychological and cerebral perfusion study. *Journal of Neurology Neurosurgery and Psychiatry* **51**, 1269–1276.

Walker-Batson D., Unwin H., Curtis S. *et al.* (1992) Use of amphetamine in the treatment of aphasia. *Restorative Neurology and Neuroscience* **4**, 47–50.

33: Surgical Rehabilitation in Tetraplegia

A. EJESKÄR AND A.-G. DAHLLÖF

Background, 482
Goals of treatment, 482
Basis for treatment, 483
Classification, 485
General principles of treatment, 485
Timing of treatment, 487
Reconstructive procedures, 488
  Elbow extensor, 488
  Hand grip reconstruction, 490
Postoperative treatment, 495
  General principles, 495
  Elbow extensor reconstruction, 496
  Hand grip reconstruction, 496
Results, 498
  Elbow extensor reconstruction, 498
  Hand grip reconstruction, 498
Conclusion, 500
Appendix, 501

Surgical procedures to improve the function of the upper extremity in tetraplegic patients have evolved during the last decade as an important part of the rehabilitation of these patients. As a result a number of articles (Lamb, 1989; Moberg, 1990b; Waters *et al.*, 1990; Freehafer, 1991; Mennen & Boonzaier, 1991; Nigst, 1991) dealing with this subject have appeared in the last 3 years. Erik Moberg has greatly contributed to this spread of interest since he began his work in this special field in Göteborg in 1970. He first presented his ideas for treatment in 1975 (Moberg, 1975) and extended them in his book on this subject (Moberg, 1978). He was one of the initiators of the international conferences on this topic, the first held in Edinburgh in 1979 and the fourth at Stanford, Palo Alto, California, in 1991. These conferences have given people interested in this subject the opportunity to meet and exchange ideas, thus stimulating and disseminating this type of treatment.

Erik Moberg started his work with these patients at the neurorehabilitation unit at the Sahlgren Hospital, Göteborg. Eight years ago Arvid Ejeskär succeeded him and has since then been in charge of this service in Göteborg, Ann-Gret Dahllöf, present chief of the neurorehabilitation unit, has been able to follow the development for almost 20 years. This article presents our current policy for treating tetraplegic patients.

Background

According to statistics in Sweden, every year about 60 subjects sustain spinal cord injuries resulting in tetraplegia. These patients are usually treated at the rehabilitation units mainly localized at the university hospitals. The initial hospitalization time is usually 8–12 months.

When the patients leave hospital, they usually go home to adjusted apartments or to special apartments with 24-hour service localized in ordinary habitation areas. It is very seldom that a spinal cord-injured patient is referred to a nursing home except for very old patients (>70 years of age).

After further rehabilitation, while living at home, a majority of the tetraplegic patients (59%) return to work or studies. The good social service in Sweden, together with the possibilities for returning to work, thus enables the patients to live a relatively normal life.

After 1 year of rehabilitation in the hospital, many patients have a strong desire to stay at home and live a 'normal' life outside hospital. These facts have considerably influenced our surgical rehabilitation programme.

Goals of treatment

The primary goal of operative treatment should be to create at least one one-hand grip and active extension of the elbow(s), but each patient should be offered maximum improvement with respect to their requests and possibilities. Each patient is unique, firstly in that the remaining sensory and motor functions seldom coincide completely with those of another patient, secondly the spontaneous position of the fingers and thumb varies from patient to patient, and thirdly his/her wishes, expectations and ambitions are different from other patients. Therefore it is impossible to use a 'cookery book' approach in the decision-making process but instead each patient should have his/her own individualized operative treatment.

Basis for treatment

The basis for treatment consists of two parts:
1 The patient's remaining motor and sensory functions.
2 The wishes of the patient.
The patient's demands and performance of daily activities must be carefully considered so that the surgeon can fully analyse what an operation may mean for the patient (examination protocol, see appendix). This analysis is more important the longer the patient has adjusted to the handicap. One must also be aware that the hand is an organ used not only for gripping, but also for feeling and for human contact. The latter function is often more important for young people than one realizes and may conflict with the gripping function in a tetraplegic hand.

At the preoperative examination the surgeon should evaluate the following:
1 *Muscle strength*. All muscles from the shoulder girdle and distally should be assessed for motor function. The posterior part of the deltoid should be tested separately. The forearm muscles with a strength grade 4 or 5 on the Medical Research Council (MRC) scale (Seddon, 1954) are of special interest as they form the basis for a one-hand grip. The supinator muscle should also be tested. This can usually be done by palpating the muscle belly over the proximal part of the radius during resisted supination.

There is no clinical way of testing separately the function of the extensor carpi radialis brevis (ECRB). If one wishes to do this, it must be tested on the operating table under local anaesthesia (Fig.

33.1) before a decision is made to transfer the extensor carpi radialis longus (ECRL). If the muscle resists weight of 5 kg, it is considered strong enough to provide sufficient wrist extension. When testing wrist extension strength clinically, one should be aware that a grade 3 strength should normally mean full extension against the weight of the limb (hand). As this weight is small, it means that the wrist extension force may not be sufficient for the patient to grip an object as it increases the total weight of the hand and then the grip is no longer functional. So a grade 3 in wrist extension should be defined as full extension against a slight resistance.

2 *Sensibility*. This is evaluated in terms of two-point discrimination (2PD). A measurement of less than 10 mm, at least in the thumb, will increase the chances of achieving valuable function in the hand after reconstruction. A 2PD of less than 10 mm in one hand is a prerequisite for simultaneous use of both hands.

The presence of 2PD <10 mm means also that the patient has sufficient proprioception in that part of the hand (Moberg, 1990a).

3 *Joint contractures*. They are not very common and are caused by a shoulder–hand–finger (SHF) syndrome which has not been fully treated or by spasticity. The SHF syndrome usually results in stiffness in the shoulder joint, the metacarpophalangeal (MCP) joints and/or the interphalangeal (IP) joints. One should always make an attempt to treat these joint contractures by active exercises and various types of splints before surgery. In a few cases it might be necessary to treat contractures of the finger joints operatively.

4 *Spasticity* is evaluated above all in the arms and hands. There are at least two separate forms of spasticity, first the 'overactive' muscle, which contracts quickly if one tries to extend it, and secondly the 'stiff muscle', which only very slowly gives way. Of course, there are intermediate and/or mixed forms but unfortunately we do not have appropriate terms to describe these phenomena.

In a few cases, spasticity can be of great value for the patient by providing the ability to lift heavy objects for short periods of time or to extend the elbow. In most patients the spasticity is neither a help nor a hindrance, but in a few patients it can be a significant problem, usually by creating joint con-

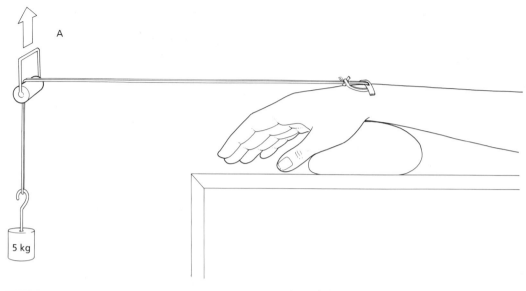

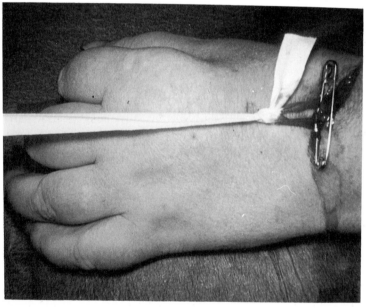

Fig. 33.1 Testing of ECRB. With local anaesthesia a safety-pin is put through the tendon of ECRB. A sterile cotton ribbon is tied round the safety pin and attached to a weight of 5 kg, passing a pulley (A) on its way. The pulley is held by an assistant while the patient is asked to dorsiflex the wrist.

tractures. These are usually located either in the elbow flexors, the finger flexors or the interossei. The worst kind gives a flexion–supination deformity of the elbows, which results in a position where the patient is completely unable to use his/her hands.

If the contracture is severe it may be an indication for surgery, and should have first priority in the treatment plan.

5 *Hyperaesthesia* can be another difficult problem, because it may completely prevent a patient from using his or her hand. Hyperaesthesia must be overcome before a reconstructive procedure is performed. If detected early after injury, it should be treated by sensibility training, which means that the patient has to be taught not to avoid contact with the hyperaesthetic skin area but instead is encouraged to softly rub it with or against a cloth.

If the hyperaesthesia is severe and above all has been present for a long time, selective nerve blocking with a long-lasting anaesthetic drug is indicated, followed by sectioning of the specific nerve responsible for the hyperaesthesia.

6 *Passive motion* in the wrist and thumb should be examined. A passive flexion greater than 45° in the MCP joint of the thumb may create problems in the construction of a good key grip. A great laxity in the carpometacarpal (CMC) joint of the thumb may also be bothersome, as well as marked dorsiflexion of the wrist joint (≥70°).

The preoperative examination, which, of course, should always be done by the surgeon, should give him/her a basis for discussion with the patient and permit an analysis whereby the patient's desires, if possible, can be fulfilled. It is also important to inform the patient what operative and postoperative stress the treatment entails, to avoid disappointment or misunderstanding. When convincing the patient of the benefits of reconstructive surgery, a patient who has undergone a similar operation can be of great assistance in describing the benefits and problems of the treatment.

Classification

The preoperative examination should lead to a classification of each arm separately. The international classification adopted for this purpose was agreed upon at the meeting in Gien in 1984 (McDowell *et al.*, 1986; Table 33.1). It does not consider the status of the shoulder but only the function in the forearm and hand. An arm may be classified as O:1 Tr− or OCu:4 Tr+, where O stands for vision or oculo, Cu for 2PD ≤ 10 mm, at least in the thumb, and the figure for the number of muscles in the forearm of minimum strength grade 4. Tr− denotes a triceps of less than strength grade 3. The majority (62/74) of our patients fell into the first five classes, O(Cu):0−4, which means that they had no active function beyond the wrist.

The distinction between group 3 (OCu:2) and group 4 (OCu:3) is difficult, due to the inability of testing the ECRB clinically. As mentioned, operative testing under local anaesthesia is necessary for this distinction in borderline cases. However, we have found reason to do such a testing in only a few patients.

Table 33.1 International classification for surgery of the hand in tetraplegia

Group	Muscle(s) with strength grade ≥ 4
O(Cu):0	No muscle
O(Cu):1	Brachioradialis (BR)
O(Cu):2	BR + extensor carpi radialis longus (ECRL)
O(Cu):3	BR + ECRL + extensor carpi radialis brevis (ECRB)
OCu:4	BR + ECRL + ECRB + pronator teres (PT)
OCu:5	BR + ECRL + ECRB + PT + flexor carpi radialis (FCR)
OCu:6	BR + ECRL + ECRB + PT + FCR + finger extensors
OCu:7	BR + ECRL + ECRB + PT + FCR + finger and thumb extensors
OCu:8	As above + partial finger flexors
OCu:9	Lacks only intrinsics
X	Exceptions

Before doing any surgery, the patient should be tested with a hand function test. We routinely examine each patient with the Sollerman hand function test* (Sollerman, 1980), a test which takes into consideration the type of grip the patient uses and the time needed for performing 20 standardized activities of daily living (ADL) tasks (Fig. 33.2 and Table 33.2). Each hand is tested separately pre- and postoperatively to evaluate the improvement after each procedure. There are other tests designed which are now undergoing evaluation.

General principles of treatment

The patients are treated at the neurorehabilitation unit during every aspect of the surgical rehabilitation except during the operations, which are performed at the hand surgical division. This is an important point, as the patients need well-trained staff to care for their many problems. Good general care is a prerequisite for a good result after surgery.

The type of anaesthesia is also important. Although many patients tolerate inhalation anaesthesia, we prefer to use various blocks. For all hand operations, an axillary plexus block is used. For the elbow extensor reconstruction, this type of

* Manufacturer of test: MITAB, S-275 00 Sjöbo, Sweden.

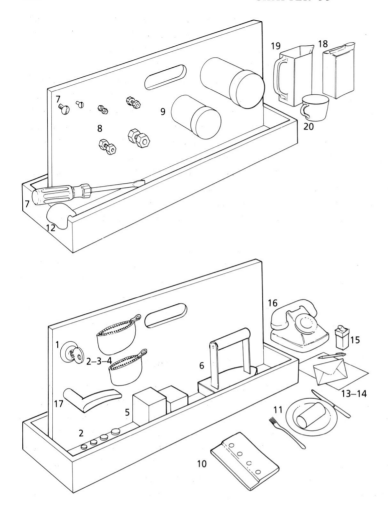

Fig. 33.2 The Sollerman test set up. The numbers in the drawing correspond to the numbers in Table 33.2.

Table 33.2 The twenty ADL tasks in the Sollerman test

1	Put key into lock	11	Cut Play-Doh
2	Pick up coins from surface and put into purse	12	Put on Tubi-grip stocking
3	Pick up coins from purse	13	Write with pen
4	Open and close zippers	14	Put on paper clip
5	Lift wooden cubes	15	Fold paper, put into envelope
6	Lift iron	16	Lift telephone receiver
7	Turn screw with screwdriver	17	Turn door handle
8	Put nuts on bolts	18	Pour water from Purepak
9	Turn lid off two jars	19	Pour water from jug
10	Button four buttons	20	Pour water from cup

block needs to be combined with a block of the axillary nerve. This is easily done posteriorly to the shoulder joint, just prior to its entry into the deltoid. Thereby we avoid the risk of pulmonary complication. The supraclavicular plexus block works as well as the interscalene plexus block.

The general principles of the operations are as follows:

1 Operate on the patient's better hand first. This is a very important rule because it is much easier for the patient to start to use the treated hand if it was the better one before the operation. If one starts treatment with the more severely affected hand, it is likely that the patient will not overcome the postoperative difficulties and will thus gain very little from the procedure. One exception to this rule is if the better hand is so good that the patient is satisfied with it and wants to have the other hand improved. This type of patient is rare.

2 Perform the elbow extensor reconstruction before the hand. Generally, it is wise to start proximally to stabilize the elbow and thereby achieve maximal gain from the later procedure in the hand. The postoperative treatment after the extensor reconstruction is longer and the patient cannot make use of a hand grip during a large portion of this period. From the psychological point of view, we therefore think it is best to start with the elbow.

The great majority of patients, who do not have active elbow extension, can benefit from a transfer of the brachioradialis (BR) for various purposes. However, to be effective the BR needs an antagonist. Several authors (Waters *et al.*, 1985, 1990; Brys & Waters, 1987; Freehafer *et al.*, 1988) have shown that, although BR works after most transfers, the effectiveness of the transfer is increased in the presence of an active elbow extensor. If the patient rejects the idea of an elbow extensor reconstruction, it does not exclude a procedure in the hand. However, if it involves a BR transfer, the patient is carefully informed on what s/he can expect to gain.

Freehafer *et al.* (1988) and Freehafer (1991) are of the opinion that the elbow extensor reconstruction should preferably be done after the hand grip operation. The reason for this is not clearly stated.

Waters *et al.* (1990) reported the results in a

few cases of simultaneous elbow extensor reconstructions and transfer of the BR to the thumb flexor. We have no experience of this procedure but only of an elbow extensor in combination with the so-called key grip (see below). The great gain for the patient with a combined operation is much shorter postoperative rehabilitation, which in some patients may be so valuable that the greater postoperative difficulties can be overcome. This must be carefully evaluated in each instance.

3 Use stainless steel tendon markers in all transfers. A suture of 5–0, or in the upper arm 3–0, stainless steel is placed on each side of the tendon anastomosis. The distance between the markers is measured during the operation and postoperatively on X-rays (Ejeskär & Irstam, 1981; Fig. 33.3). A large increase of this distance may indicate a rupture in the junction, and this knowledge is valuable when deciding on re-exploration. It is also of importance in deciding the postoperative regimen, especially in elbow extensor reconstructions.

Timing of treatment

The reconstructive treatment can be started as soon as the patient is driving a wheelchair, is well rehabilitated and has spent some time at home. This usually takes 1 year after the accident (occasionally only 7–8 months). An operation at this stage eliminates the need for the patient to relearn how to perform different activities.

One exception to this rule is the patient with a severe supination–flexion deformity of both elbows–forearms, who might be a candidate for surgery during the primary rehabilitation period.

Unfortunately, many patients are not fully informed about the possibilities offered by surgical rehabilitation. Not until they come home and meet other people with spinal cord injuries, e.g. at training centres, do they realize this. However, there is no need to hestitate to operate upon a person long after the accident. Extra care should be taken to inform the patient of what the treatment programme involves and to assure oneself that the patient accepts becoming considerably dependent on others for maybe 10–12 weeks postoperatively. The overall results in these 'old' cases are often very gratifying since the patients are usually very well motivated.

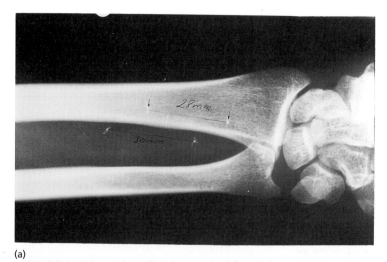

(a)

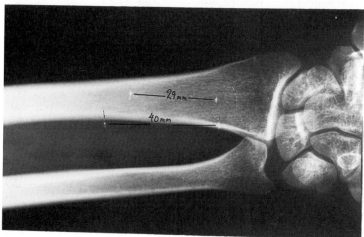

(b)

Fig. 33.3 X-rays showing tendon markers after transfer of ECRL to finger flexor and brachioradialis to flexor pollicis longus. (a) Shortly after removal of the cast. (b) Three months later, showing an increase of marker distance of 12 mm in finger flexors and a few mm in thumb flexor compared to perioperative measurements.

Reconstructive procedures

Elbow extensor

An indication for reconstruction of the elbow extensor exists in all patients who lack the ability to extend their elbows or only have muscle strength grade 1 in their triceps. The majority of the patients belong to this category. The lack of extension results in dependence on gravity for stability of the elbow, which reduces the function of the arm considerably when writing, driving a car and bringing down objects from above. When lying in bed, patients are unable to extend their elbows and, for example, read a book.

Many patients want an elbow extensor in order to facilitate or make transfers in and out of the wheelchair. However, the ability to transfer is dependent upon fixation of the shoulders to the trunk of the body and, if this function is lacking, no reconstructed elbow extensor, however perfect it may be, will help the patient to transfer. Active elbow extension, although weak, may, however, help the patient to get hyperextension in his/her elbows and by locking the joints passively it can facilitate transfers.

There are two muscles available for reconstruction of elbow extension: the posterior part of the deltoid and the biceps brachii.

Posterior deltoid transfer

Moberg described initially the transfer of the posterior deltoid, which he connected to the triceps by means of tendon grafts taken from the toe extensor tendons (Moberg, 1975, 1978). Postoperatively a cast was worn for 6 weeks with the elbow in 10° of flexion. Flexion was then slowly taken up with approximately 10° increase per week during a 6-week period.

In a trial to shorten the postoperative rehabilitation time, Castro-Sierra & Lopez-Pita (1983) introduced the idea that the posterior deltoid is detached with a piece of bone from the humerus. The central third of the triceps tendon is reflected in a retrograde fashion and the turning point is reinforced by a synthetic material. Postoperatively, a 4-week period of immobilization is followed by gradual flexion exercises for 3−4 weeks.

Both methods were used by Moberg but a follow-up study showed that the results after both methods in a great proportion of cases were unsatisfactory (Ejeskär, 1988). Therefore, we have tried various modifications. Our present method is first to do a preliminary operation (stage I), at which the deltoid insertion is reinforced by a piece of tendon (palmaris longus) in a figure of eight (Fig. 33.4). Three months after this, stage II is performed, where the posterior deltoid is detached from the humerus and connected to the olecranon by means of a tendon prosthesis (Hunter rod) and a piece of fascia lata. After stage II, the arm is immobilized in a cast for 3−5 weeks and then flexion is gradually taken up during a period of 4−5 weeks. The results of this technique are still preliminary but seem to be better than those of the original method. Although stage I gives a much stronger 'tendon' for weaving the tendon prosthesis and suturing the fascia lata, it is still this junction which is the weak point and must be protected in the postoperative phase. Otherwise it will elongate and the function will deteriorate.

One factor in the reconstruction of the elbow extensor which is seldom discussed is the shoulder joint. We have chosen not to immobilize it, which of course might be a source of stress upon the created tendon junction. The reason for this is that the patient is sent home a few days after the operation and is again taken into hospital when it is

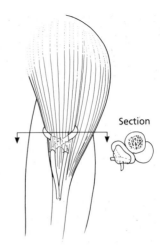

Fig. 33.4 Stage I in posterior deltoid-to-triceps transfer. The palmaris longus tendon is woven into the distal part of the muscle in a figure-of-eight configuration.

time for removal of the plaster and for the initial phase of recuperation. In other centres, the patients may stay in the hospital during the whole postoperative period. Then it is feasible to immobilize the shoulder. Differences on this point of technique might to some extent explain differences in the final results.

There are a number of other techniques described, using various materials and techniques for bridging over the distance between the posterior deltoid and the olecranon (tibialis anterior tendon: Lacey et al., 1986; dacron band: Allieu et al., 1985). No technique has really proved to be superior to the other, partly because there is no uniform method of evaluation of the results.

Biceps brachii

Transfer of the biceps brachii to the triceps tendon over the lateral aspect of the arm has been described by Friedenberg (1954) and Zancolli (1968). It can with equal ease be brought around the medial aspect of the humerus in order to avoid compromising the radial nerve. The biceps tendon can be made to reach down to the olecranon, but in my (A.E.) experience it cannot be anchored directly into the bone. Postoperatively the arm is immobilized with the elbow in 10−15° flexion for approximately 4 weeks, followed by gradual flexion exercises for 3–4 weeks.

The transfer of the posterior deltoid is the standard method. However, if the posterior deltoid does not have a strength of grade 4, or the elbow has a flexion contracture of more than 25°, a transfer of the biceps is the best choice. A prerequisite for a transfer of the biceps is that the supinator muscle is working. If there is a supination deformity, biceps transfer is mandatory.

The end result of both types of transfer is approximately the same. The majority of patients get control of the elbow, improving the function of a transferred BR, but only a minority get a strength ≥ grade 3. Some authors (Lamb & Chan, 1983; Mennen & Boonzaier, 1991) state that a proportion of their transferred posterior deltoid gave extension force grade 5! We have never seen a reconstructed extensor stronger than grade 4 and this difference is probably due to lack of a standardized method of evaluation.

Transfer of the biceps always gives full passive pronation. The postoperative phase is a little shorter than after the posterior deltoid transfer and this transfer has just one tendon junction which can elongate.

Hand grip reconstruction

Key grip

The so-called key grip is the most basic type of grip. It requires one active motor and a good passive range of motion in the wrist. Extension of the wrist closes the grip, and passive or active flexion of the wrist opens the grip. It also requires a good relationship between the thumb and the fingers, so that the thumb meets the index fingers somewhere in the region of the middle phalanx when the wrist is dorsiflexed (Fig. 33.5). The key grip has been modified several times, but the present technique involves the following steps (Fig. 33.6):

1 Temporary arthrodesis of the IP joint of the thumb.
2 Tenodesis of the flexor pollicis longus (FPL) to the radius.
3 Transfer of inactive superficialis III or IV to the abductor pollicis brevis (APB) to resist supination–flexion deformity of the thumb.
4 It may also involve one or more steps to improve the relationship between the thumb and the fingers (see below).

Transfer of brachioradialis to extensor carpi radialis brevis

The key grip requires minimum grade 3 in wrist extension. If the patient does not have that strength (belongs to group O(Cu)0–1), it might be possible to transfer a working BR to achieve sufficient wrist extension. Normally one considers that a muscle should have strength grade 4 to be used for a transfer. However, in patients with arms classified as O:0 with grade 3 in both BR and wrist extension, a transfer of the BR might increase the wrist extension force enough to make it functionally effective.

Transfer of brachioradialis to flexor pollicis longus

This transfer can be performed in patients in minimum group O(Cu):2. They have strength grade 4 in BR and ECRL. As mentioned above, this transfer works best if the patient has an active elbow extensor. The transfer replaces the tenodesis of the FPL; thus the operation includes the temporary arthrodesis of the IP joint and the passive thumb abductor transfer.

The transfer allows an active thumb flexion and is superior to the key grip if the patient has a marked dorsiflexion of the wrist (≥70°). In those cases, a tenodesis either closes the grip in an awkward wrist angle or limits the dorsiflexion of the wrist.

The Brummer winch operation

In patients in group O:0 having only supination of the forearm, a grip similar to the key grip can be made by attaching the FPL tendon to the ulna instead of the radius. By supination of the forearm, the grip is closed and released by passive pronation (Fig. 33.7).

Other methods for thumb grip reconstructions

Freehafer has described the transfer of the BR, pronator teres or ECRL to an inactive superficialis IV to create an active abduction–flexion (opponens) of the thumb (Freehafer *et al.*, 1974; Freehafer, 1991). Zancolli connects, in patients

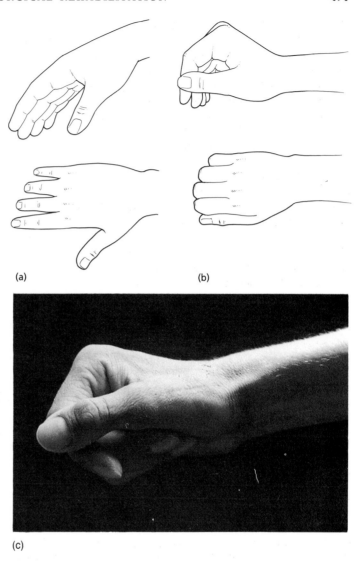

(a)

(b)

Fig. 33.5 The basis of the key grip.
(a) Opening by volar flexion.
(b) Closure by dorsiflexion of the
wrist. (c) Example of good relation
between the thumb and the fingers,
which is the most important factor
for a good function in the key grip.

(c)

with strong wrist extension, the FPL side to side with an active ECRB. Which method is the best is probably due to several factors, which may explain why there is no study comparing the results from the various methods.

Other useful procedures

Transfer of BR to give pronation

In patients in group O(Cu):1–2 with sufficient wrist extension but with difficulties of pronating

the BR can be transferred dorsally to the ulna, thereby facilitating this action.

Zancolli (1968) has described a re-routing of the biceps to achieve active pronation in cases with a supination deformity in the forearm. We have tried this technique but never achieved an active pronation. On the operating table it has been very difficult to produce pronation beyond neutral position by pulling in the distal biceps attachment after having rerouted the tendon strip. We think that the release of the biceps and elimination of its supinating power is in reality what one achieves by

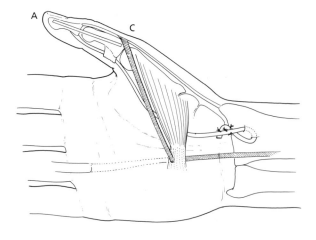

Fig. 33.6 The present modification of the key grip. A Temporary arthrodesis of the IP joint with a 2 mm Kirschner wire. B Tenodesis of the FPL. C Transfer of inactive superficialis IV or III to the abductor pollicis brevis to resist supination flexion deformity of the thumb.

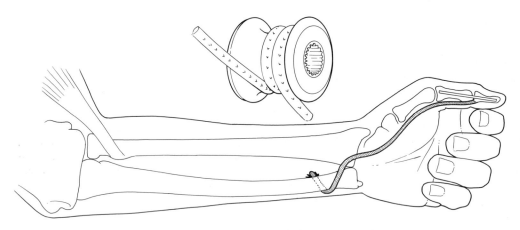

Fig. 33.7 The winch operation according to Brummer. Temporary arthrodesis of the IP joint and tenodesis of the FPL against the dorsal aspect of the ulna.

this operation. Biceps is, in our opinion, better used as a transfer to get elbow extension.

Arthrodesis of the CMC joint of the thumb

This is a useful procedure in patients with great laxity in the CMC joint, or where the thumb has an inappropriate position in relation to the fingers. Zancolli has advocated this procedure in arms classified in his group IIB – with strong wrist extension. A fusion of this joint also makes it possible to get a better opening of a thumb grip by means of a tenodesis of one of the thumb extensors. This is especially valuable in patients in the high groups

(O(Cu):0−2) by facilitating gripping of objects. A thumb with a fusion of the CMC joint gives a more predictable grip than one with a mobile CMC joint. Therefore, in patients in groups 5−7 who want to have both hands operated, fusion of the CMC joint of one thumb, leaving the other mobile, gives two different hand functions (House & Shannon, 1985), which can be very useful for the patient.

Reconstruction of finger flexor

In patients with strong wrist extension (group ≥3), finger flexion can be given to the patient by a transfer of the ECRL to the profundi. This is a simple and reliable transfer, which can made at the same time as a thumb grip. If the patient has a moderate wrist extension force and very much wants to have a finger flexor, it is wise to test the force of the ECRB, as mentioned above. In most of these cases, it is probably as well not to try to make a finger flexor but to let the patient have a fairly good wrist extension force, thereby increasing the chances of achieving a strong pinch grip. There are other muscles which can be used for finger flexion. Both BR and pronator teres have been reported for this purpose, but in our opinion the ECRL is the first option, mostly because of its length–tension characteristics and secondly because the BR is best used for other purposes, for example thumb flexion.

Intrinsic reconstruction

A transfer to give finger flexion usually results in IP joint flexion and in most patients there is a risk of getting a 'claw-hand deformity'. This means that the IP joints flex so early that the patient cannot get his/her fingers around a larger object. This risk exists in all patients who lack intrinsic muscle function, but is greatest in patients who lack finger extension and are dependent upon the wrist flexion and extensor tenodesis effect to open the hand.

Therefore a transfer to give finger flexion should, in our opinion, be accompanied by an attempt to provide intrinsic reconstruction. In the majority of tetraplegic patients, it is not possible to create an active intrinsic function but only a static or passively dynamic function. There are three different possible ways:

1 Zancolli lasso procedure (Zancolli, 1968).
2 Intrinsic tenodesis according to House (House & Shannon, 1985).
3 Transfer of superficialis to the extensor mechanism (Stiles–Bunnell transfer, Bunnell, 1942).

The Zancolli lasso procedure is indicated if the patient has an active finger extension and if passive resistance to hyperextension of the fingers improves the extension of the PIP joints.

The method involves sectioning the superficialis just proximal to the PIP joint and suturing the tendon to itself around the A1 annular ligament of each finger (Fig. 33.8). The superficialis will thus no longer flex the PIP joint but the MCP joint, and will counteract the long extensors.

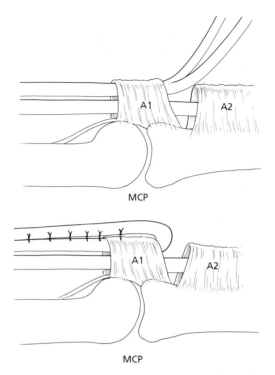

Fig. 33.8 Zancolli lasso operation. A1 and A2, first and second annular ligament of the tendon sheath. The superficialis tendon is cut distal to the A1 ligament, turned proximally and sutured to itself and to the A1 ligament with a tension which prevents hyperextension of the MCP joint.

The intrinsic tenodesis according to House and the superficialis-to-intrinsic transfers are both indicated in patients without strong active finger extension. The tenodesis is performed using a free tendon graft, which is placed from the dorsum of one PIP joint, along the lumbrical canal and volar to the axis of motion in the MCP joint, and then dorsally around the metacarpal neck and through the lumbrical canal to the dorsum of the PIP joint of the adjacent finger (Fig. 33.9). This tenodesis will work independently of the position of the wrist. The superficialis tendon transfer (Fig. 33.10) will diminish the degree of flexion of the PIP joint, as the flexion force over this joint will be eliminated. It will also give more flexion over the MCP joint, which is useful if the MCP joints have an extension contracture.

The intrinsic reconstruction is usually performed

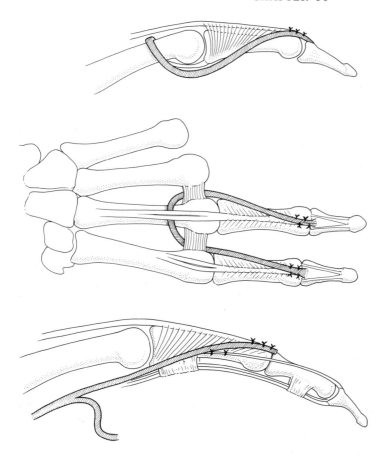

Fig. 33.9 Tenodesis according to House. The tendon transplant goes from the central slip of the index finger, through the lumbrical canal, which means volar to the intermetacarpal ligament and volar to the axis of motion in the MCP joint. It then goes dorsally round the metacarpal neck to the adjacent finger and its central extensor slip.

Fig. 33.10 Transfer of the superficialis to the extensor mechanism (Stiles–Bunnell transfer). The tendon is split into at least two parts, each part going to the lateral band and the central slip of adjacent fingers. If the superficialis is cut at the level of the PIP joint, it reaches just to the insertion of the central slip with the right tension.

at the same time as the reconstruction of the finger flexor, but can be done in the same sitting as a preceding finger extension reconstruction.

Finger extension

Patients who are given the possibility for active finger flexion will improve in function by increased gripping power. However, opening of the hand may be insufficient for gripping objects without assisting with the other hand. If they can be given some form of finger extension, the whole hand function will improve, as picking up objects will be greatly facilitated.

Finger extension can be accomplished by several means:

1 Extensor tendon tenodesis.
2 Transfer of BR.
3 Transfer of pronator teres.

The extensor tenodesis is available in most instances, but in cases without any active wrist flexion (group ≤OCu:4) the opening of the hand will be dependent upon gravity. The tenodesis should include the common extensors of the fingers, as well as at least one of the thumb extensors. However, as mentioned above, it is often very difficult to get a good tenodesis effect of the thumb without an arthrodesis of its CMC joint.

Transfer of the BR is a good method for attaining finger extension. The BR reaches down to the finger extensors and a tendon graft is used to attach it to the long or short thumb extensor. Ideally this procedure is performed before a finger flexor reconstruction, but often it is difficult to get the patient to accept the idea of having an operation from which s/he will not immediately gain anything functionally. It is not until after the flexor phase that s/he will have use for the extensor phase. Therefore, in most instances, we have performed the flexor phase first and then upon request made an extensor reconstruction. As the flexor phase might involve a BR-to-FPL transfer, one has from the start to discuss with the patient what he or she wants. According to House & Shannon (1985), the results of an extensor tenodesis and that of a transfer of the BR to the finger extensors are similar.

In patients in group OCu:4 where pronator teres is minimum grade 4, this muscle can be used for a transfer. It does not reach distally enough to be connected to the finger and thumb extensors, so an intermediate tendon transplant is needed. One of the superficialis tendons can be used for this purpose.

Other procedures

In the functional classes ≥OCu:6 the patient already has full control of the wrist and also finger extension. That means that it is possible to give the patient a still better thumb grip. Most patients in these categories have some function in the flexor carpi ulnaris and thus the flexor carpi radialis can be used for transfer to FPL. The BR can then be used to give active opponens function by means of one of the superficialis tendons. In such a case, the need for blocking the thumb IP joint is less important and the temporary arthrodesis is superfluous.

If a patient in class OCu:6 lacks sufficient thumb extension, the extensor digiti quinti might be transferred to improve this function.

In the functional classes OCu:7−9, the problems of treatment are similar to those after more isolated nerve lesions. In Table 33.3, the most commonly used procedures in the different groups are shown.

Postoperative treatment

General principles

The patient stays in the neurorehabilitation ward 2−3 days postoperatively and then goes home for 4 weeks with the arm immobilized in a cast. She then returns to the ward for 5 days after a hand operation and 12 days after an elbow extensor reconstruction.

After returning to the ward, the cast is removed and the intermarker distance is checked by X-rays. Initial training is started and the patient is taught how to train by him/herself. He or she must take the responsibility for training at home and if necessary accept the help of untrained personnel for removing and applying an orthosis. Since many patients live long distances from the hospital, we

Table 33.3 Reconstructive procedures in different groups of classification

Group	Suggested treatment									
	B−T	PD−T	Key grip	BR−ECRB	BR−pron	BR−FPL	ECRL−FF	BR−EDC	EDC−Te	INT
O(CU):0	+	(+)	(+)	(+)	−	−	−	−	−	−
O(Cu):1	+	(+)	+	+	(+)	−	−	−	−	−
O(Cu):2	(+)	+	(+)	−	(+)	+	−	−	−	−
O(Cu):3	(+)	+	(+)	−	(+)	+	(+)	(+)	(+)	(−)
OCu:4	−	(+)	(+)	−	−	+	+	(+)	(+)	+
OCu:5	−	−	−	−	−	+	+	(+)	+	+
OCu:6	−	−	−	−	−	#	+	−	−	+

B−T = biceps−triceps. PD−T = posterior deltoid−triceps. BR−ECRB = transfer of BR to ECRB. BR−pron = transfer of BR to posterior distal part of ulna. BR−FPL = transfer of BR to FPL. ECRL−FF = transfer of ECRL to finger flexor. BR−EDC = transfer of BR to thumb and finger extensors. EDC−Te = tenodesis of extensors. INT = reconstruction of intrinsics. # indicates use of another muscle for thumb flexion, e.g. flexor carpi radialis, as well as some kind of active opponens plasty.

cannot instruct the physiotherapists and occupational therapists in their local hospitals but have to rely on the patient's own learning and training capacity.

After leaving hospital the second time, they come back after another month and then usually at 3, 6 and 12 months postoperatively for follow-up examinations. At 6 and 12 months, the Sollerman test is repeated for evaluation of the functional result.

Elbow extensor reconstruction

After reconstruction of an elbow extensor using the posterior deltoid, the elbow is immobilized in a cast but the shoulder is left free. The patient is told not to adduct the arm and not to drive the wheelchair during the first postoperative period at home. When the cast is removed, intermittent flexion–extension exercises are begun (Fig. 33.11), with a splint holding the arm in slight flexion between the periods of training. The patient is allowed to flex approximately 30–40° from the start, increasing the degree of flexion by 10° per week. At 2 months the patient is left without the splint during daytime if X-rays show no or only slight increase in the intermarker distance. However, the patient wears the splint at night until 3 months postoperatively.

When starting exercises after a biceps-to-triceps transfer, the patient is instructed to flex in pronation and then to extend and at the same time supinate the elbow. As the biceps is normally a supinator, this is the easiest way for the patient to activate the biceps as an extensor. To make this easier, a biofeedback apparatus is helpful during the initial phase of training. In spite of this, it may take 2–3 months before the patient can readily activate the biceps as an elbow extensor.

If X-rays taken at the time of removal of the plaster show an increase in intermarker distance of ⩾8–10 mm, this is a warning sign. The exercises should be carried out very carefully, and another X-ray should be taken after 7–10 days to be sure that there is no further increase. A total increase in the distance of ⩾20 mm is usually equal to a failure!

Hand grip reconstruction

A hand grip reconstruction which includes a transfer of the BR or the pronator teres muscles should be protected in a cast that includes the elbow. Otherwise the risk of rupturing the tendon anastomosis is very high. In all other instances, the elbow is left free.

The patient is allowed, during the period of immobilization, to drive his/her wheelchair and use the hand as much as possible. Shoulder exercises are strongly encouraged to prevent secondary stiffness in this very important joint.

When the cast is taken off, the patient is in-

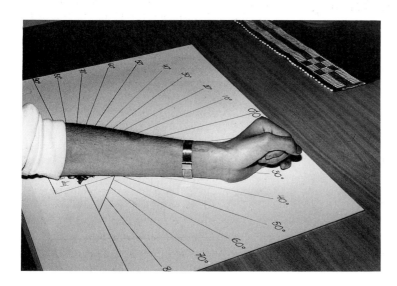

Fig. 33.11 During the early phase of training after a posterior deltoid-to-triceps transfer, a home-made protractor is useful, helping the patient to flex the elbow to the appropriate angle.

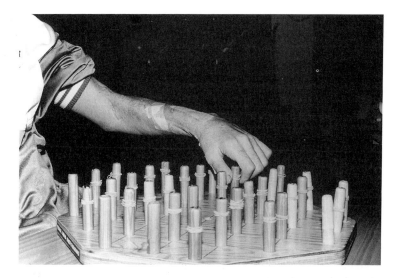

Fig. 33.12 A specially designed game is used for early exercise after a key grip. Rubber bands are wrapped around the wooden pegs to increase the friction and reduce the power needed for picking them up.

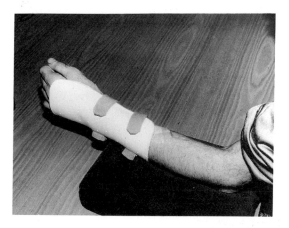

Fig. 33.13 A splint is used during the first 2–3 weeks of mobilization after a hand grip while driving the wheelchair.

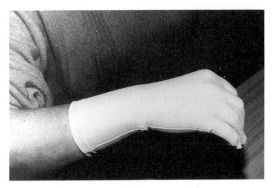

Fig. 33.14 A compression glove is often very useful during the first 4–5 days after a hand grip reconstruction to counteract the oedema.

structed to try to dorsiflex the wrist up to about 30° and at the same time practise the thumb grip by picking up lightweight objects (Fig. 33.12). The remaining dorsiflexion of the wrist should be slowly taken up during the course of 3–4 weeks in order not to stretch the tenodesis and/or tendon transfers. The patient is allowed to drive his/her wheelchair with a splint (Fig. 33.13) which protects the wrist from being forced into dorsiflexion.

During the first few days oedema of the hand is common and a compression glove is often very

useful during the first week in order to counteract this (Fig. 33.14). Continued shoulder exercises and elevation of the hand is equally important during this phase of recuperation.

In cases where the fingers have a tendency for too much extension, a flexion traction by means of rubber bands from the middle phalanxes to the wrist often helps the patient to use the thumb grip (Fig. 33.15).

If the hand grip reconstruction has included an arthrodesis of the CMC joint of the thumb, a small cast is put on around the metacarpals, protecting the arthrodesis for another 3–4 weeks (Fig. 33.16).

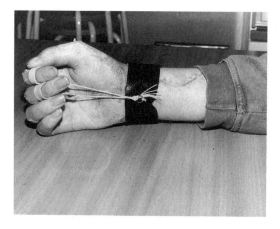

Fig. 33.15 In cases where the index and long fingers do not meet the thumb in a good position, a flexion traction by means of rubber bands from the middle phalanxes to the wrist is often very useful during the early postoperative phase.

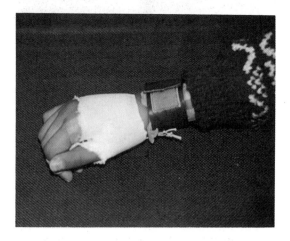

Fig. 33.16 When an arthrodesis of the carpometacarpal joint of the thumb is included in the hand grip reconstruction, the arthrodesis is protected by a small cast during the first 3 weeks of mobilization. It permits flexion of the MCP joints of the thumb and fingers, as well as extension of the wrist.

The cast must permit wrist motion and also motion in the MCP and finger joints.

In cases where a Zancolli lasso or other intrinsic reconstruction has been performed, a similar second cast is applied, but this then extends distally to the PIP joints, protecting the MCP joints from

hyperextension but allowing flexion in these joints. This type of cast, preferably made in one of the modern plastic materials (e.g. Scotch cast), is removed after 3–4 weeks.

For hand reconstructions involving transfers or tenodesis on the volar side of the forearm, the patient is instructed to refrain from making personal transfers for a period of 3 months. Such transfers induce a severe strain on the performed tendon junctions and might cause a rupture. It is important to get the patient to understand this, especially if the patient has been rather independent preoperatively.

Results

Elbow extensor reconstruction

Unfortunately, we lack a standardized and generally accepted method for objective measurement of the result of the elbow extensor reconstruction. We have measured the extension deficit in the elbow while the patient is asked to extend the elbow against the weight of the forearm. Our results after an elbow extensor reconstruction vary, but in the majority of cases the patient can extend the elbow at least in a weight-eliminating position of the arm, while 25% of patients can extend the elbow against the full weight of the forearm with a maximum of 30° lack of extension (Ejeskär, 1988). Thus a majority of the patients get an antagonist for the BR which can be used for a transfer.

Hand grip reconstruction

The effect of a hand grip reconstruction varies and depends on many factors. In most instances, a simple key grip reconstruction will give the patient an effective one-hand grip, allowing him to handle various objects with much greater ease and effectiveness than before the operation. Feeding and hygiene is facilitated, as is writing. A well-functioning thumb grip can make intermittent catheterization of the urinary bladder feasible in the male patient. Some of our young female patients have used the thumb grip to empty a continent ileum reservoir after a urinary deviation operation. They have expressed the opinion that their lives

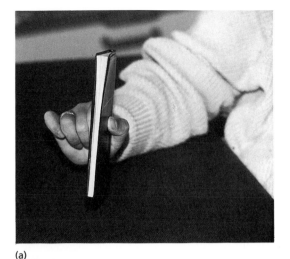

(a)

(b)

Fig. 33.17 Result of a key grip + arthrodesis of CMC I joint in an arm classified as OCu:3. Excellent position of thumb and finger. Good pinch (a) and opening of grip (b). Patient very satisfied.

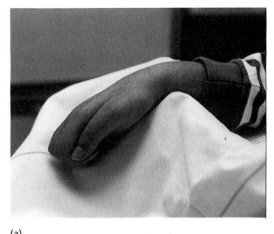

(a)

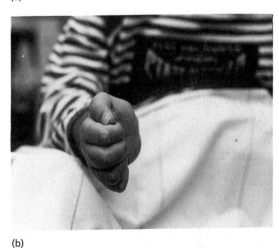

(b)

Fig. 33.18 Less satisfactory result in an arm in group OCu:3 operated upon with key grip and a transfer of ECRL to finger flexor. Postoperatively the patient was not really motivated to use his grip. He got a long-standing moderate oedema, which resulted in this flexion contracture (a). The thumb is in a supinated position (no passive opponens transfer) (b). In spite of this he had a functional improvement. This illustrates the necessity of having a well-motivated patient.

have been 'revolutionized' by these operations (Figs 33.17, 33.18 and 33.19).

The results after hand grip reconstructions can be measured in many ways, including grip strength in whole hand grip or pinch grip.

The grip strength after different thumb grip re-constructive procedures is correlated to the wrist extension force. In methods where the BR is used,

it is also related to the elbow extension force. The pinch strength after transfer of BR to FPL seems to be equal to that of a tenodesis of FPL (Waters *et al.*, 1985). The average key grip strength in the follow-up study in Göteborg was 0.7 kg in 68 hands. Similar figures have been reported by Colyer & Kappelman (1981) and Rieser & Waters (1986), who found an

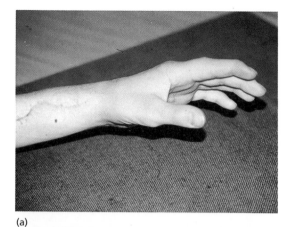

(a)

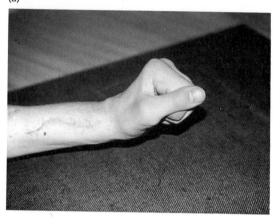

(b)

Fig. 33.19 A good end result after two-stage reconstruction of finger extension and flexion in an arm classified in group 5. In stage I: BR to finger and thumb extensors. In stage II: ECRL to profundi, key grip with passive opponens and superficialis to intrinsic. Good opening of hand (a) and good finger flexion and thumb grip (b). Patient very satisfied.

average of 0.9 kg. Kelley *et al.* (1985) have reported a value of 0.5 kg, using the technique of Freehafer. Although all these values are far below a normal pinch strength (8–12 kg), the grip strength is sufficient for many activities.

The grip strength after transfer of the ECRL to the profundi depends very much on the strength in the ECRB. The grip strength average in our patients is 0.17 kPa, as measured with the Vigorimeter, with a range from 0 to 0.48 kPa. A normal person has a grip strength in the range 0.70 to 1.8 kPa.

Results of functional testing is another way of evaluation. The use of the Sollerman test has shown that all patients, with very few exceptions, gain from reconstructive surgery. The improvement in score is dependent upon the procedure and on the functional class of the arm. The greatest increase in score is found in the intermediate groups (OCu:3–6) who have no active hand grip preoperatively. They usually increase their test score by 15–20 points, which is encouraging since the maximal test score is 80. Tests show that patients in these intermediate groups above all perform the tasks more quickly and safely and thereby increase their score.

It is also quite clear that the patients in the functional class O(Cu):0–2 often increase their wrist extension force once they get a thumb grip. A follow-up examination 1 year postoperatively after a key grip may very well show that the preoperative grade 3 wrist extension has become a grade 4, because they have been using the hand more extensively than before the operation. Functional testing also reveals that for many patients it takes more than 6 months postoperatively before they have really learnt how to use their new abilities. It is important to inform patients about this before surgery; otherwise they might become disappointed during the initial postoperative phase with ensuing psychological difficulties.

Conclusion

The majority of tetraplegic patients can benefit from reconstructive surgery, either through elbow extensor reconstruction alone or combined with a hand grip procedure. Therefore each tetraplegic patient should be examined approximately 1 year after the accident with respect to the possibility for surgical rehabilitation. If the patient at that time is not interested in a consultation, this offer should be repeated at a later date so that no single tetraplegic patient needs to say: I did not know of this possibility!

Appendix

Tetraplegia: evaluation for reconstructive arm and hand surgery

Patient: ....

Date of examination: ....

Examiner: ....

Occupation before accident:

Occupation now?

Date of accident: Type of accident: Traffic   Diving   Other

Level of skeletal injury:

Best arm before accident: Best arm after accident:

Can raise seat from wheelchair: Use manual/electric wheelchair

Can turn over completely in bed without help:

Can transfer from bed to wheelchair without help:

Can transfer from wheelchair to car and vice versa without help:

Feeding: Which hand: Which type of grip: Fork, spoon?

Hygiene: How is shaving, putting on make up, etc. performed?

How is hand writing performed?

How is stabilization in the wheelchair performed?

Spasticity?

Contractures?

Amputations of e.g. fingers?

Excessive CMC joint laxity?

Group	Right arm	Left arm
	0 Cu	0 Cu
	Tr	Tri

continued overleaf

Appendix *Continued*

Muscle function examination			Two point discrimination		
	Right	Left		Right	Left
Trapezius					
Latissimus dorsi			Thumb		
Deltoid:			Index		
1) Anterior part			Middle		
2) Posterior part			Ring		
Serratus			Little		
Outward rotators					
Inward rotators			Unusual findings or comments		
Pectorals					
1) Sternoclav. portion					
2) Costal portion					
Triceps					
Biceps brachii			Patient's own wishes		
Brachioradialis					
Supinator					
Radial wrist ext.					
Pronator teres					
Flexor carpi radialis			Suggestion for treatment:		
Finger extensors					
Finger flexors					
Extensor poll longus					
Abductor poll longus					
Flex. poll longus					
Intrinsics					

Passive joint motion:

MCPl joints:

Wrist joints:

Patient's ability to understand:

Patient's expected ability to cooperate:

References

Allieu Y., Teissier J., Triki F. *et al.* (1985) Réanimation de l'extension du coude chez le tétraplégique par transplantation du deltoïde postérieur. *Revue Chirurgique Orthopédique* **71**, 195–200.

Brys D. & Waters R.I. (1987) Effects of triceps function on the brachioradialis transfer in quadriplegia. *Journal of Hand Surgery* **12A**, 237–239.

Bunnell S. (1942) Surgery of the intrinsic muscles of the hand other than those producing opposition of the thumb. *Journal of Bone and Joint Surgery* **24**, 1–31.

Castro-Sierra A. & Lopez-Pita A. (1983) A new surgical technique to correct triceps paralysis. *Hand* **15** (1), 42–46.

Colyer R.A. & Kappelman B. (1981) Flexor pollicis longus tenodesis in tetraplegia at the sixth cervical level. *Journal of Bone and Joint Surgery* **63A** (3), 376–379.

Ejeskär A. (1988) Upper limb surgical rehabilitation in high-level tetraplegia. *Hand Clinics* **4** (4), 585–599.

Ejeskär A & Irstam L. (1981) Elongation in profundus tendon repair. *Scandinavian Journal of Plastic and Reconstruction Surgery* **15**, 61.

Freehafer A.A. (1991) Tendon transfers in patients with cervical spinal cord injury. *Journal of Hand Surgery* **16A** (5), 804–809.

Freehafer A.A., Vonhaam E. & Allen V. (1974) Tendon transfers to improve grasp after injuries of the cervical spinal cord. *Journal of Bone and Joint Surgery* **56A** (5), 951–959.

Freehafer A.A., Peckham P.H., Keith M. *et al.* (1988) The brachioradialis: anatomy, properties, and value for tendon transfer in the tetraplegic. *Journal of Hand Surgery* **13A**, 99–104.

Friedenberg Z.B. (1954) Transposition of the biceps brachii for triceps weakness. *Journal of Bone and Joint Surgery* **36A** (3), 656–658.

House J.H. & Shannon M.A. (1985) Restoration of strong grasp and lateral pinch in tetraplegia: a comparison of two methods of thumb control in each patient. *Journal of Hand Surgery* **10A** (1), 22–29.

Kelley C.M., Freehafer A.A., Peckham P.H. *et al.* (1985) Postoperative results of opponens plasty and flexor tendon transfer in patients with spinal cord injuries. *Journal of Hand Surgery* **10A** (6 Part I), 890–894.

Lacey S.H., Wilber R.G., Peckham P.H. *et al.* (1986) The posterior deltoid to triceps transfer: a clinical and biomechanical assessment. *Journal of Hand Surgery* **11A** (4), 542–547.

Lamb D.W. (1989) Upper limb surgery in tetraplegia. *Journal of Hand Surgery* **14B** (2), 143–144.

Lamb D.W. & Chan K.M. (1983) Surgical reconstruction of the upper limb in traumatic tetraplegia: a review of 41 patients. *Journal of Bone and Joint Surgery* **65B** (3), 291–298.

McDowell C.L., Moberg E.A. & House J.H. (1986) The second international conference on surgical rehabilitation of the upper limb in tetraplegia (quadriplegia). *Journal of Hand Surgery* **11A** (4), 604–607.

Mennen U. & Boonzaier A.C. (1991) An improved technique of posterior deltoid to triceps transfer in tetraplegia. *Journal of Hand Surgery* **16B** (2), 197–201.

Moberg E. (1975) Surgical treatment for absent single-hand grip and elbow extension in quadriplegia. *Journal of Bone and Joint Surgery* **57A** (2), 196–206.

Moberg E. (1978) *The Upper Limb in Tetraplegia.* Thieme, Stuttgart.

Moberg E. (1990a) Two-point discrimination test. *Scandinavian Journal of Rehabilitation Medicine* **22**, 127–134.

Moberg E. (1990b) Surgical rehabilitation of the upper limb in tetraplegia. *Paraplegia* **28** (5), 330–334.

Nigst H. (ed.) (1991) *Motorische Ersatzoperationen der oberen Extremität.* Bibliothek für Handchirurgie, Hippokrates Verlag, Stuttgart.

Rieser T.V. & Waters R.L. (1986) Long-term follow-up of the Moberg key grip procedure. *Journal of Hand Surgery* **11A** (5), 724–728.

Seddon H.J. (ed.) (1954) *Peripheral Nerve Injuries.* Special Report Series, Her Majesty's Stationery Office, London.

Sollerman C. (1980) Assessment of grip function – evaluation of a new test method. (Handens greppfunktion.) Thesis, Göteborg, Sweden.

Waters R., Moore K.R., Graboff S.R. *et al.* (1985) Brachioradialis to flexor pollicis longus tendon transfer for active lateral pinch in the tetraplegic. *Journal of Hand Surgery* **10A** (3), 385–391.

Waters R.L., Stark L.Z., Gubernik I. *et al.* (1990) Electromyographic analysis of brachioradialis to flexor pollicis longus tendon transfer in quadriplegia. *Journal of Hand Surgery* **15A**, 335–339.

Zancolli E. (1968) *Structural and Dynamic Bases of Hand Surgery.* J.B. Lippincott, Philadelphia and Toronto.

Zancolli E. (1975) Surgery for the quadriplegic hand with active, strong wrist extension preserved. *Clinical Orthopedics* **112**, 101–113.

34: Engineering Solutions for Patients with Neurological Disability

P.H. CHAPPELL AND I.D. SWAIN

Basic control engineering, 505
Control of a hand prosthesis, 506
Functional electrical stimulation (FES), 510
    Practical FES systems, 510
    Lower limb function, 511
    Upper limb function, 512
Communication aids, 513
    Communication aids for the blind, 514
    Interface requirements of communication users, 515
Conclusions, 516

The use of engineering techniques to provide missing or impaired function for the disabled is not new. Artificial limbs are described in the Rig Veda, written in Sanskrit in India between 1700 and 3500 BC (Hall, 1964). However, until recently such devices were basically simple, usually providing the desired function by adding strength or controlling position – orthoses – or by replacing missing limbs by simple peg-legs or hand hooks – prostheses. Even considering more modern devices, such as body-powered artificial hands/arms or hip replacements, all are essentially purely mechanical systems and as such are not applicable to patients with neurological deficit.

It is only with the development of computers over the past 20 years that it has been possible to incorporate 'intelligence' into engineering solutions, so that lost neurological function can be replaced, in addition to lost mechanical function. The effect that such devices can have on the quality of life of the neurologically disabled is enormous.

Applications for such systems are now becoming widespread, although by no means common in clinical practice. Most products have been developed as part of fixed-term, university-based, research projects and only a few have reached the market-place. Thus it is not even possible to guarantee participating subjects continued use or technical support of the prototype device at the end of the trial period.

There are a number of areas in which modern control/computer engineering techniques can make a significant contribution to the disabled. As well as offering increased function and mobility by applying such techniques to artificial limbs, it is also possible to provide missing function by electrically stimulating the muscles and nerves of patients who have intact reflex arcs but lack central motor control, e.g. patients with head injury or stroke and those with higher-level spinal cord injuries. In addition, the concept of computer-controlled artificial limbs can be extended to the design of robotic devices to provide some function for high-level tetraplegics or late-stage multiple sclerosis sufferers (Davies, 1984; Hillman et al., 1991; Preising et al., 1991; van Vliet & Wing, 1991). Unfortunately, space does not permit a review of work in the field of robotics in this chapter and those readers requiring further information should read the above articles.

However, computer control techniques are not only applicable to the control of mechanical systems. One of the major impacts that such techniques can make is in the field of communication aids: for the visually impaired in the form of talking word processors, for the hearing-impaired in terms of speech recognition and conversion to text, and for the speech-impaired in terms of speech synthesis.

This chapter will consider the use, implementation and limitations of technology in all of these areas and will, in particular, concentrate on the use of computer/control engineering techniques to optimize function while placing a minimum of conscious effort on the user. This can be achieved by the control system undertaking some of the automatic actions usually associated with the lower levels of the central nervous system (CNS).

Basic control engineering

From an engineering point of view, improving the physical function of a patient with a neurological disability can be described in terms of the block diagram shown in Fig. 34.1. On the left side of the figure is the aim of the improved function. A study of the existing function is required to identify how best to make improvements. This action requires measurements to be made, using sensors or special instruments. These measurements are subjected to errors from noise during the measuring process and to personal errors which are peculiar to an individual. Technology can help remove some of the latter errors using automatic or semiautomatic equipment. For example, the use of a personal

computer to gather data under program control is a well-established technique in science and engineering. Obtaining unbiased data results in the removal of the subjective assessment of a patient. An analysis of the functional data can then indicate a course of appropriate treatment, which then improves the human function or performance. By comparing the desired function with the existing function, improvements can be made to the patient's performance each time round the loop. However, this model is idealistic, since identifying the variable to be measured can be a very difficult, if not almost impossible, task, due to the complex nature of the human function.

Conceptually this structure is very similar to the physical interconnections of a typical engineering control system. For example, the common temperature-controlled room using a thermostat is shown in Fig. 34.2. If the temperature in the room

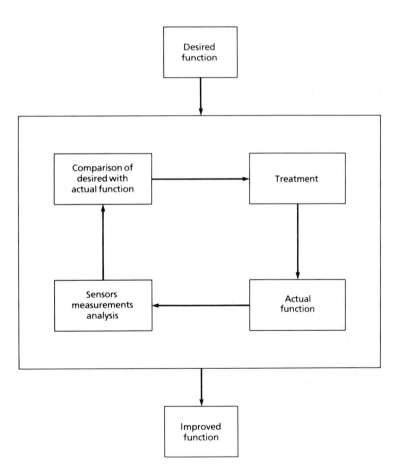

Fig. 34.1 Improved patient function.

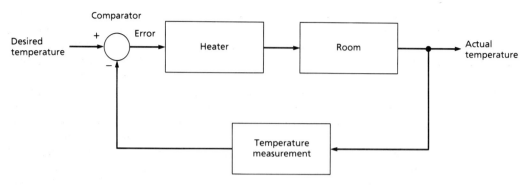

Fig. 34.2 Temperature control system.

falls below the desired temperature set on the thermostat, then there is a difference, or error, produced by the comparator, which turns the heater on to increase the room temperature. When the actual temperature is slightly above the desired temperature, the heater is turned off. In this example the control action is fully on and fully off. Most control systems, like the ones in aircraft, are of a continuous nature, where the desired output, actual output and error vary continuously. These systems are subjected to noise and disturbances, for example in the aircraft systems, where wind turbulence affects the direction of travel of the aircraft.

In order to improve function it is necessary to use technology which has been fully developed into a marketable product. Electronic technology moves on rapidly, with new devices like the single integrated-circuit microcontroller, which is now commonly found in car engines, and software tools like neural nets finding wide applications (Miller *et al.*, 1990). In engineering, neural networks are those computer systems which are based on the learning and behavioural faculties of the natural CNS. For example, a mobile robot can interact with its environment and gain information about both its surroundings and the objects it has to grasp and manipulate. It has to learn how to operate using data from sensors and in a closed loop, without a human to specify a desired behaviour. In contrast, the application of these technologies to rehabilitation is slower. A reason for this lack of pace in some areas of rehabilitation is the lack of market forces to drive the development of appropriate systems. A company will invest large amounts of capital into the development of a new analgesic,

especially if it can be made cheaply, as the international market is very large. To research, and subsequently develop, a new device for the disabled, using the latest technologies, is not seen as being profitable as usually the market size is small.

Control of a hand prosthesis

The design of an artificial hand for a below-the-elbow amputation is a challenging and an intimidating task for several reasons. The mechanical parts have some obvious design targets. The device must be robust and lightweight and of a good cosmetic appearance. Also a hand should be able to grasp an object with a reasonable force as wearers may wish to pick up heavy objects like suitcases. A natural hand is capable of very good force generation, despite an overall mechanical disadvantage. To generate a reasonable force of say 20 N (approximately 2 kg load) at the fingertips requires a force from the actuator of about 140 N for a mechanical disadvantage of 7 : 1. This high force in a small frame leads to the use of pneumatic power. Plettenburg (1989) has proposed a design suitable for children using disposable CO_2 gas containers, which are normally used in soda siphons and beer taps. However, commercial hands which are myoelectrically controlled use electric motors and gearboxes, as small modern batteries are readily available, rechargeable and hold sufficient energy for a day's usage. Also the electrical solution does not require a pneumatic/electrical interface if the input signal to the system is electrical.

Another problem is to design the mechanical parts to be reasonably natural in their actions. This is a very difficult criterion as the natural hand has many articulations and uses many muscles. For a hand to convey a formal sign language using a deaf and dumb code requires a large number of muscles and joints and the fine control of flexion, extension, adduction and abduction. An artificial hand with this capability would have limited reliability and robustness. For robotics applications, a mechanical finger which adapts to the object shape leads to a stable grip. This design would help the disabled patient gain confidence in holding irregular-shaped objects but in action the device is not anthropomorphic and can be rejected.

For any system, the man–machine interface always presents problems in terms of what information to convey and how best to convey it. It might seem reasonable to find suitable muscles on the patient's stump and to use the generated muscle activity to control one part of the artificial hand. This technique is reasonable for a single simple operation like 'open/close', but if, say, there are six channels required then the system becomes very difficult to use effectively and further is very tiring, as it requires conscious effort. For this reason the Southampton approach has been to use a single channel with serial information to instruct an artificial hand with natural commands like 'hold' and 'squeeze'. This hierarchical control method mimics the natural system. Thus the low-level spinal reflexes of the natural hand are dedicated to an electronic controller. Accommodating the artificial device within the natural hierarchy results in increasing user confidence, as patients then feel that they are in control of the prosthesis and not the other way round. A natural hand has many sensors for touch (force), position (joint angle), object slip and temperature. A sophisticated artificial hand could contain all of these sensors, using electronic devices. However, there is a large difference between the resolution of the natural system and that of the artificial system. For example, a natural fingertip has a touch spatial resolution of 2–3 mm whereas an electronically usable resolution is one site per fingertip. New sensors are capable of finer resolution than this, but it is not clear that they would benefit a disabled person. The pattern information generated from a large number of sensors could be used to distinguish the shape of an object. To detect that an artificial hand is holding

a sphere and not a cube would be possible. However, to convey the information about different objects would require a vocabulary and hence a speech system. A talking hand would be unacceptable.

Commercially available myoelectric hands are open-loop devices where there is no sensor information to feed back from the hand to the controller. Small electrical signals (electromyographic (EMG) voltages) from muscles in the wearer's stump are picked up by surface electrodes, electronically amplified and conditioned so that power from a battery is fed to a single electric motor. This action causes the thumb and fingers to move apart. The EMG signals control the hand to close round an object for it to be held. To obtain a secure grip requires overtightening, which may result in damage to the object. Some rough information about the strength of the grip can provide feedback to the wearer by the changes in mechanical vibrations (and acoustic noise) of the hand mechanism when it tightens on an object. This information can be used to gain confidence about object stability, as the motor is being subjected to its maximum torque output, which resonates the mechanical structure.

Improved performance of a commercial hand can be obtained using sensors and an electronic controller (Chappell et al., 1987). The same physical structure as the open-loop system is used except that the low-level control functions of object grip and stability are given to an electronic controller. Figure 34.3 shows the basic physical elements of the scheme. Information about the force on an object is sensed using a device mounted in the fingertip. When the open hand closes on an object, the force sensor detects when finger contact is made and the controller automatically adjusts the power to the motor so that a small and predetermined force is applied to the object. The EMG signal is bipolar (positive and negative), corresponding to the activity from two antagonistic muscles (e.g. extensor and flexor carpi radii), as shown in Fig. 34.4. Should the amputee wish to open the hand and release the object, then he/she generates an extensor signal beyond the 'relax' band. The amount of opening of the hand is proportional to the EMG signal and is under closed-loop control, using a position sensor mounted at the base of the fingers. Closing the hand around the object by

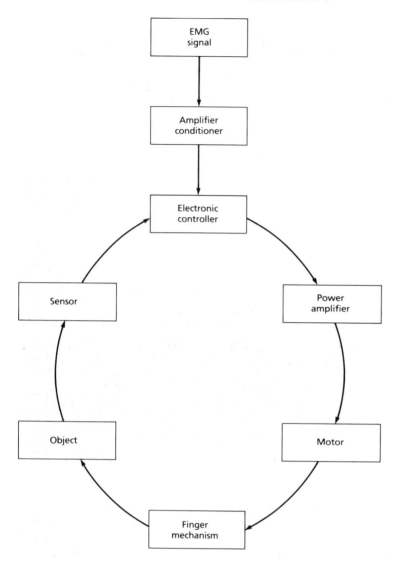

Fig. 34.3 Block diagram for the closed-loop control of an artificial hand.

decreasing the extensor signal causes the touch sensor to become active, as before.

A natural sequence of events is that the amputee wishes to hold the object steady. Here a flexor signal is generated beyond the 'hold' threshold (Fig. 34.4). The controller is now receiving information from the slip sensor mounted in the fingertip. Should the object begin to slide, then the controller feeds more power to the motor to tighten the grip. In this way the system moves from state to state and the amputee simply instructs the con-

troller. These states are 'position', 'touch', 'hold', 'squeeze' and 'release'.

Use of a single motor allows for a very limited number of hand postures. For this reason a prototype, multifunctional hand has been developed which has four motors to allow for rotation of the thumb and flexion and extension of the thumb, the index finger and the other three fingers as a group. This hand can adopt one of seven basic postures, which allow the hand to grasp a wide range of different-shaped objects (Fig. 34.5).

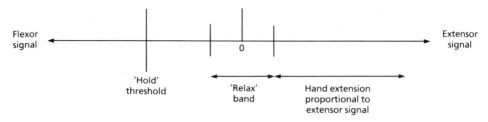

Fig. 34.4 Bipolar EMG signal and 'hold' threshold for position controller state.

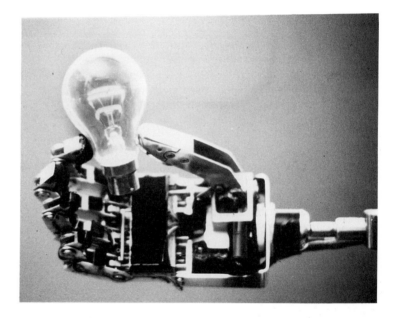

Fig. 34.5 Multifunctional hand.

Despite the greater complexity of the hand, the disabled person simply instructs the controller. The repertoire of instructions available to the user are similar to those of the single-degree-of-freedom controller. The increased co-ordination of the hand is given to the controller, thus making the device easy to use. For example, if the hand is fully open and is closing round an object, then the position sensors tell the controller that the hand should adopt the appropriate posture.

The hand has a number of touch sensors, which are mounted in the palm and along the inner surface of the fingers. In the thumb tip, a combined touch and slip sensor is mounted to allow for the automatic tightening of the grip when the object slips from the hand. The single site for slip detection results in limited operation, as not all objects touch

the thumb tip. An improved detection rate of object slip is achieved using the information from the touch sensors. A natural hand holding a tennis ball in a fist grip senses an increase in the forces on the fingertips if the ball moves out of the hand. For the artificial hand, the same force information can be conveyed to the electronic controller. As a tennis ball moves out of the hand's grasp, the tip sensors detect an increase in force while the palm sensors detect a decrease in force. An algorithm has been developed which senses the direction of object slip in the hand, so that corrective action can be taken to arrest the slide (Kyberd & Chappell, 1991).

A microcontroller is used which contains all the necessary functions for signal input, signal output, program storage and counting in a single integrated circuit. A compact and robust design is produced.

The adoption of a programmable device reflects the hierarchical nature of the control philosophy.

The programs are written for an interrupt-driven architecture, which results in a behavioural role. For example, the controller may be collecting data from the sensors while in the 'hold' state when the wearer instructs the controller to 'release' the object from the hand's grasp and return to the 'position' state. The controller suspends its data collection and executes the 'release' software before returning to data collection (Chappell & Kyberd, 1991).

Disabled people are individuals requiring individual and perhaps, therefore, special unique devices. Adopting a device with an interrupt-driven architecture allows the use of the same mechanism but different control algorithms to meet individual specifications. For example, the EMG thresholds can be set individually.

Future electronic devices will be faster (opto-electronic), with more devices in smaller packages. Better artificial hand function can then be achieved in much the same way as the natural system uses information gathered from force, joint angle, slip sensors and muscle activity. Traditional engineering techniques will still be used, but they will become integrated with new techniques, especially on the behavioural side using neural nets.

Functional electrical stimulation (FES)

The technique of electrical stimulation of muscle is not new and, as long ago as 400 BC, the torpedo fish and rubbed amber were used to treat a wide range of conditions, from headaches to asthma. However, it is only over the last 30 years that the term 'functional' electrical stimulation (FES) could be applied to the technique. This is largely due to the great advances in electronics that have occurred over that period, and today it is possible to build small multichannel stimulators to control up to 64 different muscles. Despite this potential, the number of people benefiting from FES is small and the number using complete systems on a daily basis even less. It is only over the past 2–3 years that practical systems, suitable for use in the community, have been developed. It is comparatively simple to build a stimulator with a sufficiently powerful

output, and to stand a complete paraplegic in the laboratory. However, it is a much harder problem to develop a system to enable that same person to stand safely, on demand, in a variety of locations without professional supervision.

A practical 'functional' system must therefore be reliable and safe under a wide range of operating conditions, some of which are determined by external factors and as such cannot be easily controlled. Such a system will consist of two components: firstly, a reliable and adaptable external system capable of responding rapidly to changing parameters, and, secondly, a trained user with the necessary motivation to succeed. Both parts are equally important (Swain, 1992).

Practical FES systems

The external system, consisting of stimulator circuitry and controller, must be able to provide sufficient flexibility to enable the device to be used routinely. Even when stimulating trained musculature, there is wide day-to-day and minute-to-minute variation in the stimulation parameters required to ensure safe continuous operation. In addition, although muscle fatigue can be reduced in animal studies by chronic stimulation for several months (Salmons & Henriksson, 1981), such techniques are not readily applicable to replacing complex human functions, such as walking or prehension. They are, however, applicable to replacing certain functions, such as breathing, by stimulation of the phrenic nerve (Thoma et al., 1988), diaphragm (Peterson et al., 1986) or intercostal muscles (Brindley et al., 1989), and more recently to enabling trained, fatigue-resistant muscle to be transplanted to assist the heart (see Salmons & Jarvis, 1991) or as a cure for anal incontinence (Hallan & Williams, 1989; see also Chapter 26). Even so, Thoma et al. found that fatigue was still a problem, as the microelectrodes sutured to the phrenic nerve were always stimulating the same nerve fibres. To overcome this problem, four electrodes are sutured to the nerve at 90° intervals. The control system sequences the stimulation so that different combinations of two electrodes are stimulated in turn, the four electrodes allowing 16 possible combinations. This is termed 'roundabout' stimulation. Although nowhere near as sophisticated as the CNS control system, it is successful in reducing fatigue (Thoma *et al.*, 1988).

Providing lost prehensile or ambulatory function has other problems. Although the muscle does not need to be so fatigue resistant as it does to maintain central functions such as pulmonary or cardiac operation, it does need to be able to generate sufficient force for sufficient duration to enable useful function. If, by chronic long-term stimulation, a transformation of all muscle fibres occurred so that only type I fibres were present, it is possible that insufficient force could be generated to enable the user to stand. In addition, although a spinal patient might be prepared to undergo at least 6 hours' stimulation a day to improve the fatiguability of the muscles needed to assist cardiac or pulmonary function, it is questionable if a subject would be prepared to undergo a similar training programme for all the muscles needed for walking. Such systems also need to be more flexible so that they can adapt to a variety of user demands, as well as changing environmental conditions. Only if a system safely and reliably provides its users with the ability to increase their independence will it find a place outside the laboratory.

Lower limb function

The first clinical use of an FES system was to correct foot drop in stroke patients by stimulation of the common peroneal nerve (Liberson *et al.*, 1961). This is still the most common use of FES, and today implanted (Strojnik *et al.*, 1987), as well as surface, electrode systems (Benton *et al.*, 1981) are commercially available. The timing of the stimulation is usually controlled by a foot switch in the shoe, although other feedback modalities, including accelerometers, are being considered (Willemsen *et al.*, 1990).

Standing is probably the simplest function to provide, and yet few people with spinal cord injuries have FES standing systems. Standing can be achieved by stimulating the quadriceps, with the subject supported between parallel bars. In order to stand, a torque around each knee of approximately 1 Nm per kg of body-weight is required (Taylor, 1989), although this value can be reduced to approximately 15 Nm once erect (Edwards & Marsolais, 1987). Therefore, in order to prevent

overstimulation, it is necessary to employ a closed-loop controller so that the system knows when the user is vertical and can adjust the stimulation output accordingly. A simple closed-loop control system could consist of a goniometer measuring knee angle to provide the feedback signal to the computer-based controller. Such a system would also have advantages in the actual standing up and sitting down manoeuvres as it would enable the knee angle rather than the stimulation level to be the controlled function (Ewins *et al.*, 1990). Such a system has a number of other advantages, in that it can minimize overstimulation, which can cause unwanted hip flexion and hyperextension of the knees, and also automatically adjust stimulation levels to compensate for postural changes. However, it does not substantially improve the time taken to fatigue, and standing times are usually limited to less than 10 minutes. As the stimulation level is minimized, due to the closed-loop control, the number of fibres stimulated is reduced. As these muscle fibres begin to fatigue, the stimulation output automatically increases to keep the knee locked, hence recruiting deeper fibres. However, the superficial fibres are still being stimulated as well and hence have no chance for recovery.

A number of solutions have been proposed to overcome this problem and so enable prolonged standing. These include cyclical fivefold increase in standing time if two channels are used and an eightfold improvement if three channels are used (Pournezam *et al.*, 1988). Kralj *et al.* (1986) used a system of posture switching in which either the quadriceps or the triceps surae were stimulated, depending on the patient's posture. This is possible as, when the ground reaction vector passes in front of the knee, quadriceps activity is not needed to lock the knee. Therefore, as long as dorsiflexion of the ankle is limited, the user will remain standing (Fig. 34.6).

A number of groups have adopted hybrid solutions, in which FES is used to provide the dynamic movement and an orthosis is used to provide the static support (Petrofsky *et al.*, 1986; Nene & Patrick, 1990). The majority of these devices have used simple rule-based systems rather than closed-loop control. Such hybrid solutions do increase the safety factor and reduce the energy cost of using either orthoses or FEB-based systems in isolation. How-

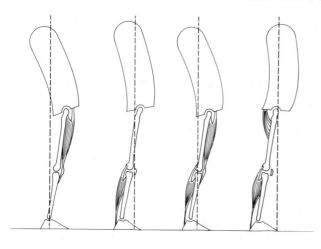

Fig. 34.6 Activity of different muscle groups for bilateral standing in different postures. (From Kralj A. & Bajd P. *Functional Electrical Stimulation – Standing and Walking After Spinal Cord Injury*. CRC Press, 1989, with permission.)

ever, they tend to be complex and bulky, take considerable time to don and doff and have inherent problems in locking and unlocking the joints of the orthosis when under load. This last point makes standing up and sitting down difficult since, if there is not perfect alignment between mechanical structures, either locking or unlocking can fail to occur.

A combination of many of these techniques has been proposed by Andrews *et al.* (1988). In this a supracondylar knee–ankle–foot orthosis is combined with a closed-loop control system with sensory feedback. This enables the user to stand with FES, without the locking problems of long leg braces, and then adopt a position so that the ground reaction vector passes in front of the knee, with the orthosis stabilizing the ankle and preventing hyperextension of the knee. As long as this posture is maintained, the FES will not be applied to the quadriceps. However, if the ground reaction vector moves behind the knee, the stimulation will be applied to the quadriceps to correct the posture. By employing such a technique, standing times can be increased up to several hours.

Although the problems of achieving suitable FES-based standing systems have not been overcome, a number of centres have been concentrating on providing walking for suitable midthoracic paraplegics. Simple · walking function can be provided by as little as two channels per leg, using quadriceps stimulation to lock the knee and stimulation of the common peroneal nerve to initiate the flexion withdrawal response (Bajd *et al.*, 1983).

Petrofsky *et al.* (1984) extended the use of surface electrodes to stimulate more channels in each leg and to use measurement of hip, knee and ankle position to provide the feedback for a closed-loop controller. The complete system was rather bulky, lacking cosmesis and restricted to the laboratory, although it did achieve greater practical usage when combined with the reciprocal gait orthosis (Petrofsky *et al.*, 1986). Marsolais & Kobetic (1987) adopted a different approach, using a 64-channel stimulator and percutaneous electrodes to achieve much greater flexibility, which made possible such activities as stair climbing, movement in a lateral direction and walking up to 330 m at half-normal walking speed. This system, although very impressive, has been limited to the laboratory by the lack of a closed-loop control system. This has resulted in lengthy setting-up procedures and an inability to automatically compensate for any changes either in the environment or in the user's physiological condition.

Upper limb function

Restoration of prehensile function to tetraplegics does not usually involve the generation of large forces, but the need for fatigue resistance is obviously of equal importance. In addition, the degree of control needed for useful function is considerable. This, combined with the complex muscular anatomy of the hand and forearm, has led to the majority of solutions employing either percutaneous or fully implanted electrodes. Peckham *et al.* (1988), Miller *et al.* (1989) and Kilgore *et al.* (1990) have developed an eight-channel system which can either work percutaneously, using intramuscular electrodes, or be fully implanted, using a radio frequency link to activate epimysial electrodes (Smith *et al.*, 1987). Both systems are controlled by movement of the opposite shoulder and can provide either a palmar or a lateral prehension grasp. At present, the control is essentially open-loop, but sensory feedback is provided for the user by two sensory substitution systems. One system uses an array of five electrodes to provide both machine status information and a spatially encoded representation of the command signal, which the tetraplegic individual generates to achieve proportional control of gripping function. The second sensory system is an integral part of an implanted FES system and utilizes a single, subdurally placed, electrode to display machine status information and a five-level frequency code for feedback of the user-generated grasp control signal (Riso *et al.*, 1991). The provision of the sensory feedback channel replaced the previous auditory feedback system and has been shown to produce a 38% energy saving in one subject.

It is possible to stimulate the muscles of the forearm to provide a functional grip using surface electrodes (Nathan, 1990), but the problems of electrode positioning become the limiting factor. This could be overcome by using an electrode array and a closed-loop controller which could automatically select the optimal electrode combination for a given movement. At present, such systems are limited to the research laboratory.

Communication aids

Speech is the most important method of human communication and is one of the major distinguishing factors between human beings and the rest of the animal kingdom. Since the invention of the gramophone, it has been possible to record and play back speech, but only recently has it been possible to generate speech. There are a number of uses for computer-generated speech, including gimmicks such as talking toys or talking instruments in cars. Alternatively, generated speech or speech synthesis can be used to great effect by providing other sensory channels of information, in stressful environments such as the flight deck of an aircraft, or as an aid for the disabled. These last two examples, although apparently unconnected, have many features in common and have led to collaboration between researchers at Dundee University, long known for their work in the field of communication for the disabled, and GEC Avionics. This is the extraordinary communication for human operators (ECHO) project (Peddie *et al.*, 1991). In both cases, the users can face impairment caused by their environment. For example, a pilot during the course of a mission may face a severe, but temporary, impairment. The requirements for the interface of his/her computer may therefore be similar to those of a permanently physically handicapped user with the interface of his/her communication device (Cairns *et al.*, 1990).

At the heart of any such system lies the computer, with a man–machine interface providing the flow of information in both directions between the user and the machine. There are problems, since computers, for all their processing power, are unintelligent and unadaptable and cannot communicate in the same way as we do (Edwards, 1991). Early machines relied on the adaptability of the user to bridge the gap of the man–machine interface. It was up to the users to find out how the computer worked and adapt themselves to make up for the inadequacies in that interface. Today, some of these limitations have been overcome. With the provision of systems on the computer such as graphic interfaces, which include 'pull-down menus', icons and the mouse input, it is possible to move a cursor around the screen, pick up the 'file' icon and place it in the 'filing cabinet' window on the screen – much as a secretary would in real life. However, computer interfaces have not been designed for the disabled. The use of a mouse and pull-down menus is perfect for those without a disability, but impossible for a person with either poor co-ordination or visual problems. These problems can be overcome if appropriate modifications are made to the man–machine interface, provided that the whole system is designed with the special needs of the user in mind. No matter how adaptive the software and how recognizable the computer-generated speech, the system will fail to increase the independence of the users if they are unable to operate the on/off switch.

Communication aids for the blind

In designing a communication aid for the blind, it is necessary to utilize other sensory channels, such as hearing or touch. The most common system to date has been braille, which although well known is not actually used by the majority of blind users. This is simply because most blind users find braille too difficult to learn, especially those with neurological disabilities where touch and fine motor skills are often also affected. For those who can use it, braille output can be obtained from a computer to provide a permanent record, although braille printers are noisy and expensive and the output occupies considerable space. Even so, a braille print-out still does not give the 'glance' facility that visual users utilize so often when working with computers. Moving braille displays do exist to give the user feedback of 'on-screen' information without the need for a permanent hard copy, but they are also expensive and unreliable due to the vast number of mechanical moving parts.

Auditory output devices also suffer the same disadvantage in that they do not have the 'at a glance' facility of visual systems, but they are more reliable and usually cheaper. Similar information can be provided by 'screen readers', which use computer-generated speech to read the information appearing on the screen. A number of devices are commercially available and are reviewed by Edwards (1991). The disadvantages of screen readers are the monotonous quality of the speech, the need to change mode to check spelling and the confusion that can occur between certain letters such as 'B' and 'P'. A block diagram showing the structure of a screen reader is shown in Fig. 34.7.

Screen readers are specifically for use with computers and as such have a limited application at present. Computer books are not common. For a blind person to be able to 'read' printed text requires

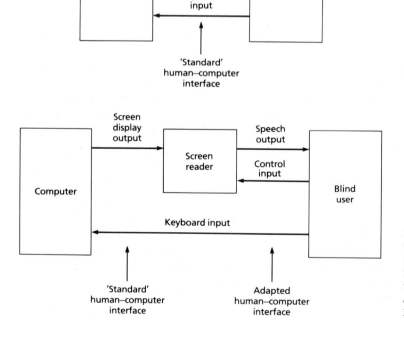

Fig. 34.7 A screen reader adapts the human–computer interface. On the left, it effectively intercepts the standard interface, transforming it such that it is accessible to blind users. (From Edwards, 1991, with permission.)

a far more complex system, in which the system is able to adapt to different typefaces. Without such a facility, any system only capable of reading a single typeface will be severely limited. The Kurzweil reading machine is capable of adapting to different typefaces and can cope with different fonts and page layouts. The machine does, however, 'give up' on encountering a picture. The principal disadvantage of the system is the cost of between £8000 and £10 000, which makes it more suitable for libraries and institutions than for individual users.

Interface requirements of communication users

The standard rate of transferring information by speech is of the order of 150 words per minute. Using a standard keyboard an experienced typist can type at approximately 60 words per minute and an experienced computer user at 30 words per minute, whereas a physically disabled user can often only type as few as 5 words per minute, given, of course, that they can cope with a standard qwerty keyboard. The only input devices capable of working at normal verbatim speeds are the Palantype and stenograph. In these devices speech is typed in syllables and converted into a code by the machine. The output is therefore not in standard English but in a shorthand code. Work by Downton, Newell and Arnott has concentrated on using a computer-based system to convert the Palantype ouput to standard English as an aid for the deaf (Arnott, 1987). However, a stenograph or Palantype requires an experienced user with a high level of manual dexterity, and therefore, although it can be of considerable use to a businessman or politician (the deaf former MP Jack Ashley used such a system in the House of Commons), it is not appropriate to the majority of users who require a communication device.

As with the visually handicapped, most neurological patients needing a communication device also lack the manual dexterity to cope with a standard keyboard, let alone a Palantype. In such cases a reduced keyboard or sequential scanning system has to be used, further reducing the speed of communication. A number of commercial systems are available and are again well reviewed by Edwards (1991). There are a number of different approaches to the problem of increasing the rate of communication. Storing complete sentences has the advantage of increasing the speed of response but has the disadvantages of restricting the user to a limited number of common phases. Alternatively, individual letter input offers great versatility, but is slow. Word and syllable level input provides intermediate solutions. Given that a large number of users will be restricted to input methods ranging from a single-switch entry to a reduced 3 × 4 keyboard, a number of solutions have been developed to increase the communication rate.

Equalizer (Edwards, 1991) is a word-based input system with an ability to expand the vocabulary to suit an individual user, who can control the scanning and selection of words using appropriate switches. The system incorporates commonly used or user-defined phrases and dynamic word anticipation. To operate the system, the user types the initial letter of a word, and a table of words starting with that letter then appears on the screen. The user can therefore select the required word, if it is present in the dictionary, or type the complete word letter by letter. An experienced user with a single-switch entry can communicate at similar speeds to an experienced computer user, 30 words a minute. The system is IBM-based and can output either to a word processor or to a speech synthesizer. Professor Stephen Hawking uses Equalizer as his communication device and with it wrote his best-selling book, *A Brief History of Time*.

Predictive adaptive lexicon (PAL) is an alternative system developed by the microcomputer centre at Dundee University. It is a word-level predictor designed for users who have difficulty with the standard keyboard. Input is via appropriate switches. PAL uses the frequency of words in the English language and the most recent use of these words by the individual to predict the required word. The user types the initial letter of the word and the computer offers the five most common choices. If none of these is correct, the user types the second letter and the computer offers the five most common words starting with those two letters. This continues until the word is completed. Using this system, the number of keystrokes can be reduced by over 50% (Swiffin *et al.*, 1987). Reduced keyboards offer another alternative (Arnott &

Javed, 1990). They used a 4 × 3 array with nine alphabetic keys (three letters per key), combined with a computer system employing disambiguation techniques to predict which letter of the three is required. If the chosen letter is not required, another letter is selected. Using this system, characters can be chosen with keying rates as low as 1.1 keystrokes per character.

Instead of using statistical techniques to improve speed, an alternative system, CHAT (Conversation Helped by Automatic Talk; Alm *et al.*, 1989), uses the fact that sentence-level utterances are needed to enable the disabled to participate in everyday conversations, e.g. the sort of conversation anyone might have in a corridor, where speed of response, rather than content, is of prime importance. The user is offered various basic feedback remarks or short utterances so that the conversation can flow at a reasonable rate.

Examples of these are:
1 Agree: e.g. Yes, All right, etc.
2 Evaluate as good: e.g. That's great, Wonderful, etc.
3 Repeat request: e.g. Pardon, etc.
The system then chooses a random phrase from its memory. These phrases are randomly selected to make the conversation more natural. Another interesting facility that CHAT offers is the ability to vary the tone or mood of the remark, enabling the user to sound angry, pleased, etc.

There are a number of other communication devices – far too many to be reviewed in this chapter. Readers requiring more information should read *Speech Synthesis – Technology for Disabled People*, by Alistair Edwards (1991). The systems described above were all selected because they used computers and predictive or adaptative techniques to increase the rate of communication, to make more natural conversations possible or to make the system easier for the user. None of the systems is ideal, but, now that the various approaches are being combined in developments such as the ECHO project, the next generation of communication devices should offer real benefits to the speech-, hearing- or visually impaired.

The use of such techniques in communication aids is analogous to the use of control engineering in prosthetics and electrical stimulation, where computers use related (but different) control techniques to reduce the conscious strain on the user.

Conclusions

Recent developments in modern electronics and computing have for the first time enabled engineers to design systems capable of replacing missing neurological function. At present, this work is in its infancy and therefore only capable of replacing lower levels of control. An engineering system requires information from a biological system, which is usually non-linear and ill-defined. The human brain is very good at making decisions with these limitations, relying on vast amounts of information from senses like sight, sound, touch and proprioception. However, technologically there is a lack of suitable robust sensors capable of feeding data back to a computer controller, which, although good at processing such data, is poor at interpreting and making decisions based on incomplete information. Therefore, in order to design future advanced systems for the neurologically disabled, it will be necessary to develop small, robust, cheap and reliable sensors and to exploit new software techniques, such as neural networks and artificial intelligence.

References

Alm N., Arnott J.L. & Newell A.F. (1989) Discourse analysis and pragmatics in the design of a conversation prosthesis. *Journal of Medical Engineering and Technology* **13** (1/2), 10–12.

Andrews B.J., Baxendale R.H., Barnett R. *et al.* (1988) Hybrid FES orthosis incorporating closed loop control and sensory feedback. *Journal of Biomedical Engineering* **10** (2), 189–195.

Arnott J.L. (1987) High-speed control of a speech synthesiser by stenotype keyboard. *Proceedings of the European Conference on Speech Technology* **1**, 335–338.

Arnott J.L. & Javed M.Y. (1990) Small text corpora in character disambiguation for reduced typing keyboards. RESNA 13th Annual Conference, Washington DC, pp. 181–182.

Bajd T., Kralj A., Turk R., Benko H. & Sega J. (1983) The use of 4 channel electrical stimulation as an ambulatory aid for paraplegic patients. *Physical Therapy* **63** (7), 1116–1120.

Benton L., Baker L.L., Bowman B.R. & Waters R.L. (1981) *Functional Electrical Stimulation – a Practical Clinical Guide*, 2nd edn. Rehabilitation Engineering Centre, Rancho Los Amigos Hospital, Downey, California.

Brindley G.S., Donaldson N.D'N. & Perkins T.A. (1989) A breathing implant to stimulate intercostal nerves. *Biological Engineering Society Publication Conference Proceed-*

ings: the Electrical Stimulation of Muscle. Hexham.

Cairns A.Y., Peddie H., Filz G., Arnott J.L. & Newell A.F. (1990) ECHO: a multimodal workstation for ordinary and extra-ordinary human computer interaction. *Digest of IEE Colloquium on Multi-Media: the Future of User Interfaces*, pp. 6/1–6/3. IEE, London.

Chappell P.H. & Kyberd P.J. (1991) Prehensile control of a hand prosthesis by a microcontroller. *Journal of Biomedical Engineering* **13**, 363–369.

Chappell P.H., Nightingale J.M., Kyberd P.J. & Barkhorder M. (1987) Control of a single degree of freedom artificial hand. *Journal of Biomedical Engineering* **9**, 273–277.

Davies B.L. (1984) The use of robots to aid the severely disabled. *Electronics and Power* **30** (3), 211–214.

Edwards A.D.N. (1991) *Speech Synthesis – Technology for Disabled People*. Paul Chapman, Baltimore.

Edwards B.G. & Marsolais E.B. (1987) Quadriceps muscle response to functional neuromuscular stimulation during isokinetic exercise and walking. Resna 10th Annual Conference, San Jose, California, pp. 605–607.

Ewins D.J., Taylor P.N. & Swain I.D. (1990) A functional closed-loop stand/sit system for mid–low thoracic paraplegics. *XR International Symposium on External Control of Human Extremities*. Dubrovnik, Yugoslavia Committee for Electronics and Automation, Belgrade.

Hall M.J. (1964) *Artificial Limbs – a Brief Historical Survey*. Report 64/4, Department of Mechanical Engineering, University College, London.

Hallan R.I. & Williams N.S. (1989) Transforming skeletal muscle. *British Medical Journal* **298**, 389.

Hillman M.R., Pullin G.M. & Gammie A.R., Stammers C.W. & Orpwood R.D. (1991) Clinical experience in rehabilitation robotics. *Journal of Biomedical Engineering* **13** (3), 239–243.

Kilgore K.L., Peckham P.H., Keith M.W. & Thrope G.B. (1990) Electrode characterization for functional application to upper extremity FNS. *IEEE Transactions in Biomedical Engineering* **37** (1), 12–21.

Kralj A., Bajd T., Turk R. & Benko H. (1986) Posture switching for prolonged FES standing in paraplegic patients. *Paraplegia* **24**, 221–230.

Kyberd P.J. & Chappell P.H. (1991) Object-slip detection during manipulation using a derived force vector. *Mechatronics* **1** (2).

Liberson W.T., Holmquest H.J. & Scott D. (1961) Functional electrotherapy: stimulation of the common peroneal nerve synchronised with the swing phase of gait. *Archives of Physical Medicine and Rehabilitation* **42**, 101–105.

Marsolais E.B. & Kobetic R. (1987) Functional electrical stimulation for walking in paraplegia. *Journal of Joint and Bone Surgery* **69A** (5), 728–733.

Miller L.J., Peckham P.H. & Keith M.W. (1989) Elbow extension in the C5 quadriplegic using functional neuromuscular stimulation. *IEEE Transactions in Biomedical Engineering* **36** (7), 771–780.

Miller W., Sutton R.S. & Werbos P.J. (1990) *Neural Networks for Control*. MIT Press, Cambridge, Massachusetts.

Nathan R.H. (1990) FES of the upper limb: targeting the forearm muscles for surface stimulation. *Medical and Biomedical Engineering and Computing* **28**, 249–256.

Nene A.V. & Patrick J.H. (1990) Energy cost of paraplegic locomotion using a parawalker – electrical stimulation 'hybrid' orthosis. *Archives of Physical and Medical Rehabilitation* **71**, 116–120.

Peckham P.H., Keith M.W. & Freehafer A.A. (1988) Restoration of functional control by electrical stimulation in the upper extremity of the quadriplegic patient. *Journal of Joint and Bone Surgery* **70A**, 114–148.

Peddie H., Fitz G., Cairns A.Y., Arnott J.L. & Newell A.F. (1990) *Extraordinary Computer Human Operation (ECHO)*. Proceedings of the 2nd joint BAF/RAF/USAF workshop on human electronic crew teamwork. Ingoldstadt, Germany. September 1990, pp. 501–508.

Peterson D.K., Nochomovitz M., DiMarco A.F. & Mortimer J.T. (1986) Intramuscular electrical activation of the phrenic nerve. *IEEE Transactions in Biomedical Engineering* **33** (3), 342–351.

Petrofsky J.S., Phillips C.A. & Heaton H.H. (1984) Feedback control systems for walking in man. *Computers in Biology and Medicine* **14** (2), 139–149.

Petrofsky S., Phillips C.A., Douglas R. & Larson P. (1986) A computer controlled walking system: the combination of an orthosis with functional electrical stimulation. *Journal of Clinical Engineering* **11** (2), 121–133.

Plettenburg D.H. (1989) Electric versus pneumatic power in hand prostheses for children. *Journal of Medical Engineering and Technology* **13**, 124–128.

Pournzam M., Andrews B.J., Baxendale R.H., Phillips G.F. & Paul J.P. (1988) Reduction of muscle fatigue in man by cyclical stimulation. *Journal of Biomedical Engineering* **10** (2), 196–200.

Preising B., Hsia T.C. & Mittelstadt B. (1991) A literature review – robots in medicine. *IEEE Engineering in Medicine and Biology* 13–22.

Riso R., Ignagni A.R. & Keith M.W. (1991) Cognitive feedback for use with FES upper extremity neuroprostheses. *IEEE Transactions in Biomedical Engineering* **38** (1).

Salmons S. & Henriksson J. (1981) The adaptive response of skeletal muscle to increased use. *Muscle and Nerve* 94–105.

Salmons S. & Jarvis J.C. (eds) (1991) *Harnessing Skeletal Muscle Power for Cardiac Assistance*. Proceedings of the Expert Meeting under EC Concerted Action HEART. Commission of the European Communities. (Also included in *Annals of the Concerted Action HEART* 1989–1990.)

Smith B., Peckham P.H., Keith M.W. & Roscoe D.D. (1987) An externally powered, multichannel implantable stimulator for versatile control of paralysed muscle. *IEEE Transactions in Biomedical Engineering* **BME 34** (7), 499–508.

Strojnik P., Acimovic R., Vavken E., Simic V. & Stanic U. (1987) Treatment of drop foot using an implantable peroneal underknee stimulator. *Scandinavian Journal of Rehabilitation Medicine* **19**, 37–43.

Swain I.D. (1992) Conditioning of skeletal muscle by functional electrical stimulation – implications for the development of practical systems. In Illis L.S. (ed.) *Spinal Cord Dysfunction*, Vol. 3. Oxford Medical Press (in press).

Swiffin A.L., Arnott J.L., Pickering J.A. & Newell A.F. (1987) Adaptive and predictive techniques in a communication prosthesis. *AAC Augmentative and Alternative Communication* **3** (4), 181–191.

Taylor P.N., Fox B.A., Ewins D.J., Biss S.J. & Swain I.D. (in press) Exercise procedure and treatment regime for prepararation of paraplegics prior to standing using functional electrical stimulation. In Clifford Rose F.,

Jones R. & Vbrova G. (eds) *Neuromuscular Stimulation: Basic Concepts and Clinical Implications*. Demos, New York.

Thoma H., Gerner H., Girsch W., Holle J., Mayr W. & Stohr H. (1988) Implantable neurostimulators, the phrenic pacemaker, technology and rehabilitation strategies. In Wallinga W., Boom H.B. & de Vries J. (eds) *Electrophysiological Kinesiology*, pp. 143–152. Elsevier Science Publishers. Amsterdam.

van Vliet P. & Wing A.M. (1991) A new challenge – robotics in the rehabilitation of the neurologically motor impaired. *Physical Therapy* **71** (1), 39–48.

Willemsen A.R.M., Bloemhof F. & Boom H.B.K. (1990) Automatic stance – swing phase detection from accelerometer data for peroneal nerve stimulation. *IEEE Transactions on Biomedical Engineering* **37** (12), 1201–1207.

35: Functional Electrical Stimulation (FES) in the Rehabilitation of Patients with Paraplegia and Hemiplegia

A. KRÄLJ, T. BAJD, U. STANIČ, R. AČIMOVIĆ-JANEŽIČ
AND R. TURK

FES training of atrophied paralysed muscles, 519
  Training modalities and assessment of training, 519
  Effects of exercise on strength, 520
  Effects of exercise on fatigue and dynamic muscle
    response, 520
  Effects of exercise on incomplete SCI subjects, 522
  Effects of exercise on contralateral untrained extremity,
    522
  FES-assisted locomotion in paraplegic subjects, 523
  Some theoretical and practical aspects, 523
  Preventing the development of secondary pathology,
    524
  Clinical experience, 527
Enhancement of hemiplegic patients' rehabilitation by
  means of FES, 528

The current achievements, clinical results and research efforts in functional electrical stimulation (FES) are reviewed. Particular attention is given to the following aspects of FES:

1 FES training of atrophied paralysed muscles and the highlighting of training modalities.

2 FES-assisted locomotion in paraplegic subjects, where clinical experience is reviewed and some theoretical and practical aspects of stimulation sequence composition are discussed, with particular emphasis on preventing the development of secondary pathologies.

3 The enhancement of hemiplegic patients' rehabilitation by means of FES, including the application of FES to stroke patients. The results of the last 10 years' experience of more than 2000 patients undergoing FES treatment are reviewed. The statistical outcomes are presented together with methods. Further developments and the future of FES are discussed.

FES training of atrophied paralysed muscles

Training modalities and assessment of training

Several training modalities can be applied to spinal cord-injured (SCI) patients with upper motor neuron lesions in order to strengthen their atrophied and paralysed muscles – for example, isotonic, isometric or isokinetic training, together with the exercise bicycle approach and biofeedback exercising. The strengthening programme, as usually applied in Ljubljana Rehabilitation Center consists of 30 min of daily sessions of cyclic surface electrical stimulation. The duty cycle is 4 s of stimulation followed by 4 s of pause. The stimulation frequency is 20 Hz and pulse duration 0.3 ms. The type of training is isotonic, as described by Kralj & Bajd (1989).

There are several approaches to the assessment of the effects of skeletal muscle exercise, including biomechanical, anthropometric, histological and histochemical measurements. In our center isometric joint torques are assessed using measuring devices built in our research laboratories.

Different characteristic muscle properties can be extracted from isometric joint torque measurements. First, the recruitment curve, being the relationship of isometric knee joint torque versus stimulation amplitude, can be recorded. The weakness of electrically stimulated paraplegic muscles can be further assessed through programmed stimulation responses, as proposed by Edwards (1978). Here, the isometric knee joint torque is measured at four different frequencies: 10 Hz, 20 Hz, 50 Hz and 100 Hz. Fatiguing of an electrically stimulated muscle can be studied during a con-

tinuous train of stimuli. The fatigue is then evaluated by means of the fatigue index, defined as
the difference between initial moment and a joint
moment after 30 seconds of stimulation. This difference is normalized by the initial moment and
expressed as a percentage. The dynamic muscle
properties can be evaluated by eliciting a muscle
twitch through a single electrical stimulus. The
delay time between electrical stimulus and the peak
of the isometric joint torque is then assessed.

Effects of exercise on strength

Positive effects of FES training were found in all
properly selected SCI subjects. The most important
criterion for patient selection is the presence of an
upper motor neuron lesion. Other criteria may
include the following: adequately preserved skin,
good psychosocial condition, motivation and co-
operation. Up to a fivefold increase in joint torque
is often observed after 2 months of training.

The strength of electrically stimulated knee extensors was studied in three groups of subjects:
untrained and trained paraplegic patients, and
neurologically intact subjects. The recruitment
curves, such as found in all three groups, are presented in Fig. 35.1. The results in untrained paraplegic subjects (group A) are shown in Fig. 35.1(a).
The average curve is plotted with a thicker line. In
untrained SCI subjects the average isometric knee
joint torque of about 25 Nm was assessed. In a
few patients (subjects 2, 8 and 10), noticeably
higher maximal joint torque values were found.
The strength of their stimulated knee extensors
exceeded 50 Nm. In our experience (Kralj & Bajd,
1989), knee joint torques over 50 Nm permit the
performance of functional FES activities, such as
standing up, standing and reciprocal walking. In
these patients, no introductory strengthening of
atrophied muscles is necessary. It is presumably
the spastic activity which preserves the satisfactory
condition of their paralysed muscles.

Considerably higher knee joint torques resulting
from FES of completely paralysed knee extensors
were found in trained paraplegics from group B
(Fig. 35.1(b)). Here, the maximal average values
reached 60 Nm, indicating the success of the FES
exercise programme. Again, noticeably higher joint
torques were found in some subjects from group B

(subjects 5, 8 and 9). Paraplegic subjects 4 and
6 had been using FES very efficiently already
for several years, but displayed knee joint torque
values considerably below the average of the B
group.

In Fig. 35.1(c) the recruitment curves found
in neurologically intact subjects (group C) are
presented. Here, the saturation values were not
assessed because of pain sensation. Nevertheless, it
can be seen that knee joint torques up to 200 Nm
can be obtained. These values are well above the
maximal strength of the trained SCI subjects, even
after extensive training and several years of daily
use of FES for restoration of simple locomotion
patterns.

Programmed stimulation response also appears
to be an efficient approach in evaluation of
the condition of the spastic atrophied paralysed
muscles. Significantly different frequency patterns
were found in untrained and trained paraplegic
patients and neurologically intact subjects.

Effects of exercise on fatigue and
dynamic muscle response

The type of FES training used in Ljubljana Rehabilitation Center, is not as effective in increasing muscle
endurance as it is in improving muscle strength.
Electrically stimulated muscle fatigue is not improved in all paraplegic subjects treated. When
studying fatigue in untrained and trained paraplegic patients and healthy subjects, the differences
among the three groups were small. No effect of
FES muscle restrengthening was observed. Average
fatigue indices of healthy subjects were statistically
significantly lower than in both groups of paraplegic subjects.

The dynamic properties of electrically stimulated
muscle were evaluated from the time delays occurring between electrical stimulus and provoked
muscle twitch. Here again, the differences among
the three groups of subjects were rather low. Nevertheless, it appears that paralysed untrained muscle
responds to electrical stimulation somewhat faster
than the restrengthened or normal muscle. This
result is in accordance with the results obtained by
Fischbach & Robbins (1984). The FES training programme results in slowing of electrically stimulated
muscle.

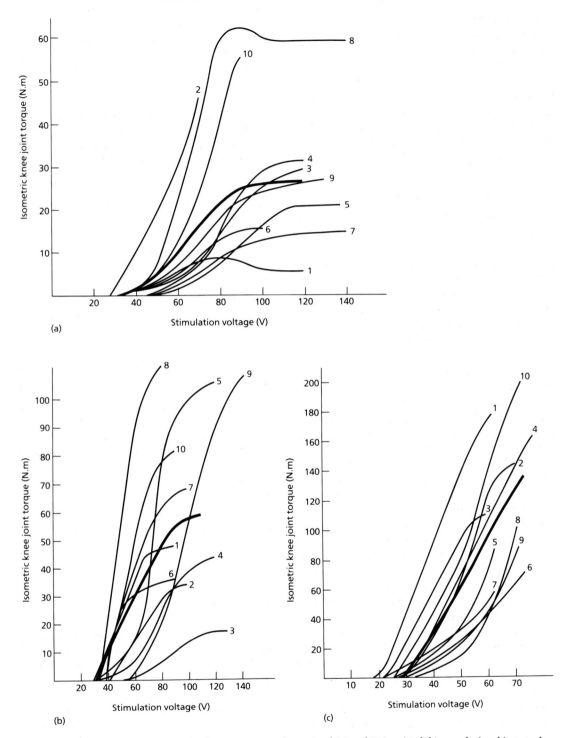

Fig. 35.1 Recruitment curves assessed in knee extensors of untrained (a) and FES-trained (b) paraplegic subjects and healthy persons (c).

Effects of exercise on incomplete SCI subjects

In addition to positive therapeutic effects, FES training also has a diagnostic value when applied to
incomplete SCI subjects. After completion of FES
training, three groups of patients were identified:
those in whom an improvement of both voluntary
and stimulated muscle force was observed, those
with an increase in stimulation response only,
and those patients in whom no effect of electrical
stimulation training could be recorded (Bajd *et al.*,
1989). The candidates for permanent orthotic
use of electrical stimulators come from the second
group, as well as those patients from the first group
whose functional levels of voluntary joint torques
were not reached. Such an outcome of the FES
rehabilitation process cannot be predicted when
the patients are first admitted to the spinal unit
very soon after an accident.

The present technological levels of both surface
and implanted stimulation seem to be appropriate
for use in restoration of walking in incomplete SCI
patients. Most of these patients can, with the help
of FES, be turned into community walkers. They
can effectively use the stimulator throughout the
day, and not only for an hour or two as is the
case in completely paralysed paraplegic subjects. In
addition, whatever exteroception or proprioception
level they have preserved, it is considerably more
efficient than that provided by artificial or restored
natural sensors.

Effects of exercise on contralateral untrained extremity

Significant increase in the strength of knee extensors was observed in the non-stimulated leg as a
result of FES knee extensor training of the contralateral leg. Three clinically completely paralysed
subjects were included in the study (D.A., thoracic-
2,3; K.D., cervical-5; D.P., cervical-5). The patient
K.D. was 5 years post-injury while the two other
patients were only several months post-injury. All
patients were in bed and did not receive any other
FES exercising. The rate of muscle torque increase
was very similar in both extremities. The maximal
response, after about 2 months of FES training, was
increased almost three times in all three cases (Fig.
35.2).

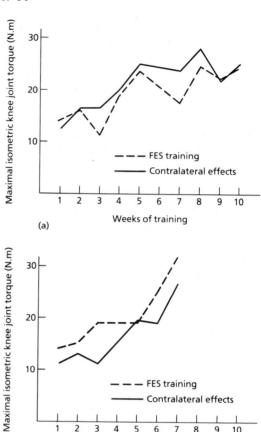

(a)

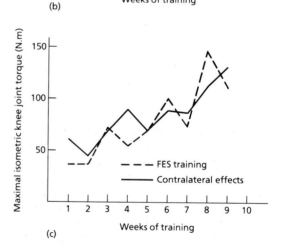

(b)

(c)

Fig. 35.2 Significant increase of strength in stimulated
and non-stimulated knee extensors in T-2,3 (a), C-5 (b)
and C-5 (c) SCI subjects.

A possible explanation for this 'cross-education' effect could be improved blood flow occurring because of local vasodilatation in the stimulated extremity spreading to the non-stimulated limb. Blood flow, heart rate and blood pressure were found to be unaffected after FES exercise performed in a group of healthy subjects (Walker *et al.*, 1988). However, there were increased central haemodynamic effects observed after FES training of paraplegic subjects (Phillips *et al.*, 1984). An adaptation of the spastic non-trained contralateral muscle via electrically elicited functions of the central nervous system cannot be excluded. It is believed that the differences in FES-induced exercise are also influenced by the autonomic nervous system, which is itself damaged as a consequence of most spinal cord injuries.

FES-assisted locomotion in paraplegic subjects

Some theoretical and practical aspects

In current FES research for enhanced systems, the functional aspect of muscle activation is considered to be the most important (Thoma *et al.*, 1983; Marsolais & Kobetič, 1987, 1989; Kralj & Bajd, 1989). From a biomechanical point of view, an SCI patient may be considered as consisting of three regions: the upper body, under normal neural control, the paralysed lower body and the connecting region, which may be considered as an additional joint. The latter is in many cases bridged to some extent by long body muscles with partially intact innervation. The three-part model is shown diagrammatically in Fig. 35.3.

FES is a means of providing functioning of the lower body part in a way which can be integrated with upper body function, in order to restore near-normal motor function and lost locomotor functions. By doing so, the lower body part is controlled according to the voluntary commands and needs of the patient and the upper body. The normal neural control in man has three levels: cortical control, supraspinal reflexes and spinal reflexes. The cortical control provides intention with high-level planning, while the supraspinal level provides additional planning and co-ordination, and final execution is carried out at the spinal level in accordance

with the limitations imposed. Thus, control information expands from higher to lower spinal levels and sensory information flowing in the opposite direction is compressed, as is depicted in Fig. 35.4. The voluntary command from the patient can be considered as the input command information which needs to be expanded, by some, at present, unknown algorithm, in such a way as to result in activation patterns for each FES muscle, thus providing appropriate timing and amplitude modulation.

The pattern of FES in some current systems proposed by Marsolais & Kobetič (1989) and Thoma *et al.* (1983) is tailored to follow the natural activity of muscles in normals, and is then subjectively modified by trial and error to provide adequate function. When it is recognized as adequate, it is stored in the stimulator memory, thus providing the means of modulating amplitude as well. The patient's commands, elicited by hand switches, simply trigger the stored FES sequences. In other systems, such as that described by Kralj & Bajd (1989), the patient composes the timing of FES sequences. S/he is limited to the selection of on and off states of muscle activity, while the amplitude has to be preset and remains fixed at a functional level. Obviously such an arrangement has no amplitude control. However, the timing is entirely under the patient's control and hence adaptative.

To some extent this second control mode gives the patient better autonomy, but it is harder to master and consequently the learning time is longer. At present, the composition of the muscle activation pattern, which is called the stimulation sequence, is subjective, and does not take into account quantitative biomechanical data. In addition, such FES sequences do not consider physiological requirements with biological elements and criteria. This is valid regardless of the control mode applied and regardless of the FES execution control, whether of a direct or closed-loop design. This presentation follows our study and is concentrated on the design of an FES system utilizing subconscious, 'natural', control, incorporating mathematically and physiologically based quantitative and formal on-line stimulation sequence synthesis (Kralj *et al.*, 1987, 1989a,b,c). Such mathematically based and formalized stimulation sequence synthesis, taking into account biophysical data and

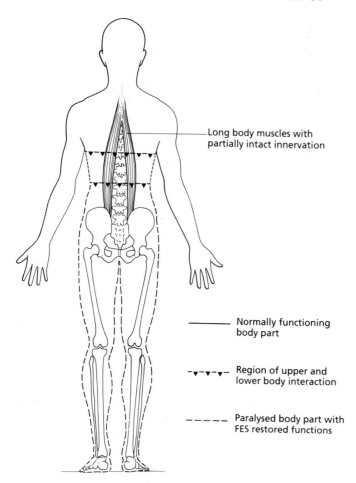

Long body muscles with
partially intact innervation

——— Normally functioning
body part

-▼-▼-▼- Region of upper and
lower body interaction

— — — — Paralysed body part with
FES restored functions

Fig. 35.3 Functional body regions in SCI subject.

physiological limitations and criteria, represents the basis for software and algorithm development, as expressed in Fig. 35.4. For each level, given algorithms, limitations and criteria apply. In this presentation, we are considering the lowest level where local co-ordination and physiological criteria are obeyed in a manner designed to prevent secondary pathology developments due to overstressing of joints, cartilage, ligaments or long bones, which may result in fractures. The latter should be minimized and should result in safety comparable to the established level of widely utilized prosthetic devices. The spinal reflexes are, when considering movement execution, responsible for determining the required safe muscular activation which must result in the desired joint torque and also ensures acceptable physiological

bone and joints stress. The underlying biomechanical and physiological aspects of such muscular activation are discussed below.

Preventing the development of secondary pathology

For minimizing or even preventing the development of secondary pathology in joints and bones, stressing of these structures is of essential importance. It must follow biophysical and physiological principles, and the natural and evolutionary developed biomechanical principles must be understood and obeyed in the composition of FES stimulation sequences. In the first instance, the principles of muscular activity in the normal must be understood. The important rule (Pauwels, 1980) that

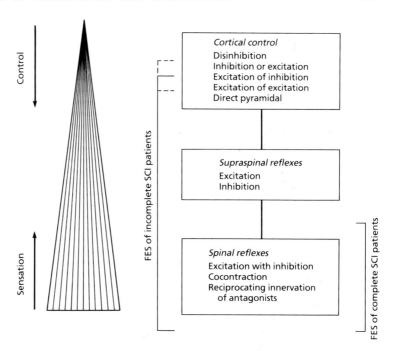

Fig. 35.4 Schematic presentation of neural control.

must be obeyed is that muscular action and torque are needed for counterbalancing external forces and loading torques caused by body weight. Thus, minimal loading requires minimal muscle activation, and long-lasting maximal muscle force is never exerted in the absence of external forces or weight. Excessive bone loading might cause bone fracture. Because bone tissue is susceptible to bending stress, in the normal person active muscle force is used to reduce it. By doing so, the compressive stress is slightly increased. The latter has no consequence because bones can sustain very high compressive stress. This principle was proved within this project, and we utilize this principle for FES sequence synthesis (Kralj & Bajd, 1989; Kralj *et al.*, 1987). This principle is one of the key elements in the muscular action selection in time, strength and also with regard to muscular co-ordination (Draganich *et al.*, 1989). By considering biomechanics and the prevention of overstressing of ligaments, joints and cartilage tissue, additional formal criteria are obtained for quantitative FES stimulation pattern synthesis, and the development of secondary joint pathology is prevented.

There are two main possibilities for provoking pathological developments in joints:
1 Overstressing of joint surface cartilage.
2 Overstressing of ligament structure, which is mostly caused by improper FES activation of muscles and may lead to 'loose joints', which are themselves pathological.
With time such a state may be aggravated by allowing overstressing of cartilage, leading to additional damage and pathology. Regardless of the causes which may result in overstressing of cartilage, the joint pathology sets in rapidly and its severity depends on many factors, such as the magnitude and duration of stress, followed by the onset of inflammation and later ossification and limited range of motion (ROM) in the joint. This is one of the major problems.

The following explanation and illustration indicate that properly selected muscular action for ensuring proper joint loading is vital for joint integrity and prevention of secondary pathology developments in joints. Figure 35.5 presents a structure composed of three segments and two joints, where element 1 transfers body weight (BW) across the

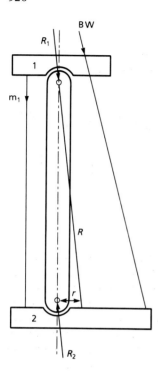

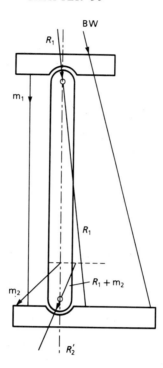

Fig. 35.5 Two-joint structure displayed during static standing.

first joint to the long bone and down to the ground. The action of muscle m_1 reduces the long bone bending stress and stabilizes the upper joint, and as a result the resultant R_1 loads the joint in a compressive way. At the same time, it should be noted that R_1 passes through the centre of the joint and that there is a large range of possible angles for the R_1 force. For all of these angles, the resultant does not pass the upper joint at the edge of its structure. The lower joint 2 is loaded by R_1' force, being the sum of R_1 and BW increased for the segment load. R_1' is nearly equal to R_1. R_1' passes the lower joint and creates a torque of

$$rR_1' = rR_1$$

Therefore, the lower joint is not stable and must be stabilized by additional muscular action, such as m_2 (Fig. 35.5), thus ensuring that the resultant

$$R_2 = R_1 + m_2$$

passes through the central region of the second joint and causes compressive stress of the lower joint. In the case of insufficient m_1 or m_2 muscle force, the joint may be bent until the forces pro-

duced and the ligamentous stress stabilize the joint. By doing so, it can happen, depending on the magnitude of the structure and the supported weight and the extent of muscular force deficit, that the joint is loaded by a resultant force passing the joint border region, as depicted in Fig. 35.6b.

Centrally located and perpendicular force loading of a joint results in low compressive stress of joint cartilage, because the joint surfaces are large enough on both sides of the resultant force, R, for sharing the load. According to equation (1), the joint surface area is proportional to the actively involved surface area resisting exactly half of the compressing force:

$$\int_0^\alpha p \, dS = \int_0^{\alpha'} p \, dS = \frac{1}{2} R \qquad (1)$$

where p is compressive pressure and dS an element of the joint surface. When the resultant force passes through the joint, as in Fig. 35.6b (Pauwels, 1980), the stressed region is very small, but has to provide support for R'. This small joint area compressive stress increases because the area represented by S may be very small. This is illustrated in Fig. 35.6b.

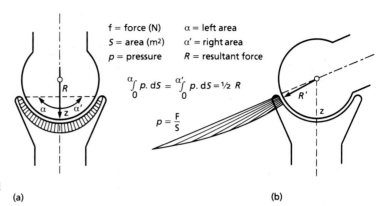

Fig. 35.6 Normal stressing and possible overstressing of the joint and ligaments.

(a)   (b)

Such high stressing will sooner or later damage the joint cartilage tissue and consequently result in the development of secondary joint pathology. Excentric loading, as depicted in Fig. 35.6b, also causes a disruption force which tends to pull out the upper joint segment and thus dislocate the joint.

Clinical experience

Standing and walking after SCI has traditionally relied on bilateral knee–ankle–foot orthoses (KAFOs) and crutches, or other walking aids. The literature indicates a high rejection rate for this technique (Natig & McAdam, 1978; Coughlan *et al.*, 1980; Mikelberg & Reid, 1981; O'Daniel & Hahn, 1981). A recent study has shown that only 26% of patients who were prescribed braces continued to use them for any purpose, with only 4% using them as their sole means of mobility (Heinemann *et al.*, 1987). Reasons for the high rejection rate include difficulties in orthotic device donning and doffing and the significant high energy expenditure for walking (Fisher & Gullickson, 1978).

In nearly all patients who regularly use FES, we have so far observed intact joints, even after 10 years of using FES, and the ROM is preserved almost as in normals and is far better than in patients not using FES. A biomechanical study of long-bone bending stress in patients utilizing FES of m. quadriceps for standing and walking was undertaken and the results partly published (Munih *et al.*, 1989). These results indicated measures of

risks for the development of secondary pathology (Munih *et al.*, 1989, 1990). Figures 35.7(a) and (b) compare long-bone bending stress in the normal and paraplegic. SCI patients, while standing by means of FES of m. quadriceps, use hands for balance. The provoked hand force is represented in Fig. 35.7 by F_y and creates the M_h bending stress to bones. An SCI patient while standing by means of FES uses an almost identical posture to normal man, except that the posture is maintained by m. quadriceps force and stabilized by F_y force against falling (locking of the ankle joint). In FES standing, the resultant bone bending stress is, in shape and magnitude, very similar to that in normal man. This can be recognized by comparing Fig. 35.7(a) with Fig. 35.7(b). The findings presented in Fig. 35.7 correlate with our clinical observations that, in a group of nearly 100 SCI patients utilizing FES as a rehabilitation means in their daily activities, no joint problems have yet occurred. Some patients have used FES for many years, and it can be concluded that FES, as currently used, does not provoke rapid development of secondary joint pathology. In addition, if the bending stress of the bones during FES standing is in shape and magnitude similar to that of normal man, then to a large extent safe and acceptable joint stress occurs. Of course, this is a subjectively derived hypothesis which needs evaluation in quantitative terms and was not the matter of this study. Quantitative evaluation is a difficult task and should be considered in further FES research planning.

The theoretical and fundamental aspects discussed here highlight the lack of knowledge which

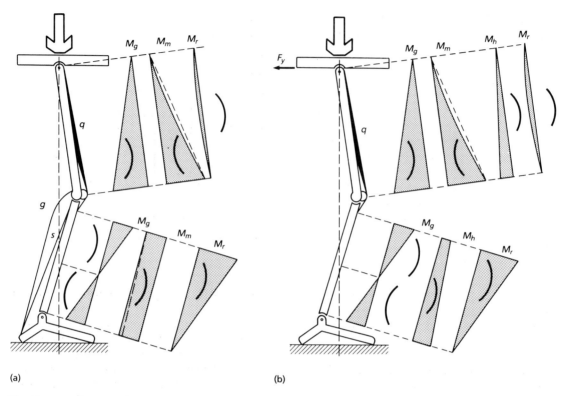

Fig. 35.7 Long-bone bending profiles in healthy subjects (a) and paraplegic patients (b).

is necessary for the development of the next generation of FES systems. We believe that the missing knowledge and principles discussed are important for the software development, particularly in regard to stimulation sequence composition, which will be the basis for improved function and safety. The aspects of FES sequence generation are important; we have discussed some issues but have left open the questions of balance control, energy recuperation in gait, the minimization of fatigue by means of posture switching, etc. We are undertaking efforts to develop new-generation FES systems following the presented lines.

Enhancement of hemiplegic patients' rehabilitation by means of FES

In the Ljubljana University Rehabilitation Institute, FES has for the past 20 years been a routine additional treatment to the standard and established therapy for rehabilitation (Ačimović-Janežič, 1989; Stanič *et al.*, 1990). At present, about 80% of all admitted patients participate in the FES therapeutic and subsequent orthotic FES programme. With the help of electrical stimulation, different muscles can be activated and strengthened, the joint ROM actively maintained, the blood circulation augmented and pain reduced. FES is a convenient and effective means for enhancement of sensory awareness. In many instances, mobilization is easier and reached in a shorter time when radically activating the patients' preserved and voluntary resources by FES, which provides afferent and indirectly induced proprioceptive and exteroceptive sensory inflow. Particularly in hemiplegia, the facilitation effect is important, 'reminding' the patient to exert the movement correctly and produce maximal effort to perform it, and hence leading to earlier restoration of function. Repetitive movement stimulation reduces contractures and, in many instances, moderates spasticity.

Typical FES application indications are: to replace the lost central control of movement by artificial FES control, to augment and teach a movement or to achieve a functional selective response of stimulated muscle groups, to break synergistic movement patterns, to prevent development of contractures, to reduce spasticity, and to augment circulation. The early induced FES-controlled pattern is selected in a manner which will: (i) resist and prevent the development of pathological synergistic patterns; (ii) produce a functional movement free of anomalies; and (iii) exert such movement in as normal away as possible. The therapist aims to produce a gait which will be repetitive, cyclical and symmetrical by using surface stimulation of the muscle groups governing flexion, extension and eversion of the ankle; knee flexion and extension; hip extension and abduction and, by careful placement of electrodes, also hip flexion (m. rectus femoris, m. tensor fasciae latae and m. sartorius). The number of FES channels is determined and the triggering mode selected according to the patient's neurological deficit and his/her independence in standing. In the most severe cases, where the patient has insecure standing and is unable to make a step, usually four or up to six channels are applied and the therapist manually triggers the preset pattern of muscle activation. As the patient improves and repetitive stepping is achieved, the triggering can be accomplished by heel switches. Hardware provisions are made for swing- and stance-phase triggering, as well as for walking rate adjustment of the set activation pattern. For patients either with less marked initial neurological deficit or who have improved with treatment, the number of stimulation channels is gradually reduced to two or even only one. The typical recovery starts in proximal joints and muscle groups and gradually progresses distally.

In Fig. 35.8 the epidemiological data for Slovenia (population 2.3 million) are presented. In the last 10 years, 2500 patients have been screened and 1575 hemiplegic or hemiparetic cases treated by FES. In the FES programme, 2000 patients were included and 425 patients received upper extremity FES and 1575 were candidates for the lower extremity FES programme.

The treatment used and selection of patients with regard to the applied number of FES channels are shown in Fig. 35.9. In 60% of cases, only one

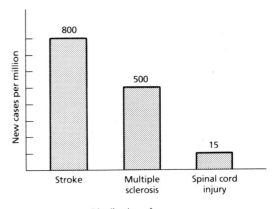

Fig. 35.8 Epidemiological data for Slovenia.

channel of FES was indicated, with two channels in 30%, and only in 10% of cases was multichannel or up to six-channel FES applied. It is interesting to see the outcome for the single-channel (Ačimović-Janežič et al., 1987; Ačimović-Janežič & Kljajić, 1990) FES applications in respect of later chronic use. Figure 35.10 summarizes the last 10 years' experience of screened and treated patients for equinovarus correction, using single-channel (peroneal brace) FES. A sample of 670 applications shows that 80% of patients required only therapeutic FES, while 20% remained chronic users (FEPA® – 10 applications). In the last few years, a smaller and more cosmetic system, MICROFES®, was applied (Ačimović-Janežič et al., 1987) and a sample of 120 patients showed that 80% of these patients decided to use the system as a home chronic assistive device and only 20% have used it only for therapy. This reversal of chronic users is also seen with two-channel FES systems after the introduction of improved patient selection (Bogataj et al., 1990). In some patients, after they have used the surface unit for about a year and expressed the wish for an implantable system, the appropriate screening and testing was performed. Finally, in only 75 patients out of 1000 cases was the implant (Ačimović-Janežič et al., 1987; Ačimović-Janežič & Kljajić, 1990) surgically placed, with a functional success of 96%. Due to various reasons 30 patients did not receive an FES assistive device and were treated by conventional methods.

In the last few years, the methodology for aug-

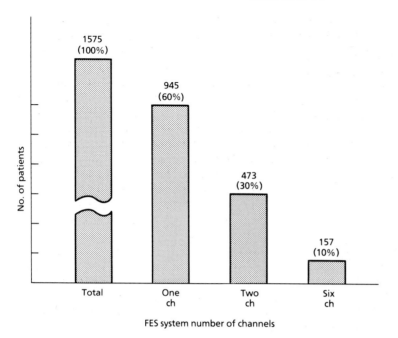

Fig. 35.9 Statistical distribution of patients in regard to number of FES channels applied.

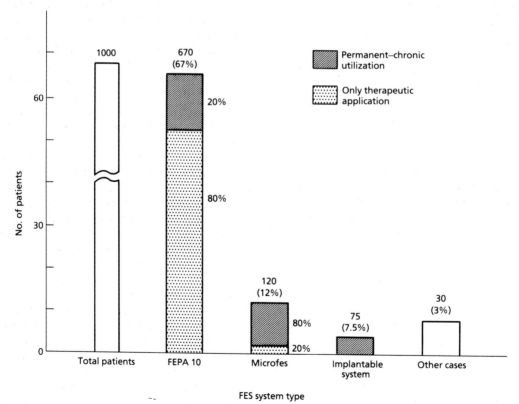

Fig. 35.10 Single-channel FES applications for equinovarus correction, indicating the device applied and the outcome.

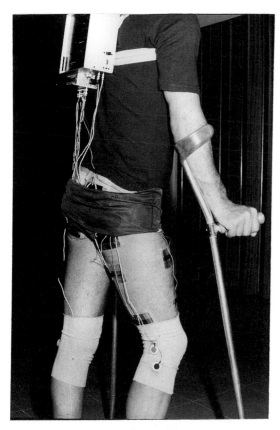

Fig. 35.11 The patient equipped for six-channel FES therapy. The electrode locations are shown.

mentation of standing and walking in patients with severe neurological deficit using six-channel FES has been refined (Stanič *et al.*, 1990). The goal of this treatment is to mobilize the patient as soon as possible and, in the case of bilateral involvement, two additional channels of FES are sometimes added. Figure 35.11 shows a patient equipped with six-channel FES in a later stage when he is already using bilateral crutches and shoe insole-mounted switches for triggering. The stimulation unit has controls for adjusting the polarity, timing, amplitude and triggering for each selected channel in regard to the function of a particular muscle. This radical therapeutic stimulation programme is applied for 2–3 weeks and later the number of channels is gradually reduced, usually to two (Bogataj *et al.*, 1990) or even just a single peroneal

stimulator. The six-channel unit and the new two-channel unit incorporate advanced software, drawing on the knowledge collected over the last 15–20 years. In Fig. 35.12 the clinical two-channel stimulation unit is shown, consisting of two main parts, the stimulator itself and the programmer–stride analyser unit (Bogataj *et al.*, 1990). The shoe insoles and the stimulation electrodes are not shown. This unit is usually used to activate a large muscle group like the m. quadriceps for knee extension, hamstring muscles for knee flexion or gluteus maximus for hip extension, and the second channel is applied for peroneal nerve stimulation of the pretibial muscle group for ankle dorsiflexion.

The six-channel and two-channel microprocessor-based units also monitor and store data about patient gait performance. The measurements are based on shoe insole switches. The statistical and average data of performance can be recalled at any instant after the gait run. Included in the assessment are the number of steps and the average heel-on and off durations for both legs, including the standard deviations (Bogataj *et al.*, 1990).

The programming unit allows user-friendly determining of the stimulation on and off time for each particular channel in regard to the selected stance- or swing-phase trigger. The walking rate-dependent (WRD) mode of stimulation or cyclical mode may be used. At the beginning of therapy, the cyclical mode is applied, while later the WRD mode allows the patient to choose his own preferred speed of gait and the stimulation sequence selected is then adjusted accordingly. The adaptation of the stimulation sequence timing to the patient's gait is based on a linear or weighted extrapolation of the previous four stride times. As a result of improved functional ability after sixchannel and later two-channel treatment, most cases end with a single peroneal stimulator, even in cases where a two-channel or even three-channel device would be preferred. This is because no such three-channel or two-channel FES units for chronic use are at present available. Of course, for skilled and motivated patients the two-channel unit can be prescribed, but in general the daily multielectrode placement and fixation is too clumsy and time-consuming, and not practical. It is expected that in the future a suitable implanted system will be developed.

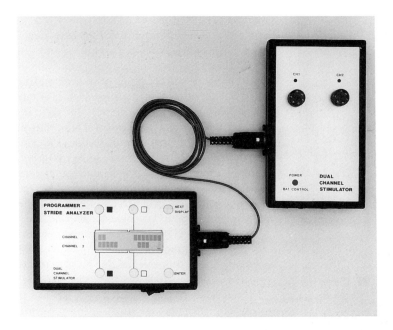

Fig. 35.12 Two-channel FES unit consisting of the stimulator and programming unit. The shoe insoles and electrodes are not displayed.

The FES therapy and methodology as described are effective and are carried out over a period of 8–10 weeks. Using comparative studies (Maležič *et al.*, 1984), it was concluded that intensive FES therapy advances the patient's recovery faster and to a higher functional level for nearly the same treatment cost. This is summarized in Fig. 35.13, which compares the FES-treated group with those receiving conventional therapy. In summary, the FES group showed faster improvement, a higher functional level, and a shorter time in hospital, demonstrating that FES is overall a cost-effective form of treatment.

Over the last 10 years, the research interest for hemiplegic hand function restoration observed in the 1970–80 decade has mostly faded out. FES was applied at the end of the 1970s as a means of improving the range of wrist and finger extension and to prevent the development of contractures caused by flexor spasticity. The application of cyclical isotonic FES of wrist and finger extensors decreases spasticity and connects wrist and finger flexion deformities (Baker *et al.*, 1979). It was concluded that two to three 30–40 minute stimulation sessions per week can substitute for all other ROM techniques. Discomfort from stimulation can be overcome by using a gradually increasing length

of stimulation. The majority of patients learn to tolerate the sensation produced by stimulation and tolerate settings which produce isometric activation of wrist and finger extensors. Bowman *et al.* (1979) have proposed position feedback for automated treatment for the hemiplegic wrist by means of FES. The only commercially available FES chronically applicable to the wrist and finger extension system which is still available here in Ljubljana was first proposed nearly 15 years ago (Reberšek & Vodovnik, 1975). Due to donning and doffing clumsiness and only minor improvement of wrist and finger function, the unit never reached the popularity of the similar one-channel peroneal stimulator. Nevertheless, the unit is still available and in therapeutic use. An implantable unit for hand function restoration in hemiplegic patients has, to our knowledge, not yet been produced or marketed. However, there are developments in the area of FES, especially progress along the line of multichannel implants, which may be suitable for hand function restoration.

The application of FES to hemiplegic patients for gait assistance and gait restoration has proved to be effective (Maležič *et al.*, 1984; Stanič *et al.*, 1990). At present, the most suitable patients for FES are those who need simple equinovarus correction. For

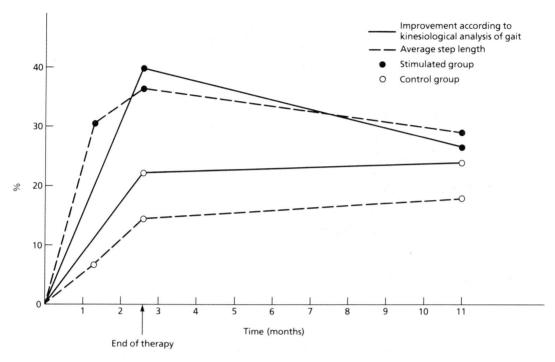

Fig. 35.13 The course of functional progress using the six-channel FES system compared with classical rehabilitation therapy.

this group of patients, the single-channel FES unit is suitable. In principle, the equinovarus deficiency needs a balanced control of equinus and varus. The latter requires in essence a two-channel unit. The research results obtained within the last few years suggest that substantial progress can be expected toward the development of totally implantable systems which are more acceptable cosmetically and eliminate the handling problems of external devices.

The recently refined recording techniques from sensory peripheral nerves (Hoffer & Sinkjaer, 1985; Johansson, 1991) indicate that, with minimal circuitry for signal recognition, it may be possible to develop very selective trigger and even control signals for arbitrary movement restoration by means of FES. This development is complemented by chronically implantable intrafascicular recording electrodes (Lefurge et al., 1991). The future looks optimistic for hand and gait function restoration in hemiplegic patients, with safe and reliable controls with trigger signals in implanted systems. Chronic

recording from peripheral nerves is very important as these nerves transmit information detected by natural undamaged sensors. For instance, a heel contact in gait can be detected from skin receptors and used for a trigger source.

Interesting developments have begun with regard to improving the motor activation of muscles by FES, and this is directly applicable to hemiplegic patients (Waters et al., 1988; Marsolais et al., 1990), including the use of epimysial electrodes for therapeutic electrical stimulation of the lower limb. The epimysial electrodes are inserted surgically and connected via percutaneous wires, as used for nearly two decades in the Cleveland Rehabilitation Center upper extremities programme (Peckham, 1987). In patients with inadequate hip stability preventing them from balancing on one limb in order to take a step, FES with implanted epimysial electrodes produces stimulation of hip joint extensor and abductor muscles (Waters et al., 1988). The results obtained indicate that the stimulation was effective for producing deep muscle contractions and that the percutaneous stimulation was safe. A similar approach (Marsolais *et al.*, 1990) uses percutaneous wire electrodes for activating muscles to produce functional improvement and progression from standing to stepping or walking. Muscle groups such as m. erector spinae for torso control, m. gluteus maximus and medius, m. tensor fasciae latae and m. posterior adductor for hip control and biceps femoris with quadriceps for knee function were implanted. In addition, the muscles of the ankle joint were stimulated to obtain the desired functional level. In all five implanted patients, improved walking was demonstrated (Marsolais *et al.*, 1990). Patients have complained about both the wires connecting the shoe-insole switch and the electrode wires. They have also complained about the problems of maintaining the electrode sites where the percutaneous wires penetrate the skin.

The same technology as so far described and used for the lower extremities, utilizing percutaneous wires and epimysial electrodes for the FES programme, can be introduced for the restoration of hand function and grasp in hemiplegic patients. The percutaneous system for hand function restoration in quadriplegic patients (Peckham, 1987) has already advanced to an implanted epimysial electrode system and only the control signal set-up prevents the development of totally implanted hardware. In Japan, Hoshimiya *et al.* (1985) report the development of a multichannel FES system for paralysed upper extremities using percutaneous wire electrodes. The design of the system is similar to that used in Cleveland, with external hardware for trigger and control signals.

This short review indicates the present trends and exciting new possibilities for the future development of FES hand function restoration hardware, as well as the present use in quadriplegic patients. We believe that these advances may be of particular benefit for hemiplegic hand rehabilitation. There are also promising trends for the FES programme in general, particularly because of the recent accomplishments in peripheral afferent signal detection, which enables the recording of signals from natural receptors, using this as an ideal control and trigger source for lower extremity FES. These developments are realistic, and supported also by exciting designs of multichannel implantable FES systems fostered by cochlear implants.

These implants have an already proved safety and functional record. There is a gradual recognition that for the entire FES field the vital technological problems are approaching a state where the hardware of the system will no longer present a problem. Difficulties are more likely to arise because of poorly developed knowledge about particular clinical applications, and this will be the most limiting and costly factor in the FES rehabilitation of hemiplegia.

References

Ačimović-Janežič R. (1989) Verwendung von FES bei Hemiplegie. *Physic und Technik in der Traumatologie Intensivmedizin und Rehabilitazion.* 14. Jahrestagung der Österreichischen Gesellschaft für BME, Wissenschaftliche Berichte, pp. 255–258. Klosterneuburg bei Wien.

Ačimović-Janežič R. & Kljajić M. (1990) *Klinische Erfahrungen mit der Applikation von implantierbaren Systemen zur Korrektur des Gehens bei hemiparetischen Patienten,* pp. 65–66. Biomedizinische Technik Band, Ergänzungsband.

Ačimović-Janežič R., Gros N., Maležič M., Strojnik P., Kljajić M., Stanič U. & Simič V. (1987) A comparative study of the functionality of the second generation of peroneal stimulators. *RESNA 10th Annual Conference,* pp. 621–623. Resna Press, San Jose, California.

Bajd T., Kralj A., Turk R., Benko H. & Šega J. (1989) Use of functional electrical stimulation in the rehabilitation of patients with incomplete spinal cord injuries. *Journal of Biomedical Engineering* **11**, 96–102.

Baker L.L., Yeh C., Wilson D. & Waters R.L. (1979) Electrical stimulation of wrist and fingers for hemiplegic patients. *Physical Therapy* **59**, 1495–1499.

Bogataj U., Kelih B., Maležič M., Filipič D. & Kljajić M. (1990) Dual-channel electrical stimulator for correction of gait. *Advances in External Control of Human Extremities* **10**, 327–333.

Bowman B.R., Baker L.L. & Waters R.L. (1979) Positional feedback and electrical stimulation: an automated treatment for the hemiplegic wrist. *Archives of Physical Medicine and Rehabilitation* **60** (11).

Coughlan J.K., Robinson C.E., Newmarch B. & Jackson G. (1980) Lower extremity bracing in paraplegia – a follow-up study. *Paraplegia* **18**, 25–32.

Draganich L.F., Jaeger R.J. & Kralj A.R. (1989) Coactivation of the hamstrings and quadriceps during extension of the knee. *Journal of Bone and Joint Surgery* **71A**, 1075–1081.

Edwards R.H.T. (1978) Physiological analysis of skeletal muscle weakness and fatigue. *Clinical Science and Molecular Medicine* **54**, 463–470.

Fischbach G.D. & Robbins N. (1984) Changes in contractile

properties of disuse soleus muscle. *Journal of Physiology* **210**, 305–320.

Fisher S.V. & Gullickson G. (1978) The energy cost of ambulation in health and disability: a literature review. *Archives of Physical Medicine and Rehabilitation* **59**, 124–133.

Heinemann A., Magieva-Planey R., Schiro-Geist C. & Gimenes G. (1987) Mobility for persons with spinal cord injury: an evaluation of two systems. *Archives of Physical Medicine and Rehabilitation* **3**, 68–90.

Hoffer J.A. & Sinkjaer T. (1985) A natural 'force sensor' suitable for closed loop control of functional neuromuscular stimulation. *Proceedings of the 2nd Vienna International Workshop on FES*, pp. 47–50.

Hoshimiya H., Iijima K., Futami R., Handa Y. & Ichie M. (1985) A new FES system for the paralyzed upper extremities. *IEEE/Seventh Annual Conference of the Engineering in Medicine and Biology Society*, pp. 327–330.

Johansson R.S. (1991) How is grasping modified by somatosensory input? In Humphrey D.R. & Freund H.J. (eds) *Motor Control: Concepts and Issues*. John Wiley & Sons Ltd, New York.

Kralj A. & Bajd T. (1989) *Functional Electrical Stimulation: Standing and Walking After Spinal Cord Injury*. CRC Press, Inc., Boca Raton, Florida.

Kralj A., Bajd T., Turk R. & Munih M. (1987) Mathematical synthesis of FES sequences. *Proceedings of the International Symposium on Advances in External Control of Human Extremities*, pp. 249–260. Yugoslav Committee for Electronics and Automation, Belgrade.

Kralj A., Bajd T. & Turk R. (1989a) FES control aspects and augmenting of subconscious natural like control. *Proceedings of Seminar on Biomechanics*, International Centre of Biocybernetics of the Academy of Sciences, Warsaw.

Kralj A., Bajd T. & Turk R. (1989b) FES control and second pathology development. *Osaka International Workshop on Functional Neuromuscular Stimulation*, pp. 113–126. Osaka.

Kralj A., Bajd T., Turk R., Munih M. & Benko H. (1989c) FES is preventing the development of secondary pathologies in joints. *3rd Vienna International Workshop on Functional Electrostimulation*, pp. 25–28. Department of Biomechanics and Physics, University of Vienna, Vienna.

Lefurge T., Goodall E., Horch K., Stensaas L. & Schoenberg A. (1991) Chronically implanted intrafascicular recording electrodes. *Annals of Biomedical Engineering* **19**, 197–207.

Maležič M., Stanič U., Kljajić M., Ačimović-Janežič R., Krajnik J., Gros N. & Stopar M. (1984) Multichannel electrical stimulation of gait in motor disabled patients. *Orthopedics* **7**, 1187–1195.

Marsolais E.B. & Kobetič R. (1987) Functional electrical stimulation for walking in paraplegia. *Journal of Bone and Joint Surgery* **69A**, 728–733.

Marsolais E.B. & Kobetič R. (1989) Design considerations for a practical functional electrical stimulation (FNS) system for restoring gait in the paralyzed person. Presented at 3rd Vienna International Workshop on Electrical Stimulation.

Marsolais E.B., Kobetič R., Barnicle K. & Jacobs J. (1990) FNS application for restoring function in stroke and head-injury patients. *Journal of Clinical Engineering* **15** (6), 489–495.

Mikelberg R. & Reid S. (1981) Spinal cord lesions and lower extremity bracing: an overview and follow-up study. *Paraplegia* **19**, 379–385.

Munih M., Kralj A., Bajd T. & Jaeger R. (1989) Bone bending profiles in standing. *12th Annual Conference RESNA*, pp. 175–176. Resna Press, New Orleans.

Munih M., Kralj A. & Bajd T. (1990) Calculation of bending moments unloading femur and tibia bones. *Proceedings of the Xth International Symposium on Advances in External Control of Human Extremities*, p. 67. Yugoslav Committee for Electronics, Telecommunication and Automation, Beograd.

Natig H. & McAdam R. (1978) Ambulation without wheelchairs for paraplegics with complete lesions. *Paraplegia* **16**, 142–146.

O'Daniel W.E. & Hahn H.R. (1981) Follow-up usage of the Scott–Craig orthosis in paraplegia. *Paraplegia* **19**, 373–378.

Pauwels F. (1980) *Biomechanics of the Locomotor Apparatus*. Springer-Verlag, Berlin.

Peckham P.H. (1987) Functional electrical stimulation: current status and future prospects of applications to the neuromuscular system in spinal cord injury. *Paraplegia* **24**, 279–288.

Phillips C.A., Petrofsky J.S., Hendershot D.M. & Stafford D. (1984) Functional electrical exercise: a compenehsive approach for physical conditioning of the spinal cord injured patient. *Orthopedics* **7**, 1112–1123.

Reberšek S. & Vodovnik L. (1975) Proportionally controlled functional electrical stimulation of the hand. *Archives of Physical Medicine and Rehabilitation* **54**, 378–382.

Stanič U., Ačimović-Janežič R., Gros N., Kljajić M., Maležič M., Bogataj U. & Rozman J. (1990) FES in lower extremity orthosed in hemiplegia. *Journal of Neurologic Rehabilitation* **5**, 23–55.

Thoma H., Frey M., Hole J., Kern H., Reiner E., Schwanda G. & Stohr H. (1993) Paraplegics should learn to walk with fingers. *Proceedings of the Conference of IEEE Frontiers of Engineering and Computing in Health Care*, pp. 579–582.

Walker D., Currier D. & Threlkeld A. (1988) Effects of high voltage pulsed electrical stimulation on blood flow. *Physical Therapy* **68**, 481–485.

Waters R.L., Campbell J.M. & Nakai R. (1988) Therapeutic electrical stimulation of the lower limb by epimysial electrodes. *Clinical Orthopaedics and Related Research* **233**.

36: Stimulation Procedures

L.S. ILLIS AND E.M. SEDGWICK

Experimental studies, 536
Clinical application, 538
Spinal cord stimulation, 539
  'Carry-over' effect, 540
  Spinal cord stimulation in neurological disease, 540
  Method of stimulation, 541
  Pain, 541
  Spasticity, 542
  Bladder dysfunction, 543
  Placebo effect, 545
  Peripheral vascular disease, 547
  Spinal cord injury, 548
  Spasmodic torticollis, 549
Conus and sacral root stimulation, 549
Phrenic nerve stimulation, 550
Stimulation of muscle, 551
Safety of electrical stimulation of nervous tissue, 551
Hardware complications, 552
Surgical complications, 552
Conclusion, 553

The earliest accounts of the use of electricity or electrical stimulation in the treatment of disease date back to the first century. The ancient descriptions are of historical interest and are sometimes of great entertainment value. Unfortunately, the techniques were of little or no therapeutic value. However, physiologists and neurologists used electrical stimulation techniques to good effect in the investigation of the central nervous system. Beginning with Fritsch & Hitzig's demonstration of the electrical excitability of the motor cortex in 1870 and culminating in Sherrington's (1906) exposition of the integrated action of the nervous system, electrical methods of stimulation resulted in the accumulation of a vast body of knowledge about the responses of nervous tissue to electrical currents. The major therapeutic application of electrical stimulation began with Melzack & Wall's (1965) theory of the gate control

of pain. More recent advances in electronics have brought reliability, miniaturization, economy of power consumption, the possibility of programming stimulation parameters and the capability of total internalization. Engineering solutions and functional electrical stimulation are dealt with in Chapters 34 and 35, and stimulation for faecal incontinence in Chapter 26.

Although the use of many stimulation techniques stems directly from Melzack & Wall's work there was a parallel and unrelated type of research which has relevance to central functional stimulation.

Experimental studies

Injury to the central nervous system produces a partial deafferentation with demonstrable neuroanatomical and neurophysiological changes. These changes may have a sudden onset, but the subsequent alteration is progressive and not static. Reorganization and possibly regeneration occur at a synaptic level and follow more or less predictable patterns. Although these changes may form part of the basis for recovery and eventually for the development of a logical programme of rehabilitation, there remains a possibility that the opposite is true and that the changes contribute to the disability and dysfunction following the lesion. The changes do, however, provide a theoretical basis for attempting to improve function in patients who have a partial lesion in the central nervous system and suggest that the problem of rehabilitation of such patients should be via active procedures aimed at the intact but poorly functioning central nervous system.

Experimental studies of the long-term effect of repetitive stimulation on the morphology and function of the central nervous system are relatively few. Most of such studies, particularly those involving physiological experiments, have been related directly or indirectly to learning theory. The major theories involve either activation of reverberatory neural networks and altering the state of excitability or inhibition in the central nervous system; or the possibility of repetitive stimulation of nerve fibres and synapses producing some long-lasting change in structure with a resultant increase in efficiency and an easier transmission of subsequent impulses along previously relatively unused pathways. These two theories are not mutually exclusive.

It should be emphasized that, although there is good evidence for environmental changes producing a demonstrable alteration in neural structure and response to stimulation, the precise part this alteration plays in neurological function remains unclear (see Chapter 5).

Morphological changes following repetitive stimulation have been reported in terms of synaptic size, synaptic vesicle change and changes in dendrite branching. This brief review is confined to vertebrates and, unless otherwise stated, to mammals. The term *synapse* refers to the site of chemical transmission in the central nervous system, but is sometimes used in this sense in peripheral ganglia and at neuromuscular junctions. The swollen or dilated ends of axon terminals where they make contact with other nerve cells have various terms, such as *end-feet, terminal knobs, boutons terminaux*, etc. The term synapse includes the terminal swelling of an afferent axon, containing mitochondria, synaptic vesicles and, in most sites, neurofibrils, and the specialized ultrastructural thickenings at the junction of the swollen terminal and the postsynaptic cell. The synaptic vesicles are minute structures containing the chemical transmitter.

De Robertis & Ferreira (1957) stimulated the splanchnic nerve and looked at the endings of this nerve in the adrenal medulla. They demonstrated an increase in synaptic vesicles. However, faster rates of stimulation (over 400/s) led to a decrease in synaptic vesicles. Similar results were found by Feher *et al.* (1972), who found an increase in vesicles in reticulocortical endings with auditory stimulation, but with a concomitant decrease in the endings of thalamocortical pathways. Rats reared in

an 'enriched environment', when compared with litter-mates, showed an expansion of visual cortex, probably due to an increase in dendritic branching, an increase in glia, an increase in cholinesterase and a possible increase in blood supply (Diamond *et al.*, 1964). Bazanova *et al.* (1965) found that peripheral nerve stimulation in the frog produced enlargement of synapses which persisted for hours after stimulation and with an increase in the uptake of silver stains. This enlargement of synapses with repetitive stimulation was confirmed by Illis (1969) in the spinal cord of adult cats, following repetitive stimulation of a single posterior root. Synapses showed a shift towards larger sizes and with an increased staining with silver stains. The size and the morphology of the synapses were similar to the normal 'giant' synapses found on Clarke's column cells. In the synaptic zones of Clarke's column, there is normally a system by which synaptic transmission is much more readily accomplished than at the anterior horn cells (Lloyd & McIntyre, 1950). Perhaps the enlarged synapses seen after repetitive stimulation could be responsible for the changes of post-tetanic potentiation. Jorgensen & Bolwig (1979) investigated the effect of electroconvulsive stimulation in rats, using protein markers of various components of the synapse and synapse organelles. They found changes which indicated an increase in synaptic vesicles and also synaptic remodelling. Rutledge (1978) reviewed the effect of cortical denervation and stimulation in cats: chronic stimulation of the cortex resulted in larger boutons, an increase in dendritic synapses and longer synaptic contacts. Repetitive stimulation of cortex (monkey) produced an increase in synaptic vesicles, which reversed after cessation of stimulation (Siegesmund *et al.*, 1969). In the hippocampus (rat), repetitive stimulation produces changes in the number of spine synapses, and alteration in bouton shape and bouton mitochondrial area (Chang & Greenough, 1984); stable potentiation of evoked responses (Lee *et al.*, 1979); and increase in glutamate receptors (Baudry *et al.*, 1980).

Structural changes and the number of synaptic vesicles in central synapses, as well as peripheral endings, may increase or decrease as a result of repetitive stimulation. The rise or fall depends on the functional state, the rate of stimulation and the metabolic climate.

Rats exposed to daylight only after weaning differ significantly from litter-mates reared totally in the dark (Cragg, 1967). In the superficial half of the visual cortex the synapses are larger, while in the deeper half of the cortex the distribution of synaptic profiles is towards the smaller sizes compared with the dark-reared rat. Experiments which involve comparing animals subjected to an enriched environment or reared in the light as opposed to reared in the dark are perhaps more 'physiological' than those involving isolation and preparation of individual nerves or nerve roots and repetitively stimulating with an artificial impulse. Tetanus toxin poisoning is an interesting example of a natural experiment. Tetanus toxin produces a progressive depression of inhibition and the most likely explanation is that the toxin acts on inhibitory synapses (Eccles, 1965). The clinical and experimental changes seen are those of increased excitation, for example repeated convulsions. Clinical follow-up of survivors from tetanus indicates an increase in irritability, sleep disturbance, myoclonus, epileptic fits and electroencephalographic abnormalities (Illis & Taylor, 1971). Clinically, therefore, one may look at tetanus poisoning as a type of central nervous system stimulation experiment. Experimentally, tetanus toxin produces an increase in synaptic vesicles (Yates & Yates, 1966) and an enlargement of boutons terminaux, with no evidence of degeneration (Illis & Mitchell, 1970).

Physiological experiments of disuse indicate a depression of monosynaptic reflexes compared with the control side (Eccles & McIntyre, 1953). Another way of reducing afferent impulses is by tenotomy (see Eccles, 1964), but surprisingly this results in more powerful monosynaptic action than on the control side. This has been explained as due to an actual increase of afferent impulse in tenotomized muscle; unfortunately, this increase is in the small afferent nerves and not the muscle spindle afferents which make monosynaptic connections, or by increased supraspinal activation of gamma motoneurons with a consequent increase in group 1a (the appropriate fibres) discharge. A further way of producing long-term change in synaptic activity is by denervating all the muscles but one of the synergic group (Eccles et al., 1962). Both the tenotomy and the denervation of muscle experiments demonstrate an increase in synaptic potency, but they do not definitely indicate that it is a consequence of excessive use. There is a further complication in that synapses at different functional levels of the central nervous system have quantitative differences. For example, frequency potentiation is powerful in cortical cells but is very poorly developed in interneurons of the spinal cord. Experiments designed to look at the effect of excess use of repetitive stimulation in higher centres such as the cortex are subject to technical difficulties, but Morrell (1961) has shown that prolonged activity in a cortical area produces hyperexcitability, which continues in the homologous area of the other hemisphere long after its isolation from the original focus. The two areas are, of course, connected by a commissural pathway.

While frequency potentiation has been observed in many sites in the nervous system, it is not ubiquitous. Recent work has concentrated on the hippocampus, where synaptic transmission is greatly enhanced by stimulation of afferents at rates above 0.2 Hz. Potentiation by a factor of 4 and with the total duration lasting many hours or even days has been observed (Bliss & Gardner-Medwin, 1973; Andersen, 1978). The interest in the hippocampus and its afferents lies partly in its anatomical arrangement, which makes specific biochemical and pharmacological experiments possible, and partly because of its proposed role in memory processes. A number of biochemical changes have been noted in association with frequency potentiation, and at present potentiation is explained by an enhanced release of transmitter substance at the synaptic terminal rather than by any change in excitability of the postsynaptic neuron. It is of interest that the greatest potentiation is seen at stimulus rates of 10–20 Hz, which are physiological rates of impulse firing. Higher and lower rates produce less potentiation. There has been no demonstration of frequency potentiation in man, but few would doubt that it occurs. It is just possible that the enhanced cervical somatosensory evoked potential seen in multiple sclerosis patients undergoing spinal cord stimulation is a reflection of frequency potentiation (Sedgwick et al., 1980).

Clinical application

The first important clinical use of electronic technology was that of cardiac pacing in the 1960s, with the advent of therapeutically useful, reliable and eventually implantable stimulators. In neurology, the clinical therapeutic application of electrical stimulation began with Melzack & Wall's (1965) illuminating theory of gate control of pain. Melzack & Wall summarized the established physiological, psychological and clinical facts and theories concerning pain, and put forward the suggestion of a gate which opens and shuts according to the balance of activity between small and large afferent fibres, with large-fibre activity tending to close the gate to nociceptive impulses. It was well known that large nerve fibres are easily stimulated by an electrical current without stimulating small fibres and, once the suggestion had been made, it was easy to see the application of electrical stimulation for the relief of pain. Electrical stimulation can be applied by electrodes on the skin (transcutaneous nerve stimulation), directly to the nerve (peripheral nerve stimulation), implanted in the central nervous system, usually over the dorsal column of the spinal cord (spinal cord stimulation), or in other places in the central nervous system. Stimulator devices were first used by Shealy et al. (1967a, b), and since that time peripheral nerves, phrenic nerves, spinal cord, cerebellum, midbrain, thalamus and cerebrum have been subjected to stimulation to reduce pain, improve diaphragmatic function and bladder function, reduce neurological deficit, alter peripheral blood flow, aid the blind and the deaf and treat intractable epilepsy. Some of the more careful studies which have been published show clear evidence of both clinical improvement and objective physiological change. Clinical improvement has occurred in chronic untreatable conditions and has produced alteration in function surpassing that achieved by any previous techniques or methods of treatment. In addition, the use of stimulation techniques has opened a new phase in the understanding of how the nervous system reacts to disease or injury and how this may be modified in order to improve function.

Spinal cord stimulation

In the experimental animal, a number of objective changes have been reported with spinal cord stimulation. These include alteration of evoked responses (Bantli et al., 1975), increase in Renshaw cell activity and inhibition of monosynaptic reflex activity (Thoden et al., 1977; Siegfried et al., 1978) and evidence for postsynaptic inhibition (Foreman et al., 1976). In decerebrate cats, stimulation of a dorsal column produces depression of tonic stretch responses in all four limbs. The effect may persist for up to 20 minutes after 1–10 minutes of spinal cord stimulation. In contrast, the phasic stretch reflex is only consistently seen in the forelimb and rarely lasts longer than the period of stimulation (Chapman et al., 1983). In man, spinal cord stimulation produces changes in auditory brain stem evoked responses as well as cervical somatosensory evoked responses with stimulation at mid and high thoracic levels (Sedgwick et al., 1980). Possibly the spinocervical tract may be inhibited by spinal cord stimulation relayed via the brain stem and cerebellum. Segmental mechanisms may interact with long propriospinal circuits to produce stronger and longer inhibition (Wagman & McMillan, 1974). Single-pulse dorsal column stimulation produces an effect on dorsal horn neurons: a brief discharge followed by inhibition lasting up to 100 mseconds, which is not influenced by rostral block or spinal cord section (Hillman & Wall, 1969). The inhibitory effect is, therefore, presumably segmental. Repetitive (several minutes) spinal cord stimulation at 50 Hz had a prolonged effect on about one-third of dorsal horn cells, with inhibition up to 30 minutes (Lindblom et al., 1977). Linderoth et al. (1991a, b), in a study on rats, demonstrated that spinal cord stimulation with a stimulation frequency between 0.5 and 50 Hz was associated with an increase in peripheral skin blood flow. They showed that the effect depends mainly on spinal mechanisms rather than the supraspinal loop and gave circumstantial evidence for inhibition of sympathetic vasoconstrictor control.

In man, objective neurophysiological data on spinal cord stimulation include a decrease in tonic stretch reflex (Siegfried et al., 1978), improvement in cervical and brain stem evoked responses (Sedgwick et al., 1980), changes in cerebrospinal fluid and blood catecholamines (Levin & Hubschmann, 1980), changes in H reflex (Illis et al., 1976; Thoden et al., 1977; Siegfried et al., 1978; Feeney & Gold, 1980), improvement in urodynamic studies (Abbate et al., 1977; Hawkes et al., 1980; Illis et al., 1980; Meglio et al., 1980; Read et al., 1980), and an increase in skin and muscle blood flow (see below).

'Carry-over' effect

In some patients the effectiveness of spinal cord stimulation persists after stimulation has been stopped. Observations include a lasting after-effect in pain relief (Nashold & Friedman, 1972; Sweet & Wepsic, 1974; Nielson *et al.*, 1975). Meglio *et al.* (1980) investigated a group of patients with non-progressive spinal cord disease with bladder dysfunction and controls with spinal cord disease but with no bladder dysfunction, and demonstrated a progressive improvement with stimulation and persistence of the beneficial effect on bladder dysfunction for up to 22 months. The decay of response from stopping stimulation to reaching prestimulation level begins from about 1 day to 8 weeks and patients reach their prestimulation level from 1 day to 6 months (Illis *et al.*, 1980).

Clinical studies use prolonged stimulation and are, therefore, not strictly comparable with acute animal experiments. Although the carry-over effect is well recognized in clinical spinal cord stimulation, animal experiments usually only show brief inhibition of dorsal horn neurons after dorsal column stimulation (Hillman & Wall, 1969; Handwerker *et al.*, 1975). Chapman *et al.* (1983) found persistence of depression of tonic stretch reflexes in decerebrate cats with spinal cord stimulation, lasting for up to 20 minutes after 1–10 minutes of spinal cord stimulation. Similar carry-over effect in the decrease of monosynaptic reflexes in the cat was reported by Siegfried *et al.* (1978) and Thoden *et al.* (1977), with a carry-over effect lasting for up to 10 minutes.

Although some electrophysiological phenomena such as post-tetanic potentiation may outlast the duration of stimulation, no change in synaptic function has ever been demonstrated which persists as long as the therapeutic benefits seen in clinical studies.

The carry-over effect suggests that the artificial signals induced by electrical stimulation do not simply reproduce afferent stimulation but are integrated by the existing spinal neuronal network, possibly producing an increase in inhibition or altering neurotransmitter patterns in a way which outlasts the period of stimulation.

Spinal cord stimulation in neurological disease

Until Cook & Weinstein's report in 1973, spinal cord stimulation was used exclusively in the treatment of chronic pain. Any changes in neurological function with spinal cord stimulation had been interpreted as complications or untoward effects. Cook & Weinstein reported that repetitive stimulation of the spinal cord in patients with multiple sclerosis produced marked improvement in neurological function. The original patient had multiple sclerosis and was stimulated to relieve pain and her neurological state improved. Instead of disregarding these changes as untoward effects, Cook & Weinstein carefully treated other patients with multiple sclerosis and demonstrated improvements related to the procedure of spinal cord stimulation.

Unrelated experimental work on the effects of partial lesions on the central nervous system and the subsequent processes of reorganization and regeneration, together with studies of the effects of repetitive stimulation on synaptic boutons, had suggested that patients with chronic neurological deficit may respond to attempts to influence the intact nervous system by 'active re-education' (Illis, 1973).

In 1976 the first cases of spinal cord stimulation in multiple sclerosis outside the USA were reported, and the first objective neurophysiological data which ruled out any possibility of the so-called placebo effect were demonstrated (Illis *et al.*, 1976). The effect of spinal cord stimulation in improving neurological function in patients with multiple sclerosis was further reported from Cook's group (Abbate *et al.*, 1977), who showed that, in 40 patients with multiple sclerosis and urinary symptoms, there was a 77% subjective improvement in sphincter control and a 42% objective improvement as shown by cystometry and sphincter electromyography. Improvement in peripheral blood flow has been reported (Cook *et al.*, 1976; Dooley & Kasprak, 1976). Improvement in neurological function has been observed in spinal injury and Friedreich's ataxia (Dooley, 1977; Campos *et al.*, 1978; Richardson & McLone, 1978).

At the Wessex Neurological Centre, Southampton, we applied spinal cord stimulation in order primarily to investigate the effects of central functional stimulation on neuroplasticity. The spinal cord was stimulated via epidural needles in the normal (patients with peripheral vascular disease), patients with multiple small lesions of the spinal cord (multiple sclerosis) and patients with a single massive lesion of the spinal cord (spinal cord injury).

Method of stimulation

The procedure is carried out with normal sterile techniques, with the patient prone on an X-ray table. Local anaesthesia is infiltrated around the interspinous ligament in the lower thoracic area. Under X-ray control, an epidural needle is introduced in the interspinous space to reach the epidural space in the midline. The stylet of the needle is removed and it is ascertained that there is no leakage of cerebrospinal fluid. An electrode is then passed through the needle pointing rostrally and advanced under X-ray control to the mid or high thoracic levels (about T10 to T12 in peripheral vascular disease) and positioned in the midline in the epidural space. Several centimetres of electrode lead should be within the epidural space since a short lead gives a greater risk of displacement. The needle is removed and a second electrode is introduced in the same way, so that the two electrodes are positioned in the midline about one to three vertebral bodies apart, or a unipolar system is used. The stimulator is connected and, if necessary, the electrodes moved until a bilateral tingling sensation is felt. For pain, the stimulation sensation must cover the painful area. The electrodes are fixed to the skin either with sutures or with Steri-strips, and anteroposterior and lateral X-rays are obtained to document the position of the electrodes. Either a totally implantable system is used or the loop antenna from the stimulator is placed over the receiver and a sterile dressing applied to secure the electrodes and the receiver. There are many minor variations of this technique, but the principles remain the same. Some centres use antibiotic cover routinely.

In a trial of spinal cord stimulation carried out in Southampton, patients were not told precisely what type of sensation they would feel and eventually the patients were grouped into those who had had stimulation symmetrically into the legs and those who had had other kinds of sensation. It was quite clear that, for clinical improvement to occur, patients must receive symmetrical sensation (Illis *et al.*, 1980).

Stimulation is carried out at about 33 Hz with 200 µs width pulses at a voltage adjusted by the patient to give a pleasant warm tingling sensation. Most centres carry out 10 days of stimulation, and if a good response is obtained clinically and physiologically then the electrodes are implanted subcutaneously and connected to a subcutaneous receiver, or a fully implantable system is used.

Pain

As indicated earlier, the rationale for the use of spinal cord stimulation in the treatment of pain arose from the gate theory of the control of pain (Melzack & Wall, 1965). Although the original theory has been modified, it has proved enormously fruitful in the area of pain research. One of the earliest clinical applications of the gate control theory was spinal cord stimulation. Since the original report from Shealy *et al.* (1967a,b), there have been numerous reports of the beneficial effect of spinal cord stimulation on patients with intractable pain: Krainick *et al.* (1975), Long & Erickson (1975), Nashold (1975), Long *et al.* (1981), Erickson & Long (1983), Koeze *et al.* (1987), Meglio *et al.* (1989) and Simpson (1991). By 1985 more than 10 000 patients had undergone spinal cord stimulation for intractable pain as indicated by published reports (Maiman *et al.*, 1985), and in many countries this technique is regarded as standard treatment. The earlier reports of the use of spinal cord stimulation in pain were optimistic but not very critical. It is now clear that the initial success rate of some 70%–80% falls rapidly within about 2 years. Gybels & Sweet (1989) reviewed 1219 patients treated with spinal cord stimulation and reported from various centres between 1972 and 1986. Good screening techniques including trial stimulation, and evaluation of psychological factors seemed important.

Clinical classification of pain

Unfortunately, many published reports on the effect of any kind of treatment for pain do not describe the type of pain in any great detail. For most clinical syndromes the relative importance of peripheral and central components is not known. The complexity of central mechanisms has meant that most workers retain a certain degree of flexibility as regards rigid classification. Nociceptive pain is pain produced by tissue damage, and neuropathic pain is pain secondary to peripheral neurological mechanisms (deafferentation pain) or central mechanisms (central pain). However, the classification breaks down since the mechanisms may include disturbance of function (increase or decrease of afferent input) as well as structural lesions. Peripheral lesions may alter ongoing signal traffic and produce central pain rather than deafferentation pain.

Neuropathic pain

Neuropathic pain or neurogenic pain is pain which is not due to tissue damage and, therefore, does not arise as a result of stimulation of nociceptors. It occurs because of dysfunction in the nervous system and this kind of pain includes the pain of post-herpetic neuralgia, causalgia (reflex sympathetic dystrophy), the pain of trigeminal and glossopharyngeal neuralgia (these are assumed not to be due to direct nociceptor stimulation), pain in multiple sclerosis, phantom limb pain, thalamic syndrome, and perhaps the pain of some peripheral neuropathies. Neurogenic pain is usually of a burning or lancinating type, sensory deficit is nearly always present (not in trigeminal or glossopharyngeal neuralgias), and it is usually resistant to morphine and to all conventional analgesics. There may be changes in sweating and vasoconstriction, suggesting an autonomic component, and allodynia (the production of pain by a non-noxious stimulus) is common. This kind of pain usually responds to spinal cord stimulation.

Pain in spinal cord injury (see also p. 548)

There are several types of pain associated with spinal cord injury and these include root pain, visceral pain, musculoskeletal pain, late pain associated with syringomyelia and the phantom body pain felt in the area of complete sensory loss—a type of central deafferentation pain.

Spinal cord stimulation is not an effective technique for the relief of chronic deafferentation pain projected below the level of complete spinal cord injury (Cole et al., 1991).

Spasticity (see also Chapter 24)

Spasticity is not a single phenomenon but is the complex result of alteration of an integrated control system. Spasticity may act as a stabilizing factor on otherwise uncontrolled joints, but excessive spasticity is associated with excessive co-activation of muscles, fatigue and severe walking difficulties. Therefore, improvement in spasticity and spasms is likely to result in improved motor control. The exact relationship between spasticity and motor control remains the subject of an unresolved debate. It has been argued that motor control and function cannot be altered by procedures which reduce spasticity. Landau & Hunt (1990) cite variations in spasticity and motor disability in relation to acute and chronic lesions and during recovery, and the abolition of stretch reflexes without loss of strength. They also state that pharmacological depression of spasticity has never been shown to improve functional motor performance. However, Peacock & Standt (1991) contest this and point out that spasticity has been implicated as an interfering factor in gait as well as other functional tasks, and it is a common clinical experience that improvement in spasticity frequently results in improvement in gait, posture and transfer.

Surface stimulation with electrodes placed over the belly of the muscle may give some improvement in spastic conditions. The strength of the stimulus used must be below that which would elicit hypertonia or spasms. Spasticity may respond to stimulation of affected muscles or of cutaneous nerves, usually at 20–50 Hz for up to 20 minutes twice a day until skin tolerance has developed. If spasticity is severe, then stimulation may be gradually increased up to 3 hours two or three times per day (Bajd et al., 1985; Dimitrijevic et al., 1987).

Spinal cord stimulation may alter spinal segmental reflexes (Illis et al., 1976; Thoden et al., 1977; Dimitrijevic & Sherwood, 1980; Feeney & Gold, 1980; Shimoji et al., 1982). Laitinen & Fugl-Meyer (1981), using isokinetic dynamometry, showed a reduction in spasticity and inhibition of spasms with concomitant electromyelogram changes. Dimitrijevic et al. (1986a, b) demonstrated an improvement in spasticity in two-thirds of patients with spinal cord injury. The effects were more marked in those patients with incomplete injuries, and better results were found with stimulation below the lesion rather than above. In some cases the effect on spasticity was immediate; in others it took several days or weeks before benefit was seen. Maiman et al. (1987) carried out experimental spinal cord stimulation in cats who had received a spinal impact injury at T8, producing paraplegia and spasticity. Stimulation above the lesion aggravated spasticity, but it was relieved with stimulation below the lesion.

After a careful and comprehensive study of 15 patients with multiple sclerosis, Read et al. (1980) concluded that:

> Voluntary reduction of spasticity in MS must be regarded as almost impossible. We were impressed by the remarkable decrease in leg spasticity . . . and the frequent reports of the abolition of nocturnal flexor spasms.

Barolat et al. (1988) made a careful study of 16 patients with spasticity and spasms refractory to medical and physical therapy. All patients had been on large doses of diazepam and baclofen for at least 6 months, with no significant benefit or with intolerable side-effects. Fifteen of the patients were traumatic and one had cervical myelopathy. Assessment included EMG polygraphic recordings, H-reflex and H-reflex recovery curves, recording of movements and spasms with the Cybex isokinetic dynamometer, videotape recording and urodynamic measurements. In 14 of the 16 patients there was significant therapeutic benefit. In eight cases there was an immediate response on stopping and starting stimulation, but in some cases response took several days, and in one patient benefit was not seen until after several weeks of stimulation. In most cases there was concomitant improvement in voluntary motor function as spasms were controlled.

Koulousakis et al. (1987) demonstrated quantitative changes in spasticity (and bladder function) in 12 patients with multiple sclerosis. Where technical breakdown of stimulation occurred, there was an increase in spasticity and deterioration of gait.

Krainick et al. (1988) assessed patients by measuring walking speed, H reflex, polygraphic electromyography, electrogoniometer and joint compliance. The use of objective measurements of assessment, as in this study, is obligatory. This study demonstrated objective evidence of improvement.

The mode of action remains controversial. In the large group of patients studied by Dimitrijevic et al. (1986a), there was a much greater chance of improvement in those patients with incomplete lesions. The best effects were in those patients reporting stimulation-induced paraesthesiae in the limbs with spasticity. This suggests that partial preservation of long tracts is essential for a good response, and that long-loop spine–brain–spine mechanisms are involved. Possibly stimulation modulates brain stem activity, which in turn suppresses segmental excitability. Saade et al. (1984) showed, in decerebrate adult cats, modulation of segmental mechanisms by activating the dorsal column–brain stem–spine loop.

There is a great deal of evidence for the effect of spinal cord stimulation on spinal cord reflex activity in experimental animals and in man. Spinal cord stimulation is a method of treating spasticity and spasm secondary to myelopathy. It is safe and effective, particularly in those patients where medical treatment and physiotherapy are ineffective or drug dosage produces unacceptable side-effects. Abnormal hyperactivity to cutaneous stimuli is reduced, pathological spread of activity to other muscle groups is reduced, clonus is reduced, spastic bladder disturbance may be reduced and voluntary motor activity may be enhanced as spasms and spasticity are controlled. However, intrathecal drug delivery may be even more effective.

Bladder dysfunction

Disturbance of bladder control is probably more distressing than any other neurological symptom. Urinary tract infection adds to the morbidity and the mortality of spinal lesions such as multiple sclerosis and spinal injury, and the problems of bladder control create depressing social effects.

Cook & Weinstein (1973) were the first to report on the beneficial action of spinal cord stimulation on bladder dysfunction. In their original report on five patients, bladder dysfunction was not emphasized but at least one of the reported patients, with no bladder sensation and with incontinence, regained bladder sensation and continence with spinal cord stimulation. Abbate *et al.* (1977) in a study of spinal cord stimulation in 40 patients with multiple sclerosis and bladder dysfunction reported that 77.5% of patients had subjective improvement in bladder control. In 42.5% of patients there was documented improvement in cystometry and sphincter electromyography, and in 35% there was subjective improvement but no change in cystometry or electromyography. Withdrawal of stimulation resulted in reversal to prestimulation state. Since that time, nearly all groups investigating spinal cord stimulation have found improvement in bladder control, particularly in reduction of frequency and urgency. Meglio *et al.* (1980) studied seven patients with non-progressive spinal cord disease, including trauma and spina bifida, and two controls – patients with spinal cord disease but with no bladder disturbance. This study confirmed the beneficial effect of spinal cord stimulation on bladder and sphincter function: complete or almost complete relief of bladder spasticity, marked increase of bladder capacity and reduction or abolition of residual urine were recorded. The beneficial effect was strictly dependent on the stimulation, although the effect could outlast the stimulation and often required some weeks to reach its maximum. Concomitant urodynamic changes were demonstrated. Spinal cord stimulation had no effect on patients with normal bladder function. Kiwersky (1979) reported on cases with spinal injury compared with control. Both groups had surgical decompression and 44 cases had simultaneous implantation of electrodes. Bladder 'automatism' was achieved twice as rapidly in the stimulated patients.

Illis *et al.* (1980) investigated 19 patients with multiple sclerosis. Sixteen of these patients had bladder symptoms and 75% showed improvement. Hawkes *et al.* (1980) studied 19 patients with multiple sclerosis. Fourteen patients had urodynamic studies. Symptomatic changes included improvement in urinary stream, urgency, hesitancy, frequency and incontinence. Residual urine decreased in five of 10 patients studied. Two out of 13 patients showed a significant reduction in detrusor instability and videocystourethrography showed improvement in three patients. Five of seven patients showed changes in urethral pressure profile. Hawkes *et al.* (1980) concluded that 'the changes in bladder function are convincing'. Read *et al.* (1980) studied 15 patients with multiple sclerosis and one patient with neurogenic bladder dysfunction of unknown cause. The combined group had an average duration of bladder dysfunction of 7 years (3–15 years). Careful assessment included mictiography (which records flow pattern, maximum flow rate, total voiding time and voided volume for each individual act of micturition) and urodynamic assessment. Twelve out of 16 patients reported improvement in bladder function, including return to full continence. Objective changes in bladder function included increased bladder capacity, voiding at a lower detrusor pressure and reduction in maximum urethral closure. Tests of bladder function are not susceptible to voluntary control, and the objective changes described must rule out any significant placebo effect.

Berg *et al.* (1982) carried out a controlled trial of spinal cord stimulation in 11 patients with multiple sclerosis. They compared two periods of placebo, each of 4 weeks, with a 6-week period of spinal cord stimulation. The most striking effect was improvement in bladder function. On several occasions patients reported a rapid deterioration of clinical benefit, and this was invariably related to movement or dislocation of electrode. After electrode repositioning the functional improvement reappeared. Similar results had been reported by Illis *et al.* (1980).

Read *et al.* (1985) presented a very interesting single case of a patient with a 15-year history of idiopathic incontinence with detrusor instability. There had been no change with drug therapy. Spinal cord stimulation usually produces changes which takes hours or days to become apparent, but in this case Read *et al.* demonstrated changes which occurred simultaneously with spinal cord stimulation. There was a simultaneous decrease in detrusor contraction and abolition of the desire to void only when the cord was stimulated, with reappearance of uninhibited spasms in the absence of stimulation. Clinical benefit was maintained for 7 months, when electrode slippage occurred and there was a subsequent deterioration in bladder dysfunction.

A long-term follow-up in 34 cases of neurogenic bladder treated by spinal cord stimulation showed improvement (Ronzoni *et al.*, 1988). This series, followed up for 7 years, comprised four cases of spina bifida, three of traumatic paraplegia, 23 of multiple sclerosis and four of arachnoiditis. Urgency was reduced by 90% and urge incontinence by 70%. Urodynamic studies showed reduction in detrusor hyperactivity and uninhibited contractions. After 3 years the benefit was decreasing and was significantly reduced after 5 years.

Placebo effect

As already indicated, many of the reported changes effectively rule out a placebo effect.

There have been two papers reporting no improvement with spinal cord stimulation (in multiple sclerosis). One of these (Young & Goodman, 1979) could be accounted for by the fact that most of the patients had technical problems and therefore may have had difficulty in achieving technically good stimulation. Rosen & Barsoum (1979) found no improvement, on objective criteria, in a group of nine patients with multiple sclerosis. In this investigation there appears to have been no attempt to screen patients temporarily before implanting a permanent stimulator. Conversely, Hawkes *et al.* (1978) stated that changes seen with spinal cord stimulation in multiple sclerosis are due to motivation and that identical improvement could be achieved with physiotherapy. After further study, Hawkes *et al.* (1980) concluded that improved walking speed and muscle power obtained with spinal cord stimulation (over 50% improvement in some patients) could be achieved with physiotherapy and motivation alone, but improvement in bladder function, which was achieved at the same time, was due to spinal cord stimulation. Why one type of improvement is due to the procedure and the other to motivation is not clear. Nor is it clear why patients who have walking disabilities are not normally motivated to walk better.

It has been suggested that the results produced with spinal cord stimulation could be the result of a placebo response and that to demonstrate otherwise would require a double-blind trial. A double-blind trial, controlled and randomized, is a sound statistical method of testing the safety and efficiency of a new drug. The process involves the administration of the test drug to some patients while giving placebo to the rest. The patients are chosen at random and neither the physician nor the patient knows who received the test drug or the placebo and it is therefore presumed that the same care would be received by all patients in the study. Unfortunately, this type of trial, though easy to perform in drug assessment, is impossible to administer in spinal cord stimulation for the simple reason that the patients being stimulated experience a subjective sensation. One-half of the double-blind is therefore invalid. Similarly, the adjustment of voltage, pulse rate and pulse width, and the changing of batteries depend on the patients reporting sensation to the physician, who also, therefore, is aware of which patient is undergoing stimulation. The other half of the double-blind is also invalid.

There are three main reasons for carrying out a randomized double-blind trial in clinical medicine.
1 To determine which of two apparently equal methods of treatment is the better.
2 To compare an untested method of treatment with standard care. However, where the patient's previous course is known, and where the disease has been stationary for 6–12 months, there is no reason why the patient should not act as his own control, particularly if periods of treatment (spinal cord stimulation) are compared with periods of non-treatment (i.e. without spinal cord stimulation) with objective physiological measurements. The primary purpose of studying spinal cord stimulation is to determine effectiveness of one treatment rather than comparison of two types of treatment.
3 To determine toxic effects or unknown side-effects. Spinal cord stimulation has been used for years in the treatment of pain and the incidence and nature of unwanted effects are well known.

There are strong ethical reasons for not placing electrodes in the epidural space of patients unless they are to receive stimulation. A trial which is sound sense in drug testing is inapplicable in this kind of study.

The double-blind trial is not a suitable method for studying stimulation just as it is not suitable for studying surgical procedures. It is mandatory, however, to design a study with an adequate control group and with reference to the possibility of placebo reactions. The trial of Illis *et al.* (1980) used patients as their own controls and made a number of observations pertinent to the placebo phenomenon.

Improvement did not *precede* spinal cord stimulation, as might be expected if hospitalization and motivation were the causes of improvement. The patients had been neurologically stable for at least 9 months prior to spinal cord stimulation, so any spontaneous improvement would be unlikely to coincide with the stimulation. It is even less likely that a further episode of improvement would coincide with a second period of stimulation unless the improvement and the stimulation were causally related (in the Wessex Neurological Centre trial most patients had at least two periods of stimulation separated by 3–6 months without stimulation). Patients with severely disturbed bladder function, in 75% of cases, showed marked improvement and this is considerably more than any reported placebo effect, as well as being greater than any reported improvement with other therapy.

Two patients were 'stimulated' without batteries and three had surface stimulation. None of these showed any improvement, though they received the same treatment as the patients undergoing epidural stimulation. When spinal cord stimulation was begun, they all responded. Nine patients in the Wessex Neurological Centre study had stimulation which produced sensation in the chest, shoulder or into one leg only. There was no clinical change in these patients. Sixteen patients had symmetrical sensation into both legs and 11 showed clinical response. Some of the patients who had shown no clinical response with unilateral stimulation responded to symmetrical stimulation. This indicates that it is not the *fact* of stimulation which produced improvement but the *type* of stimulation – namely, that which produced bilateral sensation into the legs. A further example of the importance of the type of stimulation was shown in one of our patients who responded well and had a permanent implant but began to deteriorate after 4 months. This coincided with an alteration in stimulator sensation. Radiology showed that one electrode had moved 5 mm from the midline. After this electrode was replaced he again improved (Fig. 36.1). There were also objective neurophysiological changes associated with spinal cord stimulation, which cannot be attributed to a placebo effect (Sedgwick *et al.*, 1980). The neurophysiological responses, with the exception of the contingent negative variation (CNV), are not under voluntary control and it is difficult to see how they could be placebo-mediated. The CNV is a cortical evoked response which *can* be altered by the patient's motivation, but the CNVs in our patients were not altered by spinal cord stimulation (Sedgwick *et al.*, 1980).

In the Wessex Neurological Centre trial the patient's stimulation requirements were carefully monitored (Jobling *et al.*, 1980). The current requirements of patients who showed a good clinical response tended to lie in the range 6–12 mA for a pulse duration of 0.2 ms. Some of the 'unsuccessful' patients had a very much higher current requirement. Although not all patients choosing a current in the 6–12 mA range were successful, all of those consistently choosing a higher current have been unsuccessful. The lower current requirement was frequently associated with a satisfactory bilateral sensation down the legs, but patients choosing a higher current usually only experience a tight and unpleasant sensation in the chest. Presumably the choice of current and response is dependent upon stimulation of the dorsal columns themselves. When the dorsal columns are refractory to stimulation, possibly because of extensive damage or badly sited electrodes, the patient would continue increasing the stimulus amplitude until the spinal roots were stimulated, with resultant discomfort in a local distribution. Such patients did not respond well to spinal cord stimulation. The findings can be summarized as follows: a good stimulator sensation and a low current requirement implied a successful stimulation of the dorsal columns and the probability of a good response; a low current requirement accompanied by a bad sensation suggests that the electrodes were badly sited so that dorsal roots were stimulated instead of the dorsal columns; a high current requirement accompanied by a bad sensation is probably associated with damaged dorsal columns and a good response was most unlikely.

Date	10·11·76	15·4·77	15·5·77
Stimulator sensation	Bilateral into legs	Narrow band round chest (radicular)	Bilateral into legs
X-ray of electrodes			
Bladder function	Normal	Severe frequency, urgency, nocturia, incontinence, impaired sensation	Normal

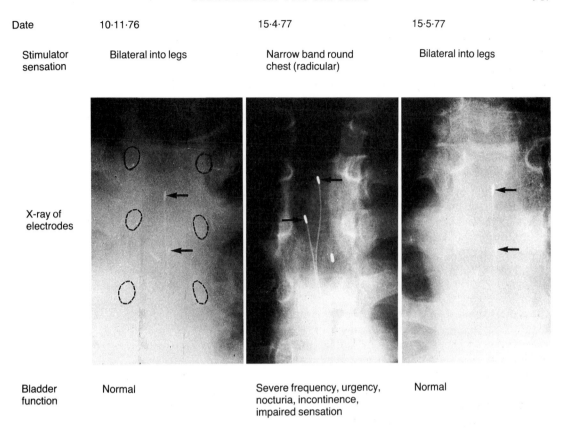

Fig. 36.1 A series of three radiographs showing the position of a pair of epidural electrodes. 10.11.76 – Original position with bilateral stimulator sensation in the legs and a good clinical result. 15.4.77 – At a time of clinical deterioration with a change in stimulator sensation. The lower electrode has shifted 5 mm to the right of the midline. 15.5.77 – Electrode replaced now giving bilateral sensation in the legs and a clinical improvement in bladder function.

Peripheral vascular disease

Bayliss, in 1901, described hindlimb vasodilator nerves in the cat. In 1933 Foerster demonstrated that stimulation of dorsal roots in humans could produce vasodilatation of the skin in the appropriate dermatome. Foerster suggested that this was due to stimulation of efferent fibres from the spinal cord and was not due to antidromic stimulation of afferent fibres.

In our experience, at the Wessex Neurological Centre, patients receiving spinal cord stimulation frequently describe a sensation of warmth in the feet. The limbs feel warmer to the touch and the sensation of warmth is not associated with pain or relief of pain, and it is postulated, therefore, that the sensation is not due to spinothalamic stimulation. In addition, those patients with discoloration of the feet, due to stagnant anoxia associated with poor peripheral circulation, show improvement in the colour. One of our patients with arteriographically demonstrated peripheral vascular insufficiency and severe claudication was receiving spinal cord stimulation for multiple sclerosis. Claudication ceased to be a problem although his mobility increased as a consequence of spinal cord stimulation. He also noted regrowth of distal hair and accelerated toe-nail growth. Another patient, with severe peripheral vascular disease and an indolent ulcer, constant rest pain and night pain, and a claudication distance of 50 yards (45 m), showed marked improvement with spinal cord stimulation:

complete relief of pain, healing of the previous
indolent ulcer, and an increased claudication distance of 350 yards (320 m). In 1974 Friedman *et al.*
reported an increase in skin temperature in the
region of analgesia during spinal cord stimulation
for pain. Cook *et al.* (1976) described eight patients
with arterial disease 'unresponsive to sympathectomy or by-pass' who developed increased temperature and blood flow with spinal cord stimulation. In
addition, these patients showed healing of ulcers,
which broke down again when stimulation was
stopped.

Dooley & Kasprak in 1976 reported increased
peripheral blood flow as measured by pulse
plethysmography with epidural stimulation.
Ebershold *et al.* (1977) found no change in skin
temperature on transcutaneous nerve stimulation
and no alteration in skin impedance. However,
Owens *et al.* (1979), using infrared thermography
in healthy volunteers, demonstrated an increase
in skin temperature with transcutaneous nerve
stimulation, which they interpreted as indicating
indirect evidence of decreased sympathetic tone.
Since that time, there have been numerous clinical
trials, including those of Augustinsson (1981,
1987), Meglio *et al.* (1981), Tallis *et al.* (1983a, b),
Broseta *et al.* (1985, 1986), Broggi *et al.* (1987),
Galley *et al.* (1988) and Jacobs *et al.* (1990). Stimulation increases the microcirculation in the diseased
limb (see Jacobs *et al.*, 1990).

In peripheral ischaemic patients the electrodes
are usually placed at about T10 to T12 and the
aim is to cover the ischaemic area with induced
paraesthesiae.

Linderoth *et al.* (1989, 1991a, b) have carried out
a series of animal experiments, monitoring peripheral blood flow with the laser doppler technique, and have suggested that the mechanism is
segmental, the spinal cord stimulation inducing a
change in sympathetic activity, or activating vasodilator fibres and local release of vasoactive
substances.

Augustinsson *et al.* (1992) have reviewed the
whole subject of spinal cord stimulation in various
ischaemic conditions. They conclude that the
best indication is Fontaine grade 3 patients (the
Fontaine classification is the generally accepted
way of grading the severity of peripheral vascular
disease: grade 1 are patients with no symptoms,

grade 2 are those with intermittent claudication,
grade 3 are those with rest and night pain, and grade
4 are those with rest and night pain and trophic
ulcers). About 80% of patients experience excellent or good pain relief with spinal cord stimulation.
Augustinsson *et al.* (1985) have reported on the
improved amputation rate in patients with spinal
cord stimulation, and this review is the most comprehensive summary to date.

Spinal cord injury (see also p. 542)

Spinal cord stimulation has been used in patients
with spinal cord trauma (Dooley, 1977; Campos
et al., 1978; Richardson & McLone, 1978; Waltz
& Pani, 1978; Meglio *et al.*, 1980). Many of the
reports are incomplete and the total number of
patients is still small, but there appears to be a
definite neurological and functional improvement
in patients with partial lesions of the spinal cord.
The improvement is seen in spasticity and autonomic hyper-reflexia. Many patients appreciate the
increased sense of alertness and freedom from
drowsiness which follows reduction or cessation of
antispastic medication (Dimitrijevic *et al.*, 1986a,
b). In our small series of spinal cord injury (four
paraplegics and two tetraplegics), we have seen no
pain relief (Cole *et al.*, 1991).

One of the severe complications of high spinal
cord injury is the autonomic abnormality known
as autonomic hyper-reflexia or dysreflexia. This
produces an acute hypertension with severe throbbing headache. There is sweating above the level of
the lesion with peripheral vasoconstriction below,
dilatation of the pupils, bradycardia and syncope.
Factors which may precipitate the rise in blood-
pressure and associated features include bladder
distension (outlet obstruction or catheter obstruction); pelvic and rectal manipulation; painful
stimuli in the perineal area; and distension of
any hollow viscus. This syndrome occurs most
frequently in patients with a lesion above T6 and
the mechanism is probably due to an exaggerated
reflex sympathetic activity in the isolated spinal
cord. Standard treatment includes the use of
ganglion-blocking agents and carotid artery compression, as well as treatment of the precipitating
cause. Prophylactic therapy is frequently disappointing. Richardson *et al.* (1979) reported the

use of percutaneous epidural stimulation in five patients with autonomic dysreflexia secondary to spinal cord injury. In four of the patients no further episodes of autonomic dysreflexia occurred during the period of spinal cord stimulation. In the fifth patient the changes of dysreflexia occurred when the voltage was rapidly reduced.

Spasmodic torticollis

Medical and surgical treatment of this condition is unsatisfactory. Medical treatment includes the use of levodopa, bromocriptine (dopamine receptor agonist), haloperidol (dopamine receptor blocker) and tetrabenazine (dopamine-depleting agent). Psychotherapy and biofeedback methods have been used. Surgical treatment includes anteriocervical rhizotomy, with section of the spinal accessory nerve and bilateral stereotactic thalamotomy. For the majority of sufferers, the condition is intractable.

Gildenberg (1978) reported the use of spinal cord stimulation in 20 patients with torticollis and two patients with dystonic musculorum deformans. Twelve of these patients were rejected after a trial of transcutaneous stimulation and percutaneous dorsal column stimulation (either because of poor response or patient refusal). Of the remainder, there was one 'excellent' and one 'good' result. The stimulating electrode was placed inconsistently in front or behind the spinal cord at C5/6 level. Waltz & Pani (1978) carried out spinal cord stimulation in 17 patients with spasmodic torticollis with an age range of 30–61 years and with a duration of symptoms from 8 months to 11 years (mean ±4.2 years). The follow-up was from 6 months to 3 years. During a period of trial stimulation of 7–10 days, 29% showed no effect. These cases were stimulated at multiple levels and with varying stimulation parameters. Of the remaining 12 cases, satisfactory response was achieved with initial stimulation; five showed marked improvement, four showed moderate improvement and one case showed mild improvement. The best results were obtained in those patients who were stimulated in the C2/3 area. The best improvement was obtained in young female patients. In addition, Waltz & Pani carried out spinal cord stimulation in 25 patients with dystonia musculorum deformans. There is still

no consensus view of the value of stimulation techniques in this condition, and botulinum toxin probably gives better results.

Conus and sacral root stimulation

Friedman et al. (1972) implanted a spinal neuro-prosthesis over the sacral cord at various levels, but usually at S2. The electrode tips were located within the intermediolateral column of the central grey matter of the sacral cord – the so-called 'sacral micturition centre'. Experiments were carried out on normal and paraplegic animals and they obtained good results in terms of an increased bladder pressure and an increased volume expelled. After most stimulation episodes there was no residual urine in the bladder and the authors emphasize the importance of a sterile bladder. During the periods of bladder infection the volume voided decreased, but with treatment the volume of urine voided increased. In 1972, Nashold et al. reported the use of this type of stimulation in four paraplegic patients, and further cases were reported in 1975 (Grimes et al., 1975). The authors emphasize careful screening and selection of patients. Those patients with marked reflex or with trabeculated and rigid bladders are excluded, as are those in whom intermittent catheterization or external sphincterotomy would be sufficient to keep them free from infection. It is essential that the conus and cauda equina are undamaged and that the patients have been clinically stationary for a period of at least 12 months since the traumatic paraplegia occurred. Patients with neuropathic bladders, as in multiple sclerosis, are probably not candidates for this kind of procedure. The authors use a psychological screening test to rule out any serious psychiatric disturbances. The patients have a careful neurological examination, as well as the normal physical examination, and urinary function and urine culture are performed. The lower urinary tract is evaluated with cystometrography and endoscopy. Myelography was carried out to evaluate the exact level of the spinal cord lesion. Percutaneous flexible electrodes, placed through a spinal needle, were used to evaluate the bladder response to sacral cord stimulation. Following this, the patients were subjected to a laminectomy and bipolar electrodes were used to determine the cord level producing the highest bladder pressure. The depth electrodes were then positioned at this level and held in place with a Dacron mesh strip and metallic clips. Electrode leads were tunnelled subcutaneously to an implanted receiver in the same way as for spinal cord stimulation in multiple sclerosis. Optimal bladder emptying occurred with stimuli of $200\,\mu s$ at about $15-20\,Hz$ using $10-15$ volts for $20-30$ seconds.

Most of the patients who have had this procedure carried out void with the stimulation and maintain a low residual urine and reduced incidence of infection. If the urine does become infected, the residual urine (usually less than $10\,ml$ with stimulation) rises promptly until the infection is treated. There appear to be two types of response: either sphincter relaxation with detrusor contraction and voiding; or the sphincter and bladder neck contract with the onset of stimulation, but as soon as the stimulus is stopped the vesical neck and urethra open and the patient voids. Associated or autonomic responses of piloerection occur and increased skin temperature. Occasionally penile erection is a problem. Adductor spasm and diffuse pelvic pain may also occur.

A technique for stimulating sacral ventral roots (S3, 4) to effect bladder emptying has been developed by Brindley (1977) and used chronically in man. Stimulation caused contraction of the detrusor and the external sphincter and pelvic striated muscles, but emptying occurred during 2-second gaps in the stimulus train when the striated muscle relaxed abruptly but the slowly responding smooth detrusor muscle maintained tension, thus forcing urine through the urethra. More than 300 patients have now been treated with Brindley's technique and the majority achieve urinary continence. For an up-to-date review of this highly specialized field, see Talalla & Bloom (1992), who discuss various types of stimulation, including conus, pelvic nerve and sacral nerve.

Phrenic nerve stimulation

Apnoeic quadriparesis and Ondine's curse* are the two indications for phrenic nerve stimulation.

Glenn *et al.* (1976) reviewed respiratory pacing by phrenic nerve stimulation in 37 quadriplegics, and they, and others with experience, point out that to switch from positive-pressure ventilation to phrenic nerve stimulation takes many weeks and requires a skilled and dedicated multidisciplinary team of workers. The benefit to an otherwise totally paralysed patient may seem marginal at first sight, but this is not so; even small reductions in the dependency of these more seriously disabled patients can make a great difference to their lives and morale. This is one stimulation procedure which is life-preserving, and even the most successfully stimulated patient must never be without an alarm and back-up system in case of failure.

In the case of spinal trauma at C4 or higher, phrenic stimulation should not be considered until at least 3 months after injury, and then only if other rehabilitation problems, such as the bladder, are under control and there has been no improvement in respiratory function despite appropriate physiotherapy. Respiratory function can recover significantly during the first $3-4$ months after trauma. The patients should be trained in positive-pressure respiration or whatever system is to be used as a back-up. Before implanting the phrenic nerve stimulator investigations should establish the functional integrity of both phrenic nerves by percutaneous or needle electrode stimulation, with fluoroscopic observation of the diaphragm and measurement of the vital capacity.

Each side is usually implanted separately, with a 2-week interval. Current thresholds and current for maximum effect should be measured at the time of implantation. Muscle relaxants should not be used at surgery. After recovery a long period of rehabilitation of the diaphragm is begun, with a programme of gradually increasing periods of stimulation and checks on blood gases. In Glenn *et al.*'s series, 13 of 37 patients were satisfactorily paced for 100% of the time and a further 10 for 50% of the time. Phrenic nerve damage, when it occurred, was probably sustained at the time of surgery and did not happen as a result of chronic stimulation. Glenn *et al.* (1976) claim that, after

---

* A Germanic mythological water-nymph, Ondine, deprived her deserting husband of all automatic function so that he had to remember to breathe. When he finally fell asleep, he died. The term Ondine's curse has been applied to any patient whose respiratory centre has lost its responsiveness to CO_2.

successful pacing has been achieved, the incidence of chest infection is no more than in the general population. This and the normalization of haemo-dynamics by restoring a negative intrathoracic pressure must be in itself sufficient justification for the procedure. Lee *et al.* (1989) note that more than 700 phrenic nerve pacers have been implanted to provide ventilatory support in patients with central hypoventilation, chronic obstructive pulmonary disease and high quadriplegia.

Stimulation of muscle

Electrical stimulation of muscle may alter muscle phenotype (see Vrbova & Lowrie, 1992, for review) and the technique may possibly replace neural-induced activity which is absent as a result of either upper or lower motor neuron lesions.

This clinical application is at an early stage, but has already shown potential in the alteration of the extreme fatiguability in muscles of patients with neurological disability, including spinal cord injury and multiple sclerosis.

Safety of electrical stimulation of nervous tissue

The aim of electrical stimulation is to excite reliably the appropriate tissue without causing damage or other adverse effect.

Materials used for the electrode are usually platinum with small amounts of iridium or rhodium. Tests in artificial serum or cerebrospinal fluid show that these materials can carry appropriate electrical currents for many years without corrosion, but corrosion over durations longer than a decade or so remains uninvestigated. A new type of electrode made from tantalum pentoxide is being studied and may prove superior to platinum as it does not pass electrons across the electrode–tissue interface and oxidation–reduction reactions are said not to occur (Donaldson, 1974).

Electrochemical reaction at the metal–tissue interface is a potential problem. All stimulators should be capacitance-coupled and some workers use only alternating-phase stimulators. This means making one electrode the anode for one pulse and the cathode for the next so that the algebraic sum of current flow is zero. These techniques reduce but

do not eliminate the risks of electrochemical reaction. Further safety is offered by constant-current stimulators and a short-duration pulse which is not permitted to reach a constant voltage (Bergveld, 1976). In some situations the electrochemical reaction products, if produced, could be satisfactorily removed by dilution, but with depth electrodes and electrodes pressed on to the surface of the brain there is minimal 'mixing' and toxic concentrations could quickly build up.

Biological changes due to the passage of current through the tissues are well known to occur. In the extreme, there is heat generated by passing a current through a resistance (nervous tissue), but this would take much greater currents than are employed for neurostimulation.

The stimulus strength or current passed is reported in different ways in the literature. The experimental studies of Pudenz (1977) indicate that the critical stimulation parameters are charge and charge density per pulse, which is more correctly called the electric flux density per pulse. Charge is expressed in coulombs (C) and electric flux density as coulombs per square metre (Cm^{-2}). For stimulation purposes, a flux density expressed in μCmm^{-2} appears a more sensible scale, but the numerical value is the same. Workers in the field of cerebellar stimulation now consider $0.4\,Cm^{-2}$ a safe electric flux density per phase when using alternating-phase stimulators. If the electrodes are of unequal size, then tissue damage will occur first beneath the smaller. The rate of pulses (within the physiological range of rates up to 200/s) does not seem to relate to damage, but safety is increased by a factor up to 10 by using pulses of alternating polarities. Pulse width does not relate directly to damage, but neurologically effective stimuli need to be 0.1–0.4 ms in duration. Longer or shorter pulses are less effective and long pulses obviously increase the charge passed (Girvin, 1978; Jobling *et al.*, 1980).

The first evidence of damage is said to be breakdown of the blood–brain barrier, which can be reversible. Charges of >0.45 μC/phase were needed to produce damage in the cerebral cortex of cats (Mortimer *et al.*, 1970; Pudenz *et al.*, 1975).

Morphological changes in stimulated cortex are the accumulation of glycogen and astrocytosis. Dendrites appear to be most sensitive, but oligodendrocytes are resistant to high currents (Brown *et al.*, 1977; Girvin, 1978).

Early and alarming reports of damage caused by cerebellar stimulation in monkeys (Gilman *et al.*, 1975) have not been substantiated by later work. There are few autopsy observations of patients undergoing cerebellar stimulation; in one case a very local change involving loss of Purkinje cells beneath the electrodes was seen, but this was attributed to pressure rather than electrical current. Another case showed no lesion while others have shown slight and localized changes, which appear to relate more to physical effects of the implant rather than to the passage of current. Many of the patients receiving cerebellar stimulation for epilepsy have pre-existing pathological change in the cerebellum (Cooper, 1978).

It is clear that stimulation can be accomplished without causing significant neuronal damage, but one must be vigilant and take every opportunity to study the stimulus parameters used and to check on changes seen at autopsy should material become available.

Pulse parameters used for stimulation should be quoted in full, including duration, current, frequency, whether monophasic or alternating, etc. Electrode geometry must be considered, as possibly only a fraction of the current actually passes through nervous tissue. The current passed is frequently known only approximately, as the radio-frequency coupling to implanted devices is dependent upon the distance between the antenna and receiver and their spatial relationship. Some form of calibration is necessary and can be done directly if the electrodes are led out through the skin, implantation being delayed until after the clinical effectiveness of stimulation has been confirmed. Spinal cord stimulation produces a sensation which becomes unpleasant at high stimulus strengths, but cerebellar stimulation gives no sensation until current spread excites nerves of the dura or neighbouring brain stem structures such as the trigeminal nerve. In these situations it is easy for excessively high or low currents to be used inadvertently. Devices could be modified to limit their outputs, but none of those presently available have a current-limiting circuit which could be preset by the physician. Low currents due to poor coupling between transmitter and receiver also occur. Both these problems could be partially solved by feedback control from the receiver to the transmitter so that constant-strength stimuli would be delivered to the electrode tips. Some warning device could be incorporated to warn if too high or too low a stimulus was being induced.

Hardware complications

The most troublesome complication is electrode slippage. Periodic radiological checks should be carried out, though slippage is more frequent in the initial 2 weeks. At later times the electrodes can break or lose their insulation and reimplantation is required. Diagnosis of a broken lead is aided by mapping the distribution of amplitude of the stimulus potential at the skin surface soon after implantation. Any change on remapping, particularly a high-amplitude potential appearing along the course of the lead, indicates a breakage.

We have not seen a failure of an implanted receiver, but the transmitter and antennae fail due to wear and tear. There is a built-in test to check the function of stimulators and their antennae, but further checks can be accomplished simply by replacing the battery and listening for the pulse on a radio placed next to the device.

Nothing is known of possible harmful effects during pregnancy. The placing of electrodes involves radiology and therefore stimulation cannot be recommended during pregnancy. Stimulation procedures of any sort cannot be used in patients with cardiac pacemakers. The 'on-demand' pacemakers can interpret the stimulation field as of cardiac origin and will not deliver a pulse. Pulsed radio-frequency fields are a potential source of unintentional stimulation. Such fields can occur in the vicinity of radar transmitters, badly serviced electric motors and poorly screened microwave ovens.

Surgical complications

Patients are exposed to the usual surgical risks, but those specific to stimulation are nervous tissue damage at the time of implantation, cerebrospinal fluid leak when the dura has been opened, and infection. Infection has been rare but, especially when leads are left passing through the skin, constant vigilance is essential. Our practice has been to remove the implant if a superficial infection proves resistant to one course of antibiotics. Cerebrospinal fluid leaks are common but frequently self-limiting.

It is said that surgical procedures can trigger a relapse in multiple sclerosis. The evidence seems to be anecdotal and we have not observed such an occurrence. Allergy to implanted silastic has been reported but is very rare.

Conclusion

Neurostimulation producing modulation of neuro-logical activity is non-destructive and has shown therapeutic benefit. The technique is reversible. This chapter has concentrated largely on spinal cord stimulation. Siegfried (1992) has summarized and reviewed the use of deep-brain stimulation and thalamic stimulation for pain and movement disorders.

References

Abbate A.D., Cook A.W. & Attalah N. (1977) The effect of electrical stimulation of the thoracic spinal cord on function of the bladder in multiple sclerosis. *Journal of Urology* **117**, 285–288.

Andersen P. (1978) Long-lasting facilitation of synaptic transmission. In *Functions of the Septo-Hippocampal System*, pp. 87–102. Ciba Symposium 58, Elsevier, Amsterdam.

Augustinsson L.E. (1981) Indications for spinal cord stimulation. In Hosobuchi Y. & Corbin T. (eds) *Proceedings of a Symposium, 7th International Congress of Neurological Surgery, Munich*, pp. 72–75. Excerpta Medica, Amsterdam.

Augustinsson L.E. (1987) Epidural spinal electrical stimulation in peripheral vascular disease. *Pacing and Clinical Electrophysiology* **10**, 205–206.

Augustinsson L.E., Holm J., Carlsson C.A. & Jivegard L. (1985) Epidural electrical stimulation in severe limb ischaemia: evidences of pain relief, increased blood flow and a possible limb-saving effect. *Annals of Surgery* **202**, 104–111.

Augustinsson L.E., Linderoth B. & Mannheimer C. (1992) Spinal cord stimulation in various ischaemic conditions. In Illis L.S. (ed.) *Spinal Cord Dysfunction, Vol. 3, Function Stimulation*, pp. 270–293. Oxford University Press, Oxford.

Bajd T., Gregoric M., Vodovnick L. & Benko H. (1985) Electrical stimulation in treating spasticity due to spinal cord injury. *Archives of Physical Medicine* **66**, 515–517.

Bantli H., Bloedel J.R., Long D.M. & Thienprasit P. (1975)

Distribution of activity in spinal pathways evoked by experimental dorsal column stimulation. *Journal of Neurosurgery* **42**, 290–295.

Barolat G., Myklebust J.B. & Wenninger W. (1988) Effects of spinal cord stimulation on spasticity and spasms secondary to myelopathy. *Applied Neurophysiology* **51**, 29–44.

Baudry M., Oliver M., Creager R., Wieraszko A. & Lynch G. (1980) Increase in glutamate receptors following repetitive electrical stimulation in hippocampal slices. *Life Sciences* **27**, 325–330.

Bayliss W. (1901) On the origin from the spinal cord of the vasodilator fibres of the hind limbs and the origin of these fibres. *Journal of Physiology* **26**, 173–209.

Bazanova I.S., Evdokimov S.A., Maiorov V.N., Merkulova O.S. & Chernigovskii V.N. (1965) Morphological and electrical changes in interneuronal synapses during passage of rhythmic impulses. *Federation Proceedings* **25**, T187–T190.

Berg V., Bergmann S., Hovdal H. *et al.* (1982) The value of dorsal column stimulation in multiple sclerosis. *Scandinavian Journal of Rehabilitation Medicine* **14**, 183–191.

Bergveld P. (1976) Simple test for electrophysiologically tolerable parameters of artificial stimulation. *Medical and Biological Engineering* **14**, 479–482.

Bliss J.V.P. & Gardner-Medwin A.R. (1973) Long-lasting potentiation of synaptic transmission in the dentate area of the unanaesthetised rabbit following stimulation of the perforant path. *Journal of Physiology* **232**, 357–374.

Brindley G.S. (1977) An implant to empty the bladder or close the urethra. *Journal of Neurology, Neurosurgery and Psychiatry* **40**, 358–369.

Broggi G., Servello D., Franzini A. *et al.* (1987) Spinal cord stimulation for treatment of peripheral vascular disease. *Applied Neurophysiology* **50** (1–6), 439–441.

Broseta J., Garcia-March G., Ingelmo A. *et al.* (1985) Chronic spinal cord stimulation in peripheral arterial insufficiency: comparative study. *Angiologia* **37** (2), 70–86.

Broseta J., Barbera J., De Vera J.A. *et al.* (1986) Spinal cord stimulation in peripheral arterial disease: a co-operative study. *Journal of Neurosurgery* **64**, 71–80.

Brown W.J., Babb T.L., Sloper H.V., Lieb J.P., Ottino C.A. & Crandall P.H. (1977) Tissue reaction to long-term electrical stimulation of the cerebellum in monkeys. *Journal of Neurosurgery* **47**, 336–376.

Campos R.J., Dimitrijevic M.M. & Sharkey P.C. (1978) Clinical evaluation of the effects of spinal cord stimulation on motor performance in patients with upper motor neurone lesions. *Proceedings of the VIth International Symposium on the External Control of Human Extremities, Dubrovnik, Yugoslavia*, pp. 569–574.

Chang F.-L.F. & Greenough W.T. (1984) Transient and enduring morphological correlates of synaptic activity and efficacy change in the rat hippocampal slice. *Brain Research* **309**, 35–46.

Chapman C.E., Rvegg D.G. & Wiesendanger M. (1983) Effects of dorsal cord stimulation on stretch reflexes. *Brain Research* **258**, 211–215.

Cole J.D., Illis L.S. & Sedgwick E.M. (1991) Intractable central pain in spinal cord injury is not relieved by spinal cord stimulation. *Paraplegia* **29**, 167–172.

Cook A.W. & Weinstein S.P. (1973) Chronic dorsal column stimulation in multiple sclerosis: preliminary report. *New York State Journal of Medicine* **73**, 2868–2872.

Cook A.W., Oygar A., Baggenstos P., Pacheco S. & Klerigo E. (1976) Vascular disease of extremities. *New York State Journal of Medicine* **76**, 366–368.

Cooper I.S. (1978) *Cerebellar Stimulation in Man*. Raven Press, New York.

Cragg B.G. (1967) Changes in visual cortex on first exposure of rats to light. *Nature* **215**, 251–253.

De Robertis E. & Ferreira A.V. (1957) Submicroscopic changes of the nerve endings in the adrenal medulla after stimulation of the splanchnic nerve. *Journal of Biophysics, Biochemistry and Cytology* **3**, 611–614.

Diamond M.C., Krech D. & Rosenzweig, M.R. (1964) The effects of an enriched environment on the histology of the rat cerebral cortex. *Journal of Comparative Neurology* **123**, 111–120.

Dimitrijevic M.R. & Sherwood A.M. (1980) Spasticity: medical and surgical treatment. *Neurology* **30**, 19–27.

Dimitrijevic M.M., Dimitrijevic M.R., Illis L.S., Nakajima K., Sharkey P.C. & Sherwood A.M. (1986a) Spinal cord stimulation for the control of spasticity in patients with chronic spinal cord injury. I. Clinical observations. *Central Nervous System Trauma* **3**, 129–144.

Dimitrijevic M.R., Illis L.S., Nakajima K., Sharkey P.C. & Sherwood A.M. (1986b) Spinal cord stimulation for the control of spasticity in patients with chronic spinal cord injury. II. Neurophysiological observations. *Central Nervous System Trauma* **3**, 145–152.

Dimitrijevic M.M., Dimitrijevic M.R., Verhagen-Metman L. & Partridge M. (1987) Modification by muscle tone in patients with upper motor neuron dysfunctions by electrical stimualtion of the sural nerve. *American Academy of Clinical Neurophysiology, Abstracts* **2**, 9.

Donaldson P.E.K. (1974) The stability of tantalum-pentoxide films in vivo. *Medical and Biological Engineering* **12**, 131–135.

Dooley D.M. (1977) Demyelinating, degenerative and vascular disease. *Neurosurgery* **1**, 220–224.

Dooley D.M. & Kasprak M. (1976) Modification of blood flow to the extremities by electrical stimulation of the nervous system. *Southern Medical Journal* **69**, 1309–1311.

Ebershold M.J., Laws E.R.J. & Albers J.W. (1977) Measurements of autonomic function before, during and after transcutaneous stimulation in subjects with chronic pain and in control subjects. *Mayo Clinic Proceedings* **52**, 228–232.

Eccles J.C. (1964) *The Physiology of Synapses*. Springer-Verlag, Berlin.

Eccles J.C. (1965) Pharmacology of central inhibitory synapses. *British Medical Bulletin* **21**, 19–25.

Eccles J.C. & McIntyre A.K. (1953) The effects of disuse and of activity on mammalian spinal reflexes. *Journal of Physiology, London* **121**, 492–516.

Eccles R.M., Kozak W. & Westerman R.A. (1962) Enhancement of spinal monosynaptic reflex responses after denervation of synergic hind-limb muscles. *Experimental Neurology* **6**, 451–464.

Erickson D.L. & Long D.M. (1983) Ten-year follow-up of dorsal column stimulation. In Bonica J.J., Lindblom U. & Iggo A. (eds) *Advances in Pain Research and Therapy*, pp. 583–589. Raven Press, New York.

Feeney D.M. & Gold G.N. (1980) Chronic dorsal column stimulation: effect of H reflex and symptoms in a patient with multiple sclerosis. *Neurosurgery* **6**, 564–566.

Feher O., Joo F. & Halasz N. (1972) Effect of stimulation on the number of synaptic vesicles in nerve fibres and terminals of the cerebral cortex of the cat. *Brain Research* **47**, 37–48.

Foerster O. (1933) The dermatomes in man. *Brain* **56**, 1–39.

Foreman R.D., Beall J.E., Applebaum A.E., Coulter J.D. & Willis W.D. (1976) Effects of dorsal column stimulation on primate spinothalamic tract neurons. *Journal of Neurophysiology* **39**, 534–546.

Friedman H., Nashold B.S. & Senechal P. (1972) Spinal cord stimulation and bladder function in normal and paraplegic animals. *Journal of Neurosurgery* **36**, 430–437.

Friedman H., Nashold B.S. & Somgen G. (1974) Physiological effects of dorsal column stimulation. *Advances in Neurology* **4**, 764–773.

Fritsch G. & Hitzig E. (1870) Über die electrische Erregbarkeit des Grosshirns. *Archives of Anatomy and Physiology* **37**, 300–332. Translation by Bonin G. von. In *The Cerebral Cortex*, pp. 73–96. C.C. Thomas, Springfield, Illinois.

Galley D., Elharrar C., Scheffer J. *et al.* (1988) Intérêt de la neurostimulation épidurale dans les artériopathies des membres inférieurs. *Artères et Veines* **7**, 61–71.

Gildenberg P.L. (1978) Treatment of spasmodic torticollis by dorsal column stimulation. *Applied Neurophysiology* **41**, 113–121.

Gilman S., Dauth G.W., Tennyson V.W. & Kremzner L.T. (1975) Chronic cerebellar stimulation in the monkey. *Archives of Neurology* **32**, 474–477.

Girvin J.P. (1978) A review of basic aspects concerning chronic cerebral stimulation. In Cooper I.S. (ed.) *Cerebellar Stimulation in Man*, pp. 1–12. Raven Press, New York.

Glenn W.W.C., Holcomb W.G., Shaw R.K., Hogan J.F. & Holschuk K.R. (1976) Long term ventilatory support by diaphragm pacing in quadriplegia. *Annals of Surgery* **183**, 566–577.

Grimes J.H., Nashold B.S. & Anderson E.E. (1975) Clinical application of electronic bladder stimulation in paraplegics. *Journal of Urology* **113**, 338–340.

Gybels J.M. & Sweet W.H. (1989) *Neurosurgical Treatment of Persistent Pain*, pp. 293–302. Karger, Basle.

Handwerker H.O., Iggo A. & Zimmermann M. (1975) Segmental and supraspinal actions on dorsal horn neurons responding to noxious and non-noxious skin stimuli. *Pain* **1**, 147–165.

Hawkes C.H., Wyke M., Desmond A. *et al.* (1978) Epidural stimulation in twenty one patients with multiple sclerosis. *Proceedings of the 6th International Symposium on External Control of Human Extremities, Dubrovnik, Yugoslavia*, pp. 603–607. Committee for Electronics and Automation, Belgrade.

Hawkes C.H., Wyke M., Desmond A., Bultitude M.I. & Kanegaonkar G.S. (1980) Stimulation of dorsal column in multiple sclerosis. *British Medical Journal* **1**, 889–891.

Hillman P. & Wall P.D. (1969) Inhibitory and excitatory factors influencing the receptive fields of lamina V spinal cord cells. *Experimental Brain Research* **9**, 284–306.

Illis L.S. (1969) Enlargement of spinal cord synapses after repetitive stimulation. *Nature* **223**, 76–77.

Illis L.S. (1973) Regeneration in the central nervous system. *Lancet* **i**, 1035–1037.

Illis L.S. & Mitchell J. (1970) The effect of tetanus toxin on boutons termineaux. *Brain Research* **18**, 283–295.

Illis L.S. & Taylor F.M. (1971) Neurological and electro-encephalographic sequelae of tetanus. *Lancet* **i**, 826–830.

Illis L.S., Sedgwick E.M., Oygar A.E. & Awadalla M.A.S. (1976) Dorsal column stimulation in the rehabilitation of patients with multiple sclerosis. *Lancet* **i**, 1383–1386.

Illis L.S., Sedgwick E.M. & Tallis R. (1980) Spinal cord stimulation in multiple sclerosis: clinical results. *Journal of Neurology, Neurosurgery and Psychiatry* **43**, 1–14.

Jacobs M.J.H.M., Jorning P.J.G., Beckers R.C.Y. *et al.* (1990) Foot salvage and improvement of microvascular blood flow as a result of epidural spinal cord electrical stimulation. *Journal of Vascular Surgery* **12**, 354–360.

Jobling D.T., Tallis R.C., Sedgwick E.M. & Illis L.S. (1980) Electronic aspects of spinal cord stimulation in multiple sclerosis. *Medical and Biological Engineering and Computing* **18**, 48–56.

Jorgensen O.S. & Bolwig T.G. (1979) Synaptic proteins after electroconvulsive stimulation. *Science* **205**, 705–707.

Kiwersky J. (1979) Preliminary evaluation of epidural electric stimulation of the spinal cord. *Neurology-Neurochirurgia, Poland* **13** (5), 511–516.

Koeze T.H., Williams A.C. de C. & Reiman S. (1987) Spinal cord stimulation and the relief of chronic pain. *Journal of Neurology, Neurosurgery and Psychiatry* **50**, 1424–1429.

Koulousakis A., Buckhaas U. & Nittner K. (1987) Application of spinal cord stimulation for movement disorders and spasticity. *Acta Neurochirurgica (Suppl.)* **39**, 112–116.

Krainick J.-U., Thoden U. & Riechert T. (1975) Spinal cord stimulation in post-amputation pain. *Surgical Neurology* **4**, 167–170.

Krainick J.-U., Waisbrod H. & Gerbershagen H.U. (1988) The value of spinal cord stimulation (SCS) in treatment of disorders of the motor system. In Müller H., Zierski J. & Penn R.D. (eds) *Local Spinal Therapy of Spasticity*, pp. 245–252. Springer-Verlag, Berlin.

Laitinen L.V. & Fugl-Meyer A.R. (1981) Assessment of function effect of epidural electrostimulation and selective posterior rhizotomy in spasticity. *Applied Neurophysiology* **45**, 331–334.

Landau W.M. & Hunt C.C. (1990) Dorsal rhizotomy, a treatment of unproven efficacy. *Journal of Child Neurology* **5**, 174–178.

Lee K., Oliver M., Schottler F., Creager R. & Lynch G. (1979) Ultrastructural effects of repetitive synaptic stimulation in the hippocampal slice preparation: a preliminary report. *Experimental Neurology* **65**, 478–480.

Lee M.Y., Kirk P.M. & Yarkony G.M. (1989) Rehabilitation of quadriplegic patients with phrenic nerve pacers. *Archives of Physical Medicine and Rehabilitation* **70**, 549–552.

Levin B.E. & Hubschmann O.R. (1980) Dorsal column stimulation: effect on human cerebrospinal fluid and plasma catecholamines. *Neurology* **30**, 65–71.

Lindblom U., Tapper D.N. & Wiesenfield Z. (1977) The effect of dorsal column stimulation on the nociceptive response of dorsal horn cells and its relevance for pain suppression. *Pain* **4**, 133–144.

Linderoth B., Fedorcsak I. & Meyerson B.A. (1989) Is vasodilatation following dorsal column stimulation mediated by antidromic activation of small diameter afferents? *Acta Neurochirurgica Suppl.* **46**, 99–101.

Linderoth B., Fedorcsak I. & Meyerson B.A. (1991a) Peripheral vasodilatation after spinal cord stimulation: animal studies of putative effector mechanisms. *Neurosurgery* **28**, 187–195.

Linderoth B., Gunasekera L. & Meyerson B.A. (1991b) Effects of sympathectomy on skin and muscle microcirculation during dorsal column stimulation: animal studies. *Neurosurgery* **29**, 874–879.

Lloyd D.P.C. & McIntyre A.K. (1950) Dorsal column conduction of group I muscle afferent impulses and their relay through Clarke's column. *Journal of Neurophysiology* **13**, 39–54.

Long D.M. & Erickson D.E. (1975) Stimulation of the posterior columns of the spinal cord for relief of intractable pain. *Surgical Neurology* **4**, 134–141.

Long D.M., Erickson D., Campbell J. & North R. (1981) Electrical stimulation of the spinal cord and peripheral nerves for pain control – 10 years experience. *Applied*

Neurophysiology **44**, 207–217.

Maiman D.J., Larson S.J. & Sances A. (1985) Spinal cord stimulation for pain. In Myklebust J.B., Cusick J.F., Sances A. & Larson S.J. (eds) *Neural Stimulation*, pp. 148–154. CRC Press, Florida.

Maiman D.J., Myklebust J.B. & Barolat-Romana G. (1987) Spinal cord stimulation for amelioration of spasticity: experimental results. *Neurosurgery* **21**, 331–333.

Meglio M., Cioni B., d'Amico E., Ronzoni G. & Rossi G.F. (1980) Epidural spinal cord stimulation for the treatment of neurogenic bladder. *Acta Neurochirurgica* **54**, 191–199.

Meglio M., Cioni B., Del Lago A., De Sandis M., Pola P. & Serricchio M. (1981) Pain control and improvement of peripheral blood flow following epidural spinal cord stimulation. *Journal of Neurosurgery* **54**, 821–823.

Meglio M., Cioni B. & Rossi G.F. (1989) Spinal cord stimulation in management of chronic pain. *Journal of Neurosurgery* **70**, 519–524.

Melzack R. (1975) The McGill pain questionnaire: major properties and scoring methods. *Pain* **1**, 277–299.

Melzack R. & Wall P.D. (1965) Pain mechanisms: a new theory. *Science* **150**, 971–979.

Morrell F. (1961) Lasting changes in synaptic organisation produced by continuous neuronal bombardment. In Delafresnaye J.F. (ed.) *Brain Mechanisms and Learning*, pp. 375–392. Blackwell Scientific Publications, Oxford.

Mortimer J.T., Shealy C.N. & Wheeler C. (1970) Experimental non-destructive electrical stimulation of the brain and spinal cord. *Journal of Neurosurgery* **32**, 553–559.

Nashold B.S. (1975) Dorsal column stimulation for control of pain: a three year follow-up. *Surgical Neurology* **4**, 146–147.

Nashold B.S. & Friedman A.H. (1972) Dorsal column stimulation for control of pain: preliminary report on 30 patients. *Journal of Neurosurgery* **36**, 590–597.

Nashold B.S., Friedman H., Glenn J.H., Grimes J.H., Barry W.F. & Avery R. (1972) Electromicturition in paraplegia. *Archives of Surgery* **104**, 195–202.

Nielson K.D., Adams J.E. & Hosobuchi Y. (1975) Experience with dorsal column stimulation for relief of chronic intractable pain. *Surgical Neurology* **4**, 148–152.

Owens S., Atkinson E.R. & Lees D.E. (1979) Thermographic evidence of reduced sympathetic tone with transcutaneous nerve stimulation. *Anaesthesiology* **50**, 62–65.

Peacock W.J. & Standt L.A. (1991) Selective posterior rhizotomy: further comments. *Journal of Child Neurology* **6**, 173C–174C.

Pudenz R.H. (1977) Adverse effects of electrical energy applied to the nervous system. In Burton C.V., Ray C.D. & Nashold B.S. (eds) Symposium on the Safety and Clinical Efficacy of Implanted Neuro-augmentive Devices. *Neurosurgery* **1**, 186–232.

Pudenz R.H., Bullara L.A., Dru D. & Talalla A. (1975) Electrical stimulation of the brain. II. Effects on the blood–brain barrier. *Surgical Neurology* **4**, 37–42.

Read D.J., Matthews W.D. & Higson R.H. (1980) The effect of spinal cord stimulation on patients with multiple sclerosis. *Brain* **103**, 803–833.

Read D.J., James E.D. & Shaldon C. (1985) The effect of spinal cord stimulation on idiopathic destrusor instability and incontinence: a case report. *Journal of Neurology, Neurosurgery and Psychiatry* **48**, 832–834.

Richardson R.R. & McLone D.G. (1978) Percutaneous epidural neurostimulation for paraplegic spasticity. *Surgical Neurology* **9**, 153–155.

Richardson R.R., Cerullo L.J. & Meyer P.R. (1979) Autonomic hyper-reflexia modulated by percutaneous epidural neurostimulation: a preliminary report. *Neurosurgery* **4**, 517–520.

Ronzoni G., De Vecchis M., Rizzotto A., Raschi R. & Cuneo L. (1988) Long-term results of spinal cord electrostimulation in the treatment of micturition disorders associated with neurogenic bladder. *Annals of Urology (Paris)* **22**, 31–34.

Rosen J.A. & Barsoum A.H. (1979) Failure of chronic dorsal column stimulation in multiple sclerosis. *Annals of Neurology* **6**, 66–67.

Rutledge L.T. (1978) Effects of cortical denervation and stimulation on axons, dendrites and synapses. In Cotman C.W. (ed.) *Neuronal Plasticity*. Raven Press, New York.

Saade N.E., Tabet M.S., Atweh S.F. & Jabbur S.J. (1984) Modulation of segmental mechanisms by activation of a dorsal column brainstem spinal loop. *Brain Research* **310**, 180–184.

Sedgwick E.M., Illis L.S., Tallis R.C. *et al.* (1980) Evoked potentials and contingent negative variation during treatment of multiple sclerosis with spinal cord stimulation. *Journal of Neurology, Neurosurgery and Psychiatry* **43**, 14–24.

Shealy C.N., Taslitz N., Mortimer J.T. & Becker D.P. (1967a) Electrical inhibition of pain: experimental evaluation. *Anaesthesia and Analgesia* **46**, 299–305.

Shealy C.N., Mortimer J.T. & Reswick J. (1967b) Electrical inhibition of pain by stimulation of the dorsal column: preliminary clinical reports. *Anaesthesia and Analgesia* **46**, 489–491.

Sherrington C.S. (1906) *The Integrative Action of the Nervous System*. Charles Scribner's & Sons, New York.

Shimoji K., Shimizu H., Maruyama Y., Matsuki M., Kurirayashi H. & Rjioka H. (1982) Dorsal column stimulation in man: facilitation of primary afferent depolarization. *Anaesthesia Analgesia* **61**, 410–413.

Siegesmund K.A., Sances A. & Larson S.J. (1969) Effects of electroanaesthesia on synaptic ultrastructure. *Journal of Neurological Sciences* **9**, 89–96.

Siegfried J. (1992) Neurostimulation methods for correcting functional imbalances. In Young R.R. &

Delwaide P.J. (eds) *Principles and Practice of Restorative Neurology*, pp. 166–176. Butterworth, Heinemann, Oxford.

Siegfried J., Krainick J.U., Haas H., Adoriani C., Meyer M. & Thoden U. (1978) Electrical spinal cord stimulation for spastic movement disorder. *Applied Neurophysiology* **41**, 134–141.

Simpson B.A. (1991) Spinal cord stimulation in 60 cases of intractable pain. *Journal of Neurology, Neurosurgery and Psychiatry* **54**, 196–199.

Sweet W.H. & Wepsic J.G. (1974) Stimulation of the posterior columns of the spinal cord for pain control: indications, technique and results. *Clinical Neurosurgery* **21**, 278–310.

Talalla A. & Bloom J.W. (1992) Sacral electrical stimulation for bladder control. In Illis L.S. (ed.) *Spinal Cord Dysfunction*, Vol. 3. Oxford University Press.

Tallis R.C., Illis L.S., Sedgwick E.M., Hardwidge C. & Garfield J.S. (1983a) Spinal cord stimulation in peripheral vascular disease. *Journal of Neurology, Neurosurgery and Psychiatry* **46**, 476–484.

Tallis R.C., Illis L.S., Sedgwick E.M., Hardwidge C. & Kennedy K. (1983b) The effect of spinal cord stimulation upon peripheral blood flow in patients with chronic neurological disease. *International Rehabilitation Medicine* **5**, 4–9.

Thoden U., Krainick J.-U., Strassburg H.M. & Zimmerman H. (1977) Influence of dorsal column stimulation on spastic movement disorders. *Acta Neurochirurgica* **39**, 233–240.

Vrbova G. & Lowrie M.B. (1992) Experimental nerve–muscle stimulation. In Illis L.S. (ed.) *Spinal Cord Dysfunction, Vol. 3, Functional Stimulation*, pp. 93–109. Oxford University Press, Oxford.

Wagman I.H. & McMillan J.A. (1974) Relationships between activity in spinal sensory pathways and 'pain mechanisms' in spinal cord and brainstem. In Bonica J.J. (ed.) *Advances in Neurology, 4*, pp. 171–177. Raven Press, New York.

Waltz J.M. & Pani K.C. (1978) Spinal cord stimulation in disorders of the motor system. In *Proceedings of the VIth International Symposium on the External Control of Human Extremities*, pp. 545–555. Dubrovnik, Yugoslavia Committee for Electronics and Automation, Belgrade.

Yates J.C. & Yates R.D. (1966) An electronmicroscopic study of the effects of tetanus toxin on motoneurones of the cat spinal cord. *Journal of Ultrastructural Research* **16**, 382–394.

Young R.F. & Goodman S.J. (1979) Dorsal spinal cord stimulation in the treatment of multiple sclerosis. *Neurosurgery* **5**, 225–230.

Appendices
Assessment Schedules

Appendix 1: Neurological Assessment: Kurtzke Functional Systems (FS)

Descriptors have been added to the Kurtzke items for additional clarification and are given in parentheses.

Pyramidal functions   ☐

0 Normal
1 Abnormal signs without disability
2 Minimal disability
3 Mild to moderate paraparesis or hemiparesis (detectable weakness but most function sustained for short periods, fatigue a problem); severe monoparesis (almost no function)
4 Marked paraparesis or hemiparesis (function is difficult), moderate quadriparesis (function is decreased but can be sustained for short periods); or monoplegia
5 Paraplegia, hemiplegia or marked quadriparesis
6 Quadriplegia
9 Unknown

Cerebellar functions   ☐ ☐

0 Normal
1 Abnormal signs without disability
2 Mild ataxia (tremor or clumsy movements easily seen, minor interference with function)
3 Moderate truncal or limb ataxia (tremor or clumsy movements interfere with function in all spheres)
4 Severe ataxia in all limbs (most function is very difficult)
5 Unable to perform co-ordinated movements due to ataxia
9 Unknown
Record #1 in small box when weakness (grade 3 or worse on pyramidal) interferes with testing.

Brain stem functions   ☐

0 Normal

1 Signs only
2 Moderate nystagmus or other mild disability
3 Severe nystagmus, marked extraocular weakness or moderate disability of other cranial nerves
4 Marked dysarthria or other marked disability
5 Inability to swallow or speak
9 Unknown

Sensory functions   ☐

0 Normal
1 Vibration or figure-writing decrease only in one or two limbs
2 Mild decrease in touch or pain or position sense and/or moderate decrease in vibration in one or two limbs; or vibratory (c/s figure writing) decrease alone in three or four limbs
3 Moderate decrease in touch or pain or position sense, and/or essentially lost vibration in one or two limbs; or mild decrease in touch or pain and/or moderate decrease in all proprioceptive tests in three or four limbs
4 Marked decrease in touch or pain or loss of proprioception, alone or combined, in one or two limbs; or moderate decrease in touch or pain and/or severe proprioceptive decrease in more than two limbs
5 Loss (essentially) of sensation in one or two limbs; or moderate decrease in touch or pain and/or loss of proprioception for most of the body below the head
6 Sensation essentially lost below the head
9 Unknown

Bowel and bladder functions   ☐
(Rate on the basis of the worse function, either bowel or bladder)
0 Normal

561

1 Mild urinary hesitancy, urgency or retention
2 Moderate hesitancy, urgency, retention of bowel or bladder or rare urinary incontinence (intermittent self-catheterization, manual compression to evacuate bladder, or finger evacuation of stool)
3 Frequent urinary incontinence
4 In need of almost constant catheterization (and constant use of measures to evacuate stool)
5 Loss of bladder function
6 Loss of bowel and bladder function
9 Unknown

Visual (or optic) functions

0 Normal
1 Scotoma with visual acuity (corrected) better than 20/30
2 Worse eye with scotoma with maximal visual acuity (corrected) of 20/30 to 20/59
3 Worse eye with large scotoma, or moderate decrease in fields, but with maximal visual acuity (corrected) of 20/60 to 20/99
4 Worse eye with marked decrease of fields and maximal visual acuity (corrected) of 20/100 to 20/200; grade 2 plus maximal acuity of better eye of 20/60 or less
5 Worse eye with maximal visual acuity (corrected) less than 20/200; grade 4 plus maximal acuity of better eye of 20/60 or less
6 Grade 5 plus maximal visual acuity of better eye of 20/60 or less

9 Unknown
Record #1 in small box for presence of temporal pallor.

Cerebral (or mental) functions

0 Normal
1 Mood alteration only (does not affect DSS score)
2 Mild decrease in mentation
3 Moderate decrease in mentation
4 Marked decrease in mentation (chronic brain syndrome – moderate)
5 Dementia or chronic brain syndrome – severe or incompetent
9 Unknown

Other functions
(Any other neurological findings attributable to MS)

Spasticity

0 None
1 Mild (detectable only)
2 Moderate (minor interference with function)
3 Severe (major interference with function)
9 Unknown

Others:

0 None
1 Any other neurological findings attributed to MS: Specify ....
9 Unknown

Appendix 2: Neurological Assessment: Kurtzke Disability Status Scale (DSS)

Note 1: DSS steps 1 to 4 refer to patients who are fully ambulatory, and the precise step number is defined by the Functional System score(s). DSS steps 5 to 9 are defined by the impairment to ambulation and usual equivalents in Functional System scores are provided. Note 2: The usual equivalents for defects in the Functional Systems are listed in parentheses.

☐ ☐

0   Normal neurological examination (all grade 0 in functional systems*)
1   No disability and minimal signs such as Babinski sign or vibratory decrease (grade 1 in functional systems)
2   Minimal disability, for example, slight weakness or mild gait, sensory, visuomotor disturbance (one or two functional systems, grade 2)
3   Moderate disability though fully ambulatory (for example, monoparesis, moderate ataxia or combinations of lesser dysfunctions) (one or two functional systems, grade 3, or several, grade 2)

* Excludes cerebral function grade 1.

4   Relatively severe disability though fully ambulatory and able to be self-sufficient and up and about for some 12 hours a day (one functional system, grade 4, or several, grade 3 or less)
5   Disability severe enough to preclude ability to work a full day without special provisions. Maximal motor function: walking unaided no more than several blocks (one functional system, grade 5 alone, or combination of lesser grades)
6   Assistance (canes, crutches or braces) required for walking (combinations with more than one system, grade 3 or worse)
7   Restricted to wheelchair but able to wheel self and enter and leave chair alone (combinations with more than one system, grade 4 or worse; very rarely pyramidal system, grade 5 alone)
8   Restricted to bed but with effective use of arms (combinations usually grade 4 or above in several functional systems)
9   Totally helpless bed patients (combinations usually grade 4 or above in most functional systems)
10 Death due to multiple sclerosis

Appendix 3: Neurological Assessment: Kurtzke Expanded Disability Status Scale (EDSS)

Note 1: EDSS steps 1.0 to 4.5 refer to patients who are fully ambulatory, and the precise step number is defined by the Functional System score(s). EDSS steps 5.0 to 9.5 are defined by the impairment to ambulation, and usual equivalents in Functional System scores are provided. Note 2: EDSS should not change by 1.0 step unless there is a change in the same direction of at least one step in at least one FS. Each step (e.g. 3.0 to 3.5) is still part of the DSS scale equivalent (i.e. 3). Progression from 3.0 to 3.5 should be equivalent to the DSS score of 3.

□ □ □

0   Normal neurological exam (all grade 0 in FS*)

1.0   No disability, minimal signs in one FS* (i.e. grade 1)

1.5   No disability, minimal signs in more than one FS* (more than one FS grade 1)

2.0   Minimal disability in one FS (one FS grade 2, others 0 or 1)

2.5   Minimal disability in two FS (two FS grade 2, others 0 or 1)

3.0   Moderate disability in one FS (one FS grade 3, others 0 or 1) or mild disability in three or four FS (three or four FS grade 2, others 0 or 1) though fully ambulatory

3.5   Fully ambulatory but with moderate disability in one FS (one grade 3) and one or two FS grade 2; or two FS grade 3; or five FS grade 2 (others 0 or 1)

4.0   Fully ambulatory without aid, self-sufficient, up and about some 12 hours a day despite relatively severe disability consisting of one FS grade 4 (others 0 or 1), or combinations of lesser grades exceeding limits of previous

*Excludes cerebral function grade 1.

steps; able to walk without aid or rest some 500 metres

4.5   Fully ambulatory without aid, up and about much of the day, able to work a full day, may otherwise have some limitation of full activity or require minimal assistance; characterized by relatively severe disability usually consisting of one FS grade 4 (others 0 or 1) or combinations of lesser grades exceeding limits of previous steps; able to walk without aid or rest some 300 metres

5.0   Ambulatory without aid or rest for about 200 metres; disability severe enough to impair full daily activities (e.g. to work a full day without special provisions) (usual FS equivalents are one grade 5 alone, others 0 or 1; or combinations of lesser grades usually exceeding specifications for step 4.0)

5.5   Ambulatory without aid or rest for about 100 metres; disability severe enough to preclude full daily activities (usual FS equivalents are one grade 5 alone, others 0 or 1; or combination of lesser grades usually exceeding those for step 4.0)

6.0   Intermittent or unilateral constant assistance (cane, crutch, brace) required to walk about 100 metres with or without resting (usual FS equivalents are combinations with more than two FS grade 3+)

6.5   Constant bilateral assistance (canes, crutches, braces) required to walk about 20 metres without resting (usual FS equivalents are combinations with more than two FS grade 3+)

7.0   Unable to walk beyond approximately 5 metres even with aid, essentially restricted to wheelchair; wheels self in standard wheelchair and transfers alone; up and about in wheelchair some 12 hours a day (usual FS equivalents are combinations with more than one FS grade 4+; very rarely pyramidal grade 5 alone)

7.5   Unable to take more than a few steps; restricted to wheelchair; may need aid in transfer; wheels self but cannot carry on in standard wheelchair a full day; may require motorized wheelchair (usual FS equivalents are combinations with more than one FS grade 4+)

8.0   Essentially restricted to bed or chair or perambulated in wheelchair, but may be out of bed itself much of the day; retains many self-care functions; generally has effective use of arms (usual FS equivalents are combinations, generally grade 4+ in several systems)

8.5   Essentially restricted to bed much of day; has some effective use of arm(s); retains some self-care functions (usual FS equivalents are combinations, generally 4+ in several systems)

9.0   Helpless bed patient; can communicate and eat (usual FS equivalents are combinations, mostly grade 4+)

9.5   Totally helpless bed patient; unable to communicate effectively or eat/swallow (usual FS equivalents are combinations, almost all grade 4+)

10.0 Death due to MS

Appendix 4: Minimal Record of Disability: Summary Record of Clinical Scores and Notes (Sample)

Demographic information

1 Patient code   `2` `4` `6` `8` `1` `0`

2 Today's date   `0` `3` `0` `9` `8` `5`

3 Date of onset (month, year)   `1` `2` `8` `1`

4 Date of diagnosis (month, year)   `0` `2` `8` `2`

5 Sex (1−male, 2−female)   `2`

6 Date of birth   `1` `0` `3` `0` `5` `0`

7 Total number of years of education: `1` `8`
   Elementary − 1−8
   High school − 9−12
   College − 13−16
   Masters − 17−18
   Doctorate − 19−20

8 What is your marital status?   `1`
   1 − Married
   2 − Cohabiting
   3 − Separated
   4 − Divorced
   5 − Widowed
   6 − Single (never married)
   7 − Other: ....

9 Who lives with you at the present time?   `1`
   (1 − Yes, 2 − No)

   (a) Spouse

   (b) Children   `1`

   (c) Parent(s)   `2`

   (d) Brother(s) and/or sister(s)   `2`

   (e) Other relative(s)   `2`

   (f) Friends   `2`

   (g) Live alone   `2`

10 Have you ever held a job?
    (1 – Yes, 2 – No)   1

11 What is your current employment status?   3
    1 – Employed outside the home
    2 – Home-bound employment
    3 – Homemaker
    4 – Sheltered workshop
    5 – Volunteer work
    6 – Retired
    7 – Unemployed
    8 – Student or trainee

12 (If employed) What kind of work do you do?

Neurological Assessment (Kurtzke)

Functional Systems

1 Pyramidal   3

2 Cerebellar   3   ☐

3 Brain stem   1

4 Sensory   1

5 Bowel and bladder   1

6 Visual   1   ☐

7 Mental   0

8 Other functions
   (a) Spasticity   3

   (b) Other................................

Disability Status Scale   0   6

Expanded Disability Status Scale   0   6   5

Incapacity Status Scale   2   1

   1 Stair climbing

   2 Ambulation   2   1

   3 Transfers   1   1

   4 Bowel function   1

   5 Bladder function   1

   6 Bathing   1   1

  7 Dressing   [1] [1]

  8 Grooming   [1] [1]

  9 Feeding   [1] [1]

 10 Vision   [1] [1]

 11 Speech and hearing   [0] [1]

 12 Medical problems   [0]

 13 Mood and thought   [1]

 14 Mentation   [0]

 15 Fatiguability   [2]

 16 Sexual function   [1]

Sexual Concern Inquiry

  1 Does not feel like sex   [1]

  2 Can't find partner   [2]

  3 Can't keep partner   [2]

  4 Can't satisfy partner   [2]
     (sexual problems)

  5 Can't satisfy partner   [1]
     (physical problems)

  6 Can't satisfy self   [2]
     (sexual problems)

  7 Can't satisfy self (physical problems)   [2]

  8 Can't become a father or   [2]
     mother

  9 Can't be like a man or   [2]
     a woman

 10 Partner doesn't feel like sex   [2]

 11 Genitourinary hygiene   [2]

 12 Lack of privacy   [2]

 13 Other concerns, specify . . . .

Which is the area of greatest concern?   [0] [5]

Environmental Status Scale

  1 Work   [3]

  2 Financial   [0]

  3 Home   [0]

4 Personal assistance   3

5 Transportation   3

6 Community assistance   0

7 Social activity   3

Clinical comments

. . . .
. . . .
. . . .
. . . .
. . . .

Signature . . . .

Appendix 5: Demographic Information

1 Name: . . . . Code: ☐☐☐☐☐☐

2 Today's date:

   Month ☐☐ Day   ☐☐   Year ☐☐

3 When did you have your first symptoms of MS?

   Month ☐☐   Year ☐☐

4 When were you first diagnosed as having MS?

   Month ☐☐   Year ☐☐

5 Sex: (1 – male, 2 – female)   ☐

6 Birth date:

   Month ☐☐ Day   ☐☐   Year ☐☐

7 Total number of years of education: ☐☐
   Elementary – 1–8
   High school – 9–12
   College – 13–16
   Masters – 17–18
   Doctorate – 19–20

8 What is your marital status?   ☐
   1 – Married
   2 – Cohabiting
   3 – Separated
   4 – Divorced
   5 – Widowed
   6 – Single (never married)
   7 – Other: . . . .

9 Who lives with you at the present time?
   (1 – Yes, 2 – No)

   (a) Spouse

   (b) Children   ☐

   (c) Parent(s)   ☐

(d) Brother(s) and/or sister(s)   ☐

(e) Other relative(s)   ☐

(f) Friend(s)   ☐

(g) Live alone   ☐

10 Have you ever held a job?   ☐
    (1 – Yes, 2 – No)

11 What is your current employent status?   ☐
    1 – Employed outside the home
    2 – Home-bound employment
    3 – Homemaker
    4 – Sheltered workshop
    5 – Volunteer work
    6 – Retired
    7 – Unemployed
    8 – Student or trainee

12 (If employed) What kind of work do you do?

Index

Page numbers in **bold** refer to tables, those in *italic* refer to figures.

accommodation, post-brain injury
151–2
acetylcholinesterase 91
acquired immune deficiency
syndrome, *see* AIDS
activities of daily living (ADL)
function, post-stroke 161
agitation, pharmacologically
mediated improvement in
475–6
AIDS 57, 269–81
anxiety states 277
CNS infection 269–73
opportunistic infections 271–3
Candida albicans 272–3
cryptococcal infection 272
toxoplasmosis 271–2
depressive disorders 277–8
HIV-associated dementia 273–7
clinical/pathological features
273
environmental restructuring
275–6
epidemiology and natural history
274–5
evaluation 273–4
general support 275
provision of services 275
psychoactive medication
276–7
motor and sensory disorders
278–9
myelopathy 278
myopathy 279
peripheral neuropathy 278–9
patient care 279–80
aids and adaptations
elderly patients 323, **324**
availability of 324
principles of provision 323–4
problems 324
post-brain injury 152
alcohol, interruption of reflex arc by
342
Alzheimer's disease 57
and Down's syndrome 448
epilepsy in 181–2

genetic management 448
see also dementia
amantadine, in treatment of
Parkinson's disease 172
anal reflex 357
anocutaneous reflex 357
anticholinergics 171
anticonvulsant drugs, *see* epilepsy,
drug therapy
antidepressants, in treatment of
chronic fatigue syndrome
288
antiviral agents, in treatment of
chronic fatigue syndrome
288
anxiety states, in AIDS 277
aphasia 409, **410**, 411, **412**–15,
416–19, 420
definitions **410**
diagnosis 411, **412**
effect of treatment 415, **416–19**,
420
management 412–15
clinician's role 414
patient's role 414–15
pharmacologically mediated
improvement in **477**, *478*
apomorphine, in treatment of
Parkinson's disease 172
arm, post-stroke recovery 161
assessment **83**–4
bladder function 357–63
brain injury 149–50
chronic fatigue syndrome
289–90
elderly patients 320, **321**–2
Parkinson's disease 173
progressive neuromuscular
disorders 240–1
stroke 158–60
see also assessment schedules; audit
assessment schedules 561–71
demographic information 571
Kurtzke disability status scale 563
Kurtzke expanded disability status
scale 564–5
Kurtzke functional systems
561–2
minimal record of disability
566–9

ataxias, inherited, genetic
management of 448–9
audit 113–30
aims of rehabilitation 113–14
Barthel ADL index **123**
case-mix measures **118**–19
clinical 119
Frenchay activities index **129**
life satisfaction questionnaire
124
measures for use in 120, **121**–2
disability 122
handicap 122
impairment 120, 122
pathology 120
motricity index and trunk control
test **127**
Nottingham extended ADL
assessment **128**
outcome **117**–18
process **116**–17
Rivermead mobility index **125**
service 119, **120**
short orientation, memory and
concentration test **126**
structure **115**–16
autonomic dysreflexia 236–7,
377
axillary nerve injury 251
axonotmesis 250–1
axons
clinical neurophysiology 91–2
degeneration 54

baclofen, in treatment of spasticity
340
ballistic movements *98–9*
Barthel ADL index **123**, **321**
Becker muscular dystrophy, genetic
management of 449–50
behavioural problems, post-brain
injury 152–3
biological models of CNS lesions 35,
36–7
bladder
function
multiple sclerosis 216–17
spinal cord lesions 223,
231–3

intermittent catheterization
232–3
spinal cord stimulation
543–5
hyperactivity 367–8
hypoactivity 368–70
neuropathic 349–81
central nervous influences
352–3, 354
brain centres 353, 354
efferent tracts 353
sacral micturition centre
353–4, 355
sensation 352–3
classification of 363–4
functional 364
neurological condition
363–4
symptoms 364
clinical assessment 355–7
anal reflex 357
anocutaneous reflex 357
bulbocavernous reflex 357
clinical examination 356–7
urological history 355, 356
complications of 376–7
autonomic dysreflexia 377
chronic bacterial infection
376
intramural ureteric
obstruction 376
urinary calculi 376–7
vesico-ureteric reflux 376
functional considerations
354–5
investigation 357–63
assessment of vesico-urethral
function 357
detrusor function 358, 359
electromyography 363
pharmacological tests 361
post-micturitional residual
urine 358
sacral evoked potentials 363
urethral pressure profilometry
361, 362–3
urinary infection 357–8
urodynamic results 360, 361
uroflow measurement 359,
360
management of 364, 365–76
bladder hyperactivity 367–8
bladder hypoactivity 368–70
detrusor stimulation/urethral
relaxation 369
enhancement of detrusor
activity 368–9
sacral anterior root stimulator
369
surgical techniques 369–70
catheterization 372–4
indwelling urethral 372–3
intermittent 373–4
suprapubic 374
cutaneous urinary diversion
375–6

general/social factors 364–5,
366
hyperactive urethra 370–2
midline outflow obstruction,
surgical management
370–2
reduction of outlet
resistance 370
long-term vesico-urethral
neuropathy 366–7
urethral incompetence
374–5
palliation of incontinence
377–8
incontinence appliances
377–8
theoretic considerations
349–55
vesico-urethral structure and
innervation 350, 351, 352
detrusor 350
receptor sites 351–2
urethral smooth muscle 350,
352
urethral striated muscle
350–1
peripheral innervation 355
blind patients
communication aids 514–15
tactile vision substitution system
459–61, 462–4
Bobath method 126–7
botulinum toxin, in treatment of
spasticity 340–1
bowel function
multiple sclerosis 216–17
spinal cord lesions 224, 233–4
see also faecal incontinence
brachial plexus injury 257–61
clinical picture 257
electrodiagnostic techniques 266
neurotmesis 251
pain in 259–61
treatment 258–9
brain
cellular organization 46
cortex
somatotopic remapping in 72,
73
sprouting in 71
development 45–6
diseases of 50, 51–3, 54, 55–6, 57
AIDS 57
elderly patients 57
epilepsy 52–3
head injury 50–1, 52
multiple sclerosis 53–4
Parkinson's disease 51–2
progressive neuromuscular
diseases 54, 55, 56–7
stroke 51, 53
see also individual conditions
lesions of, see brain injury
stimulation, in chronic pain
403–4
volume transmission in 457–8

see also central nervous system;
spinal cord
brain injury 50, 51, 141–56
acute phase 144
assessments 149–50
recordable 150
relevance of 149–50
repeatable 150
retrievable 150
causation 143, 144
community rehabilitation teams
148
definitions 141–2
discharge home 148
incidence of 142, 143
long-stay care 148–9
need for research 155
outcomes 150–2
accommodation 151–2
aids and adaptations 152
dependency 152
employability 150, 151
financial status 151, 152
pharmacotherapy 469–81
animal models 469–75
noradrenergic mediation of
recovery 473, 474–5
sensorimotor functions
469–70, 471, 472–3
visual functions 473
humans 475–9
agitation and cognition
475–4
aphasia 477, 478
motivation 475
sensorimotor function 476–7
mechanisms underlying 478–9
post-acute phase 144
prognosis 154
rehabilitation 145
relevant disciplines 145–8
carers and relatives 147
case managers 147
clinical psychologists 146
disablement resettlement officers
147–8
doctors 145
nursing staff 146–7
occupational therapists 145
physiotherapists 145–6
social workers 146
speech therapists 146
technical instructors 148
voluntary organizations 148
severity of 142
specific problems 152–4
behavioural 152–3
epilepsy 152
memory and concentration
153–4
post-traumatic syndrome 154
pre-injury personality 154
bromocriptine, in treatment of
Parkinson's disease 172
Brummer winch operation 490,
492

Brunnstrom method   137
bulbocavernosus reflex   357

callosotomy   195
Candida albicans, and AIDS   272–3
carbamazepine, in treatment of
    epilepsy   **185**
carers
    AIDS patients   279–80
    elderly patients   327–9
    in multiple sclerosis   27–8
    role in rehabilitation, brain injury
        147
case managers, role in rehabilitation
    of brain injury   147
catheterization, bladder   372–4
    indwelling urethral   372–3
    intermittent   373–4
    suprapubic   374
causalgia   264
central functional stimulation in
    spasticity   343, **344–5**
    mode of action   345
central nervous system
    diseases of   50–7
        AIDS   57, 269–73
            Candida albicans   272–3
            cryptococcal infection   272
            opportunistic infections
                271–3
            toxoplasmosis   271–2
        elderly patients   57
        epilepsy   52–3
        head injury   51–2, *53*
        see also brain injury
        multiple sclerosis   53–4
        Parkinson's disease   51–2
        progressive neuromuscular
            diseases   54, 55, 56–7
        stroke   51, *53*
        see also individual conditions
    dysfunction   34–5
    lesions of   35
        altered synaptic transmission/
            effectiveness   39, *40*
        biological models   35, *36–7*
        neuropathological   50, *51*
        pharmacological changes   37–9
        sprouting of intact fibres   39
        unmasking of existing synapses
            39
        see also brain injury; spinal cord
            lesions
    organization of   45–6, *47*
        cellular organization of brain
            46
        development of brain and spinal
            cord   45–6
    pathology   46, *47–50*
        cerebral oedema,
            space-occupying lesions and
            raised intracranial pressure
            47, *49–50*
        interference with neuronal
            function   46–7

plasticity in
    modulation of synaptic efficacy
        72, *73*
    sprouting   70–2
    role in micturition   353, *354*
    see also brain; spinal cord
central pattern generator   34–5
cerebral oedema   47, *49–50*
cerebrospinal fluid   46
cerebrovascular disease, *see* stroke
Charcot joints   234
Charcot–Marie–Tooth disease   55,
    243
    genetic management   447–8
children
    chronic fatigue syndrome in
        293
    neuromuscular disorders in
        295–312
        Duchenne muscular dystrophy
            302, *303*, **304**, *305–6*, *307–9*,
            310
        intermediate spinal muscular
            atrophy   295, *296*, *297–9*,
            300, *301–2*
chronic fatigue syndrome   282–94
    aetiology   284–6, **287–8**
        effects of inactivity   286
        hyperventilation   286
        immune dysfunction   285
        muscle dysfunction   285
        psychiatric disorder   285–6
        psychological factors   286
        sleep disorder   286
        social factors   286
        viruses   285
    clinical description   284
    definitions   282, **283**
    future research   293–4
    prevalence and prognosis   284
    rehabilitation   289–92
        assessment   289–90
        evaluation of   292
    service implications of   293
    treatment   288–9, 290–2
        antidepressant drugs   288
        antiviral agents   288
        cost of   292
        immunological agents   288
        initiation of   290, 292–3
        planned activity and rest
            288–9
        problems in   292–3
        psychological treatments   289
        role of family   291
        specific techniques   291–2
chronic pain syndrome, *see* pain,
    chronic
claw hand, reconstructive surgery
    256–7
clinical audit   119
clinical neurophysiology   82–102
    assessment   **83–4**
    axons   91–2
    future of   100
    higher nervous function   99–100

motor unit   91
movement   95–9
    anatomy of   96, *97*, *98–9*
        ballistic movements   *98–9*
        ramp movements   *97–8*
    corticospinal tract   95
    magnetic stimulation   95–6
    muscle spindles   92–3
    plasticity of somatotopic maps
        89–90
    progress   84
    research   84
    techniques   84, **85–9**
        polyelectromyography   84–5,
            86, 87
        spinal cord inhibition   86–7,
            88–9
    trophic factors   90–1
    walking   *93, 94–5*
clinical psychologists, role in
    rehabilitation of brain injury
    146
clinical trials   106–7
    interpretation of results   107–8
clobazam, in treatment of epilepsy
    185–6
clonazepam, in treatment of epilepsy
    186
cognition, pharmacologically
    mediated improvement in
    475–6
cognitive-affective concept of
    pain   395
common peroneal nerve injury
    251
communication aids   513–16
    for blind patients   *514–15*
    interface requirements   515–16
communications   11–12
    effective   **15–16**
    failure in   22–3
communication and swallowing
    disorders   409–27
    language disorders   409, **410**–11,
        412–15, **416–19**, 420
        definitions   **410**
        diagnosis   411, **412**
        effect of treatment   415,
            416–19, 420
        management   412–15
            clinician's role   414
            patient's role   414–15
    motor speech disorders   425–6
    swallowing disorders   420, **421–2**,
        423–5
        evaluation and treatment
            423–4
        muscular and neural control
            420, 423
community rehabilitation team
    brain injury   148
    stroke   164
competition   65–6
conductive education   137–8
conservation   66
conus stimulation   549–50

co-ordination   12–13
cortex
    somatotopic remapping in   72, **73**
    sprouting in   71
cortical blindness   73–4
corticospinal tract   95
cost–benefit analysis   110
cost-effectiveness analysis   110
cost–utility analysis   110–11
counselling   138–9
Creutzfeldt–Jakob disease   57
cryotherapy, in treatment of
        spasticity   339
Cryptococcus neoformans, and AIDS
    272
cutaneous sensory substitution   463,
    464
cutaneous urinary diversion   375–6

dantrolene, in treatment of spasticity
    340
decubitus ulcers, in multiple sclerosis
    218–19
definitions   8
dementia
    genetic management   448
    HIV-associated   273–7
        clinical and pathological features
        273
        environmental restructuring
        275–6
        epidemiology and natural history
        274–5
        evaluation   273–4
        psychoactive medication
        276–7
        service provision   275
        support   275
    Parkinson's disease   174
demographic information   570–1
demyelination   47, *48*
denervation   55
    supersensitivity   69–70
    trophic function   90–1
dependency, post-brain injury   152
depression
    AIDS   277–8
    Parkinson's disease   174
detrusor muscle   350
    enhancement of activity   368–9
    function tests   358, *359*
    inhibition of activity
        pharmacological   367
        surgical   367–8
    stimulation of   369
diagnosis   120
    aphasia   411, **412**
    epilepsy   183–4
    language disorders   411, **412**
    pain   398–9
    Parkinson's disease   169, **170**
diaschisis   60, 73–4
diazepam
    in treatment of epilepsy   **186–7**
    in treatment of spasticity   339–40

disability
    definition of   8, 142
    measurement of   122
    prevalence of in elderly patients
    314
disablement resettlement officers,
        role in rehabilitation of brain
        injury   147–8
discharge home
    brain injury   148
    stroke   164
doctors, role in rehabilitation
    brain injury   145
    language disorders   414
domiciliary care   327
dopamine agonists   172
L-dopa, in treatment of Parkinson's
        disease   171
driving, and epilepsy   203–4
Duchenne muscular dystrophy
    241–2
    in children   302, *303*, **304**, 305–6,
        307–9, 310
        management   305–6, *307–9*,
        310
        natural history   302, *303*, **304**,
        305
    genetic management of   449–50
    natural history   241
    prevention   242
    treatment   241–2
dynamic sphincter supplementation
    387
dysarthria, in multiple sclerosis   218
dyskinesia   173–4
dysphagia   420, **421–2**, 423–5
    evaluation and treatment   423–4
    in multiple sclerosis   218
    muscular and neural control   420,
    423
dystonia   174
dystrophies
    limb-girdle, genetic management
        of   451
    muscular   241–3
        Becker type, genetic
        management of   449–50
        Duchenne type   241–2
            in children   302, *303*, **304**,
            305–6, *307–9*, 310
            facioscapulohumeral type
            242–3
            genetic management of
            449–50
        facioscapulohumeral type,
        genetic management of   451
        myotonic, genetic management
        446–7

economic analysis of treatment
    109–11
    cost–benefit/cost-effectiveness
        analysis   110
    costs and benefits   109–10
    cost–utility analysis   110–11

ectopic neural firing   69
education, and epilepsy   201–2
elbow extensor reconstruction
        488–90
    biceps brachii   489–90
    posterior deltoid transfer   *489*
    postoperative treatment   *496*
    results   498
elbow, trick movements   252–3
elderly patients
    adverse social circumstances   316
    brain damage in   57
    chronic disabling disease in   313,
        314–15, 316
    medication as cause of   322–3
    geriatric rehabilitation   329–30
    global impact of focal disease in
        315
    immobility in   315–16
    neurological rehabilitation
        313–32
        aids for   323, **324**
            availability of   324
            principles of provision
            323–4
            problems   324
        definition of   316, *317*
        long-term care   329
        multidimensional assessment
        320, **321–2**
        multidisciplinary team   318,
        319–20
        multiple pathology   315
        needs of carers   327–9
        principles of   317, *318*
        service organization   324–7
            domiciliary care   327
            geriatric day hospitals   326–7
            hospital admission   325–6
            progressive patient care   325
electrodiagnostic techniques   264–7
    brachial plexus injury   266
    facial nerve injury   267
    root lesions   266–7
electromyography, in assessment of
        urethral function   363
electrotherapy   135
EMG feedback   137
emotional recovery, post-stroke
        161–2
employment
    and epilepsy   199, **200–1**
    post-brain injury   150, **151**
engineering solutions   504–18
    basic control engineering   **505**,
    506
    communication aids   513–16
        for blind patients   *514–15*
        interface requirements   515–16
    control of hand prosthesis
        506–7, *508*, *509–10*
    functional electrical stimulation
        510–13
        lower limb function   511, *512*
        practical systems   510–11
        upper limb function   512–13

ephedrine, in treatment of urethral
    incompetence 374
epilepsy 177–211
    accidental injury 196–7
    diagnosis 183–4
    drug therapy 184, **185–90**,
        191–2
        acute dose-related toxicity 190
        acute idiosyncratic toxicity
            190–1
        choice of drug 184, **185–90**
        chronic toxicity **191**
        long-term management 192
        starting therapy 194
        teratogenicity 191–2
    and education 201–2
    and employment 199, **200–1**
    epidemiology *178, 179*
    explanation of 19–20
    and family relationships 202–3
    mortality from 196
    pathology 52–3
    post-brain injury 152
    prognosis *182,* **183**
    and psychiatric disorders 198–9
    as psychosocial handicap 197–8
    remote symptomatic causes of
        178–82
        cerebrovascular disease 181
        CNS infections/infestations 181
        head injury 179–80
        hypoxic-ischaemic cerebral
            insults 178–9
        neurosurgical conditions
            180–1
    seizures 195–7
    service provision for 205–6
        assessment centres 205–6
        epilepsy clinics 205
        residential care 206
    surgical treatment 192–5
        callosotomy 194
        hemispherectomy 194–5
        temporal lobe surgery 193, **194**
    and travel 203–4
        abroad 204
        driving 203–4
        fare concessions 204
    voluntary associations 206
ethosuximide, in treatment of
    epilepsy **187**
exercise therapy 135–6
explanation 16, **17**–22
    epilepsy 19–20
    genetic disorders 20
    head injury 21–2
    motor neuron disease 17–19
    multiple sclerosis 19
    strokes 20–1

facial nerve injury, electrodiagnostic
    techniques 267
facioscapulohumeral muscular
    dystrophy 242–3
    genetic management of 451

faecal incontinence 382–93
    aetiology 384–5
    anatomy/physiology of pelvic floor
        muscles 382–3
    idiopathic 384
    pathogenesis of **383–4**
    prevalence of 382
    treatment 385–90
        continence aids 385
        electrical stimulation of anal
            sphincter 388, **389**–90
        medical 385
        surgical 386–8
            postanal repair 386
            repair of divided anal
                sphincter 386–7
            supplementation of weak anal
                sphincter 387–8
            dynamic sphincter
                supplementation 387
            gracilis sling procedure
                387–8, *389*
            Thiersch procedure 387
failure, causes of 22–3
family care 138
fatigue
    definition of 282–3
    in multiple sclerosis 217–18
femoral nerve injury 251
fertility, and spinal cord lesions
    434–5
fibre–fibre interaction 65
fibre–substrate affinity 65
financial status, post-brain injury
    151, *152*
Frenchay activities index **129**
Friedreich's ataxia, genetic
    management of 448–9
functional electrical stimulation
    510–13, 519–35
    effects of exercise
        contralateral untrained
            extremity 522–3
        fatigue and dynamic muscle
            response 520
        incomplete SCI subjects *522*
        strength 520, *521*
    hemiplegic patients 528, *529–33,*
        534
    lower limb function 511, *512*
    paraplegic patients 523–8
        clinical experience 527, *528*
        prevention of secondary
            pathology 524–5, *526, 527*
        theoretical and practical aspects
            523, *524, 525*
    practical systems 510–11
    training modalities and assessment
        of training 519–20
    upper limb function 512–13

genetic disorders
    DNA analysis 440, **441**, *442–3*
    explanation of 20
    mechanisms of 439–40

Glasgow Coma Score 142
gracilis sling procedure 387–8, *389*
gradients 65
Guillain–Barré syndrome 54, *55*

hand
    prosthesis 506–7, *508, 509*–10
    trick movements 253
hand grip reconstruction 490–5
    arthrodesis of CMC joint of thumb
        492
    brachioradialis transfer
        to extensor carpi radialis brevis
            490
        to flexor pollicis longus 490
        to give pronation 491–2
    Brummer winch operation 490,
        492
    finger extension 494–5
    intrinsic reconstruction *493, 494*
    key grip 490, *491, 492*
    postoperative treatment 496, *497,*
        498
    reconstruction of finger flexor
        492–3
    results 498, *499, 500*
handicap
    definition of 8, 142
    measurement of 122
head injury
    and epilepsy 179–80
    explanation of 21–2
    pathology 50–1, *52*
    and sexual disabilities 431
    see also brain injury
heat treatment 135
hemiplegia, functional electrical
    stimulation in 528, *529–33,*
        534
hemispherectomy 194–5
hereditary motor sensory neuropathy
    55, 243
    genetic management 447–8
hereditary spastic paraplegia, genetic
    management of 449
H reflex 87
human immunodeficiency virus, *see*
    AIDS
Huntington's disease 20
    genetic management 444–6
hydrocephalus 50
hyperalgesia, secondary (neurogenic)
    74
hyperventilation, in chronic fatigue
    syndrome 286, 292
hypoxic-ischaemic cerebral injury,
    and epilepsy 178–9

ice therapy 135
immune dysfunction, and chronic
    fatigue syndrome 285
immunoglobulin, in treatment of
    chronic fatigue syndrome
        288

impairment, definition of 120, 122, 141–2
improvements
  in management 23–4
  potential for 9–10
incontinence
  faecal 382–93
    aetiology 384–5
    anatomy/physiology of pelvic floor muscles 382–3
    idiopathic 384
    pathogenesis **383**–4
    prevalence 382
    treatment 385–90
      electrical stimulation of anal sphincter 388, **389**–90
      medical 385
      surgical 386–8, *389*
  urinary 377–8
    drainage appliances 377–8
    occlusive devices 377
    pants and pads 377
induction 66
infarct, *see* stroke
International Classification of Diseases 8
intramural ureteric obstruction 376
intrathecal drug treatment
  in chronic pain 403–4
  in treatment of spasticity 341–2

Kurtzke disability status scale 563
Kurtzke expanded disability status scale 564–5
Kurtzke functional systems 561–2

language disorders 409, **410**–11, **412**–15, **416–19**, 420
  definitions **410**
  diagnosis 411, **412**
  effect of treatment 415, **416–19**, 420
  management 412–15
    clinician's role 414
    patient's role 414–15
lateral olfactory tract, plasticity of in newborn 63–4
leg
  reconstructive surgery 256–7
  splintage *255*
  trick movements 253
Lewy bodies 51–2
life satisfaction questionnaire **124**
limb-girdle dystrophy, genetic management of 451
long-stay care, following brain injury 148–9
lysuride, in treatment of Parkinson's disease .172

magnetic stimulation 95–6
Mair Report 7
massage 135

measurement of function 10–11
median nerve injury
  neurotmesis 251
  reconstructive surgery 256
  splintage 253
  trick movements 253
medication, and chronic disability in old age 322–3
memory and concentration, post-brain injury 153–4
micturition, *see* bladder
minimal record of disability 566–9
mitochondrial disorders, genetic management of 451–2
mononeuritis multiplex, in AIDS 278
motivation, pharmacologically mediated improvement in 475
motor control, and spasticity 338
motor neuron disease 245–6
  explanation of 17–19
motor speech disorders 425–6
motor unit 91
motricity index and trunk control test **127**
movement 95–9
  anatomy of 96, 97, 98–9
  ballistic movements 98–9
  corticospinal tract 95
  magnetic stimulation 95–6
  ramp movements 97–8
multiple sclerosis 212–20
  carer's viewpoint 27–8
  explanation of 19
  genetic management of 453
  pathology 53–4
  patient evaluation 212–13
  patient's viewpoint 25–7, 28–30
  and sexual disabilities 216–17, 432
  symptoms 213
    primary
      bladder, bowel and sexual dysfunction 216–17
      dysarthria 218
      dysphagia 218
      fatigue 217–18
      gait disturbance 213–16
      upper extremity involvement 217
    secondary
      decubitus ulcers 218–19
      fibrous contractures 219
    tertiary 219
muscle
  spindles 92–3
  stimulation 551
musculocutaneous nerve injury 251
mutual dependence 66
myelopathy, in AIDS 278
myelotomy 342
myopathy 55, *56*–7
  in AIDS 279
myotonic dystrophy, genetic management 446–7

nerve cells
  communication
    disturbance of 47, *48*
    neurohormonal 37
    neuromodulation 37
    point-to-point 37
    volume transmission 37–8
    see also synapses
  regeneration, *see* sprouting
neurasthenia, and chronic fatigue syndrome 283
neurohormonal transmission 37
neurological disorders
  genetic management 438–54
    basic genetics 439–40
    Charcot–Marie–Tooth disease 447–8
    dementias 448
    DNA analysis 440, **441**, *442–3*
    Duchenne and Becker muscular dystrophies 449, *450*–1
    facioscapulohumeral dystrophy 451
    Friedreich's ataxia 448–9
    hereditary spastic paraplegia 449
    Huntington's disease 444–6
    limb-girdle dystrophy 451
    mitochondrial disorders 451–2
    multiple sclerosis 453
    myotonic dystrophy 446–7
    prion diseases 452–3
  spinal cord stimulation in 540–1
neurological service
  elderly patients 318, **319**–20, 324–7
    domiciliary care 327
    geriatric day hospitals 326–7
    hospital admission 325–6
    progressive patient care 325
  functions of 14–15
neuromodulation 37
neuromuscular disorders 54, *55–6*, 57, 239–49
  assessment 240–1
  in children 295–312
    Duchenne muscular dystrophy 302, *303*, **304**, *305–6*, *307–9*, 310
    intermediate spinal muscular atrophy 295, **296**, *297–9*, **300**, *301–2*
  epidemiology **240**
  hereditary motor and sensory neuropathies 243
  motor neuron diseases 245–6
  muscular dystrophies 241–3
    Duchenne type 241–2
    facioscapulohumeral type 242–3
  post-polio syndrome 246–7
  spinal muscular atrophies 243–5
  see also neurological disorders
neuromuscular stimulation, in treatment of spasticity **343**
neuropraxis 250

neurosurgical conditions, and
    epilepsy 180–1
neurotmesis 251–2
newborn, neural plasticity in 62,
    63–5
  critical periods 62
  lateral olfactory tract 63–4
  superior colliculus 62–3
  visual cortex 64–5
NMDA receptors, and synaptic
    modulation 74–5
noradrenergic mediation in
    rehabilitation of brain lesions
    473, 474–5
Nottingham extended ADL
    assessment **128**
nursing staff, role in rehabilitation of
    brain injury 146–7

occupational therapists, role in
    rehabilitation of brain injury
    145
occupational therapy 139
out-patient appointments, problems
    arising from **17**

pain
  in brachial plexus injury 259–61
  chronic 394–408
    behavioural approach 395
    brain stimulation in 403–4
    clinical features 396–7
    cognitive-affective concept 395
    diagnostic procedures 400
      diagnosis of pain-producing
        problem 398–9
      diagnostic blocks 399–400
      diagnostic/therapeutic
        individualization 397–8
      testing 399
    in-patient programme 402–3
    intrathecal narcotics in 403–4
    medical model 394–5
    patients complaining of **396**
    psychosocial examination
      400–1
    reparative surgery and specific
      treatment 403
    spinal cord stimulation in
      403–4, 541–2
      neuropathic pain 542
      spinal cord injury 542
    therapeutic plan 401–2
  clinical classification of 541–2
  neuropathic 542
  in peripheral nerve injury 263–4
  in spinal cord lesions 235–6, 542
paraplegia 221
  functional electrical stimulation in
    523–8
    clinical experience 527, *528*
    prevention of secondary
      pathology 524–5, *526*, 527

theoretical and practical aspects
    523, *524*, *525*
Parkinson's disease 169–76
  case history 169–70
  diagnosis 169, **170**
  epidemiology and organization of
    services 176
  natural history 170, *171*
  pathology 51–2
  sexual disabilities 433
  treatment
    approach to 173–5
      constipation, urinary
        difficulties and sexual
        function 175
      dyskinesia 173–4
      management of fluctuations
        173
      neuropsychiatric problems
        174
      pain and dystonia 174
      patient assessment 173
      sleep 175
    drug therapy 170–3
      L-dopa and decarboxylase
        inhibitor 171
      amantidine 172
      anticholinergics 171
      apomorphine 172
      bromocriptine 172
      dopamine agonists 172
      lysuride 172
      pergolide 172
      selegiline 172–3
    non-drug 175–6
      Parkinson's Disease Society
        175–6
      therapists 175
Parkinson's Disease Society 175–6
pergolide, in treatment of Parkinson's
    disease 172
peripheral nerve disorders 250–68
  axonotmesis 250–1
  brachial plexus lesions 257–61
    clinical picture 257–8
    pain in 259–61
    treatment 258–9
  electrodiagnostic techniques
    264–7
    brachial plexus lesions 266
    facial nerve 267
    root lesions 266–7
  future research 267
  neuropraxia 250
  neurotmesis 251–2
  pain in 263–4
    causalgia 264
  reconstructive surgery 255–7
  re-education 261–3
    motor 261
    sensory 261, **262**–3
  splintage 253, *254*, *255*
  treatment 252
  trick movements 252–3
peripheral nervous system

disorders of, *see* peripheral nerve
    disorders
  plasticity in 66–70
    arrested regeneration and
      ectopic firing 69
    collateral/reactive sprouting 69
    denervation supersensitivity
      69–70
    regenerative sprout outgrowth
      66–7
    response to injury 66
    target/modality selectivity
      68–9
peripheral neuropathy
  in AIDS 278–9
  diabetic 432
  and sexual disabilities 216–17,
    432
peripheral vascular disease, spinal
    cord stimulation in 547–8
pharmacology of CNS lesions 37–9
pharmacotherapy in brain damage
    469–81
  animal models 469–75
    noradrenergic mediation of
      recovery 473, *474*–5
    sensorimotor functions
      469–70, *471*, *472*–3
    visual functions 473
  humans 475–9
    agitation and cognition 475–6
    aphasia **477**, *478*
    motivation 475
    sensorimotor function *476*–7
  mechanisms underlying 478–9
phenobarbitone, in treatment of
    epilepsy **187**–8
phenol, interruption of reflex arc by
    342
phenylpropanolamine hydrochloride,
    in treatment of urethral
    incompetence 374
phenytoin, in treatment of epilepsy
    188
phrenic nerve
  functional assessment 83–4
  stimulation 550–1
physiotherapy 134–8
  brain injury 145–6
  early intervention 134–5
  Parkinson's disease 175
  in spasticity 339
  specific procedures 136, **137**–8
  types of 135–6
Pick's disease
  epilepsy in 182
  genetic management 448
plasticity, neural 59–81
  adult central nervous system
    modulation of synaptic efficacy
      72, *73*–5
    NMDA receptors 74–5
    secondary hyperalgesia 74
    somatotopic remapping 72,
      73

spinal shock, cortical blindness and diaschisis 73–4
sprouting 70–2
adult peripheral nervous system 66–70
  arrested regeneration/ectopic neural firing 69
  collateral/reactive sprouting 69
  denervation supersensitivity 69–70
  regenerative sprout outgrowth 66–7
  response to injury 66
  target and modality selectivity 68–9
ineffective synapses, modulation of 75–8
  use dependence of synaptic efficacy 75, *76–7*
newborn versus adults 62–5
  lateral olfactory tract *63–4*
  superior colliculus 62–3
  visual cortex 64–5
principles of 65–6
somatotopic maps 89–90
varieties of 60–2
  diaschisis 60
  sprouting *61*
  substitution 60–1
  synaptic modulation 61–2
point-to-point transmission 37
polyelectromyography 84–5, *86, 87*
position markers 65
POSSUM apparatus 23
post-polio syndrome 246–7
post-traumatic amnesia 142
post-traumatic syndrome 154
pre-injury personality 154
primidone, in treatment of epilepsy **189**
prion disorders, genetic management of 452–3
procaine, interruption of reflex arc by 342
progabide, in treatment of spasticity 340
prognosis in brain injury 154
proprioceptive neuromuscular facilitation 137
psychiatric disorders
  and chronic fatigue syndrome 285–6
  and epilepsy 198–9
psychological factors in chronic fatigue syndrome 286
PULHEEMS classification 10
pyramidal hypertonia 337–8

radial nerve injury
  neurotmesis 251
  reconstructive surgery 256
  splintage 254–5
ramp movements *97–8*
reconstructive surgery 255–7

re-education in peripheral nerve injury 261–3
  motor 261
  sensory 261, **262**–3
reflex arc, chemical interruption of 342
rehabilitation theory 33–44
  CNS dysfunction 34–5
  effects of CNS lesions 35
  feasibility of 42–3
  nature of dysfunction and recovery 35–40
    altered synaptic transmission/effectiveness 39, *40*
    biological models 35, *36–7*
    pharmacological changes 37–9
    sprouting of intact fibres 39
    unmasking of existing synapses 39
  spinal shock 40–2
reinnervation 55
relatives, role in rehabilitation of brain injury 147
remedial therapy 133–40
  counselling 138–9
  family/social care 138
  and improved functional ability 134
  occupational therapy 139
  physiotherapy 134–8
    early intervention 134–5
    specific procedures 136, **137**–8
    types of 135–6
  stimulation techniques 139
  untreated patients 133–4
remyelination 54–5
Renshaw neurons 89
response to injury 66
rhizotomy 342
Rivermead mobility index **125**
root lesions, electrodiagnostic techniques 266–7

sacral anterior root stimulator 369
sacral micturition centre 353, *354*
sacral root stimulation 549–50
Schiff–Sherrington phenomenon 96
sciatic nerve injury 251–2
segmental demyelination 54
seizures, *see* epilepsy
selegiline, in treatment of Parkinson's disease 172–3
sensorimotor function, pharmacological rehabilitation of
  animal models 469–71, *472–3*
  humans *476–7*
sensory substitution 459–61, *462–4*
  cutaneous sensory substitution in leprosy patients *463, 464*
  tactile vision substitution system *459–61, 462, 463, 464*
    practical applications 460–1,

462–3
    theoretical aspects 460
service audit 119, **120, 121**
sexual disability 428–37
  anatomy and physiology 428–30
  clinical conditions 430–3
    head injury 431
    multiple sclerosis 216–17, 432
    Parkinson's disease 433
    peripheral neuropathies 432
    spinal cord lesions 224, 433
    stroke 431–2
  specific difficulties 433–5
    erection 433–4
    fertility 434–5
    sexual intercourse 434
short orientation, memory and concentration test **126**
short-wave diathermy 135
shoulder
  reconstructive surgery 256
  trick movements 252
sleep disturbance
  chronic fatigue syndrome 286, 292
  Parkinson's disease 175
social care 138
social factors in chronic fatigue syndrome 286–7
social recovery, post-stroke 161–2
social workers, role in rehabilitation of brain injury 146
sodium valproate, in treatment of epilepsy **189**
Sollerman hand function test *486*
somatotopic maps 89–90
space-occupying lesions 47, *49*–50
  effects of 49–50
spasticity 335–48
  clinical features 336–8
    interference with movement 338
    primary motor/internal capsule lesions 337–8
    transverse lesion of spinal cord 336–7
  multiple sclerosis 219
  muscle tone and movement 335–6
  spinal cord lesions 234–5
  spinal cord stimulation in 542–3
  treatment 338–45
    central functional stimulation 343, **344**–5
    chemical interruption of reflex arc 342
    cryotherapy 339
    drug therapy 339–42
      baclofen 340
      botulinum toxin 340–1
      dantrolene 340
      diazepam 339–40
      intrathecal 341–2
      progabide 340
      tizanidine 340

general management   339
peripheral functional stimulation
      343
physiotherapy   339
surgical   342–3
speech therapists, role in
      rehabilitation of brain injury
      146
spinal cord
   development   45–6
   inhibition in   86–7, *88–9*
   injury, *see* spinal cord lesions
   local circuit sprouting   70–1
   somatotopic remapping in   72, *73*
   stimulation   539–49
      bladder dysfunction   543–5
      'carry-over' effect   540
      method   541
      in neurological disease   540–1
      pain   541–2
         chronic   403–4
         clinical classification   541–2
         neuropathic   542
         spinal cord injury   542
      peripheral vascular disease
         547–8
      placebo effect   545–6, *547*
      spasmodic torticollis   549
      spasticity   542–3
      spinal cord injury   548–9
   see also brain; central nervous
      system
spinal cord lesions   50, *51*, 221–38
   autonomic dysreflexia   236–7
   causes of   **222–3**
   Charcot joints   234
   and fertility   434–5
   natural history   223–4
      bladder function   223
      bowel function   224
      motor function   223
      sensory function   223
      sexual function   224
      untreated patients   224
      vascular changes   224, *225*
   pain in   235–6, 542
   para-articular ossification   234
   pathological fractures   234
   prognosis   224–5, *226–7*
   rehabilitation
      active phase   228, **229, 230,
         231–4**
         bladder care   231–3
         bowel training   233–4
         skin care   230–1
      early phase   227–8
         care of joints and soft tissues
            227–8
         mobilization   228
         position   227
   and sexual disabilities   224, 433
   skeletal complications   234
   spasticity in   234–5, 336–7
   special equipment   237
   spinal cord stimulation in   548–9
   sport   237–8

terminology   221–2
spinal muscular atrophies   243–5
   in children   295, **296,** *297–9,* **300,**
      301–2
   natural history   243–4
   prevention   245
   treatment   244–5
spinal shock   73–4
   rehabilitation model   40–2
splintage   253, *254, 255*
sport, post-spinal cord lesion   237–8
sprouting   39, 54, *61*
   central nervous system   70–2
      cortex and cortical projections
         71
      fine-fibre pathways   71–2
      spinal cord   70–1
   compensatory   *61*
   compensatory stunting   *61*
   peripheral nervous system   66–7
      arrested   69
      collateral/reactive   69
      ectopic neural firing   69
      target and modality selectivity
         68–9
   reactive   *61*
   regenerative   *61*
stabilization   66
Stiles–Bunnell transfer   *494*
stimulation techniques   139,
      536–57
   clinical application   538–9
   complications
      hardware   552
      surgical   552–3
   conus/sacral root stimulation
      549–50
   experimental studies   536–8
   muscle stimulation   551
   phrenic nerve stimulation   550–1
   safety of   551–2
   spinal cord stimulation   539–49
      bladder dysfunction   543–5
      'carry-over' effect   540
      method   541
      in neurological disease   540–1
      pain   541–2
      peripheral vascular disease
         547–8
      placebo effect   545–6, *547*
      spasmodic torticollis   549
      spasticity   542–3
      spinal cord injury   548–9
stroke   157–68
   assessment   158–60
   definitions   157–8
   epidemiology   158
   and epilepsy   181
   explanation of   20–1
   home rehabilitation   464–5
   incidence   158
   model service   165
   organization of care   162–5
      community support   164
      home discharge   164
      hospital   162, **163**

in-patient rehabilitation units
      163
   residual disability   164–5
   pathology   51, *53*
   prevalence   158
   recovery from   160–2
      arm recovery   161
      daily living activities   161
      influence of 'therapy' on   160
      intensity and timing of treatment
         160–1
      social and emotional recovery
         161–2
      walking   161
   and sexual disabilities   431–2
   stages of   162
   substitution   60–1
superior colliculus, plasticity of in
      newborn   62–3
swallowing disorders, *see* dysphagia
synapses
   altered transmission/effectiveness
      39, *40*
   central nervous system,
      modulation of   72, *73–5*
   efficacy, use dependence of   75,
      76–7
   modulation of   61–2
      and adaptation   77–8
      central nervous system   72,
         73–5
      NMDA receptors   74–5
      relatively ineffective synapses
         75, *76–8*
   relatively ineffective, modulation
      of   75, *76–8*
   unmasking of   39

tactile vision substitution system
      459–61, *462–4*
   practical applications   460–1,
      462–4
   theoretical aspects   460
technical instructors, role in
      rehabilitation, brain injury
      148
teratogenicity of anticonvulsant
      drugs   191–2
tetraplegia   221, 482–503
   background   482
   basis for treatment   483, *484–5*
   classification   **485,** *486*
   evaluation   *501–2*
   general principles of treatment
      485, 487, *488*
   goals of treatment   482–3
   postoperative treatment   495–8
      elbow extensor reconstruction
         496
         hand grip reconstruction
            496, *497, 498*
      general principles   495–6
   reconstructive procedures
      488–95
      elbow extensor   488–90

biceps brachii 489–90
  posterior deltoid transfer *489*
  postoperative treatment 496,
    497
  results 498
hand grip reconstruction
    490–5
  arthrodesis of CMC joint of
    thumb 492
  Brummer winch operation
    490, *492*
  finger extension 494–5
  intrinsic reconstruction *493,
    494*
  key grip 490, *491*
  postoperative treatment 496,
    497, 498
  reconstruction of finger flexor
    492–3
  results 498, *499, 500*
  transfer of brachioradialis
    to extensor carpi radialis
      brevis 490
    to flexor pollicis longus
      490
    to give pronation 491–2
results of treatment 498–500
  elbow extensor reconstruction
    498
  hand grip reconstruction 498,
    499, 500
  timing of treatment 487
Thiersch procedure 387

thyrotropin-releasing hormone 38
timing 65
tizanidine, in treatment of spasticity
    340
torticollis, spasmodic, spinal cord
    stimulation in 549
Toxoplasmosis gondii, and AIDS
    271–2
traction 136
treatment evaluation 105–12
  clinical trials 106–7
    interpretation of results 107–8
  economic 108–11
    cost–benefit/cost-effectiveness
      analysis 110
    costs and benefits 109–10
    cost–utility analysis 110–11
  efficacy, effectiveness and
    efficiency 106
  implementation 108
trick movements 252–3
trophic function 90–1

ulnar nerve injury
  neurotmesis 251
  splintage 253, *254*
  trick movements 253
ultrasound 135
unconsciousness, definition of 142
urethra
  hyperactive 370–2
  incompetence of 374, *375*

peripheral innervation *355*
  smooth muscle 350
  striated muscle 350, *351, 352*
urethral pressure profilometry 361,
    362–3
urinary calculi 376–7
urinary infection 357–8
  chronic 376
uroflow assessment 359, *360*

vesico-ureteric reflux 376
vigabatrin, in treatment of epilepsy
    190
viral infection, and chronic fatigue
    syndrome 285
visual cortex, plasticity of in newborn
    64–5
visual function, pharmacological
    rehabilitation of 473
volume transmission 37–8
  in brain 457–8
voluntary organizations, role in
    rehabilitation of brain injury
    148
walking *93, 94*–5
  multiple sclerosis, disturbances of
    213–16
  post-stroke 161
  see also movement

Zancolli lasso operation *493*